McILWRAITH & TURNER'S
EQUINE SURGERY
Advanced Techniques
SECOND EDITION

McILWRAITH & TURNER'S
EQUINE SURGERY
Advanced Techniques

SECOND EDITION

C. Wayne McIlwraith
BVSc, MS, PhD, FRCVS, Drhc (Vienna)

Diplomate, American College of Veterinary Surgeons
Diplomate, European College of Veterinary Surgeons
Professor of Surgery
Department of Clinical Sciences
College of Veterinary Medicine and Biomedical Sciences
Colorado State University
Fort Collins, Colorado

James T. Robertson, DVM

Diplomate, American College of Veterinary Surgeons
Associate Professor of Surgery
Veterinary Teaching Hospital
Ohio State University
Columbus, Ohio

Illustrations by:

Tom McCracken, MS
Biographics Inc.

Williams & Wilkins
A WAVERLY COMPANY

BALTIMORE • PHILADELPHIA • LONDON • PARIS • BANGKOK
BUENOS AIRES • HONG KONG • MUNICH • SYDNEY • TOKYO • WROCLAW

Editor: Carroll Cann
Managing Editor: Paula Brown
Marketing Manager: Diane Harnish
Project Editor: Karen Ruppert

351 West Camden Street
Baltimore, Maryland 21201-2436 USA

Rose Tree Corporate Center
1400 North Providence Road
Building II, Suite 5025
Media, Pennsylvania 19063-2043 USA

Printed in the United States of America

First Edition, 1987
Second Edition, 1998

Library of Congress Cataloging-in-Publication Data

McIlwraith, C. Wayne.
McIlwraith & Turner's equine surgery : advanced techniques / C. Wayne McIlwraith, James T. Robertson ; illustrations by Tom McCracken. —2nd ed.
p. cm.
Rev. ed. of: Equine surgery. 1987.
Includes bibliographical references and index.
ISBN 0-683-05770-7
1. Horses—Surgery. I. Robertson, James T., DVM. II. Equine surgery. III. Title.
SF951.M46 1998
636.1'0897—dc21 98-15576
CIP

98 99 00 01 02
1 2 3 4 5 6 7 8 9 10

PREFACE TO SECOND EDITION

It is with some sadness that I note the departure of my friend and colleague, Dr. Simon Turner, from authorship of this second edition of *Equine Surgery: Advanced Techniques.* Dr. Turner has moved to a career in orthopaedic research. His loss to the teaching of large animal surgery to veterinary students and residents was and is considerable. We partnered two editions of *Techniques in Large Animal Surgery* and the first edition of this textbook. He was the instigator and provided major drive in these past efforts, and he is missed. His lack of participation is probably the reason why the second edition has taken so long to come to fruition!

In that regard, Carroll Cann has been extremely patient in awaiting the second edition, and I thank him for that. A fair amount of the textbook is retained in its original form, but changes have been made to keep the book current, some techniques have been changed, and new techniques have been added. At the same time, we have tried to retain the character of the book as a "how-to" book rather than an exhaustive review of literature.

It is a pleasure to welcome Dr. James Robertson to authorship of this book. His prominence in soft tissue surgery is well recognized, and he has made excellent modifications and additions to soft tissue surgeries in this text. I would also like to thank Tom McCracken for continuing to participate in the illustrations and Helen Mawhiney for secretarial assistance.

C. Wayne McIlwraith
Fort Collins, Colorado

PREFACE TO FIRST EDITION

This book follows the excellent response to our previous textbook, *Techniques in Large Animal Surgery.* Because of the popularity of that format and the requests that more advanced techniques be similarly presented, this book has been produced. Again, the techniques are designed to be brief, and each discussion is accompanied by appropriate illustrations. The book is not meant to replace more detailed treatises on pathogenesis, clinical signs, and treatment alternatives published elsewhere.

In general, the surgical procedures are more complex than in the previous book and demand more surgical expertise and specialized training. Some techniques that have evolved since the last book or have not reached the stage of being "time honored" are simple, however. With a fair degree of consistency, we have presented techniques that are currently being performed. Some readers will be disappointed that certain procedures are not presented (two examples are cleft palate repair and esophageal anastomosis). Such procedures were omitted usually because follow-up results raised questions of how often they were of real value. On the other hand, some of the techniques presented may be abandoned in the future as results are evaluated more critically and better alternatives are found. In some procedures, a certain amount of expertise is assumed regarding basic approaches and principles presented in our previous text.

All of the drawings in the book are original and based on rough sketches and photographs taken at various points during actual surgery. Dissections on cadavers were also performed in some instances.

To try best to represent techniques currently performed and favored, we have asked and received critical review of these procedures from a number of colleagues. These people include Dr. Ted Stashak and Dr. Gayle Trotter, our surgical colleagues at Colorado State University, as well as Dr. Larry Bramlage, Dr. Charlie Boles, Dr. Joe Foerner, Dr. Peter Haynes, Dr. Doug Herthel, Dr. Tom Montgomery, Dr. Jim Robertson, Dr. Mike Shires, and Dr. John Stick. We are also grateful to our colleagues Dr. Robert Kainer for checking the manuscript and illustrations with regard to nomenclature, Dr. Richard Park for help with radiographs, and Dr. Robert Jones for his help and expertise in the sections on prophylactic antibiotics and nosocomial infections.

Of primary importance, we wish to acknowledge the work of Tom McCracken and John Daugherty, who have provided us with the excellent illustrations. We also would like to thank Al Kilminister for taking photographs during the various procedures and dissections to aid the art work. We also wish to thank Ms. Helen Acevedo for typing the manuscript.

The idea for this book was conceived in 1983 based on requests and encouragement from Mr. George Mundorff, executive editor, Lea & Febiger, and Mr. Christian F. Spahr Jr., veterinary editor of Lea & Febiger. We appreciate their continuing assistance.

C. Wayne McIlwraith
A. Simon Turner
Fort Collins, Colorado

CONTENTS

1

CASE SELECTION, CLIENT COMMUNICATION, AND INSURANCE POLICIES FOR EQUINE SURGICAL PATIENTS

Good surgical principles and skillful technique are important to successful equine surgery. State-of-the-art techniques are paramount to maintenance of standards. Two other principles, however, are equally important to a successful surgical practice: sound surgical judgment and client communication. We must be more than just good technicians. Opinions vary widely regarding whether certain conditions should be surgically treated. Some of this divergence is based on differing experiences and some on a lack of prospective and retrospective data to give us definitive results. Unfortunately, closed-mindedness on the part of some clinicians is a factor in some situations. Diverging opinions among competent and experienced surgeons regarding important surgical decisions is real and needs to be accepted. Surgical decision making is not an exact scientific process, and it is unreasonable to expect exact answers to clinical problems.

CASE SELECTION

Analyses of second-opinion programs in human surgery indicate that the number of consultants needed to provide a reliable clinical decision probably exceeds those who are logistically available and whom the patient is willing to visit (1). Many aspects of surgical decision making are subjective because of the lack of controlled data, but this situation has improved in recent years. Differences among surgeons regarding their inclination to operate are associated with many factors, and some of these differences are not easily resolved.

Conversely, a surgeon *who has had experience* with a particular condition might consider a certain treatment clearly appropriate or inappropriate. "Reinvention of the wheel" remains a problem with some surgical residents and clinicians who are overaggressive, inadequately trained and supervised, or whose skills are not sufficiently updated. There are too many good training programs, continuing education courses, textbooks, and published papers available today to justify many of the needless or futile surgical interventions that take place. The old cliches "if in doubt, cut it out" and "a chance to cut is a chance to cure" are still with us, and both of us admit having used these at times to justify surgical intervention. It should be recognized, however, that any surgical intervention should be based on good judgment, not on mere enthusiasm to perform surgery.

Yet, conservatism based on ignorance or closed-mindedness is equally unacceptable. The statement "surgery won't do any good"—which is sometimes heard when the speaker has no experience with a technique, has never handled such a case, or is unaware of data supporting a given technique—is also unfortunate and sometimes prevents horses from receiving the best chance they deserve. A surgical decision should be based on data of cases handled up to the present time. When such data are not available, the decision to operate should be based on an open-minded evaluation of all options. This entails not only an awareness of what has been done in the past but also, in many cases, consultation with other surgeons. In addition, no individual should be defensive about obtaining a second opinion, whether seeking it oneself or at a client's request. Adherence to the above principles is not only conducive to optimal standards but also increasingly important for protection from litigation.

CLIENT COMMUNICATION

In tandem with the foregoing principles, communication with clients (owners or trainers) is critical for ensuring that one's practice is both successful and litigation-free. Many clinicians, ourselves included, believe that legal problems are commonly related to poor communication between clinician and client. This includes communication with owners and trainers regarding options, costs, prognoses, likely complications, and recommendations. In addition, communication regarding postsurgical care is critical and should be accelerated when complications develop. To minimize problems, good communication must be linked to good judgment. Any communication should be as honest and realistic as possible. All clients need to be warned of potential problems, but exaggerating the difficulty of surgery or the gravity of the potential consequences to protect oneself, or to make oneself look good when a successful result is obtained, is inappropriate.

Direct communication with the person paying the bill is ideal, as is keeping written records of the quoted fees. Providing written aftercare instructions is also a good, if not necessary, practice and later minimizes the time spent in telephone contact. Such principles are part of an increased need for written documentation of everything we do, as reflected by the adage "if it isn't written down, it hasn't been done." We must be "business-like" to some extent. These communications become easier as the clinician acquires experience in his or her clinical expertise, surgical judgment, and interaction with clients.

INSURANCE POLICIES FOR THE EQUINE SURGEON

The potential threat of a malpractice claim is well recognized. The legal profession continues to make us "malpractice defensive." Adherence to the principles outlined previously in this chapter as well as throughout the book can help prevent some malpractice claims but cannot protect us completely. Subsequent chapters provide relevant material for our optimal performance and do not give further consideration to the subject of malpractice.

Several insurance policies are available to the horse owner, but the ones that principally concern surgeons are equine mortality insurance, loss of use insurance, and major medical and surgical insurance. Loss of use policies are uncommon.

Equine Mortality Insurance

Policies affect equine surgeons regularly and should be addressed. Guidelines published by the American Association of Equine Practitioners (AAEP) help clarify a number of points and are a useful source of information and reference (2). Equine mortality insurance policies provide coverage for loss from accident or disease. The policy does not cover minor injuries, depreciation of value, or failure of an animal to perform certain functions. Destruction because of unsuitability for a particular use is not covered. Three areas are relevant to our role as equine surgeons:

1. **Veterinary Examination for Mortality Insurance.** The veterinarian's responsibilities in conducting an examination prior to a horse's being insured are well laid out in the AAEP guidelines. The responsibilities to the insurance company include identifying the animal beyond a reasonable doubt and noting sex, color, breeding, age, markings, tattoos, and brands. The veterinarian is required to report the medical facts to the best of his or her knowledge and belief by answering all questions on the application, but is not required to attest to the insurability of the horse or to its current value. Despite an owner's reluctance, the examination should be thorough. Looking at a horse in the horse trailer, for example, does not constitute a legitimate examination.
2. **Performance of Surgery on an Insured Horse.** Insurance companies have several options regarding elective surgery to be performed on an insured animal. The client must first notify the insurance company, which in turn may (*a*) permit the surgery and issue a premium charge for the additional exposure, (*b*) permit the surgery, issuing no premium charge and accepting no liability for the surgical procedure, or (*c*) permit the surgery, issuing no premium charge but accepting liability for the surgical procedure. Deciding which of these options to follow is the concern of the insurance company and the client only. The surgeon's concern is that permission for surgery has been obtained and that the insurance company is aware the surgery to be performed is elective. We believe that it is always up to the client to perform this notification.

   The situation for emergency surgery is somewhat different. Virtually all insurance companies will support a veterinarian's decision to proceed with surgery, or even euthanasia subsequent to the surgery, if necessary. It is important to make a positive identification of the animal, however, and communicate with the insurance company as soon as possible.
3. **Performance of Euthanasia on Humane Grounds.** This area can create difficult decisions for the equine surgeon. We have all found ourselves in the situation of treating a valuable horse that is rendered useless for its proposed career and being pressured by the owner when the need for euthanasia on humane grounds is debatable. In this regard, the guidelines for recommending euthanasia set up by the AAEP Equine Insurance Committee, with the concurrence of all insurance industry representatives, are highly useful. The committee suggests that the following criteria be considered when evaluating the immediate necessity for intentional destruction of a horse: (*a*) Is the condition chronic and incurable? (*b*) Does the immediate condition have a hopeless prognosis for life? (*c*) Is the horse a hazard to himself or his handlers? (*d*) Will the horse require continuous medication for the relief of pain for the remainder of his life? If these guidelines are followed, difficult decisions can be more easily made.

Another problem regularly arises. On some occasions, a condition may be present that potentially could be treated by surgery but for which the prognosis is debatable and its success or failure not evident for some time in the future. To complicate matters, the insurance policy is shortly due to expire and the animal may be found insufficiently acceptable for insurance renewal beyond a 30-day extension clause.

As an example, we will use a horse having a comminuted fracture of the various carpal bones following a race. Although such a horse could be potentially salvaged for breeding by attempting primary repair with lag screw fixation augmented by cast immobilization, it was known that this operation could be unsuccessful, and a continued collapse of the carpus might occur several months later, requiring euthanasia. In such a case, expiration of the insurance policy in 1 month allows insufficient time for a fair decision to be made.

Such situations still pose problems, and it is important that the veterinarian knows what can be done and that the prognosis represents the interests of the parties concerned. It would be unfortunate, in such situations, if euthanasia were performed on a horse because the insurance company could not assure that the policy would not lapse before the situation was resolved.

Loss of Use Insurance

This insurance usually takes the form of a "loss of use endorsement" to a mortality insurance program. For an additional premium, the insurer would usually pay a percentage (60% is one figure quoted) of the value of the animal at the time of injury or of the insurance company's liability as specified in their schedule (or 50% of the value and the owner keeps the animal). Loss of use is determined if a horse (*a*) is injured by sudden external, accidental, and violent means; (*b*) becomes totally and permanently unfit for the use as specified in the declarations or schedule as a result of such injury; and (*c*) does not require destruction for humane reasons. There are caveats, however, including "lameness not brought about by a sudden external accidental and violent means, including but not limited to navicular disease, arthritis, degenerative joint disease, Lyme's disease, or bone spavins, which means careful preinjury evaluation is necessary" (3).

Major Medical or Surgical Insurance

There are two forms of "surgical" insurance that take the form of either major medical endorsements or surgical endorsements to mortality policies. Major medical carries a higher premium but a higher reimbursement. The policy would usually reimburse for all reasonable fees for surgery or medical expenses resulting from injury, illness, or disease. It will also pay 50% of any diagnostic test, but if a covered surgical or medical procedure is performed, they will pay 100% of that test or treatment. Of relevance to surgeons is that they pay all reasonable associated fees for both the actual surgery and the aftercare. However, aftercare is limited to 50% of the cost of surgery and does not extend beyond 20 days postsurgery. There is no deductible. Surgery must be performed under general anesthesia.

Other policies such as the surgical endorsement may limit reimbursement to a certain limit per animal. There are many options regarding liability limits.

REFERENCES

1. Rutkaw IM, Gittelsohn AN, Zuidema GD. Surgical decision making. The reliability of clinical judgement. Ann Surg 1979;190:409.
2. American Association of Equine Practitioners: The Veterinary Role in Equine Insurance. Golden, CO: 1985.
3. American Bankers Insurance Company of Florida, Miami. Livestock Mortality Program Loss of Use Endorsement in 1996.

2

GENERAL CONSIDERATIONS IN PREPARING THE EQUINE SURGICAL PATIENT

Numerous steps are involved in preparing a horse for surgery. Guidelines rather than hard and fast rules are presented because each case must be treated individually and because protocols vary, depending on whether surgery is emergency or elective. In emergency cases, certain procedures in the preoperative preparation must be omitted.

FOOD RESTRICTION AND GROOMING

In elective cases, all food (but not water) should be withheld. The duration of withholding varies, depending on the case. The authors withhold feed for 12 hours in cases of simple, relatively short procedures such as arthroscopic surgery and cryptorchidectomy. The night before surgery, the animal is muzzled. Some procedures require a longer period of food restriction (e.g., 24 hours) to produce more complete emptying of the intestinal tract, but such a requirement is rare in our experience.

Although food restriction is even more important in the ruminant, it is essential for surgical preparation of the horse. The most frequent problem the authors encounter in patients that were not sufficiently withheld from food is tympany of the large colon and cecum. We have seen a few cases in which the horse required celiotomy and intestinal decompression because respiratory embarrassment was so severe. Certainly, pressure on the diaphragm and inadequate ventilation represent the biggest threat to the horse's life. As a short-term remedy, the horse is first placed on mechanical ventilation. If bloating is persistent and severe, decompression of the distended large intestine can be achieved by trocharization via the flank. If the small bowel is distended, trocharization offers little value. It is most useful when the needle (e.g., 18 g, 3 inches) can be placed on a large gas cap of the cecum or large colon. Nasogastric intubation before anesthetic induction may be valuable in emergency cases in which the patient must be anesthetized on a full intestinal tract.

Oral antibiotics have been used in humans and in small animals to decrease bloating, but they are not used routinely in horses. The risk of altering the flora of the intestinal tract and producing a case of salmonellosis is far too great. The use of preoperative medications, including antibiotics and nonsteroidal anti-inflammatory drugs, is discussed elsewhere throughout the text.

The authors prefer to muzzle the horse rather than strip the bedding out of the stall. Without bedding, the horse often lies in feces overnight, which makes grooming the next morning a difficult chore. If the horse is muzzled, the muzzle must be applied securely so that the horse does not remove it and feed on the bedding material.

Horses that are dirty or shedding a winter coat must be thoroughly groomed before surgery. Some horses may require a bath to remove dirt and feces from their coats. Vacuuming of the hair coat with one of the commercially available vacuums used for show animals is also useful.

CLIPPING OF THE SURGICAL SITE

Unless the horse is unruly or must be anesthetized on an emergency basis, the authors clip the surgical site the night before surgery or early the same day of surgery. With a busy surgical practice it may be impractical to clip immediately before surgery, as is recommended for human patients. Clipping can produce microlacerations of the dermis, which, if inflicted the night before surgery, have a greater opportunity to become colonized by normal skin flora. Clipping a horse before surgery requires good technical support and communication between the surgeon and whoever will be clipping. A no. 40 blade is used in most instances, but the procedure can be expedited in horses with a heavy winter coat by using the coarser no. 10 clipper blade initially. The surgical area should always be clipped in a neat square or rectangle, with sharp, well-defined edges. (Owners often judge the success of the surgery by the neat clipping job and a neat suture line in the skin incision.) Horses undergoing surgery of the limbs should have hair removed around the limb's entire circumference. Some surgical sites are virtually impossible to clip until the animal has been anesthetized and is in dorsal recumbency. With most horses about to undergo celiotomy, it is possible to do most of the steps involved in clipping the ventral abdomen without anesthesia. Occasionally, depilatory creams are indicated to remove hair. The dense, coarse hair of the mane can be removed in patients undergoing laminectomy for dorsal decompression of the spinal cord.

The authors routinely shave for all equine surgery. It is important to note that any shaving used is done in the immediate preoperative period. However, this precaution does not necessarily avoid rapid growth of bacteria in injured sites during the operative procedure (1). Evidence in human surgery suggests that clipping is as good as or perhaps better than shaving for reducing potential contamination of the surgical wound and eliminates the need for skilled personnel to do the shaving. In a 1-year study in humans, hair was removed from the operative site with clippers (high quality clippers are necessary) instead of shaving or using depilatories. The study involved the comparison of clean (class I) wound infection rates in 2580 patients that were clipped with 17,424 patients in the 7 preceding years that were shaved and had depilation (1). There was no significant change in the wound infection rate (1%).

The use of chlorhexidine gluconate as an alternative to povidone-iodine has increased recently. One hundred seventeen cattle undergoing surgery were assigned randomly to two preoperative skin preparation protocols. Group I (60 animals) skin preparation was with povidone-iodine, soap, and isopropyl alcohol; group II (57 animals) had skin preparation with chlorhexidine gluconate and isopropyl alcohol. A significant decrease in colony-forming units (CFU) occurred postscrub for both skin preparations. Chlorhexidine and alcohol preparation resulted in significantly few CFUs and a greater percent reduction in CFUs postscrub than povidone-iodine and alcohol (2). Group II had a significantly higher percentage of negative cultures postscrub (49.1%) than did group I (18.3%). The number of postoperative CFUs was not significantly different between the two treatment groups. Also, wound infection frequency for clean surgical procedures was not significantly different between the two skin preparation protocols, although in this study a higher infection rate for ventral abdominal procedures compared with flank or orthopaedic procedures was noted.

In another study in dogs comparing povidone-iodine with chlorhexidine gluconate, there were no significant differences between povidone-iodine and chlorhexidine gluconate except that acute contact dermatitis was observed more frequently after skin preparation with povidone-iodine.

The authors concluded that both preparations were equally effective for up to 1 hour in the preoperative skin preparation of dogs (3). In a clinical trial of 100 dogs, there were no significant differences in percentages of bacterial reduction for surgical times of up to 8 hours, but there were fewer negative cultures after chlorhexidine plus 70% isopropyl alcohol rinse compared with povidone-iodine with saline or alcohol and chlorhexidine gluconate with saline. The authors concluded that chlorhexidine gluconate with alcohol may actually be inferior to povidone-iodine residual antimicrobial activity (4). However, in an experimental model (5), chlorhexidine was noted to be more effective as an irrigating solution in deep wounds when blood or plasma are added to muscle specimens before disinfection.

Immediately before the induction of anesthesia, the horse's mouth should be washed out. Catheterization of the jugular vein and cleaning of the feet should also be done at this time.

POSITION OF THE HORSE

Once the horse is anesthetized, the correct positioning of the horse on the operating table is ultimately the responsibility of the surgeon. A good support team, however, that knows not only how to position the horse but also understands the idiosyncratic demands of the surgeon is invaluable. Such a team allows the surgeon to proceed with scrubbing, gowning, and opening instruments, reducing much of the time the horse needs to be under the anesthetic. The surgeon should check the final position of the horse and suggest any "fine tuning" of the animal's position. The important part of positioning is ensuring that the surgical site does not require the surgical team to adopt an awkward fatiguing position throughout the procedure. Surgeon fatigue always compromises technique.

Padding of the horse must be adequate and correctly positioned to avoid pressure-related injuries to dependent muscle groups. The authors use commercially available water mattresses made to a size dictated by our table dimensions. Studies using Wick catheters to measure intracompartmental muscle pressures have shown that supporting a horse on a water mattress causes the least dramatic pressure elevation of the lower limb muscles (e.g., the triceps muscle), while foam padding produced the most (6). Careful selection of protective padding therefore reduces the severity of muscle damage (6). Water mattresses are surprisingly robust and if cared for will last 1 to 2 years. Small holes can be quickly repaired, but they do not withstand the ravages of towel clamps or scalpel blades. The water temperature within the waterbed can be controlled. Foals, especially those in various degrees of circulatory collapse, can be assisted in maintaining body temperature by using warm water. Adults can have cold water placed in the waterbed. Both authors have operated on many horses on foam-based padding; avoidance of prolonged surgery times obviates pressure-related problems.

All areas of concentrated pressure on the horse should be avoided, if possible. Limbs overhanging the table edge must be in contact with suitable padding. Horses in dorsal recumbency should not hang off the edge of the table. A standard-size operating table made for a 450- to 500-kg horse may not be suitable for one of the large draft or European breeds. Horses in lateral recumbency should have the upper hind limb raised by a suitable leg stand so that the medial thigh muscles are not compressed. Raising the upper hind limb also ensures that venous return is not compromised. The "down" forelimb should be pulled forward in extension, to reduce intracompartmental muscle pressures to acceptable levels (6). In particular, triceps and gluteal muscle groups should be adequately padded. The authors have found that diligent padding, positioning, and adequate blood pressure maintenance during surgery, combined with a short anesthetic time, are the best precautions against postanesthetic rhabdomyolysis ("tying-up").

SKIN PREPARATION

The aim of skin preparation is to remove debris and to reduce the bacterial population to levels that can be handled by the patient's natural defenses (7). Complete sterilization of the skin is impossible because many bacteria are harbored in the hair follicles. A wide area of skin should always be prepared in case the skin incision has to be lengthened or modified. Limbs subjected to surgery should be scrubbed around their entire circumference. Many methods of applying the numerous germicidal agents have been documented. Little difference has been shown between spraying or painting methods of application. Because of the density of the hair follicles in domestic animals, however, scrubbing with a germicide that has detergent properties has become accepted practice. The actual mechanical scrubbing of the skin is more important than the killing ability of the germicidal agent used.

The choice of germicide is commonly one of personal preference and tradition. At Colorado State University, three povidone-iodine scrubs (Betadine scrub) alternated with three (70%) alcohol rinses, performed by a gloved, trained veterinary technician, are used. After each alcohol application, the surgical site is dried with sterile hand towels. Alcohol rapidly kills microorganisms, and it defats the skin at the same time. Defatting the skin helps plastic surgical adhesive drapes adhere better. During their application, both the povidone-iodine and alcohol are applied with gauzes held either in the hand or with sponge forceps. The povidone-iodine is applied by vigorous scrubbing, while the alcohol is wiped on with firm pressure. In areas near open wounds or mucous membranes of the eye, sterile saline solution can be substituted for alcohol.

If one of the commercially available plastic surgical adhesive drapes is used, the final drying of the alcohol must be thorough; otherwise, the drape will not adhere. If plastic drapes are not being used, the surgical site can be sprayed with a suitable germicidal spray such as povidone-iodine (Betadine).

SURGICAL DRAPING

Plastic surgical adhesive drapes are used routinely in equine animal surgery. Their purpose is to prevent skin bacteria from gaining access to the surgical wound by immobilizing them. Controversy exists over their actual role in reducing wound infection. The adhesive drapes are useful in surgery of the limbs because surrounding anatomic landmarks can be identified, which is a difficult task if they are buried by an excessive amount of draping material. Some parts of the horse are unsuitable for draping with these products because of their uneven configuration or because the hair is too dense and coarse. A major drawback occurs when poor application of the drape allows blood and irrigation fluids to seep under it. The authors use films containing iodophor (Ioban, 3M Company, Medical Products Div., Minnesota Mining Company, St. Paul, MN)(also used in human surgery), which seem to adhere better. There have been no controlled studies proving their microbiologic efficacy in the horse.

For limb surgery on horses, the hoof must be diligently isolated from the surgical field. Several disposable gloves can be stretched over the foot. Plastic adhesive drapes can be used over the gloves to prevent the gloves from becoming dislodged. Alternatively, the plastic adhesive drapes can be used to isolate the hoof.

There are reams of literature regarding the advantages and disadvantages of disposable (single-use) or reusable drapes. The majority of the literature leans in favor of disposable drapes and gowns (i.e., a complete system) (8–11). Regardless the type of drape used, it must resist penetration by microorganisms. With the large variety of woven and nonwoven materials, the choice is often difficult. The old traditional draping material is muslin (140 threads per inch). It is capable of bacterial penetration when it becomes wet with any aqueous fluid, allowing microorganisms to travel freely in both directions (8, 9). The surgeon must keep this risk in mind, especially in lengthy wet operations such as abdominal surgery or repair of long bone fracture. These findings have prompted a finer type of drape (280 threads per inch) to be produced, but moisture is still a problem (8). An autoclaved orthopaedic stockinette, commonly used by human orthopaedic surgeons, does not have the recommended thread density and offers less resistance to bacterial strike than does the traditional muslin. In orthopaedic cases, such as repair of long bone fracture for which surgical time is long and the extent of surgical manipulation extreme, the use of a stockinette as a barrier should be discouraged. Bacterial penetration can occur even with dry drapes because of mechanical pressure.

Disposable drapes made of a nonwoven material resembling paper or synthetic polymers should now be accepted as the surgical drape of choice. Many veterinary hospitals now use them exclusively. They are waterproof, can be sterilized, and many are available prepackaged. Some manufacturers (Gepco, General Econopack, Inc., Philadelphia, PA) now cater entirely to the veterinary profession and will design a system that includes all the appropriately sized drapes for a particular operation. The authors currently have such a system for arthroscopic surgery and abdominal surgery.

One disadvantage of disposable drapes is that they are easily torn by towel clamps, as might occur when clamping an x-ray cassette to a limb for intraoperative radiographs.

The actual sequence of draping varies tremendously, depending on how the surgeon was trained. We have both been surprised at the different standards of draping seen at various surgical facilities throughout the world. Because virtually all the surgical procedures discussed in this book must be done under strict aseptic conditions, *isolation of a sterile field and its maintenance must be given the highest priority.* Although fast skillful surgery makes up for deficits in aseptic technique, such deficits should not be condoned. Before draping, the gowned surgeon should don two pairs of gloves because a break in aseptic technique is likely to occur at this time in the procedure. The drapes must be firmly anchored so that any inadvertent movement by the horse does not dislodge them and expose them to contaminated areas. The first drape should cover most of the horse (except for surgical site area). Projecting areas that the surgical team might brush against, such as table edges or the animal's limbs, must be covered.

Careful draping of the limb to be operated on requires good coordination and cooperation among surgeon, assistants, and operating room personnel. The limb can be suspended by white adhesive tape or a wire attached to an intravenous fluid stand, or it may be supported with a special leg stand that is part of the operating table.

To apply a plastic adhesive drape correctly, a sterile assistant should see that it is seated, without wrinkles, directly on the surgical site. The logical time to place the plastic adhesive drape is after the surrounding drapes are in position. This ensures that fluids are carried across the top of the drapes and are not allowed to flow under them (9). A method for additional draping, which is useful in long bone fracture repair, is the "toweling-in technique," performed after the skin incision is made. To secure drapes to the skin edge, a simple continuous suture of no. 1 or no. 2 nylon can be used. Michel clips or skin staples are also useful. Skin staples can be used to secure skin towels in areas that are difficult to drape (12).

For abdominal surgery, drapes to protect the wound edges are available. These consist of a flexible plastic ring attached to an opening of similar size in a plastic vinyl drape. After the abdomen is entered and hemostasis achieved, the drape is spread over the wound, and the ring is inserted into the abdomen and allowed to expand into its circular shape under the body wall. The plastic sheet is then tautly drawn and secured with towel clamps.

REFERENCES

1. Olson MM, MacCallum J, McQuarrie DG. Preoperative hair removal with clippers does not increase infection rate in clean surgical wounds. Surg Gynecol Obstet 1996;162:181–182.
2. Desrochers A, St-Jean G, Anderson DE, et al. Comparative evaluation of two surgical scrub preparations in cattle. Vet Surg 1996;25:336–341.
3. Osunu DJ, De Young DJ, Walker RL. Comparison of three skin preparation techniques in the day. Part 1: Experimental trial. Vet Surg 1990;19:14–19.
4. Osunu DJ, De Young DJ, Walker RL. Comparison of three skin preparation techniques. Part 2: Clinical trials in 100 days. Vet Surg 1990;19:20–23.
5. Taylor DJ, Leeming JD, Bannister GC. Effect of antiseptics, ultraviolet light and lavage on airborne bacteria in a model wound. J Bone Joint Surg 1993;75-B:724–730.
6. Lindsay WA, Pascoe PJ, McDonell WN, et al. Effect of protective padding on forelimb intracompartmental muscle pressures in anesthetized horses. Am J Vet Res 1985;46:688.
7. Kaul AF, Jewett JF. Agents and techniques for disinfection of the skin. Surg Gynecol Obstet 1981;152:677.
8. Ha'eri GB, Wiley AM. Wound contamination through drapes and gowns: a study using tracer particles. Clin Orthop 1981;154:181.
9. Beck WC. Aseptic barriers in surgery. Arch Surg 1981;116:240.
10. Cole WR, Bernard HR. Wound isolation in the prevention of postoperative wound infection. Surg Gynecol Obstet 1967;133:1.
11. Moylan JA, Kennedy BV. The importance of gown and drape barriers in the prevention of wound infection. Surg Gynecol Obstet 1980;151:465.
12. Morris DM. The use of skin staples to secure skin towels in areas difficult to drape. Surg Gynecol Obstet 1984;159:387.

3

USE OF PROPHYLACTIC ANTIBIOTICS IN EQUINE SURGERY

Surgical antibiotic prophylaxis, in the practical sense, refers to the administration of antibiotics to patients without clinical evidence of infection in the operative field (1). The objectives of prophylaxis are to prevent naturally occurring organisms in one site from proliferating in a normally sterile site, to prevent organisms that are contaminating a normally sterile site from producing disease, and to prevent infection by exogenous organisms. Antibiotic prophylaxis is indicated in the surgical patient when there is a high risk of postoperative infection, or when there is a low risk but the consequences of infection could be devastating or lethal.

It is now well-recognized that in the majority of "clean" surgical procedures, the use of antibiotic prophylaxis is unnecessary. However, there are no controlled studies in horses to define the differences made by using antibiotics in preventing infection of surgical sites. Clearly, the wide use of antibiotics in association with surgery has not eliminated surgical infection as a threat to the patient. There is evidence that widespread, and often indiscriminate, use of these antibiotics may be responsible for the changing sensitivity patterns of bacteria implicated in nosocomial infections and for the emergence of bacterial species (amphibionts) that were previously considered nonpathogenic. (Nosocomial infections are discussed elsewhere in this book.) The emergence of pathogenic species combined with the selection of resistant organisms is of great concern.

WOUND INFECTIONS

The first step in the development of an infected wound is bacterial contamination of surgically manipulated tissue. Bacterial contamination, a component of every surgical wound, arises from two sources: exogenous contamination from the surgery room or endogenous contamination from the skin or from the gastrointestinal, respiratory, or urogenital tracts of the patient. Whether the bacterial contamination produces infection depends on the number and virulence of the organisms, the patient's defense mechanisms, and the condition of the disrupted tissue. Exogenous habitats of potential pathogens include water, soil, fodder, fomites, and nonequine animal reservoirs. Obviously, these sources should be restricted in the surgery room. The majority of the microorganisms of veterinary importance are not true free-living organisms. Contaminated water, however, is a common source of enterobacteria, and *Salmonella* persists in tap water for 87 days and in pond water for 115 days (2). The most noteworthy equine pathogen found to be free-living in many bodies of water is *Pseudomonas aeruginosa*, which is also found in the intestinal tract and on mucous membranes.

For endogenous infection, indigenous microflora are found throughout the GI tract, upper respiratory tract, genitourinary tract, skin, and visible mucous membranes (2). There is no evidence of permanent resident microflora in muscle, the lower respiratory tract, or organs outside the GI tract.

The risk of staphylococcal infection from the patient's skin, an endogenous source of infection, must be considered. It is of major concern in antibiotic prophylaxis in humans during insertion of implants. Bacteremia, particularly in foals, also represents a source of infection (it is considered capable of seeding prosthetic materials). Another group of patients of concern are those that have a foci of infection remote to the intended operative site. Three areas that may be infected before surgery are the skin, lungs, and genitourinary tract (3). Patients with infection in these sites have been reported as having three times the normal surgical infection rate.

People are the major source of contamination in the hospital environment; therefore, the shedding potential must be controlled. Thirty percent of the population are carriers for *Staphylococcus aureus* (4). Persons shedding more than 1000 bacteria per minute are classified as shedders. In a conventional operating room, the more complete the surgical attire worn by everyone in the room, the better the control of shedding potential. This applies to the use of body exhaust equipment for the anesthesiologist and scrub nurse as well as for the surgeon. Other effective environmental controls purported to reduce wound contamination are laminar airflow systems and the use of ultraviolet light.

Whether a bacterial contamination becomes an infection depends on critical events in the early inflammatory phase following surgery, which is a "decisive period" in wound infection. If the occurrence of inflammation is inappropriate and phagocytosis is overwhelmed, the patient develops an infection. Necrosis, ischemia, hemorrhage, and the presence of debris impair local host defense mechanisms and decrease the number of bacterial organisms required to cause infection. If a host is compromised, there is an increased risk for infection (1). If an appropriate antimicrobial agent is present in adequate concentrations, an infection in the contaminated wound is less likely. Antibiotics must be present in the tissues in the early decisive period to effectively prevent bacterial invasion and proliferation. If they are given later, when the bacteria are well established, the antibiotics will have no prophylactic effect. For example, in a clinical study involving human patients undergoing gastric, biliary, or colonic surgery, it was found that cefazolin, administered 1 hour before surgery, significantly decreased the incidence of postoperative infection in comparison with a placebo. If the cefazolin was begun 1 to 4 hours after the operation, however, no reduction occurred in the postoperative infection rate (1).

The probability of surgical wound infection can be ascertained by estimating the microbial density in the wound. Because this method may not be practical for a given surgical procedure, a method of clinical classification that predicts the incidence of wound infection has been established (5, 6). In our text, this classification scheme refers to surgical wounds. Some authors apply this classification to surgical procedures.

CLASSIFICATION OF SURGICAL WOUNDS

Clean Surgical Wounds

Clean surgical wounds are produced when procedures are performed on a noncompromised host under ideal operating room conditions. Such procedures are elective, and no entry is made into the oropharyngeal cavity or lumen of the respiratory, alimentary, or genitourinary tracts. Inflammation is not encountered, there is no break in the sterile technique, and the incision is primarily closed without placement of a drain. Examples of such procedures in the horse include elective joint surgery for removal of chip fragments and osteochondritis dissecans debridement.

Clean-Contaminated Surgical Wounds

Clean-contaminated surgery involves controlled opening of the oropharyngeal cavity or the lumen of the respiratory, alimentary, or genitourinary tracts without significant contamination from these sites. This category also includes wounds that are otherwise clean in which surgery is performed on an urgent or emergency basis; a wound created in an area that has received blunt trauma with intact skin; reoperation within 7 days through a previously clean incision; and those surgical sites where a minor break in the sterile technique occurs. Because the mucosa of the oropharyngeal, respiratory, alimentary, and genitourinary tracts harbor diffuse and dense microbiologic flora, some contamination of the wound is inevitable. Procedures involving the upper respiratory tract are good examples of this situation.

Contaminated Surgical Wounds

Contaminated surgical wounds involve surgery at a site where there has been a penetrating trauma of less than 4 hours' duration; a major break in sterile technique; nonpurulent inflammation at the operative site; major spillage from a hollow viscus; and chronic open wounds that are being grafted, revised, or debrided.

Dirty Surgical Wounds

Surgical wounds are classified as dirty if there is purulence or abscessation, penetrating trauma greater than 4 hours' duration, or preoperative perforation of the alimentary, urogenital, or respiratory tracts.

In humans, infection rates for clean, clean-contaminated, and contaminated and dirty surgical wounds are < 2%, < 10%, 20%, and 40%, respectively (6).

PROPHYLACTIC VALUE OF ANTIBIOTICS

Any specific recommendations regarding antibiotic prophylaxis in equine surgery are difficult because of a lack of controlled retrospective studies. We often extrapolate information from human studies and then apply it to our own situation. In doing so, the following general principles should be recognized.

It is unequivocally accepted that prophylactic antibiotics are most effective when given before the inoculation of bacteria at the surgical site. A full therapeutic dose should be delivered, preferably intravenously, before surgery at such a time as to ensure appropriate tissue levels at the time of incision. The half-life of the antibiotic should be long enough to maintain effective tissue levels for the duration of the procedure. Should the procedure last more than 3 hours or two times the half-life of the selected antibiotic, the antibiotic should be redosed (7).

Prophylactic antibiotics should be selected with a knowledge of the most likely pathogens, their antimicrobial susceptibilities, and the minimum inhibitory concentrations of antibiotics that are necessary. Effective hospital surveillance for surgical site infections and current data regarding the wound isolates and their sensitivities are essential for identifying new pathogens or any significant changes in the patterns of resistance. The antibiotics selected for prophylaxis should be safe for the patient and cost effective.

Combinations of antibiotics may be advantageous if the combination provides a broader spectrum of coverage than any single antibiotic, if the selected antibiotics have different mechanisms of action, and if the antibiotics act synergistically (8). Inappropriate antibiotic combination therapy, however, can produce the following problems: (*a*) drug interactions at receptor sites, (*b*) changes in elimination of drugs because of competition for elimination routes, (*c*) potential for greater disruption of normal flora, (*d*) adverse drug reactions, and (*e*) increased costs with little or no benefit (9).

It has been shown in humans and in dogs that prophylactic antibiotics are not necessary for most clean procedures (10, 11). Exceptions would be a clean operation in which an implant is placed or in which there are patient risk factors that would increase the likelihood of surgical infection. In these instances prophylactic antibiotics are recommended. Prophylactic antibiotics are indicated in clean-contaminated, contaminated, and dirty procedures.

There is an inherent risk, however, in recommending that prophylactic antibiotics are not necessary or should not be used with clean operations. The risk is that many factors can be related to this so-called clean operation that increase the likelihood of surgical infection. The decision to use prophylactic antibiotics should be based on the surgeon's assessment of the patient's condition, on the likelihood of endogenous or exogenous bacterial inoculation of the wound, and on the surgeon's own level of skill and experience. In other words, the surgeon does a risk assessment for the probability of surgical site infection.

The assessment of the effects of antibiotics in surgical procedures is difficult because antibiotic prophylaxis is only one of many factors that can influence outcome. Indeed, antibiotics probably play a minor role in preventing postoperative infection when compared with the surgeon's skill in removing dead tissue and blood clots or in providing adequate drainage, or with the activities of a well-trained epidemiologist in maintaining proper infection control (9). The surgical procedure should be done properly and swiftly, and care should be taken to handle the tissues gently and maintain normal physiologic conditions. The use of closed suction drains is recommended for deep wounds in which a dead space is left. In other situations, drains are deleterious because of their potential to cause retrograde infection.

Although one cannot recommend with certainty the amount of time that an antibiotic should be continued when it is used prophylactically, there is evidence that no more than one or two additional antibiotic doses are necessary for effective antibiotic prophylaxis in the normal host (1). In a retrospective study, no difference in infection rates was observed between patients receiving antibiotics for 1 day after surgery and those receiving antibiotics for 7 days after surgery (12). This finding is important because antibiotics are expensive, can involve drug-related side effects, and may unfavorably influence the local and hospital microflora. (This last problem is further discussed in the section "Nosocomial Infections" in Chapter 4.) In addition, disturbing the endogenous microflora is considered to be particularly important in the induction of postoperative complications such as salmonellosis in the horse.

STUDIES IN EQUINE AND HUMAN PATIENTS

The use of perioperative antibiotics for equine gastrointestinal surgery is well accepted, although their general use in human abdominal surgery has been challenged (13). Studies in humans have emphasized that they should be used in a sufficient dose to provide coverage of the endogenous or exogenous pathogens anticipated and that they should be given for short periods only. In general, short-term perioperative antibiotic prophylaxis is believed to be useful (14).

The authors recommend potassium or sodium penicillin G (22,000 IU/kg IV, q.i.d.) and gentamicin (2.2 mg/kg IV, t.i.d. or 6.6 mg/kg IV, s.i.d.) as prophylactic antibiotics for gastrointestinal surgery in the horse (15). This drug combination provides effective protection against both aerobes and anaerobes with the exception of *Bacteroides fragilis.* Metronidazole (15–25 mg/kg per OS or per rectum, q.i.d.) can also be added to this antibiotic combination to provide more coverage against anaerobic bacteria (16, 17).

Aminoglycosides can have toxic effects that include neuromuscular blockade, cardiovascular depression, nephrotoxicity, and inhibition of gut motility, and the surgeon should keep these in mind when selecting an aminoglycoside for prophylaxis. If the use of an aminoglycoside is extended beyond 3 days, particularly in a critically ill patient, the dosage and treatment intervals may need to be modified based on monitoring of plasma concentrations and renal function. These drugs can also affect the normal bacterial population of the GI tract of the patient with an acute abdomen, and have some potential to contribute to postoperative complications such as diarrhea (which may or may not be caused by salmonellosis).

In human orthopaedics, many elective musculoskeletal procedures, especially those of short duration, do not require antibiotics. The one exception, however, is the large group of procedures involving implantation of foreign bodies, for which the results of infection can be catastrophic. Antibiotic prophylaxis is therefore considered justifiable and necessary in such cases. *Staphylococcus aureus* and *S. epidermidis* are the organisms implicated in more than 90% of the infections occurring after implant surgery in humans. Because first-generation cephalosporins are active against most staphylococci, their use is desirable in this situation. Cephalosporins are considered to offer protection equal to that offered by other single agents or antibiotic combinations, and the risk of side effects is minimal. Twenty-four hours or less of a first- or second-generation cephalosporin is often recommended for antibiotic prophylaxis in the normal host for clean and clean-contaminated procedures (1, 7, 18, 19).

Penicillin G is considered to have limited use in human orthopaedic surgery because of its relative lack of activity against penicillinase-producing *Staphylococcus aureus* and most Gram-negative pathogens. The semisynthetic penicillins have enhanced anti–Gram-negative activity and are useful for prophylaxis against such organisms as *Escherichia coli.* These factors must be considered when evaluating the use of prophylaxis in equine orthopaedics.

Recommendations for equine patients require knowledge of the most likely bacterial combination of surgical sites. In most human trauma centers, coverage with two antibiotics is recommended for open fractures because of the difficulty in treating Gram-negative microorganisms, which have been found with increasing frequency in posttraumatic wound infections. One author recommends administration of cefazolin and gentamicin for 4 to 5 days, with either benzyl penicillin G or clindamycin added for highly contaminated wounds in which anaerobes are expected (1).

Little information is available on the effectiveness of antibiotic prophylaxis in equine orthopaedic surgery. Information from retrospective studies of orthopaedic infections shows that the staphylococcal bacteria are the most likely organisms to be cultured from infected joints following surgery, but Enterobacteriaceae may also be recovered (20). Infections of surgically repaired fractures will usually culture more than one bacteria type, including *Staphylococcus* spp., Enterobacteriaceae, *Pseudomonas* spp., *Streptococcus* spp., and anaerobes (21).

Elective arthroscopic procedures are clean and therefore prophylactic antibiotics should not be necessary (22). However, many of these patients have been recently injected with intraarticular corticosteroids or other intraarticular agents, some of which produce synovitis. Often, the history of treatment is vague, and as a result many surgeons prefer to use prophylactic antibiotics such as penicillin and gentamicin or amikacin for routine arthroscopic surgery. Perioperative antibiotics are certainly indicated in horses undergoing fracture repair utilizing implants. A combination of penicillin G or cephalosporin and amikacin is indicated for prophylaxis in horses undergoing surgical repair of a long bone fracture (23). Frequently in these patients, antibiotics are administered for at least 4 to 5 days following surgery.

Antibiotic prophylaxis is commonly used for prosthetic laryngoplasty and mesh herniorrhaphy. Nonabsorbable material is implanted, and infection could have devastating consequences.

The use of local antibiotic treatment and intraoperative wound lavage is controversial in humans and has not been well studied in the horse. In the horse, frequent surgical site lavage with an antibiotic solution is an accepted practice during prolonged orthopaedic procedures.

The finding that aminoglycosides are chemically and microbiologically suitable for inclusion in polymethylmethacrylate (PMMA) bone cements for prevention or treatment of orthopaedic surgical infection has led to their use in human and veterinary orthopaedics, particularly in association with implant surgery. The drug has also been incorporated into PMMA beads and plaster-of-Paris pellets (24). Antibiotic-impregnated PMMA beads and cylinder-shaped implants have been used for local treatment in the horse (25, 26).

Antimicrobial-impregnated polymethylmethacrylate (AIPMMA) can be surgically implanted into a site of infection and deliver a high local concentration of antimicrobial with limited systemic absorption. This is advantageous for avoiding toxic or allergic effects of the drug. Effective local concentrations are maintained for several weeks, making the treatment cost effective. The antibiotic selection should be based on culture and sensitivity testing and on the available information of the antibiotic's elution characteristics from the PMMA. It is imperative that the AIPMMA be used in conjunction with appropriate wound management, including complete surgical debridement and the establishment of effective drainage (25, 26).

RECOMMENDATIONS

The following points are important to consider when choosing prophylactic antibiotics:

1. Prophylaxis should be directed against the most likely pathogens at a specific site. Antimicrobials cannot sterilize all possible pathogens at all sites in the animal. The surgeon must therefore consider: (*a*) susceptibility of the most likely pathogens, (*b*) activity of the drug, and (*c*) the pharmacokinetics of the drug.
2. The shorter the duration of antibiotic administration, the broader the range of organisms inhibited. A longer duration of administration is more likely to result in resistant organisms.
3. The dose of the antibiotic must be equal to the therapeutic dose and delivered before surgery at such a time as to ensure appropriate tissue levels at the time of incision.

The surgeon must select the *appropriate antibiotic*, the *effective concentration* at the site of bacterial lodgment, and the *critical time* of administration.

REFERENCES

1. Mader JT, Cierny G. The principles of the use of preventative antibiotics. Clin Orthop 1984;190:75.

2. Knight HD, Hietala S. Antimicrobial susceptibility patterns in horses. Second Equine Pharmacology Symposium. Denver, CO: American Association of Equine Practitioners, 1978:63.
3. Monson TP, Nelson CL. Microbiology for orthopedic surgeons: selected aspects. Clin Orthop 1984;190:14.
4. Ritter MA. Surgical wound environment. Clin Orthop 1984;190:11.
5. Ad Hoc Committee of the Committee on Trauma, Division of Medical Sciences, National Research Council, National Academy of Sciences. Postoperative wound infections: the influence of ultraviolet irradiation of the operating room and various other factors. Ann Surg 1964;160(Suppl):1.
6. Page CP, Bohnen JMA, Fletcher JR, et al. Antimicrobial prophylaxis for surgical wounds. Arch Surg 1993;128:79–88.
7. Meakins JL. Guidelines for prevention of surgical site infection. Surgical infections: diagnosis and treatment. Sci Am Med 1994:127–138.
8. Solomkin JS, Miyagawa CI. Principles of antibiotic therapy: surgical clinics of North America. 1994;74:497–517.
9. Quintilani R, Nightengale C. Principles of antibiotic usage. Clin Orthop 1984;190:31.
10. Guglilelmo BJ, Hohn DC, Koo PJ, et al. Antibiotic prophylaxis in surgical procedures: a critical analysis of the literature. Arch Surg 1983;118:943.
11. Vasseur PB, Paul HA, Enos LR, et al. Infection rates in clean surgical procedures. A comparison of ampicillin prophylaxis vs. a placebo. JAVMA 1985;187:825.
12. Nelson CL, Green TG, Porter RA, et al. One day versus seven days of antibiotic therapy in orthopedic surgery. Clin Orthop 1983;176:250.
13. Hurley DL, Paxton H, Hahn HH. Perioperative prophylactic antibiotics in abdominal surgery: a review of recent progress. Surg Clin North Am 1979;59:919.
14. Lewis RT, Allan CM, Goodall GR, et al. Discriminate use of antibiotic prophylaxis in gastroduodenal surgery. Am J Surg 1979;138:640.
15. Godber LM, Walker RD, Stein GE, et al. Pharmacokinetics, nephrotoxicosis, and in vitro antibacterial activity associated with single versus multiple (three times) daily gentamicin treatments in horses. Am J Vet Res 1995;56:613–618.
16. Garber JL, Brown MP, Grunwall RS, et al. Pharmacokinetics of metronidazole after rectal administration in horses. Am J Vet Res 1993;54:2060–2063.
17. Sweeney RW, Sweeney CR, Soma LR, et al. Pharmacokinetics of metronidazole given to horses by intravenous and oral routes. Am J Vet Res 1986;47:1726–1729.
18. Fitzgerald RH. Cephalosporin antibiotics in the prevention and treatment of musculoskeletal sepsis. J Bone Joint Surg 1983;65-A:1201.
19. Williams DN, Gustilo RB. The use of preventative antibiotics in orthopaedic surgery. Clin Orthop 1984;190:83.
20. Schneider RK, Bramlage LR, Moore RM, et al. A retrospective study of 192 horses affected with septic arthritis/tenosynovitis. Equine Vet J 1992;24(6):436–442.
21. Snyder JR, Pascoe JR, Hirsh DC. Antimicrobial susceptibility of microorganisms isolated from equine orthopedic patients. Vet Surg 1987;16(3):197–201.
22. McIlwraith CW, Yovich JV, Martin GS. Arthroscopic surgery for the treatment of osteochondral chip fractures in the equine carpus. JAVMA 1987;191(5):531–540.
23. Moore RM, Schneider RK, Kowalski J, et al. Antimicrobial susceptibility of bacterial isolates from 233 horses with musculoskeletal infection during 1979–1989. Equine Vet J 1992;24:450–456.
24. Whelton A. The aminoglycosides. Clin Orthop 1984;190:66.
25. Swalec-Tobias KM, Schneider RK, Besser TE. Use of antimicrobial-impregnated polymethylmethacrylate. JAVMA 1996;208:841–845.
26. Schneider RK, Andrea R, Barnes HG. Use of antibiotic-impregnated polymethylmethacrylate for treatment of an open radial fracture in a horse. JAVMA 1995;207:1454–1457.

4

COMPLICATIONS OF EQUINE SURGERY

Postoperative Rhabdomyolysis (Myopathy)

Postanesthetic myopathy (also called rhabdomyolysis) is an uncommon but serious complication of general anesthesia. It is usually associated with extended periods of general anesthesia or prolonged recumbency. The condition was originally thought to be a neurologic problem caused by nerve compression and dysfunction, but the usual cause of musculoskeletal compromise following anesthesia has since been recognized as being associated with pathologic change in the muscles (1, 2). However, peripheral myopathy can occur in conjunction with postanesthetic myopathy as well as independently (3). In addition, neurologic dysfunction at the level of the spinal cord can also result in a horse's failure to recover from anesthesia (4). Previous separation of localized and generalized myopathy entities in the first edition of this text are probably inappropriate now as investigations have revealed the generalized nature of this condition. However, a localized compartment-like syndrome has been recognized and may occur (5). The condition is most often noticed during recovery from anesthesia, but in some instances may appear later. Difficulty recovering or failure to recover from anesthesia is noted, as is an increased level of pain that in turn causes distress and excitement, as well as tachycardia, tachypnea, and sweating (6).

The muscles involved in postanesthetic myopathy in horses in lateral recumbency include the triceps brachii, supraspinatus, infraspinatus, pectorals, brachycephalic, deltoid, intercostal, masseter, hind limb extensors, and quadriceps femoris muscles. For horses in dorsal recumbency, the muscles of the back—longissimus, iliocostalis, and gluteal medius as well as the vastus lateralis and adductor (adductor pectineus and gracilis muscles) can be affected. Although the problem is usually associated with muscles in contact with the operating table, the upper limb can be involved, and the problem is usually associated with inappropriate or insufficient support to prevent compression and compromised circulation. Affected muscle groups will be swollen and painful on palpation. Muscle fasciculation may also be observed (6).

Triceps myopathy is the most commonly recognized entity for horses in lateral recumbency. An affected limb will bear little weight, and the elbow is dropped. Increased intracompartmental pressures, up to 80 mg of mercury, have been observed. Increasing intracompartmental pressure is painful. Such increase in pressure may also affect nerve transmission and can explain the confusion between the terms "triceps brachii rhabdomyolysis or myopathy" and "radial paralysis." Complete paralysis of the brachial plexus or the radial nerve causing a nonpainful lameness has been reported (7).

Horses with myopathy after dorsal recumbency anesthesia usually present with dysfunction of the hind limbs. When adductor muscles are affected, horses have difficulty standing and tend to have a wide-based crouched position in the hind limbs. The stifle, hock, and fetlock joints are flexed, with the animal attempting to bear weight on the dorsal aspect of the hooves (8). Dysfunction in the quadriceps muscles (as seen with prolonged extension of the hind limbs with femoropatellar arthroscopy) causes extensor dysfunction and similar signs. Nerve paralysis of the femoral or sciatic nerve may also cause a similar posture without pain (3). When the myopathy problem involves the longissimus dorsi and gluteal muscle groups, there is back pain and reluctance to walk (6).

Diagnosis can usually be made on evidence of clinical signs alone. However, measurement of muscle enzymes has been used to confirm the diagnosis or aid in differential diagnosis. Serum creatine kinase (CK) increases rapidly and usually peaks 6 to 8 hours after anesthesia. In cases of significant myopathy, the levels are usually above 2000 IU/L. In one study, CK activity exceeded 9000 IU/L after 6 hours of anesthesia (9). In the same study, aspartate transaminase activity (AST) increased more slowly, plateauing 24 to 48 hours after anesthesia and exceeding values of 900 IU/L. Some increase in these enzymes is usual after uncomplicated anesthesia. Gleed suggests that maximal CK and AST levels should exceed 3000 and 400 IU/L, respectively, to support a diagnosis of postanesthetic myopathy (6).

The differential diagnosis of postoperative myopathy includes traumatic fracture or luxation, myelomalacia, hemorrhagic myelopathy, and thromboembolic ischemic myelopathy. Hemorrhagic myelopathy manifests as complete hind limb paralysis with lack of nociception. The first author has encountered four cases, all involving young Warmblood horses. In no instance was anesthesia prolonged, and the causes are controversial (4).

Etiology and Pathogenesis

The pathologic changes in the muscles have been well described elsewhere (6). Extrapolating from muscle crush syndrome in humans, it has been suggested that deformation (stretch) of cell membranes by external compression permits increased cellular influx of sodium chloride, water, and calcium down their electrochemical gradients (6). At the same time, the energy available for cationic extrusion pumps is reduced by ischemic hypoxia secondary to vascular compression. As a result, the muscle cells swell and the concentration of sarcoplasmic and mitochondrial calcium increases as the pumps are overwhelmed. Increased calcium, in turn, then leads to activation of autolytic processes and further interference with cell respiration and homeostasis.

The closing pressure for muscle capillaries is approximately 30 mm Hg, and pressure greater than this for a period of time will lead to ischemic neuromuscular damage (10). Pressures above this have been reported in the weight-bearing muscles of horses under anesthesia (1, 5, 11, 12). It has been suggested that during ischemia, the energy stores of the muscle are depleted by the reduced ability to generate ATP and the continued amount of the mechanisms responsible for cellular homeostasis. More recently it has been suggested that the most significant damage occurs during reperfusion after ischemia and not during the period of ischemia itself (6). Researchers believe that during reperfusion the sodium–calcium exchange mechanism is reactivated—the sodium being exchanged for calcium—resulting in further accumulation of intracellular calcium. Excessive intracellular calcium impairs a number of cellular functions, including mitochondrial inhibition and ATP production, activation of proteinases, and proteolytic conversion of xanthine dehydrogenase to xanthine oxidase. These changes, in turn, lead to production of free radicals. Free radicals attack the unsaturated bonds of free fatty acids in the phospholipid layer of cellular membranes, causing cellular swelling, edema, and necrosis (13, 14).

Treatment

Treatment for postanesthetic myopathy should be prompt and vigorous. It is essentially symptomatic. The initial treatment should be directed at preventing further muscle damage, and this in turn involves symptomatic treatment with tranquilizers and analgesics. Mild cases may require nothing more than observation, but NSAIDs such as phenylbutazone and flunixin meglumine are used. Acetylpromazine (.04 mg/kg intravenously) will promote vasodilation in the muscle and tranquilization. Xylazine (0.1–0.3 mg/kg intravenously) or detomidine hydrochloride (10–20 μg/kg intravenously) will produce both sedation and analgesia (6). Detomidine has also been suggested as having a longer duration of effectiveness. In some instances, more potent analgesics such as meperidine may be indicated.

The relationship to pathogenic pathways previously described suggests treating with free radical scavengers such as dimethylsulfoxide (DMSO) is logical. Although cellular accumulation of calcium seems to play a role in ischemic and reperfusion muscle damage, conventional calcium entry blockers do not appear to protect against reperfusion injury (15). However, the use of potassium-sparing diuretics such as amiloride and benzamil have been reported as experimentally inhibiting sodium–calcium exchange during reperfusion and provide partial protection against reperfusion injury (6). If these drugs are being used clinically, simultaneous fluid administration is critical. The use of glucocorticoids (such as dexamethasone sodium phosphate) is also logical to reduce inflammation and inhibit prostaglandin synthesis. The latter can promote free radical production.

Equally important in the treatment is nursing care, including assistance standing and appropriate padding and nursing if the horse is not immediately able to stand. Hopefully, the horse has some ability to attempt to stand, in which case assisting with a tail rope through a wall ring as well a similar device for the head is the best option. If support of the tail and head is unsuccessful, the use of a sling is another option. However, not all animals can adapt to such support. Minimal anesthetic time and careful positioning and padding of the horse are the critical features in preventing this problem (16).

Padding should evenly distribute the weight of an animal over as large an area as possible. At Colorado State University, the authors have used commercially available waterbeds for the past 17 years. A study in 1985 showed that a water mattress produced the least traumatic increase in triceps muscle pressure when horses were in lateral recumbency. This was followed by air dunnage bag, concrete flooring, and a 10-cm thick foam mattress (11). However, another study showed foam to be superior to no padding at all (5). The authors use thick pads in the recovery stall. It is important to use waterproof pads because water leakage into the foam will decrease their ability to satisfactorily provide padding. Closed-cell mattresses are another option. Limb positioning also can help, particularly in lateral recumbency. The lower limb is always pulled forward, and the edge of the table should not be under the brachial area or the shoulder. Support of the upper limb to prevent adductor compression (particularly in the hind limb) is important. In dorsal recumbency, the hind limbs are not usually supported (unless surgery is being done on them). Avoid having the legs in extension and unsupported.

Blood pressure maintenance is important because systemic arterial hypotension induced by halothane reportedly causes myopathy (1, 17). Some researchers suggest that mean systemic arterial pressure be maintained in excess of 80 mm Hg and that a pressure below 70 mm Hg be treated by minimizing the depth of anesthesia and intravenous fluid administration. Dobutamine is commonly used to augment cardiac output or perfusion pressure (18). This is given to effect using a solution of 0.1 mg dobutamine per milliliter of 0.9% saline (6). Noninvasive indirect methods of measuring blood pressure are the most convenient, but the authors prefer direct blood pressure measurement using an arterial catheter. The use of DMSO as a prophylactic free radical scavenger in horses that are problem-prone (such as draft horses) has also been recommended.

Another potential preventive measure is the prophylactic use of the calcium channel blocker dantrolene (19). Dantrolene has been used to treat malignant hyperthermia in humans and is suggested as possibly appropriate in those horses at risk (20). The oral formulation has been used for prophylaxis, but because of risk uncertainty, evaluating its usefulness is virtually impossible. More recent reviewers have suggested it not be used. It has been associated with prolonged recumbency and is potentially hepatotoxic. There is little evidence for its effectiveness.

REFERENCES

1. Lindsay WA, Robinson GM, Brunson DB, et al. Induction of equine postanesthetic myositis after halothane-induced hypotension. Am J Vet Res 1989;50:404–410.
2. White KK, Short C. Anesthetic/surgical stress-induced myopathy (myositis). II. A postanesthetic myopathy trial. Procedures of the 24th Annual Meeting of the American Association of Equine Practitioners, Miami, FL, 1979:107.
3. Dyson S, Taylor P, Witwell K. Femoral nerve paralysis after general anaesthesia. Equine Vet J 1988;20:376–380.
4. Yovich JV, Lecouteur RA, Stashak TS, et al. Postanesthetic hemorrhagic myelopathy in a horse. JAVMA 1986;188:300–301.
5. White NA, Suarez M. Change in triceps muscle intracompartmental pressure with repositioning and padding of the lower most thoracic limb of the horse. Am J Vet Res 1986;47:2257–2260.
6. Gleed RD. Postanesthetic myopathy. In: Nixon AJ, ed. Fractures in the Horse. Philadelphia: WB Saunders, 1996:343–349.
7. Robertson SA, Green SL, Carter SW, et al. Postanesthetic recumbency associated with hyperkalemic periodic paralysis in a Quarter Horse. JAVMA 1992;201:1209–1212.
8. Dodmann H, Williams R, Court MH, et al. Postanesthetic hindlimb adductor myopathy in five horses. JAVMA 1988;193:83–86.
9. Muir WM. Complications. In: Muir WM, Hubbell JAE, eds. Equine Anesthesia: Monitoring and Emergency Therapy. St. Louis: Mosby, 1991:419–443.
10. Hargens AR, Akeson WH, Mubarak SK, et al. Fluid balance within the canine anterolateral compartment and its relationship to compartment syndromes. J Bone Jt Surg 1978;60A:499–505.
11. Lindsay WA, Pascoe PJ, McDonell WN, et al. Effect of protective padding on forelimb intracompartmental muscle pressures in anesthetized horses. Am J Vet Res 1985;46: 688–691.
12. Norman WM, Williams R, Dodman NH, et al. Postanesthetic compartmental syndrome in a horse. JAVMA 1989;195:502–504.
13. Korthuis RJ, Granger DN, Townsley MI, et al. The role of oxygen-derived free radicals in ischemia-induced increases in canine skeletal muscle vascular permeability. Circ Res 1985;57:599–609.
14. McCord JM. Oxygen-derived free radicals in postischemic tissue injury. N Engl J Med 1985;312:159–163.
15. Odeh M. The role of reperfusion-induced injury in the pathogenesis of the crush syndrome. N Engl J Med 1991;324:1417–1422.
16. Gleed RD, Dobson A. Improvement in arterial oxygen tension with change in posture in anaesthetized horses. Res Vet Sci 1988;44:255–259.

17. Grandy JL, Steffey EP, Hodgson DS, et al. Arterial hypotension and the development of postanesthetic myopathy in halothane-anesthetized horses. Am J Vet Res 1987; 48:192–197.
18. Donaldson LL. Retrospective assessment of dobutamine therapy for hypotension in anesthetized horses. Vet Surg 1988;17:53–57.
19. Valverde A, Boyd CJ, Dyson DH, et al. Prophylactic use of dantrolene associated with prolonged postanesthetic recumbency in a horse. JAVMA 1990;197:1051–1053.
20. Waldron-Mease E. Correlation of post-operative and exercise-induced myopathy with the defect malignant hyperthermia. In: Proceedings of the 24th Annual Convention of the American Association of Equine Practitioners, St. Louis, MO, 1978:95–99.

Wound Infection

Wound infection after surgery is an ever present threat, regardless the type of surgery, the duration of surgery, or the experience of the surgeon. The overall effect on the patient will vary from simply extended hospital time to loss of limb function (e.g., septic arthritis) or even death (e.g., peritonitis after intestinal anastomosis). The authors have no concrete numbers regarding the cost of wound infection as it relates to increased hospitalization, further bandages, and more antibiotics, but the cost should not be underestimated. Extended hospitalization increases the horse's chance of acquiring a nosocomial infection or acting as a source of infection for other animals. The end result of a wound infection is often also a source of client dissatisfaction.

Classification

The surgeon should be aware, through good medical records, of the incidence of infection following operations. Although the number of operations on horses is much less than those on humans, clinicians should constantly monitor infections. If the incidence of infection is unacceptably high, a thorough analysis of where a "breakdown" occurred is required. For example, was there a break in aseptic technique or a lack of proper sterilization by a malfunctioning autoclave? What constitutes an unacceptably high incidence of infection will vary depending on the type of operation. Operations are classified into four categories based on an estimate of wound contamination (1) (also discussed earlier in Chapter 3):

I. **Clean Wound.** No infection is encountered, no break in aseptic technique is discovered, and no hollow muscular organs are opened. Examples are arthroscopy, laryngoplasty, and internal fixation of a closed fracture.
II. **Clean-Contaminated Wound.** A hollow muscular organ is opened but minimal spillage of contents occurred. Examples are cystorrhaphy for ruptured bladder and laryngeal sacculectomy.
III. **Contaminated Wound.** A hollow muscular organ is opened with gross spillage of contents or, alternatively, acute inflammation without pus formation is encountered. A traumatic wound of less than 4 hours' duration falls into this group, as do operations associated with a major break in aseptic technique (e.g., large colon resection).
IV. **Dirty Wound.** Pus is encountered at operation or a perforated viscus is found. A traumatic wound of more than 4 hours' duration is put in this category. An example is guttural pouch empyema.

Definition

The surgeon must also *define* what is infection. Is an inflamed wound with serous discharge infected or possibly infected? Should the definition of infection include a purulent exudate?

In human surgery, the rate of infection for "clean wounds" using the definition above is 1.5%. In the authors' hospital, the rate of infection of certain clean operations, such as arthroscopy, is close to zero.

Prevention

Every aseptic or preventive practice should be viewed as desirable if there is a possibility, albeit slight, that it will lead to prevention of wound infection. Failure to adopt practices that might conceivably prevent infection should be considered both ethically and legally unwise (2).

Prevention of infection begins on many fronts. To avoid prolongation of operating time, the surgeon should not even attempt the surgery without a working knowledge of the local anatomy, and, where applicable, should practice on cadaver specimens. Researchers have demonstrated clinically and experimentally that the infection rate of clean wounds roughly doubles with every hour of surgery (1). There are four possible explanations for this: (*a*) dosage of bacterial contamination increases with time; (*b*) wound cells are damaged by drying and by exposure to air and retractors; (*c*) increased amounts of suture and electrocoagulation may reduce the local resistance of the wound; and (*d*) longer procedures are more likely to be associated with blood loss and shock, thereby reducing an animal's general resistance level (1).

Failure to observe the fundamental techniques for tissue handling greatly contributes to the risk of infection. These techniques include prevention of serum formation, hemostasis, and adequate debridement. Careful consideration of antimicrobial therapy is important, especially when using prosthetic implants such as mesh for herniorrhaphy or nonabsorbable sutures for laryngoplasty. In a classic study, Burke emphasized the need to give prophylactic antibiotics *before* contamination occurs and showed that if administration is delayed beyond a certain point, the benefit is lost (3).

Even simple procedures such as the use of double gloves can reduce the incidence of infection. Double gloving should be employed in *all* orthopaedic operations involving fracture manipulation because of the high risk of perforation. The authors do not advocate double gloving for all equine operations mentioned in this book, but we routinely double glove during the draping procedure because this is commonly where a break in asepsis occurs. The outer gloves are shed just before making the skin incision, or, if double gloving will be used throughout the operation, the outer gloves are then changed. Studies show that because more holes occur in the outer gloves than in the inner ones, and because contamination of outer gloves is more frequent than of inner ones, frequent changing of the outer gloves during the procedure is an important way of minimizing contamination (4).

Appropriate operating room conduct *and* attire should be considered the norm in any of the surgeries described in this textbook. Gown-over-scrub clothes (not street clothes), caps, and masks are the current standard in modern equine practice. Because draping the wound or surgical site cannot be underplayed or emphasized enough in equine surgery, an entire section is devoted to it.

The use of various substances to irrigate a wound during surgery has received extensive clinical and experimental study in human surgery (5), but controlled studies in equine surgery have not been done. Certainly, the literature is confusing, especially regarding the inclusion of various antiseptics such as povidone-iodine in the flush solution. One study, for example, demonstrated that flushing with povidone-iodine produced favorable results (6), but another showed no beneficial effects (7). A third study showed that for high-risk cases, the inclusion of a topical antiseptic such as povidone-iodine *with* prophylactic systemic antibiotics may be beneficial (8). Clinical trials to support or refute these methods to reduce infection in horses are lacking. The authors have abandoned povidone-iodine use as an abdominal cavity flush but still use it for contaminated and dirty wounds. Such flushing is always accomplished by copious volumes of irrigating fluid. The benefit of mechanical rinsing should not be underestimated. On careful analysis of the literature, inclusion of antibiotics in flush solutions *is* beneficial. Using penicillin instead of saline solution lowered the incidence of infection in sutured lacerations in humans (5), as did the inclusion of neomycin/bacitracin (9).

The potentiation of infection by foreign material (e.g., sutures) and devitalized tissue is well recognized. The *type* of suture material selected also can influence the incidence of postoperative infection (10). Studies have shown that the number of bacteria in a wound needed to establish infection can be reduced 10,000-fold by the use of a silk suture and can be reduced even further if tissue is enclosed in the suture (10).

All wounds contain bacteria, whether the wound is accidental or intentional. The source of bacteria in the "clean" surgical wound is the endogenous microbial population of normal skin. Deep within the hair follicles, microorganisms can be as numerous as 10^3 per gram of tissue. It is the normal flora of the skin that constitutes a significant source of infection to all surgical patients. The microtrauma (knicks and abrasions) produced by clippers and safety razors has been shown to increase the infection rate in human surgical patients. Because of the thickness and density of hair in animals, clipping and shaving are unavoidable, but wound infection produced by endogenous skin flora can be minimized by careful skin preparation before surgery.

Open traumatic wounds may contain bacteria in sufficient quantities such that wound closure will result in infection. Analysis of tissue samples to quantitate the number of bacteria (quantitative wound biopsy) has received considerable application in humans and is beginning to be used in veterinary surgery, notably in the horse (11, 12). Tissue sample analysis is also applicable in skin grafting to ascertain the suitability of the graft bed. The authors do not use quantitative wound biopsy routinely but encourage its use if it is available. However, the technique should not replace a thorough physical examination and sound surgical judgment (11). Wounds can be closed if the number of bacteria per gram of tissue is 10^5 or less; some sources quote 10^6 as the number (11, 12). Some bacteria may be clinically more significant at much lower levels than have been described.

Note also that joints are particularly vulnerable to infection, and studies have revealed that only 100 colony-forming units of *Staphylococcus aureus* need be present for predictable infection of a synovial joint (13). This is much lower than the 10^6 quoted for infecting an open traumatic wound and emphasizes the importance of aseptic technique when operating on joints.

The postoperative surgical wound infection rates in 452 cases of equine orthopaedic surgery over a 9-year period were reported (14). A wound was defined as infected if there was discharge of purulent material from the wound, spontaneous dehiscence in one or more wound layers accompanied by serous drainage, or if clinical signs of infection were present (erythema, pain, swelling). This study included clean and clean-contaminated wounds. The overall postoperative infection rate was 10% (45/452). Clean surgeries (N = 433) had an 8.1% infection rate; clean-contaminated surgeries (N = 19) had a 52.6% infection rate. Using univariate and multivariate analysis, significant determinants of postoperative infection included surgical classification, orthopaedic involvement, duration of surgery, administration of preoperative antibiotics, and gender. Clean-contaminated surgeries had an increased rate of infection compared with clean surgeries (odds ratio [OR] 24.3); procedures involving long bones had an increased risk of infection compared with procedures involving articular surfaces (OR 5.1); surgeries lasting 90 minutes or longer had an increased risk of infection compared with those lasting less than 90 minutes (OR 3.6); administration of preoperative antibiotics was associated with an increased risk of infection (OR 4.6); and female patients were 2.6 times more likely than male patients to develop postoperative infection. The authors noted that although these infection rates were higher than in previous human and canine studies, their definition of infection was more encompassing. That the study only included orthopaedic procedures (some of which are extensive and more prone to infection) was a factor in the overall percentage. The increased incidence with preoperative prophylactic antibiotics is not considered a direct cause-and-effect. It is more likely that the relationship indicated the surgeon recognized factors associated with high risk and then instituted prophylactic antibiotics (14).

Treatment

The key to successful treatment of wound infection is early recognition. This, in turn, is related to the standard of patient care that the horse receives. As soon as a wound infection is diagnosed or a pending wound infection suspected, a good avenue of communication between the surgeon and the person responsible for the horse must be established. The client should be informed of the seriousness of the infection and of the potential consequences.

The surgeon should wear sterile surgical gloves during any treatment of the wound itself. Such treatment should be scheduled *after* the day's surgery to reduce the possibility of spread of infection to other surgical patients.

A bacterial swab should be taken and submitted for both anaerobic and aerobic culture. The appropriate hematology samples should also be submitted when systemic involvement is likely. In the simplest of cases, removal of some ventrally located skin sutures to provide drainage may be all that is required. Other more elaborate measures, such as insertion of closed suction or Penrose drains, may be required. The wound will require daily cleaning, and scalding of the skin should be prevented by applying petrolatum to areas of ventral drainage. Sterile gloves should be worn. For infected wounds on the lower limbs of horses, some form of bandaging is usually essential. Not only does a cotton bandage protect the wound from exogenous contaminations with organisms such as *Pseudomonas* spp. and *Proteus* spp., but also it will, through capillary action, act like a wick to draw away fluids and exudates. Bandages also reduce formation of edema in the limbs.

The use of topical antimicrobial sprays are of doubtful value in the management of an established wound infection. The active ingredient in these sprays is frequently inactivated by tissue fluids and is prevented for the most part from reaching the source of infection (8). Infected wounds of the limbs of horses are frequently pruritic, and restraint in the form of a neck cradle will be necessary to prevent mutilation and dislodging of bandages and dressings.

Probably because of the large number of prosthetic hips implanted in humans, comparatively little has appeared in the veterinary literature regarding infection management following the use of implants. Buried polymerized caprolactam (Vetafil) historically has been one of the most common offenders. It is packaged in plastic dispenser bottles, chemically sterilized, and suitable for skin closure. It must be autoclaved before being buried and never used in the presence of infection. If these principles are not followed, chronic drainage and fistulation will occur, typical of infection that has become established around a foreign body. Infection after the use of a nonmetallic prosthesis (e.g., polypropylene for herniorrhaphy) and insertion of metallic orthopaedic implants will be discussed in more detail.

Despite widespread use of various types of suture material for laryngoplasty, little has been written about the management of serious postoperative infections around the prosthesis. The technique of laryngoplasty is discussed in Chapter 6. The principles of infection prevention previously discussed are all appropriate to laryngoplasty. Management of an infected laryngeal prosthesis must focus on its eventual removal. It should be removed under general anesthesia when localized swelling and edema have subsided. To salvage the horse and return it to some form of respiratory function will require arytenoidectomy.

Treatment of an infected synthetic mesh used for herniorrhaphy should follow principles similar to those used to treat an infected midline incision. Removal of one or two offending anchoring sutures will occasionally resolve the infection and is always worth a try. If the entire mesh is infected, the surgeon will find discolored, devitalized, and unhealthy tissue immediately adjacent to the mesh. This will be a strong indication that the entire mesh must be removed along with any fistulous tracts. When the wound has sterilized itself (several weeks later), the mesh is reinserted.

Following removal of the infected mesh, the wound can be closed immediately with 18- or 22-g wire in a simple interrupted vertical mattress suture, placed through all layers of the abdominal wall (15). Before such a closure, devitalized infected tissue must be removed by sharp dissection. To reduce the tendency of the wire to cut, 2.5-cm lengths of hard rubber are used in the sections of suture overlying the skin. The sutures are pre-placed, and the defect in the abdominal wall is closed by putting simultaneous tension on all sutures. Closure of the skin is optional (15) and will depend on the amount of drainage required to avoid abscessation. This method of midline closure is also applicable to an infected midline incision that has occurred *without* mesh implantation. Similar principles are followed, including removal of all previous sutures, sharp dissection of devitalized infected tissue, removal of fistulous tracts, and apposition of the body wall using the suture pattern described (15).

Infection following internal fixation of a fracture (osteomyelitis) is caused by contamination of an open fracture or contamination at the time of open reduction. Contamination can occur during surgery despite antibiotics and strict aseptic technique, especially if the operation is long. Broad-spectrum antibiotics should be given to horses with any fracture in which internal fixation devices will be implanted. The ideal duration of chemoprophylaxis in animals undergoing orthopaedic surgery has not been determined. It has been shown in humans that short-term *perioperative* regimens (24–48 hr) are as effective as regimens lasting 2 to 3 weeks (16).

The most striking clinical sign of a horse with osteomyelitis following internal fixation is reluctance to bear weight. The onset of lameness may be sudden. The limb, unless protected by a cast, will be hot and painful, leukocytosis will be present, and there may be fever. There is usually retarded wound healing over the implants or even fistula formation. Radiographically, there will be lysis at the fracture site and around the implants (along the screw threads), under the plate, or along the pin if one is used. Sequestra may be evident.

The treatment of osteomyelitis following internal fixation requires more than administration of broad-spectrum (and appropriate) antibiotics. Culturing a sinus tract may be useful (a bone sample is preferable), not so much from the standpoint of what antibiotic to use but to give the surgeon an idea as to the epidemiology of the infection.

An infected fracture must be made stable at all costs if it is to heal. Studies repeatedly show that a stable infected fracture is better than an unstable infected fracture (17). Bone union must occur before the sepsis can be overcome. In some cases, the internal fixation devices (e.g., bone plates) must be removed and replaced by another, more stable device. The existing internal fixation devices may be left in place as long as they are providing stability. Some wound infections require excision of fistulous tracts, sequestrectomy, and bone grafting. If the bone graft is used, it should be inserted in a viable bed with an abundant blood supply; otherwise, graft survival is severely compromised. External coaptation to aid in achieving stability of the fractures is often required.

Suction drains or ingress/egress systems are sometimes valuable, although the technical problems associated with the proper maintenance of such systems in an uncooperative horse make their value questionable.

Treatment of infection following internal fixation is often much more expensive than postoperative infections after other surgical procedures mentioned in this section. Any further treatment is usually fruitless if *stability* at the fracture site cannot be achieved (17). Other details on the management of osteomyelitis are available elsewhere (18).

The potential for peritonitis always exists following abdominal surgery in horses when the lumen of the bowel is entered (e.g., enterotomy anastomosis). Other contributing factors are poor technique (leaks in anastomosis), excessive tissue handling, and overzealous use of chemically irritating antiseptics (e.g., 10% povidone-iodine). Both anaerobic and aerobic bacteria are usually present. Anaerobic bacteria have been traditionally underestimated because of inadequate sampling methods at the time cultures are taken. Acute peritonitis is characterized by shock, ileus, abdominal distension, and nasogastric reflex (stomach tube). The animal may be febrile, the refill time will be poor, and there will be hemoconcentration and leukopenia. Plasma protein will decline because of its effective loss from the circulation into the inflamed peritoneal cavity (third spacing of fluid). Abdominal paracentesis after abdominal surgery as a diagnostic aid is of limited value; an invasion as small as an exploratory laparotomy in a normal healthy horse can cause high white counts in abdominal fluid (this normally resolves in a few days). In acute peritonitis, however, the neutrophil is characterized by degenerative changes, and a consistent and continued rise in the count will occur.

An aggressive, energetic attitude is required to treat acute peritonitis. Attention must be given first to fluid replacement, gastric decompression, and analgesia. Antibiotics directed at both anaerobes and aerobes are required. The usual prescription is penicillin in combination with one of the aminoglycosides. In the authors' experience, acute wound dehiscence does not appear to be a problem with acute peritonitis unless the horse is in pain and violent and a mechanical disruption of the suture line occurs. Midline incisions seem to heal even in the face of acute peritonitis.

Lavage has been widely advocated in both small animal and human cases of peritonitis, but increasing doubt has arisen over just how long an animal can tolerate continual loss of peritoneal fluid. Application of these methods to horses is logical but fraught with technical problems. Localized flushing through ventrally located catheters is, in the authors' opinion, of questionable value. Instillation of catheters in the flanks and collection through ventrally located catheters also is of limited value because the ingress fluid tends to follow several paths of least resistance without exposing the enormous surface area of the peritoneum to the benefits of the lavage.

The most effective way to lavage the horse's abdomen is to reopen the midline incision under general anesthesia and liberally expose all of the abdomen to large volumes of warmed polyionic solutions. The inclusion of antibiotics is not recommended, especially antibiotics that produce neuromuscular blockade and therefore the potential for respiratory arrest while the horse is anesthetized. The literature abounds with experimental and clinical experiences with the use of antiseptics (especially povidone-iodine) in the abdominal cavity. The authors have drifted further and further away from using antiseptics in the abdomen as current literature tends to discredit them, in opposition to the initial enthusiasm for their use in the early 1970s.

Certainly a horse with acute peritonitis is a poor anesthetic risk, and good clinical judgment is required in deciding *when* lavage under general anesthesia is indicated. Surgery should be timed to occur after stabilization (e.g., treatment of shock, endotoxemia) has been undertaken and it is becoming evident that conservative measures are failing.

REFERENCES

1. Cruse PJE, Ford R. The epidemiology of wound infection: a 10-year prospective study of 62,939 wounds. Symposium on Surgical Infections. Surg Clin North Am 1980;60: 27.

2. Garner JS, Emori TG, Haley RW. Operating room practices for the control of infection in U.S. Hospitals, October 1976 to July 1977. Surg Gynecol Obstet 1982;155:873.
3. Burke JF. The effective period of preventive antibiotic action in experimental incisions and dermal lesions. Surgery 1961;50:161.
4. McCue SF, Berg EW, Saunders EA. Efficacy of double-gloving as a barrier to microbial contamination during total joint arthroplasty. J Bone Joint Surg 1981;63A:811.
5. Lindsey D, Nava C, Marti M. Effectiveness of penicillin irrigation in control of infection in sutured lacerations. J Trauma 1982;22:186.
6. Sindelar WF, Mason GR. Irrigation of subcutaneous tissue with povidone-iodine solution for prevention of surgical wound infections. Surg Gynecol Obstet 1979;148:227.
7. de Jong TE, Vierhout RJ, Vroonhoven TJ. Povidone-iodine irrigation of the subcutaneous tissue to prevent surgical wound infections. Surg Gynecol Obstet 1982;155:221.
8. Gallard RB, Heine KJ, Trachtenberg LS, et al. Reduction of surgical wound infection rates in contaminated wounds treated with antiseptics combined with systemic antibiotics: an experimental study. Surgery 1982;91:329.
9. Benjamin JB, Volz RG. Efficacy of a topical antibiotic irrigant in decreasing or eliminating bacterial contamination in surgical wounds. Clin Orthop 1984;184:114.
10. Le Cicero J, Robbins JA, Webb WR. Complications following abdominal fascial closures using various nonabsorbable sutures. Surg Gynecol Obstet 1983;157:25.
11. Hackett RP, Dimock BA, Bentinck-Smith J. Quantitative bacteriology of experimentally incised skin wounds in horses. Equine Vet J 1983;15:37.
12. Peyton LC, Connelly MB. Evaluation of quantitative bacterial counts as an aid in the treatment of wounds in the horse. Equine Vet J 1983;15:251.
13. Gustafson SB, McIlwraith CW, Jones RL. Comparison of the effect of polysulfated glycosaminoglycans, corticosteroids and sodium hyaluronate in the potentiation of a subinfective dose of *Staphylococcus aureus* in the midcarpal joint of horses. Am J Vet Res 1989;50:2014–2017.
14. MacDonald DG, Morley PS, Bailey JV, et al. An examination of the occurrence of surgical wound infection following equine orthopaedic surgery (1981–1990). Equine Vet J 1994;26:323–326.
15. Tulleners EP, Fretz PB. Prosthetic repair of large abdominal wall defects in horses and food animals. JAVMA 1983;182:258.
16. Fitzgerald RH, Thompson RL. Current concepts review: cephalosporin antibiotics in the prevention and treatment of musculoskeletal sepsis. J Bone Joint Surg 1983;65A:1201.
17. Burri C. Post-traumatic Osteomyelitis. Bern: Hans Huber Publishers, 1975.
18. Trotter GW. Osteomyelitis. In: Nixon AJ, ed. Fractures in the Horse. Philadelphia: WB Saunders, 1996:359–366.

Nosocomial Infections

Nosocomial infections in veterinary hospitals were first noted as a major problem in 1985, and there are, unfortunately, continued reminders of their importance (1). Although the highest incidence rates are observed in large referral or teaching hospitals, nosocomial infections can occur in any veterinary practice.

Definition

Nosocomial (hospital-acquired) infections are those that occur during hospitalization but are not present or incubating at the time of admission. Such infections may become clinically apparent during hospitalization or after discharge from the hospital. As a rule, new infections occurring after 48 hours of hospitalization can be considered nosocomial (2). Nosocomial infections are frequently caused by endogenous microorganisms inhabiting the patient's flora. Bacteria are the most frequent agents involved in nosocomial infections, but viruses, *Chlamydia*, mycoplasma, fungi, and protozoa can also be involved.

Etiology and Pathogenesis

For a nosocomial infection to develop, a potential pathogen must be transmitted to a susceptible patient. The source of most endemic nosocomial infections is the endogenous flora of the patient (1, 3, 4), but a nasal carrier in an operating room staff member was the critical cause in one study in humans (3). The inanimate environment of the patient has minimal influence on the incidence of nosocomial infections that are caused by multiple drug-resistant (MDR) bacteria. The likelihood that a patient will become infected depends on a complex interaction of four major factors: (*a*) the virulence of the agent; (*b*) the patient's susceptibility to infection by the agent; (*c*) the nature of exposure to the agent; and (*d*) the effect of antimicrobial therapy. Several factors considered to be important in the nosocomial colonization of human beings with MDR bacteria include: (*a*) patient-to-patient spread, often facilitated by transient carriage of the organisms on the hands of the attending personnel; (*b*) direct spread between patients as a result of environmental contamination; and (*c*) the effect of antibiotic pressures, including suppression of susceptible flora with sequential colonization by MDR bacteria and selection of resistant subpopulations of bacteria present in the flora (4). Some factors that are not considered important for human beings but must be considered for animals include housing conditions, patient hygiene, and behavioral aspects of feeding and defecation.

The sources of the opportunistic pathogens causing nosocomial infections include people, animals, inanimate objects, air currents, and, occasionally, insects or rodents. Once bacteria gain entrance to the hospital, they become part of the "normal flora" of animals. The patient therefore becomes its own major reservoir for endogenous infections. Common sites of colonization include the upper respiratory and digestive tracts. The important source of organisms that infect the patient and sustain an endemic outbreak is the patient's own intestinal tract (1). As an example of this in the horse, a study at Colorado State University demonstrated intestinal colonization of horses by MDR bacteria during the course of hospitalization. Nineteen horses that had not been hospitalized previously at the Veterinary Teaching Hospital were cultured on admission and on the fourth day of hospitalization (1). Twelve horses became colonized with MDR organisms. One additional horse included in the study had been released from the hospital 10 weeks before readmission. This horse was colonized with MDR organisms at the time of admission. The organisms were identified as *Klebsiella* spp., *Escherichia coli*, *Enterobacter* spp., *Salmonella enteritidis*, and *Citrobacter freundii*. These bacterial isolates share a unique pattern of resistance to ampicillin, chloramphenicol, and gentamicin, which, in mating studies, was shown to be readily transferable. This study indicated that a conjugate or plasmid was probably responsible for the resistance.

Bacteria may acquire resistance as a result of the presence of extrachromosomal plasmids, or R factors, which may be transferred in total between bacteria and may contain genetic elements called transposons capable of moving from one R factor to another. Such transfer of plasmids and transposons allows resistances to spread widely among the bacterial population, crossing species and genera boundaries. Moreover, several resistant determinants may be linked on one plasmid, making it possible for resistance to multiple unrelated antibiotics to emerge together. Bacteria may also acquire resistance by spontaneous chromosomal mutation, which may be selected from a population of sensitive organisms by "antibiotic pressures." The aforementioned study in the horse demonstrated nosocomial colonization of veterinary patients in a manner similar to that observed in human patients. It is also significant that 60 to 87% colonization was detected, using only a single fecal sample of 1 to 2 grams from each subject (1). This common source of multiple drug resistance was considered to be related to an endemic plasmid problem.

Certain types of patients are known to be at high risk for bacterial colonization or infection. In an investigation of an outbreak of nosocomial *Salmonella Saint-Paul* infection in hospitalized horses at the University of California Veterinary Medical Teaching Hospital in Davis, it was found that horses receiving parenteral antibiotics were at 10 times greater risk of having *S. Saint-Paul* isolated than were horses not receiving parenteral antibiotics (5). The organism had an unusual pattern of antibiotic resistance, being sensitive to tetracycline yet resistant to most commonly used antimicrobial drugs tested, including penicillin, streptomycin, neomycin, kanamycin, gentamicin, chloramphenicol, sulfa drugs, and ampicillin. Most of the 33 horses from which *S. Saint-Paul* was isolated showed no or minimal signs of salmonellosis. In 23 horses, some degree of clinical signs were found, 2 died with acute *S. Saint-Paul* bacteremia, and 7 others were euthanized following moderate to severe diarrhea (5). In the horse, association of antibiotics with occurrence of salmonellosis is considered to be caused by selective elimination of the gut flora antagonistic to *Salmonella*. The authors believe that these cases were nosocomial for several reasons. The serotype seldom had been isolated from hospitalized animals at this clinic, and a relatively large number of cases were detected within a short period. In addition, this organism is most often isolated from turkeys and humans and is not commonly isolated from horses. Finally, the organism had an unusual pattern of antibiotic resistance.

Other associated factors were considered to influence the likelihood of infection in this hospital population (5). Horses intubated with nasogastric tubes, for example, were 3.9 times more likely to have had the organism isolated from fecal specimens than those horses not intubated, and horses with a presenting complaint of colic had 2.2 times greater risk of isolation than those horses with other presenting complaints. Based on their findings of parenteral antibiotics as an important iatrogenic risk factor in their study, the authors believe that antibiotic use should be carefully evaluated for each patient. It was also noted that further studies may suggest that certain classes of antibiotics were less likely to be associated with an increased risk of nosocomial *Salmonella* infection or disease and that it might be possible to prefer these antibiotics over others for high-risk patients (5).

With regard to this aspect, a study was carried out on the bacteriologic fecal flora of horses before and after oral doses of oxytetracycline or of trimethoprim plus sulfadiazine (6). Administration of oxytetracyclines to horses was followed by large increases in counts of coliforms, *Bacteroides*, and *Streptococcus* spp., as well as the appearance of *Clostridium perfringens* organisms in large numbers and the accumulation of watery fluid in the rectal contents. Conversely, these changes were not seen following administration of trimethoprim-sulfadiazine, and the study concluded that oral treatment of horses with this combination was unlikely to be accompanied by the same hazardous effect (7). It is to be noted that in a study of colitis in the horse, *C. perfringens* type A was the principal etiologic agent (6).

Normally the host and the anaerobic bacterial flora of the digestive tract act synergistically to limit colonization by potentially pathogenic bacteria, a mechanism known as "colonization resistance." Oral therapy with partially absorbed antimicrobials or parenteral therapy with antimicrobials excreted in the intestine in active form may lead to a decrease in colonization resistance if the anaerobic flora is susceptible to the drug. The ability of antimicrobials to affect colonization resistance has been classified for various agents. In addition to suppressing normal flora, the antimicrobial therapy promotes development of antimicrobial-resistant bacteria. Resistance to more than one agent frequently occurs and is usually plasmid mediated. Plasmid-mediated resistance is readily transferred between Gram-negative bacteria. The antimicrobial therapy therefore may result in the development of an endemic plasmid or resistance factor rather than simply a single endemic strain of bacteria.

Twenty-three isolations of *Serratia* spp. were made from 21 horses at the University of Florida over a 3½-year period. Possible nosocomial infection, variable antibiotic sensitivity, and a trend toward decreased antibiotic sensitivity after antibiotic administration were noted (8).

Control of Nosocomial Infections

The initial goal in the control of any nosocomial infection is to identify the reservoirs, which will include colonized and infected patients, as well as sources of environmental contamination. Careful microbiologic surveillance is important to detect many epidemics of two or more similar MDR isolates. Detection of certain resistance patterns, such as gentamicin resistance or multiple-drug resistance, indicate nosocomial infection. Gentamicin resistance can be considered a marker for plasmid-mediated multiple resistance (9). Precautions to control an endemic nosocomial infection include segregation, isolation, glove use, careful hand washing, and asepsis. Susceptible patients must be separated, and circumstances may sometimes warrant closure of the hospital unit to new admissions. At the same time, the host risk should be modified as much as possible. Hospitalization time should be kept to a minimum. Antibiotic use should be carefully controlled, particularly in surgical prophylaxis (discussed in Chapter 3). Topical antimicrobial therapy instead of systemic therapy could be useful in some instances. Specific antimicrobial therapy against a nosocomial isolate is an area fraught with hazard, and specific recommendations would be premature. Although agents such as amikacin and cefuroxime are effective against gentamicin-resistant *Klebsiella*, indiscriminant use of these drugs causes more antibiotic pressure.

In another study of the antibiograms of 408 *Salmonella* species isolated from horses during a 3-year period, the predominant *Salmonella* serotype isolated was group B, and a high percentage of all isolates were resistant to ampicillin and tetracycline. A pattern of increasing resistance to chloramphenicol and gentamicin was also documented for serogroup B isolates. In another group of isolates, there was a decrease in incidence of susceptibility to trimethoprim-sulfamethoxazole, but these changes are not as remarkable as the overall decrease of susceptibility to chloramphenicol and gentamicin. In summary, an increasing level of resistance to ampicillin, chloramphenicol, gentamicin, and tetracycline was observed in isolates from patients during the 3-year period. The report established that serious problems were present in these patients before receiving treatment at the particular hospital, and it was considered that these problems may have been associated with prior contact with antibiotics via food, prescription, or undirected use of drugs by an owner or manager (10).

Based on experience with nosocomial salmonellosis, the authors' clinical microbiologist has identified problem areas and set up control measures. Three major areas of concern have been identified: infected animals, physical facilities, and personnel.

Infected animals are the major source of large numbers of salmonellae. Following are some recommendations that should be established as hospital policy.

1. Any animal arriving at the hospital as a possible salmonellosis case should be placed in the isolation barn.
2. Any hospitalized animal with a positive *Salmonella* culture should be moved to an isolation area.
3. Any hospitalized animal with clinical signs consistent with salmonellosis, but without bacteriologic confirmation, may remain in the large animal barn only if all hospital personnel are aware of the case and adequate precautions are established. These precautions should include personnel assignments that limit possible spread of contamination, setting up foot baths, policies for changing clothes, and placement of rope barriers to restrict all traffic from a perimeter area, including adjacent stalls and areas of drainage in hallways.
4. Any animal placed in the isolation areas must remain there until discharged from the premises. If an animal is to be brought back into the barns from an isolation area, it must have three negative fecal cultures (24 or more hours apart) during a 1-week period and be free of clinical signs of possible contagious disease during that week.

Physical facilities must be properly cleaned so they do not serve as a reservoir.

1. *All walls and floors must be repaired and sealed* so that they can be cleaned and disinfected.
2. If loose and torn edges of floor coverings are discovered, they must be trimmed away for proper cleaning.
3. All stalls must be cleaned as if contaminated by salmonellae, regardless of the history of the animal leaving the stall.
4. Shovels, forks, and brooms must be cleaned after use in each stall.
5. Drain covers must be removed and drain bowls must be cleaned to prevent reverse flow of contamination.
6. Hard surface stalls that have been cleaned and disinfected can be reassigned the next day. Dirt floors should remain unoccupied for 1 week.
7. Cleaning personnel should wear rubber boots, which are to be disinfected after cleaning each stall.

Personnel training must continue to be a major part of any control program for nosocomial infections.

1. Boots, foot baths, and scrub brushes should be available and used in all contaminated or potentially contaminated areas. As a precaution, foot baths should be required between major areas of the barn.
2. Traffic in contaminated areas should be restricted.
3. Clothing changes and showers should be required after handling an animal with salmonellosis.
4. Handwashing and cleanliness should be emphasized.

To facilitate these recommendations at Colorado State University, a full-time Infectious Disease Control Officer was appointed in 1985. This person is a staff member who can direct cleaning crews, assign or restrict stall use, maintain liaison with the bacteriology laboratory, and set up, maintain, and enforce control measures for foot baths, traffic, and relocation of animals.

Since the above recommendations were written (published in the first edition), an outbreak of salmonellosis was encountered in 1996 at Colorado State University, necessitating closure of the clinic. The initiating source is uncertain but was presumed to be an infected horse. Even more stringent biosecurity measures are now in force to minimize any transmission between horses or via personnel or equipment.

REFERENCES

1. Jones RL, Fafoutis D, McCurnin DM. Nosocomial colonization of horses by multiple antibiotic-resistant enterobacteriaceae. JAVMA 1985;187:291–292.
2. Jones RL. Control of nosocomial infections. In: Current Veterinary Therapy. IX. Philadelphia: WB Saunders, 1986.
3. Steingold L, Dunn L, Hawksworth F, et al. The influence of ward ventilation in hospital cross infection. J Appl Bacterial 1963;26:1–6.
4. Weinstein RA, Cabins SA. Strategies for prevention and control of multiple drug-resistant nosocomial infection. Am J Med 1981;70:449–454.
5. Hird DW, Pappaioanou M, Smith BP. Case-control study of risk factors associated with isolation of *Salmonella Saint-Paul* in hospitalized horses. Am J Epidemiol 1984; 120:852–864.
6. Weirup M. Equine intestinal clostridiosis. Acta Vet Scan 1977;62(Suppl):1–182.
7. White G, Prior SD. Comparative effects of oral administration of trimethoprim-sulfadiazine or oxytetracycline on the faecal flora of horse. Vet Rec 1982;111:316–318.
8. Colahan PT, Peyton LC, Connelly MR, et al. *Serratia* spp. infection in 21 horses. JAVMA 1984;185:209–211.
9. Casewell MW, Phillips I. Aspects of the plasmid-mediated antibiotic resistance and epidemiology of *Klebsiella* spp. Am J Med 1981;70:459–462.
10. Benson CE, Palmer JE, Bannister MF. Antibiotic susceptibility of *Salmonella* spp. isolated at a large animal veterinary medical center: a 3-year study. Can J Comp Med 1985;49:125–128.

Laminitis in the Postsurgical Patient

Laminitis (or acute laminin separation) as it relates to the equine surgical patient is an ever present threat. All who perform major surgery on horses will have experienced a case of laminitis at one time or another.

The essential lesion in laminitis is damage to the laminae resulting in breakdown of the interdigitating system of primary and secondary laminae, which provide a firm bond between the wall and the lamina corium (1). Vasoconstriction within the digit, microthrombosis, perivascular edema, arteriovenous shunting of blood at the level of the coronary band, and venoconstriction are all pathophysiologic mechanisms that have been proposed to cause laminitis. These factors are thought to produce hypoperfusion of the digit, leading to ischemia, edema, and necrosis of the laminae. Venous constriction is considered to increase capillary pressure and hydrostatic movement of fluid into the interstitial space, predisposing to edema and, subsequently, poor perfusion.

Etiology

When considering postsurgical laminitis, it is appropriate to divide the syndrome into a systemic form and a mechanical form.

Systemic Laminitis

A number of systemic factors can lead to laminitis. Carbohydrate overload is the recognized cause, and much of the initial research was done with an experimental model of carbohydrate overload. It is possible to have a surgical case with an analogous clinical syndrome. Such an example would be the obese but well-cared-for show horse, such as a Quarter horse used in halter classes. When admitting such a patient for surgery, the authors are careful about the amount of concentrate the horse is fed and prefer to remove all concentrate from the diet during hospitalization, feeding grass hay only. Although this regimen and the subsequent weight loss can cause client discontent, it is preferable to an acute case of laminitis. Reduction of grain in the diet may also minimize the chance of postanesthetic myopathy.

Endotoxemia is a major factor in systemic laminitis, and the postoperative colic horse is a classic candidate for this problem (2). Laminitis after abdominal surgery is a devastating and disheartening complication that can occur after a horse has essentially recovered from colic. It is an ever-present threat whenever there is strangulation of the bowel with mucosal damage or any degree of stasis of the contents. The severity of the laminitis varies from mild to severe and can necessitate euthanasia. Other etiologic factors that can potentially cause laminitis, including severe soft tissue infection, cellulitis, retained placenta, and pneumonia, can be explained by a circulating endotoxin. Prevention is the key to avoidance and management of laminitis, with appropriate antibiotic and fluid therapy. Laminitis is always in the back of one's mind when a case of postoperative salmonellosis also occurs.

Mechanical or Support Laminitis

Mechanical laminitis is seen when a horse bears excessive weight on one limb because of a painful condition in the opposite member. Such conditions are most commonly fractures that, despite internal fixation and external coaptation, cannot provide enough pain-free support to the limb. In a number of instances, these repairs are complicated by infection. Mechanical laminitis is essentially a variation on the classic "road founder." There is no obvious metabolic component to this type of laminitis but instead a mechanical effect of the pull of the deep digital flexor tendon, with the digital cushion as a fulcrum. Distal displacement (sinkers) does not occur in the mechanical form.

Diagnosis

Laminitis has been broadly classified into acute, subacute, refractory, and chronic stages. In the instance of postoperative laminitis, it would be classified as acute. With the systemic form, it is usually bilateral (occasionally involves all four feet). The grades of lameness vary and have been classified by Obel.

Grade 1—the horse lifts its feet repeatedly, often every few seconds

Grade 2—the horse moves willingly at a walk but the gait is characteristic of laminitis and the horse does not resist lifting of the forefoot

Grade 3—the horse moves reluctantly, and vigorously resists attempts to lift a forefoot because of pain in the contralateral leg

Grade 4—the horse must be forced to move and may be recumbent

The higher the Obel grade of lameness, the greater the likelihood of permanent damage to the laminae. In the instance of systemic laminitis, the horse will initially present with increased digital pulse and increased periods of recumbency. When the problem is of the mechanical type, resulting from the limb bearing excessive weight, the two usual signs are increasing periods of recumbency and an unusual degree of weight-bearing on the limb that has been operated and which the horse should be protecting. Careful monitoring will probably elicit an increased pulse developing in the leg before any obvious clinical signs.

Diagnosis is based on increased pulse in the digital arteries, increased heat in the foot, pain over the toe on hoof tester examination, and typical lameness. As soon as laminitis is suspected, radiographs (lateral to medial views) of the feet involved should be taken. If the horse cannot walk well from the stall to the x-ray room, the radiographs should be taken with a portable machine in the stall. Two primary reasons for radiographs are to establish if a preexisting rotation of the distal phalanx is present and the current bout is a flare-up (chronic exacerbative laminitis) and to establish a baseline set of radiographs to monitor the rate and amount of rotation or distal displacement of the distal phalanx. Radiographically, laminitis can be divided into a number of categories: (*a*) no abnormalities; (*b*) distal displacement of the third phalanx (this can be evaluated by a soft tissue defect along the coronet, an increased density between the extensor process of the distal phalanx and the coronary band); (*c*) rotation of the distal phalanx; (*d*) rotation and sinking of the distal phalanx; and (*e*) rotation of the distal phalanx with secondary chronic changes (1, 3). Radiographs can provide other information, including the distance between the dorsal hoof wall and the distal phalanx (it should be less than 18 mm or less than 30% of the length of the distal phalanx measured along the palmar border from the tip of the distal phalanx to its articulation with the navicular bone). Widening of the distance between the distal phalanx and the dorsal hoof wall could be reflective of acute swelling associated with severe laminitis. The degree of rotation can be determined by subtracting the hoof angle from the angle of the dorsal surface of the third phalanx based on lateral radiographs. The degree of phalangeal rotation is a determinative prognosis, but proximity of the phalanx to penetration of the surface of the sole is a better indicator of the chance of survival (4). It is important to recognize that because the x-ray views deviate from exact lateral to medial views, distal phalangeal rotation is underestimated (5).

Treatment

It is usually more effective to prevent laminitis than to treat it once it has occurred. Preventive measures that can be taken for the systemic form of postoperative laminitis include aggressive minimization of the development or effects of endotoxemia. This includes maintaining fluid balance, treating septicemia, and administering appropriate anti-inflammatory drugs such as phenylbutazone or flunixin meglumine. Anticoagulants such as acetylsalicylic acid (aspirin) or heparin (heparin sodium) have been recommended. In one study evaluating the development of laminitis in horses with duodenitis/proximal jejunitis, the proportion among horses that received heparin (0/12) was significantly less ($P = 0.018$) than among horses that did not receive heparin (31/104). Because of the small number of horses that received heparin and the retrospective design of the study, the clinical importance of this finding is uncertain (6). In another study, evaluation of heparin for prophylaxis of equine laminitis in 71 cases showed no significant benefit (7).

The key to successful management of laminitis resulting from excessive weight-bearing is attention to the primary problem, which is the pain in the opposite limb. Has the fracture become unstable? Have efforts at rigid immobilization of the fracture failed with plates or screws? Has the surgical site become infected? These questions must be asked, and the limb may require a cast change (if present) and radiographic evaluation to assess the source of the pain. In this type of laminitis, the patient's contribution to its own successful recovery should never be underestimated. Some horses refuse to lie down and do not spare the uninjured limb. A "sensible" horse will spend a large amount of time in sternal or lateral recumbency, thereby resting the support limb. The authors have not generally used shoes and pads as a prophylaxis, but will place a horse in a sand stall.

Once laminitis is present, it must be treated aggressively. Although unlikely in a hospital situation, if there is excessive grain ingestion, 1 to 2 gallons of mineral oil orally should be administered to delay absorption of endotoxins and provide a laxative effect. Nonsteroidal anti-inflammatory drugs (NSAIDs) are used. One must remain aware of the risk of toxicosis (renal papillary necrosis, gastrointestinal ulceration, protein-losing enteropathy) with prolonged administration of high doses of phenylbutazone. Corticosteroids are contraindicated. Additional therapy for laminitis includes the administration of acetyl promazine to improve vasodilation (preferable to isoxsuprine) and DMSO (0.1 gm/kg IV) as a free radical scavenger to hopefully prevent cellular reperfusion injury. The authors do not routinely use phenoxybenzamine. Baxter outlined the goals of treatment, which are to: (*a*) correct the primary illness or remove the causative factor, (*b*) block the pain-hypertension cycle, (*c*) improve digital blood flow and laminar perfusion, (*d*) prevent or correct rotation or sinking of the distal phalanx, and (*e*) promote keratinization and healing of sole and hoof defects (in the chronic stage) (1). Pentoxifylline (8 mg/kg), a methyl xanthine derivative, is a newer vasodilating agent with enhanced activity, compared with isoxsuprine, and may have a place in laminitis control.

The authors' approach to hoof management (8) is relatively simple: using a sand stall. This is a useful way of improving weight distribution to the frog and caudal regions of the hoof. The sand also helps the ease of break over, reducing forces contributing to lamina separation. The authors prefer a sand stall over the use of a heart bar shoe or taped-on frog support pad. If sand is not available and the horse tends to have its heels off the ground, using a shoe to raise the heels has been beneficial.

The use of deep digital flexor tenotomy is controversial. In an initial report of 13 cases of chronic laminitis treated with deep digital flexor tenotomy, 5 horses returned to limited athletic endeavors, 6 horses improved and were comfortable on pasture, 1 horse improved clinically but was euthanized for economic reasons, and 1 horse improved but deteriorated 9 months after surgery and was euthanized (9). However, in a second report of midmetacarpal deep digital flexor tenotomy in the management of 20 horses with severe, acute, or chronic laminitis (unresponsive to conventional treatment), 16 horses improved within 72 hours, 1 horse worsened, and 2 horses were affected by surgery, but 11 horses survived less than 1 month after surgery and 6 horses survived longer than 6 months. Three horses surviving longer than 6 months remained lame, and no horse returned to athletic activity. It was believed that although transection of the deep digital flexor tendon at the midmetacarpus decreased the pain associated with the acute refractory stage of laminitis and could be useful as an immediate salvage procedure, the survival rate of affected horses may not be altered (10).

Prognosis

The prognosis of a horse with laminitis is guarded. Factors determining the prognosis include: (*a*) duration of acute laminitis, (*b*) number of feet affected, (*c*) amount of distal phalanx rotation, (*d*) occurrence of sinking, (*e*) severity of lameness and response to treatment, and (*f*) occurrence of secondary abscessation and osteomyelitis of the distal phalanx (1). Clinical signs are recognized as the best prognostic indicator (11). It has also been reported that horses with less than 5.5 degrees of rotation of the distal phalanx can return to performance (4). Another group reported that duration of lameness (but not body weight) was a significant risk factor for development of laminitis in the contralateral limb in horses with unilateral lameness and that horses developing this complication were more likely to be euthanized than animals that did not (12). Distal displacement of the distal phalanx warrants a poor prognosis. The type of horse at greatest risk for developing "sinking" of the distal phalanx was a large, middle-aged female that developed laminitis in all four feet subsequent to a primary septic, endotoxemic, or metabolic condition requiring intensive medical treatment. Treatment for this condition was strictly empiric and most often unsuccessful, leading to euthanasia of the most affected animals (13).

Horses with subacute or acute laminitis that respond to therapy within 7 to 10 days may recover completely (1). Horses with refractory and severe chronic laminitis are unlikely to perform again, but some are salvaged. Unfortunately, others are euthanized because of continued pain, lack of response to therapy, and severe permanent laminar and hoof wall changes.

REFERENCES

1. Baxter GM. Laminitis. In: Robinson NE, ed. Current Therapy in Equine Medicine. IV. Philadelphia: WB Saunders, 1997:737–743.
2. Kaufman JR, discussant of Chapman B, Platt GW. Laminitis. In: The Proceedings of the 30th Annual Convention of the American Association of Equine Practitioners 1984, Dallas, TX, 1985:110.
3. Stick JA, Jann HW, Scott EA, et al. Pedal bone rotation as a prognostic sign in laminitis of horses. JAVMA 1982;180:251.
4. Peloso JG, Cohen ND, Walker MA, et al. Case-control study of risk factors for the development of laminitis in the contralateral limb in equidae with unilateral lameness. JAVMA 1996;209:1746–1749.
5. Koblik PD, O'Brien TR, Coyne CP. Effect of dorsopalmar projection obliquity on radiographic measurement of distal phalangeal rotation angle in horses with laminitis. JAVMA 1988;192:346–349.
6. Cohen ND, Parson EM, Seahorn TL, et al. Prevalence and factors associated with

development of laminitis in horses with duodenitis/proximal jejunitis: 33 cases (1985–1991). JAVMA 1994;204:250–254.

7. Belknap JK, Moore JN. Evaluation of heparin for prophylaxis of equine laminitis: 71 cases (1980–1986). JAVMA 1989;195:505–507.
8. Goetz TE. Anatomic hoof and shoeing considerations for the treatment of laminitis in horses. JAVMA 1987;190:1323–1332.
9. Allen D, White NA, Foerner JF, et al. Surgical management of chronic laminitis in horses: 13 cases (1983–1985). JAVMA 1986;189:1604–1606.
10. Hunt RJ, Allen D, Baxter GM, et al. Mid-metacarpal deep digital flexor tenotomy in the management of refractory laminitis in horses. Vet Surg 1991;20:15–20.
11. Hunt RJ. A retrospective evaluation of laminitis in horses. Equine Vet J 1993;25:61–64.
12. Nixon AJ. Laminitis and contracture deformity. In: Nixon AJ, ed. Fracture Repair. Philadelphia: WB Saunders, 1996:367–370.
13. Baxter GM. Equine laminitis caused by distal displacement of the distal phalanx: 12 cases (1976–1985). JAVMA 1986;189:326–329.

Postoperative Salmonellosis

Acute equine salmonellosis has been reported in association with various factors, including hospitalization (1–4), general anesthesia (4, 5), transportation (4, 6), surgery (4, 5) (particularly abdominal surgery for colic [4, 7, 8]), anthelmintic medication (9, 10), tetracycline administration (2, 6), and hot, humid weather (1). The syndrome concerning the equine surgeon is seen during hospitalization in surgical cases and typically following surgery. It can involve many of the aforementioned predisposing factors. The source of the pathogen in many cases is unclear. Contaminated environment (7) and subclinical or inapparent infection in a resident, or newly admitted, animal (6) may be a source of the pathogen. Environmental contamination may come from horses with enteritis or from subclinical shedders admitted to the hospital for other reasons (4, 7). Alternatively, the animal may have been infected before developing the clinical signs, such as colic, which prompted its admission to the hospital. Stress associated with colic, transport to the hospital, hospitalization, anesthesia, and surgery may all compromise the immunologic status of carrier animals and initiate clinical enteritis.

The hypothesis that colicky horses may be shedding *Salmonella* organisms at the time of hospitalization even though many of these shedders do not develop other clinical signs of enteritis has been confirmed (5, 8, 11). Studies show that apparently normal horses can be *Salmonella* shedders and that such animals can develop clinical salmonellosis after entering a hospital. In one study, feces from 1451 horses entering a veterinary hospital over a 13-month period were cultured for *Salmonella* (12). A total of 46 horses (3.2%) yielded one or more *Salmonella*-positive fecal cultures. Twenty horses were found to be excreting *Salmonella* in the feces on admission, and 5 of these later had severe diarrhea associated with enteric salmonellosis. Abdominal surgery and other severe stresses were associated with all cases of severe enteric salmonellosis.

Stress of transport, hospitalization, or surgery when a horse is excreting *Salmonella* does not necessarily lead to a clinical problem, however. In one study evaluating the value of early *Salmonella* cultures in predicting the occurrence of acute salmonellosis as a complication following surgery for colic, it was found that most colic horses that shed *Salmonella* did not develop acute enteritis despite the extremely stressful conditions they were subjected to. Thirteen of one hundred horses had a positive culture for *Salmonella,* but only two developed clinical signs of salmonellosis (5). Because 12 of 13 of the culture-positive horses survived, the infection was considered to have been mild (and this should be contrasted with 28 of 87 culture-negative horses that survived overall) (5). Thus, it appears that being stressed while being exposed to *Salmonella* is not sufficient to produce acute enteritis in all cases. Whether this is caused by variability in the host's response to stress, variability in bacterial virulence, or an as yet undefined factor in the host-bacterium interaction is unclear.

Clinical evidence has also been presented to indicate that the potential for a stressed horse, which happens to be a *Salmonella* carrier, to develop diarrhea after stress may be exacerbated by tetracycline therapy (2, 6). The reason for this has been explained in terms of distribution of tetracycline in the body. Tetracyclines are removed from the blood by the liver and excreted in a concentrated form in the bile into the intestines. Biliary levels average at least 5 to 10 times higher than the simultaneous plasma concentration. This biliary concentration is greater than the minimal inhibitory concentration required against strains of E. *coli, Proteus,* and *Klebsiella aerobacter,* the most frequently detected bacterial infections of the human biliary system. The amount of tetracycline that reaches the intestine as a result of concentration by the liver could have a profound effect on the normal aerobic and anaerobic flora. Conversely, antibiotics such as penicillin, streptomycin, and chloramphenicol are excreted mainly by the kidney, and only a small portion is excreted by the liver. These antibiotics are not thought to reach sufficient concentration to cause comparable disturbances to the normal flora in the intestine. Experimental studies have also been done to demonstrate the combination of *Salmonella* infection, transportation, surgical stress, and tetracycline administration to produce a salmonellosis syndrome (6).

Various *Salmonella* spp. have been involved in clinical equine salmonellosis syndromes. The most common isolates have been *S. typhimurium* and *S. anatum* (1, 7, 13, 14). *S. enteritidis, S. newport, S. heidelberg, S. agona, S. typhimurium var. copenhagen, S. infantis, S. montevideo,* and, more recently, *S. Saint-Paul* and *S. Kreteld* (3, 11) have also been involved. Dual infections have also been reported.

The syndrome of salmonellosis in hospitalized horses was initially described as a specific entity, with clinical signs of fever and diarrhea and a neutrophil count of less than 3600 per cubic millimeter, or a rapid decline in neutrophilic numbers as specific for the disease (7). The horse apparently has a relatively small leukocyte reserve, and the hemogram was considered to be an important clinical indicator of bacterial infection and endotoxemia. Because of additional clinical and experimental studies, clinicians now believe that four clinical syndromes should be considered for a horse infected with *Salmonella* in the hospital situation (13):

1. Asymptomatic fecal shedding, intermittently or constantly (9)
2. Fever, depression, and anorexia without colic or diarrhea, and, in some cases, neutropenia and left shift (10)
3. Severe, acute fulminant diarrhea with fever, depression, anorexia, neutropenia, and dehydration (7)
4. Septicemia, fever, depression, anorexia, neutropenia, and death (15)

From these syndromes it can be seen that some infected horses may show fever, anorexia, and depression without concurrent diarrhea or any other obvious gastrointestinal abnormalities.

One report suggests that the degree of temperature rise may provide an indication of the severity of the problem (1). In this study, horses that had temperatures of 38.9 to 40°C, with diarrhea, had a 50% survival. When the temperature rise was at the 40.6 to 41.1°C level and diarrhea was present, all the patients succumbed (1). That 9 of 16 clinically ill patients in this study died is adequate indication of the severity of the problem.

In another study, where salmonellosis was experimentally produced, neutropenia occurred within 24 hours after stress and lasted 5 days, whereas the diarrhea developed between 3 and 9 days after stress. Therefore, neutropenia may not be apparent clinically at the onset of diarrhea. It is also possible for neutrophilia to be detected at the onset of diarrhea, which would be misleading (6). The authors of the study believe that if the clinician is aware of stress, regular white blood cell counts will assist in predicting where stress-induced salmonellosis with enteritis and diarrhea are likely to occur (6). For reasons cited above, however, the association between *Salmonella* infection, stress, and clinical disease is not an absolute one. Confirmation of the disease requires aggressive bacteriologic studies, and up to 5 consecutive negative cultures are considered appropriate before the presence of salmonellosis can be eliminated.

In clinical salmonellosis, fluid and electrolyte therapy is essential. The value of antimicrobial drugs in enteric salmonellosis of horses requires further study. The efficacy of antimicrobial therapy directed toward eliminating the *Salmonella* from the GI tract, lymph nodes, and major organs of the host has not been encouraging or consistent. Chloramphenicol was commonly prescribed but is used less so today because of the human health hazards. Although the isolate may show sensitivity to drugs such as gentamicin sulfate, an organism's acquired resistance to such antibiotics is a common problem, and the potential to develop nosocomial infections is a real threat. Early identification of the disease and attempts to minimize surgical and medical stresses are important. *When any hospitalized horse develops a temperature with depression, a white cell count and differential is done immediately.* Although the stress of transportation cannot be eliminated in a referral clinic, timely and fast surgery with minimal stress, both preoperatively and postoperatively, is important. The authors believe that surgery should be done within 48 hours of hospitalization to minimize the acquisition of an infection and that postoperative hospitalization should be kept to a minimum. One group recommend that surgery be done within 24 or 48 hours of hospitalization or delayed for a week (7). Although some degree of food withholding is important for general anesthesia, starvation acts as an additional stress on the gastrointestinal system and could potentially promote the disease. Avoid using tetracycline in hospitalized surgical patients.

Minimizing the chance of hospital contamination is important. Any horse that develops diarrhea is isolated from other patients. A horse is considered nonsuspect after three consecutive negative cultures. Remember that fewer *Salmonella* organisms are needed to produce the disease in a weak animal. *Salmonella* bacteria have a marked ability to survive and remain viable in places where *E. coli* quickly die out. Only a small amount of urine and/or feces in moisture is needed for good growth of *Salmonella,* and the organism will grow better in diluted urine and feces than in the normal excretions.

Salmonellosis in veterinary hospitals continues to be a major problem and, more recently, was the cause for closure of the Veterinary Teaching Hospital at Colorado State University. Recent experiences illustrate some important features of multiple cases of salmonellosis: (*a*) persistent and virulent cellular organisms can rapidly emerge, (*b*) adapted virulent organisms may predominate in a geographic area, and (*c*) clinicians at private veterinary hospitals need to implement the same degree of vigilance in preventing nosocomial infections with *Salmonella* as personnel at teaching hospitals have instituted. The latter is evidenced by a recent report of an outbreak of *S. anatum* that was initiated by two foals being referred from a private veterinary clinic (14). Because *S. anatum* cultured from the foals possessed the same pattern of resistance to multiple drugs and because both foals had been referred from the same private veterinary clinic, further information was sought and an epidemiologic investigation was begun. The veterinary clinic was confirmed as the source, and it was also demonstrated that before the spring of 1991 (the time of referral), *S. anatum* isolates at the veterinary teaching hospital were generally not resistant to antibiotics; 15 cultures from clinical environmental sources after April 1991 were resistant to multiple antimicrobial agents. The epidemiologic study supported the belief that the *S. anatum* isolates acquired antimicrobial resistance from the drug-resistant enteric bacteria detected in the private veterinary clinic environment. In the study, a failure to culture *S. anatum* from samples obtained from the veterinary medical teaching hospital environment inferred that nosocomial infections did not account for the observed affected horses.

Although careful attention to transmission within a veterinary hospital remains critical, it has also been recently emphasized that the admission of infected horses into a hospital is a critical factor. In a study at the University of California, dissemination of *S. krefeld* between stalls within the intensive care unit could not be demonstrated, but the organism was isolated from fecal samples obtained from several horses within 24 hours of hospitalization (too short a time for the acquisition and shedding within the hospital) (16). Vigilant monitoring of admitted patients is important.

REFERENCES

1. Morse EV, Duncan MA, Page EA, et al. *Salmonellosis equidae*: a study of 23 cases. Cornell Vet 1976;66:198–213.
2. Owen R ap R. Poststress diarrhoea in the horse. Vet Rec 1975;96:267–270.
3. Smith BP, Hardy AJ, Reina-Guerra M. A preliminary evaluation of some preparations of S. *typhimurium* as vaccines in horses. Proceedings of Equine Colic Research Symposium. University of Georgia: 1982:211.
4. Smith BP. Atypical salmonellosis in horses: fever and depression without diarrhea. JAVMA 1979;175:69–71.
5. Palmar JE, Benson CE, Whitlock RH. Subclinical salmonellosis in horses with colic. Proceedings of Equine Colic Research Symposium. University of Georgia: 1982:1980.
6. Owen R ap R, Fullerton J, Barnum DA. Effects of transportation, surgery and antibiotic therapy in horses infected with *Salmonella.* Am J Vet Res 1983;44:46.
7. Dorn CR, Coffman JR, Schmidt DA, et al. Neutropenia and salmonellosis in hospitalized horses. JAVMA 1975;166:65–67.
8. Palmar JE, Benson CE, Whitlock RH. *Salmonella* shed by horses with colic. JAVMA 1985;187:256–257.
9. Baker JR. Salmonellosis in the horse. Br Vet J 1970;126:100–105.
10. Dimock WW, Edwards PR, Bryner DW. The occurrence of paratyphoid infection in horses following treatment for intestinal parasites. Cornell Vet 1940;30:319.
11. Murray MJ. Salmonellosis in horses. JAVMA 1996;209:558–560.
12. Smith BP, Reina-Guerra M, Hardy AJ. Prevalence in epizootiology of equine salmonellosis. JAVMA 1978;172:353–356.
13. Bruner DW. Salmonellosis: a continual threat to New York state's cattle and horses. Cornell Vet 1985;75:93–96.
14. Hartmann FA, Callan RJ, McGuirk SM, et al. Control of an outbreak of salmonellosis caused by drug-resistant *Salmonella anatum* in horses at a veterinary hospital and measures to prevent future infections. JAVMA 1996;209:629–631.
15. Whitlock RH, Morris DD, Palmer JE, et al. Differential diagnosis of acute salmonellosis in colic. Proceedings of Equine Colic Research Symposium, University of Georgia, 1982:187.
16. Pare J, Carpenter TL, Thurmond MC. Analysis of spatial and temporal clustering of horses with *Salmonella krefeld* in an intensive care unit of a veterinary hospital. JAVMA 1996;209:626–628.

Infections of the Respiratory Tract

Many of the operations described in this book are done on racing horses or show horses. Typically, these horses are in contact with a large number of other horses, all potentially harboring a wide variety of respiratory viruses. Superimposed on viral diseases may be a poorly ventilated stall with dust and ammonia fumes capable of producing a chemical irritation in the respiratory tract. Further compounding this is the inhalation of dirt and blood during strenuous exercise (1). Endoscopy of horses involved in maximum exercise has confirmed just how "traumatic" racing is to the pulmonary tissues, as evidenced by the high incidence of blood and dirt found in the lower respiratory tract (2). A further compromise to the respiratory system occurs when a horse's head is tied up for extended periods, removing the assistance of gravity as a method of clearing exudate and debris. This list of insults to the respiratory system is also compounded by the vague syndrome of "stress," such as the stress of racing and training, changes in weather, or transport over long distances to a surgical facility. Pleuritis and pleural effusion are occasionally seen following stress from transport or general anesthesia. In one study of 153 cases of pleuropneumonia, 60 horses (39.2%) had been *transported* a long distance (3). Acute pleuritis can also be seen following general anesthesia.

When a horse is unable to lower its head, natural drainage of the respiratory tract is prevented, and secretions and exudates tend to drain back into the lungs. This hypothesis is supported by numerous anecdotes. When horses with fractures of the long bones are treated in flotation tanks to reduce the effective body weight, they are unable to lower their heads because of the design of the tank. A frequent complication of prolonged inability to lower the head has been termed flotation-induced pulmonary disease (4). Occasionally a horse must be cross-tied to an overhead wire system to prevent it from lying down and disrupting a suture line (e.g., in femorotibial arthrotomy used for approach to subchondral cysts of the distal femur; see Chapter 5 for details). These horses must be watched carefully for signs of bronchopneumonia and pleuritis because of impairment of natural drainage (gravity) of the respiratory tract. If an overt respiratory infection develops, the horse should be untied and allowed hand grazing as frequently as practical, with its head in the natural position, to aid in removal of exudate from the respiratory tract.

Other causes of postoperative respiratory tract infections are any operations to correct abnormalities of the upper respiratory tract, such as laryngoplasty or staphylectomy. In these patients, the normal function of the larynx is altered, and the chance of inhalation of foreign material is increased, especially during feeding. Surgery in the region of the guttural pouch can cause nerve dysfunction resulting in dysphagia and aspiration pneumonia. The prognosis for recovery from aspiration pneumonia is variable and has to be assessed on an individual basis. If aspiration pneumonia is suspected, appropriate doses of broad-spectrum antibiotics are indicated.

The presence of a respiratory tract infection in a surgical candidate is exacerbated by the combined effect of the general anesthetic *and* being in sternal or lateral recumbency for extended periods. Most general anesthetic agents, if used in sufficient doses to provide analgesia, will produce varying degrees of depression in respiratory function, including compromise in ciliary function (5). A horse with an infection of the lower respiratory tract has already lost varying degrees of respiratory reserve. While the horse is in lateral or sternal recumbency, there will inevitably be some degree of hypoxia and hypercapnia, both of which will be compounded by atelectasis and edema from an infectious process in the lung.

Hypoxia and hypercapnia can be most severe during anesthetic induction when there are varying degrees of apnea. To avoid these complications, the horse should be intubated immediately and placed on an oxygen-rich gas mixture. This treatment is particularly applicable to the horse with a compromised respiratory system. Intermittent positive-pressure ventilation (IPPV) should be considered in the patient at risk. The horse is vulnerable during the postsurgical period as well, when it has been disconnected from the anesthetic machine and is breathing room air (5).

Another immediate threat to the horse's life if it is anesthetized while it has a respiratory tract infection is the risk of exacerbation or flare-up of the condition, which may produce a life-threatening bronchopneumonia or pleuritis. In one study of 82 cases of pleuritis, 7 (8.5%) were postsurgical patients (6). Patients may die or develop permanent respiratory compromise. Invariably, hospitalization time is lengthened, which further increases the horse's chance of acquiring other respiratory viruses from hospitalized horses or of contracting a more serious nosocomial infection such as salmonellosis.

All surgical candidates should be carefully evaluated before surgery with respect to the respiratory system. This evaluation should begin with a complete history, including vaccination history, history of any prior illnesses of the horse or of stable mates, and any vital information that pertains to the respiratory tract, such as a history of exercise-induced pulmonary hemorrhage. A thorough physical examination is essential. Auscultation of the lungs should be done in a quiet room with the aid of a rebreathing bag. It may not be possible to hear increased bronchovesicular sounds, pleural friction rubs, etc., with the horse breathing normally at rest.

Any horse shipped to a clinic for surgery that arrives with a serous or mucopurulent nasal discharge and a spontaneous or inducible cough is carefully scrutinized. A horse with an elevation in temperature (1 to 3°F, 1 to 2°C) with no obvious involvement of other body systems is regarded with suspicion for a respiratory tract infection. Such horses should have an immediate complete blood count and a serum fibrinogen level count. A complete blood count from a horse with a respiratory infection will usually show an increased white blood cell count with relative and absolute neutrophilia with a slight shift to the left in some cases. The fibrinogen level will likely be elevated. The lungs and trachea should be carefully auscultated. An area of ventral dullness should immediately arouse suspicion of pleuritis with pleural effusion (discussed in greater detail later in this chapter). An endoscopic examination can be done to assess for upper airway inflammation and the source of any exudate and to evaluate the trachea for evidence of blood, exudate, or food contamination.

Radiographic and ultrasound examination of the chest are not part of a routine preoperative workup but should be done if bronchopneumonia or pleuritis with pleural effusion is suspected. Radiographs and ultrasonograms can also be used to evaluate the chest in horses in which it is not possible to auscultate lung sounds even with a rebreathing bag. Many practices are limited in their ability to perform chest radiographs because of lack of equipment. Most studies are limited to lateral views, and although anatomic differences exist between horses and small animals, radiographic signs of pulmonary disease are similar (7). In the authors' hospitals, it is common to find evidence of peribronchiolar infiltrates and mild increase in interstitial density in the lungs of normal horses. Chest radiographs should not be "over read." Conversely, horses, and particularly foals, can have severe radiographic changes that are reflective of advanced pulmonary disease yet on auscultation might be considered "normal." The clinical significance of the radiographic findings must be determined by the clinician in consultation with the radiologist. Ultrasonographic examination of the chest is useful for detecting pleural effusion and any underlying pulmonary parenchymal disease (8).

A horse with pleuritis will be stiff and reluctant to move—signs resembling those of acute laminitis or even "tying up." Some appear almost colicky, with

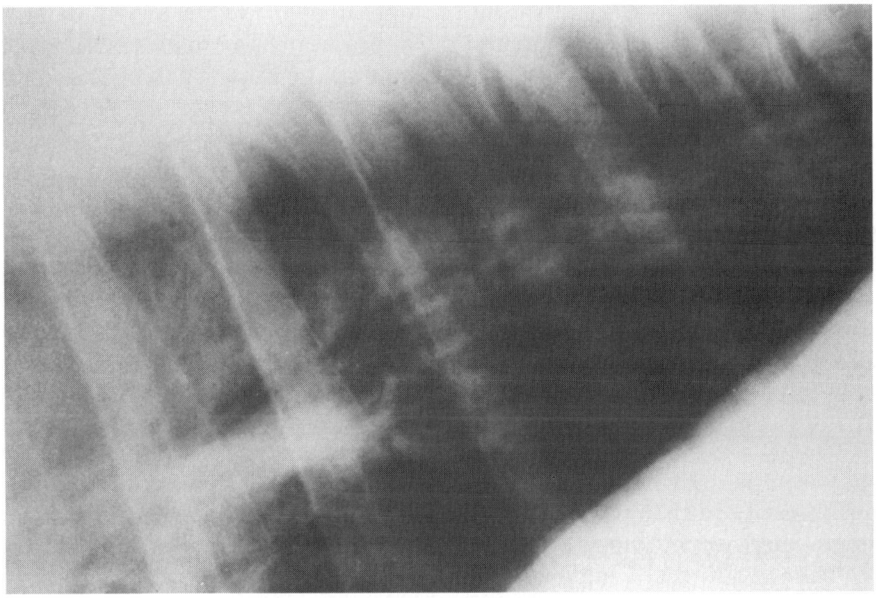

FIGURE 4.1. Lateral radiograph of a horse with pleural effusion. The pleural effusion has obliterated a portion of the diaphragm border, the caudal vena cava, and heart border. The fluid has gravitated to the ventral thorax causing the increased opacity.

an anxious expression (9). They feel pain when pushed firmly on the ribs and breathe with shallow respirations. Auscultation of the thorax may be unremarkable *early* in the disease, but as the disease progresses, respiratory sounds decrease in the ventral thorax region and normal to harsh airway sounds are heard dorsally. Radiographs may reveal a fluid line, and there may be radiographic signs of a concurrent bronchopneumonia (Fig. 4.1). Ultrasonographic examination will show pleural effusion, and if there is an anaerobic infection, gas echoes may be visible (8). If pleural fluid is detected, either in the presurgical evaluation or as a sequela to surgery and general anesthesia, pleurocentesis is indicated.

Pleurocentesis is done through surgically prepared skin between the 5th and 7th ribs, immediately dorsal to the costochondral junction (9). The skin, intercostal muscles, and sensitive parietal pleura are infiltrated with the appropriate local anesthetic solution (6). Fluid is collected with a sterile 3-inch metal teat cannula or catheter. The fluid should be collected in an EDTA tube for fluid analysis, as well as submitted for culture, cell count, cell type, and protein measurement (9). Most cases of pleuritis will have a high protein content and a high white blood cell count. Pleural fluid can best be considered identical to peritoneal fluid so far as clinicopathologic values are concerned (10).

The authors' immediate approach to a case of respiratory disease, either preoperatively or postoperatively, is to inform the owner of the nature of the condition and discuss the overall plan for management. When the horse arrives for surgery with preexisting respiratory disease, the prudent thing is to delay surgery until the horse is fully recovered. Whether to send the horse home or to hospitalize it until recovery must be decided on an individual basis; hard and fast rules cannot be laid down. To subject the horse to a long journey immediately may be more harmful than to monitor the convalescence in your hospital, where the horse could be exposed to a wider population of viruses. The delay in performing surgery will mean increased hospitalization and certainly far more expense for the owner. If there is good client communication, the end result will be a minimum of dissatisfaction and a good understanding of the seriousness of the disease and its sequela if surgery were to be performed. As a general rule, the authors believe that a horse should be operated on within 2 days of arrival, provided a physical examination and the appropriate diagnostic tests show that the horse is a good risk. To delay surgery so that the horse "can become accustomed to the hospital" and thereby be "less stressed" is a fallacy. All delay will do is increase the horse's exposure to other viruses and possible nosocomial infections.

The authors believe that a course of antibiotics is indicated for any animal with respiratory disease that may be subjected to general anesthesia. They also believe that the use of broad-spectrum intravenous perioperative antibiotics may help prevent against the development of postoperative pleuropneumonia. Certainly, cases of respiratory disease that occur postsurgically must be evaluated on an individual basis. Which antibiotic to use is a matter of personal choice. Refractory cases are placed on broad-spectrum antibiotics. Too often, clinicians change antibiotics after 1 or 2 days because the respiratory disease fails to respond completely, and then another antibiotic is chosen when there is no response. This type of therapy is one of the major factors behind the development of a chronic refractory pneumonia unresponsive to many different potent expensive antibiotics. The first drug used to treat the respiratory condition must be given a chance to be effective before a more potent antibiotic is selected. Serial white blood counts, daily auscultation of the lungs, and twice-daily monitoring of body temperature are all necessary to monitor recovery.

If pleuropneumonia is diagnosed, it may be necessary to place indwelling thoracic catheters with one-way valves to provide continuous passive drainage. These drains are generally left in place no more than 72 hours or as long as they are effectively draining fluid, and are then removed. A daily ultrasound examination of the chest is used to determine if there is significant accumulation of fluid and if further drainage is required. Provided vigorous therapeutic efforts are made, the outcome for most horses with pleuropneumonia is favorable. Most horses can be saved, and many return to athletic activities, including racing (11).

In chronic cases of pleuritis with abscess formation, surgical drainage in the form of a thoracotomy has been performed. An open thoracotomy through an intercostal incision or with a 6th or 7th partial rib resection can be done in the standing horse (12–14). Horses with pleural abscesses that are candidates for surgical drainage are identified using radiography, ultrasonography, and, possibly, pleuroscopy (3, 12, 15). There are many advantages to doing an open thoracotomy in the standing patient; however, certain criteria must be met before surgical drainage is considered. There must be an abscess that is encapsulated and walled off from the rest of the thoracic cavity, otherwise after fluid drains from the surgical incision, a pneumothorax will quickly develop. With an open thoracotomy, a bilateral pneumothorax could be fatal. The abscess must also be adherent to the parietal pleura so that when its wall is incised, the contents do not spill into the thoracic cavity. An indwelling chest tube can be placed into the abscess cavity and left open to the air. If no signs of pneumothorax develop, it can be assumed that the abscess is amenable to open thoracic drainage. The advantage of doing a partial rib resection and thoracotomy is that it allows more direct access to the abscess, enabling the surgeon to pass a hand into the abscess cavity. Necrotic contents of the abscess can be removed, and loculated abscesses can be drained more effectively (13). The incision is left open for drainage and to allow flushing of the abscess cavity. In some cases, a small fistulous tract may persist at the surgical site (13).

REFERENCES

1. Mansmann RA. The stages of equine pleuropneumonia. In: Proceedings of the 29th Annual Convention of the American Association of Equine Practitioners 1983, Las Vegas, NV, 1984:61.

2. Arthur RM. Subacute and acute pleuritis. Proceedings of the 29th Annual Convention of the American Association of Equine Practitioners 1983, Las Vegas, NV, 1984;65.
3. Byars TD, Becht JL. Pleuropneumonia. Vet Clin North Am Equine Pract 1991;7:63–78.
4. McClintock SA. Some Clinical and Physiological Effects of Floatation of Horses. MS Thesis, The University of Sydney, 1984.
5. Gillespie JR, Amis TC. Respiratory physiology of the surgical patient. In: Jennings PB, ed. The Practice of Large Animal Surgery. Philadelphia: WB Saunders, 1984:356.
6. Raphel CF, Beech J. Pleuritis and pleural effusion in the horse. In: Proceedings of the 27th Annual Convention of the American Association of Equine Practitioners, 1981. 1982:17.
7. Farrow CS. Equine thoracic radiology. JAVMA 1981;179:776.
8. Reimer JM, Reef VB, Spencer PA. Ultrasonography as a diagnostic aid in horses with anaerobic bacterial pleuropneumonia and/or pulmonary abscessation: 27 cases (1984–1986). JAVMA 1989;194:278–282.
9. Smith BP. Pleuritis and pleural effusion in the horse. A study of 37 cases. JAVMA 1977;170:208.
10. Wagner AE, Bennett DG. Analysis of equine thoracic fluid. Vet Clin Pathol 1981;11:13.
11. Seltzer KL, Byars TD. Prognosis for return to racing after recovery from infectious pleuropneumonia in Thoroughbred racehorses: 20 cases (1984–1989). JAVMA 1996; 208:1300–1301.
12. Schott HC, Mansmann RA. Thoracic drainage in horses. Compend Contin Educ Pract Vet 1990;12:251–261.
13. Shearer DC, Slone DE, Moll HD, et al. Rib resection and thoracotomy as a treatment for chronic pleuritis. In: Proceedings of the 31st Annual Conference of the AAEP, Toronto, Canada, 1985:393–397.
14. Speirs VC, Boulton CH. Lower respiratory system. In: Auer JA, ed. Equine Surgery. Philadelphia: WB Saunders, 1992:496–506.
15. Mackey VS, Wheat JD. Endoscopic examination of the equine thorax. Equine Vet J 1985;17:140–142.

5

ORTHOPAEDIC SURGERY

Lag Screw Fixation—Principles

One method to compress a fracture is to use a lag screw, a fundamental technique used routinely by carpenters and engineers. Lag screw technique in equine surgery is typically done by using cortical bone screws applied in a lag screw manner instead of using actual lag screws (1, 2). This method is particularly suited to horses with intra-articular fractures, where accurate anatomic alignment at the level of the joint surface is essential to avoid secondary degenerative joint disease (DJD). Alignment is particularly important for the racing horse, who must be 100% sound or the operation is deemed a failure.

General Considerations

A variety of fractures in horses are amenable to lag screw fixation, but the ones described in detail in this book are:

1. Slab fractures of the third carpal bone
2. Sagittal fractures of the proximal phalanx
3. Lateral condylar fractures of the third metacarpus or metatarsus
4. Midbody fractures of the proximal sesamoid bone

A single lag screw alone is used to repair certain slab fractures of the third carpal bone, but, generally speaking, two or more are used to prevent *rotation* of the fragment in fractures of the metacarpus and first phalanx. Lag screws alone are rarely used to repair long, oblique, spiral, or fissure fractures of the tubular long bones such as the femur, tibia, radius, and humerus. Lag screws are often used in combination with bone plates to repair major long bone fractures. In the repair of comminuted fractures, the fracture site is reconstructed with lag screws before applying a neutralization plate or plates. The use of lag screws to reconstruct a comminuted fracture of the third metacarpal bone is discussed in this section.

Two types of screws are available for lag screw fixation: the cortical bone screw (applied with the lag screw technique) and the cancellous screw (a true lag screw when there is a nonthreaded portion). Under most circumstances, owing to the density of equine bone, a cortical bone screw is used. Various sizes of cortical screws are available. The most commonly used size is 4.5 mm, but there are indications for 2.7-mm, 3.5-mm, and 5.5-mm diameter screws. To achieve the lag screw principle, the thread of the screw must gain purchase only in one fragment. For cortical screws this is achieved by *overdrilling* the fragment next to the screw head to such a size that the screw thread will not gain purchase on this portion of the bone. This hole is termed the *gliding hole.* If it were not overdrilled, when the screw is tightened, the gap between the fracture fragments would be maintained. Therefore, the screw should achieve purchase only in the "far" cortex or transcortex (i.e., away from the head). The hole in this cortex is the *thread hole.* A cortical screw is threaded for its entire length and has a lower ratio between the outer diameter and the core than does the cancellous screw.

In certain areas of the musculoskeletal system, particularly in the metaphyseal regions of the bone in foals, bone is too soft for 4.5-mm cortical screws and thus one option is to use a *cancellous screw* to achieve compression between the fragments. To increase the surface area of contact between the screw and bone, the ratio between the outer diameter and the core is greater than that found in a cortical screw. The cancellous screw has a smooth shank near the head and a threaded portion near the tip. When employed as a lag screw, the smooth shank must pass through one fragment and the threaded portion must gain purchase in the other; thus, as the screws tighten, the fragments are compressed. Cancellous screws have two lengths of thread at the tip, 16 mm and 32 mm. Because maximum holding power is desired during fracture repair in horses, there is little place for screws with small threads, and the cancellous screws with the longer threads (i.e., 32 mm) should be used whenever possible. Cancellous screws threaded along their entire length have also become available. There are not true lag screws.

Cancellous screws should be used with caution in dense cortical bone. If the surgeon has stripped a cortical screw as a result of overzealous tightening, however, the only way to achieve compression is to use a cancellous screw in its place or a larger diameter (e.g., 5.5 mm) of cortical screw.

During the healing process, new bone will form around the smooth shank of the cancellous screw, and, consequently, if screw removal is necessary, the cancellous thread must be able to cut its way back out of the bone. If the bone around the shank is too dense, the cancellous screw can break at the screw thread junction. Therefore, cancellous screws are used as lag screws only when cortical screws have failed. Repair of fractures in young foals with very soft bone is a possible exception to this rule.

The system of orthopaedic implants recommended is the AO-ASIF system (Arbeitsgemeinschaft Fur Osteosynthesefragen-Association for the Study of Internal Fixation). This system of implants has been used most widely in horses and, in the authors' opinion, is the most adaptable (1).

To exert the maximum amount of interfragmentary compression, a lag screw must be inserted at right angles to the fracture plane (3). If the bone is under some axial load, however, the screw ideally should be inserted at right angles to the long axis of the bone. Therefore, the ideal direction to achieve maximum interfragmentary compression and resistance to axial load is a direction between these two extremes. This is a somewhat hypothetical solution and is not always feasible in certain equine fractures. For example, in a repair of a sagittal fracture of the proximal phalanx, insertion of the screws either at right angles or parallel to the long axis of the bone usually achieves adequate compression to align the joint surface.

Mechanical testing of the holding power of orthopaedic screws shows that 5.5-mm diameter cortical bone screws provide greater holding power than 4.5-mm cortical bone screws in the diaphysis of foal bone. In addition, the 5.5-mm screw is a suitable alternative to a 6.5-mm cancellous screw (4). In adult horse bone, 5.5-mm diameter screws show greater holding power and greater tensile strength than 4.5-mm cortical screws; therefore, the larger screws should be used when available (5).

The steps in insertion of a lag screw are illustrated in the technique "Fracture of the Third Carpal Bone." The equipment used for lag screw fixation is listed in Appendix I and illustrated in Figure 5.1.

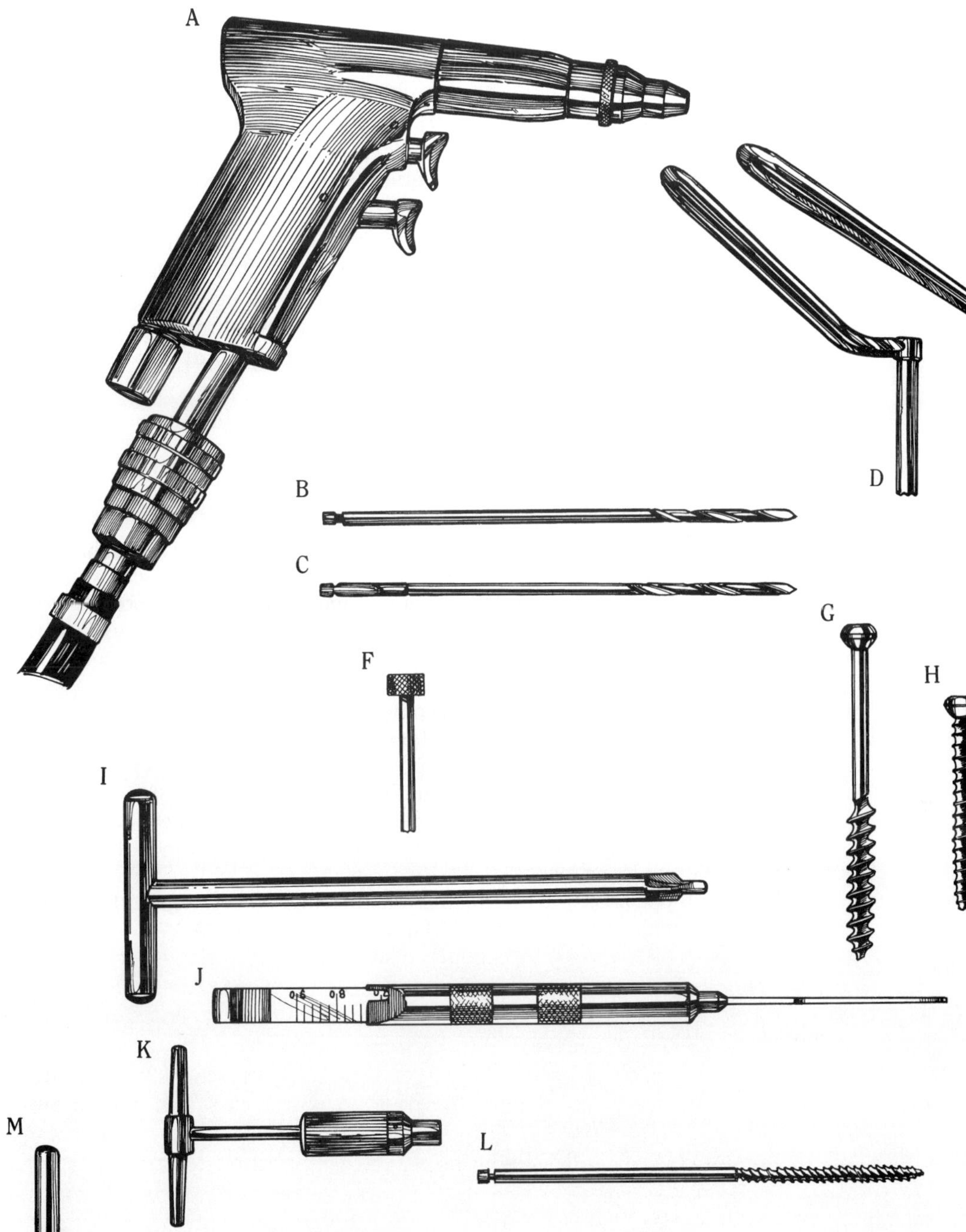

FIGURE 5.1. Instruments required for lag screw fixation. A, air drill; B, 4.5-mm drill bit; C, 3.2-mm drill bit; D, 4.5-mm tap sleeve; E, 6.5-mm tap sleeve; F, 3.2-mm drill sleeve; G, cancellous screw (32-mm thread); H, cortical screw; I, countersink; J, depth gauge; K, tap handle; L, 4.5-mm cortical tap; M, 6.5-mm cancellous tap; N, hexagonal-headed screwdriver.

Cannulated Screws

More recently, cannulated screws have been developed. The shaft of the screw is opened so that a guide pin passes through the central canal. In addition, there are reverse self-cutting threads that allow removal of the screw after fracture healing. The AO-ASIF large cannulated screw system requires a set of cannulated instruments for its insertion. A 2-mm guidewire is preplaced using a parallel wire guide, and this is used for drilling and placement of the screws.

The Herbert bone screw is also a cannulated screw. It is also headless and incorporates screw threads of two different pitches to create fracture compression. A 4.5-mm Herbert screw is available and has been used for condylar fractures and tarsal slab fractures (6, 7). Although the screw eliminates the need for a head within vital soft tissue structures, there is a suggestion that less effective compression might be obtained in some equine fractures.

REFERENCES

1. Auer JA. Screw application techniques. In: Nixon AJ, ed. Equine Fracture Repair. Philadelphia: WB Saunders, 1996:65–67.
2. Fackelman GE, Nunamaker DM. Manual of Internal Fixation in the Horse. New York: Springer-Verlag, 1982.
3. Mueller ME, Allgower M, Schneider R, et al. Manual of Internal Fixation. 2nd ed. New York: Springer-Verlag, 1979.
4. Yovich JV, Turner AS, Smith FW. Holding power of orthopaedic screws in equine third metacarpal and metatarsal bones. I. Foal bone. Vet Surg 1985;14:221.
5. Yovich JV, Turner AS, Smith FW. Holding power of orthopaedic screws in equine third metacarpal and metatarsal bones. II. Adult horse bone. Vet Surg 1985;14:230.
6. Herthel DJ, Moody JL, Lauper L. The repair of condylar fracture of the third metacarpal and third metatarsal bone using the Herbert compression screw in 9 Thoroughbred racehorses. Equine Pract 1995;17:6–12.
7. Martin F, Herthel DJ. Central tarsal bone fractures in 6 horses. Report on the use of an annulated compression bone screw. Equine Pract 1992;14:23–27.

Repair of Fracture of the Third Carpal Bone Using Arthrotomy

A slab fracture of the third carpal bone is one that extends from one articulation to the next and is most frequently located on the dorsomedial surface of the bone (radial facet) (Fig. 5.2*A*). The injury is seen most commonly in the fast-gaited horse such as the racing Thoroughbred, Quarter horse, and Standardbred. Other carpal bones such as the radial and fourth carpal bones can sustain slab fractures. The basic principles of repair apply to all fractures, however, but the following description will apply to the more common third carpal bone slab fracture.

A slab fracture of any carpal bone may begin as a hairline fissure fracture that can later displace into a more painful fracture that carries a worse prognosis. Such undisplaced fractures are difficult to diagnose, and various radiographs at oblique angles and skyline views are necessary to delineate the fracture. Prompt diagnosis is essential because continual weightbearing causes micromotion at the fracture site, resulting in DJD. The authors and other colleagues believe that many early lesions on the third carpal bone go undiagnosed and with continued exercise develop a displacing slab fracture with a much worse prognosis (1).

Occasionally, slab fractures of the carpal bones (especially the third) occur in a sagittal and not the usual frontal (or nearly frontal) plane. The majority of these fractures are managed conservatively, but some are amenable to lag screw fixation (2).

Typically, a slab fracture of the third carpal bone is more painful than the more common chip fracture. There is marked pain on carpal flexion and distension of the midcarpal (intercarpal) joint as well as pain on palpation of the fracture itself (3). Intra-articular (local) anesthesia is not required for diagnosis unless the fracture is undisplaced.

A complete set of radiographs should be taken: AP, lateral, flexed lateral, APLMO, and APMLO views. The well-known "skyline" or tangential view is mandatory when a slab fracture of any of the carpal bones is suspected (1–7). This view will show the position of the slab fracture in relationship to the tendon of the extensor carpi radialis and thereby help the surgeon decide on the correct location for the bone screw. It will also demonstrate the thickness of the slab and help the surgeon decide if removal is more appropriate or if a smaller screw or even two screws are required. This view can also demonstrate whether the slab is in one or two pieces, which would have a profound effect on the prognosis. As with any injury to the carpus in a fast-gaited horse, the contralateral carpus should be radiographed because both joints frequently are involved (4).

It has been stated regarding the indications for screw fixation of slab fractures of the equine carpus that "any fracture that is radiographically distinct will benefit from surgery" (1). When displacement occurs, the authors believe that screw fixation is indicated for all horses that are to be returned to athletic activity and for horses to be used for breeding purposes. In severe slab fractures in which there is imminent collapse of the second row of carpal bones, internal fixation is essential for salvage.

Repair of carpal slab fractures using arthrotomy has been largely superseded by arthroscopic surgery (described in the next procedure). Arthroscopy also allows complete examination of the joint and resolution of multiple problems. When experience has been gained with the arthroscope in the midcarpal joint of the horse, slab fractures can be repaired by inserting the screw through a stab incision over the fragment and monitoring fracture reduction through the arthroscope.

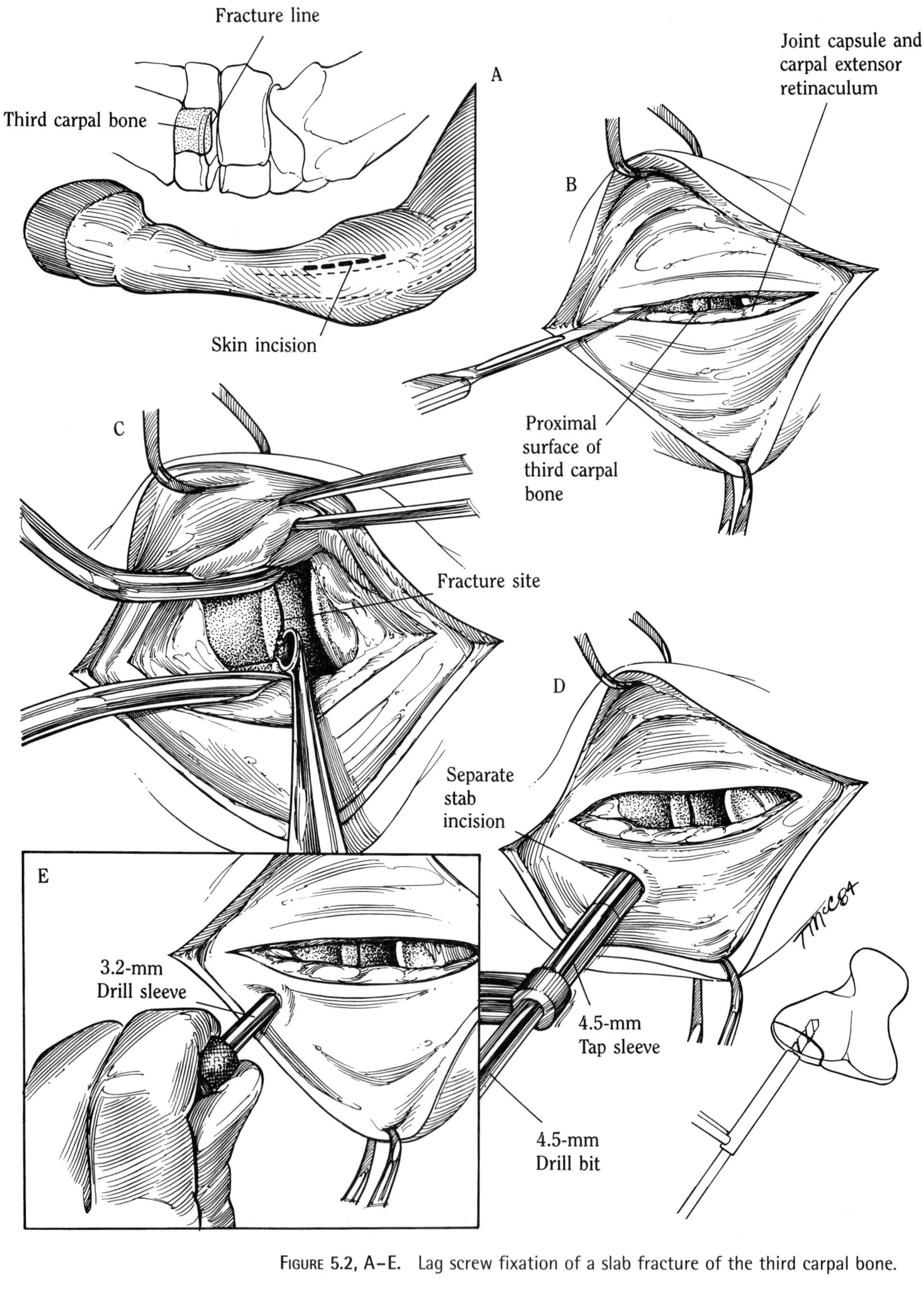

Figure 5.2, A–E. Lag screw fixation of a slab fracture of the third carpal bone.

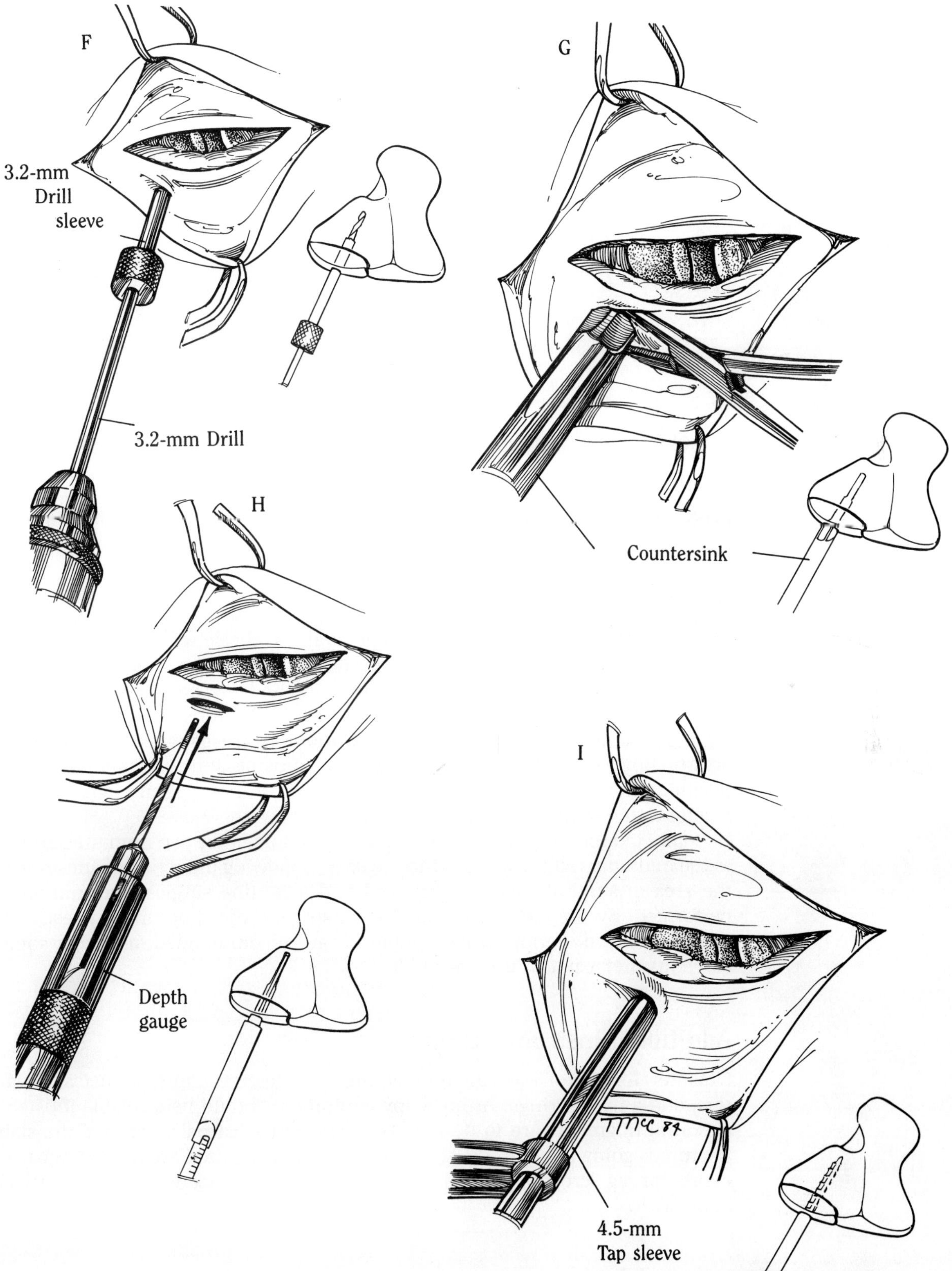

FIGURE 5.2, F–I. *(continued)* Lag screw fixation of a slab fracture of the third carpal bone.

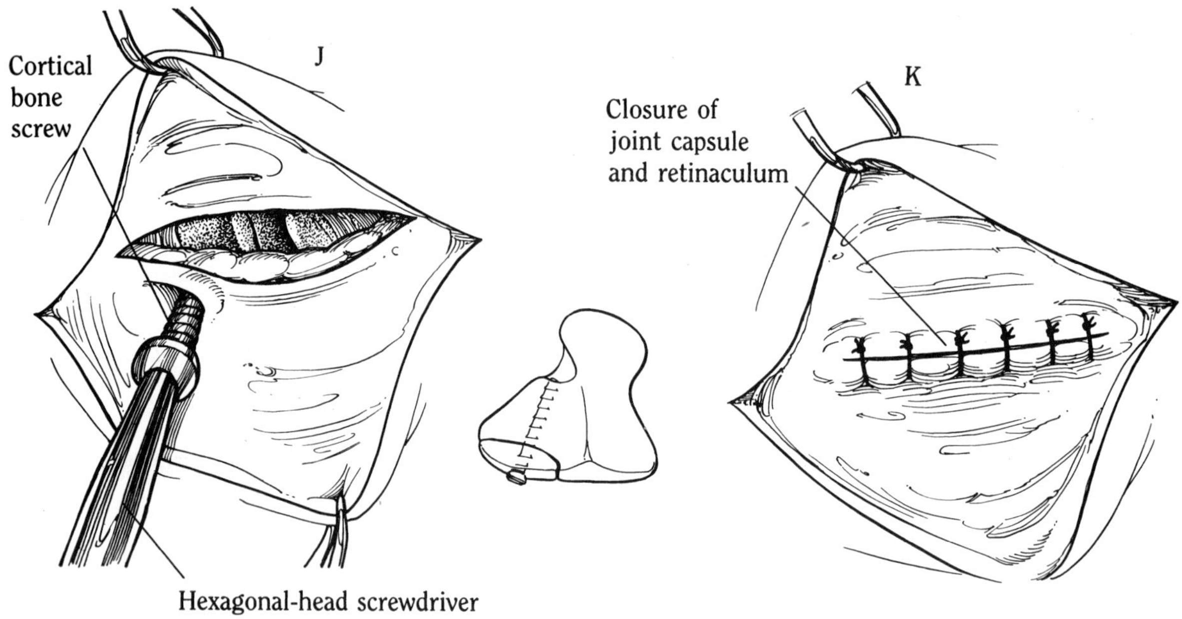

Figure 5.2, J–K. *(continued)* Lag screw fixation of a slab fracture of the third carpal bone.

Anesthesia and Surgical Preparation

The surgical procedure is done under general anesthesia with the horse placed in lateral recumbency and the affected limb down. Some surgeons prefer to operate with the horse in dorsal recumbency and the limb elevated to take advantage of natural hemostasis. Certainly, if both limbs are to be operated on (e.g., one for screw fixation with or without arthroscopy and the other for arthroscopy), the authors strongly recommend using dorsal recumbency. This position allows the surgeon to go immediately to the opposite joint without having to roll the horse over.

Before induction of anesthesia, the patient's limb is clipped from the coronet to the midradius all the way around the limb. Following induction of anesthesia, the area of surgical excision is shaved and a routine surgical preparation is performed. By preparing the limb before surgery, the time under anesthesia can be reduced. Perioperative antibiotics are recommended, although some surgeons prefer not to use any at all.

Additional Instrumentation

Lag screw fixation of a slab fracture requires curettes, retractors, periosteal elevators, and a bulb syringe. Arthroscopy equipment should be available if osteochondral fragments are to be removed from either carpal joint or if the slab fracture is going to be fixed arthroscopically. Also required are the ASIF instruments for lag screw fixation (see Appendix I) and a selection of ASIF cortical bone screws.

Surgical Technique

After draping (sterile plastic adherent drapes are recommended for this procedure), the following structures should be identified: the tendinous insertion of the extensor carpi radialis muscle, the tendon of the extensor carpi obliquus muscle, the antebrachiocarpal joint, and the midcarpal joint. Identification of these structures is facilitated by flexing and extending the carpal joint. An 8-cm straight incision is made parallel and medial to the edge of the tendon of the extensor carpi radialis (Fig. 5.2*A*). The incision extends from the middle of the face of the radial carpal bone to the middle of the face of the third carpal bone. The skin edges are then reflected from the subcutaneous fascia toward the base. A straight incision approximately 5 cm long is made through the subcutaneous fascia, carpal extensor retinaculum, and joint capsule. The incision is made parallel to the tendon of the extensor carpi radialis muscle but avoids the tendon sheath (Fig. 5.2*B*). Synovial fluid will flow from the incision when the joint is entered. Any blood vessels or their visible lumens should be cauterized at this point. Using suitable retractors, the surgeon carefully retracts the edges of the incision in the carpal extensor retinaculum and joint capsule; this retraction will expose the proximal surface of the third carpal bone and the distal surface of the radial carpal bone.

The extent of the fracture is examined, and the approximate center of the fragment (site for screw location) is estimated. Any free fragments of bone and cartilage at the fracture site are removed, as well as any osteochondral fragments on the margin of the "slab" or on the opposite surface of the radial carpal bone. Curettage is done where necessary (Fig. 5.2*C*).

Reduction of the fracture usually occurs when the limb is put in flexion. With the limb in this position, a 4.5-mm gliding hole is drilled using the 4.5-mm tap sleeve to protect the surrounding soft tissues (Fig. 5.2*D*). Frequently, the screw must be inserted through a separate stab incision through the tendon of the extensor carpi radialis if the site does not coincide with the arthrotomy incision. The stab incision should be made in a direction parallel to the fibers of the tendon. Direction of the drill bit is critical; it should be directed perpendicular to the plane of the fracture and parallel to the articular surface. In fractures that are somewhat displaced, the surgeon will "feel" when the fracture site has been entered. In the undisplaced hairline or fissure fracture, it may be impossible to feel when the 4.5-mm drill bit has arrived at or crossed the fracture site. One technique is to place a ruler on the surface of the bone parallel to the bit and monitor the depth of bone that has been penetrated (5). Most slab fractures are 6- to 10-mm thick, but the gliding (clearance) hole should be at least 12-mm deep to allow countersinking (5). Intraoperative radiographs are also useful to see that the drill bit has crossed the fracture line.

A 3.2-mm drill sleeve is inserted into the 4.5-mm gliding hole (Fig. 5.2*E*). Parting the soft tissues that tend to cover the gliding hole with the tips of a hemostat will facilitate its location. The 3.2-mm thread hole is drilled into the parent portion of the third carpal bone. It is usually not necessary to drill out the palmar surface of the bone, and such drilling should be avoided so that the contents of the carpal canal are not damaged. The drill should be cleaned frequently. A thread hole of 20 to 25 mm is recommended to provide enough length for a 4.5-mm cortical bone screw (5) to provide adequate compression (Fig. 5.2*F*).

The hole is now countersunk, again using hemostats to part the soft tissues at the entrance to the hole. The hole should be countersunk around its entire circumference. Because the tip of the countersink is 12 mm, a glide hole of adequate length must be provided to allow it to engage the bone. Inadequate countersinking results in excessive protrusion of the screw head into the soft tissues (Fig. 5.2*G*). Failure to countersink the hole increases the chance of splitting the fragment during tightening. The depth gauge is inserted to determine the appropriate size of screw (Fig. 5.2*H*). Its length is read off the scale, and 2 mm is subtracted from the measurement.

The 4.5-mm cortical tap is inserted using the 4.5-mm tap sleeve to protect the soft tissues (Fig. 5.2*I*). Care must be taken not to impact the tap in the blind ending pilot hole because it will strip the threads of bone that have been cut in the parent portion of the bone (Fig. 5.2*I*).

The appropriate-sized screw is inserted and tightened judiciously (Fig. 5.2*J*). Excessive torquing may result in splitting the fragment, which would have catastrophic results. Radiographs should be taken intraoperatively and postoperatively to ensure the correct direction and final placement of the bone screw.

The arthrotomy incision is closed in three layers. The joint capsule and retinaculum are closed with a layer of simple interrupted sutures of absorbable synthetic material or monofilament, nonabsorbable material. The sutures should not penetrate the synovial membrane. Preplacement of the sutures in the joint capsule and extensor retinaculum ensures an accurate apposition and a tight seal (Fig. 5.2*K*).

Following joint capsule closure, 4 to 5 mL of Ringer's solution is flushed into the joint with a 20-gauge needle. If any leaks are observed through the incision, additional sutures can be placed at this time. The subcutaneous fascia is closed with a simple continuous pattern using synthetic absorbable sutures. The skin is closed with a simple interrupted or vertical mattress pattern using synthetic monofilament sutures, and the limb is wrapped with a tight pressure bandage. Control of minute capillary ooze will be possible if the tourniquet is released after the pressure wrap is applied.

Postoperative Management

The limb is wrapped in a firm pressure bandage for 3 weeks, during which time the bandage is changed several times. If the carpal joint is unstable or if there is some question regarding the stability achieved with internal fixation, a full-limb cast should be applied to protect the repair while the horse recovers from the anesthetic. For example, horses with multiple slab fractures or a slab fracture causing complete joint collapse should have a cast during recovery from anesthesia as well as during a good portion of the convalescence. The cast may be cut off some weeks later when the soft tissues have healed. Skin sutures are removed at 10 to 12 days. Care must be taken when bandaging the carpal joint so as not to cause a pressure sore on the accessory carpal bone; this can be avoided by cutting a small hole in the back of the bandage over the accessory carpal bone.

During convalescence, the horse is kept in a box stall. The convalescence and aftercare will vary depending on the individual horse and on the severity of injury to the carpal bone. Generally, 6 to 12 months should elapse before the horse returns to athletic activities. Radiographic monitoring of the fracture healing is recommended. Also, the degree of periosteal proliferation can be assessed. Excessive periostitis usually points to a poorer prognosis.

The implants are usually not removed. They are frequently blamed for causing permanent disability when the real cause is concurrent DJD.

Comments

For large slab fractures of the third carpal bone, two screws should be used. This is rare in the authors' hospital but should be considered if indicated. Two screws can be used in slab fractures of the other carpal bones, such as the fourth carpal bone (6). When two screws are being used, most surgeons opt for the smaller diameter screws because two large 4.5-mm screws may weaken the bone and risk splitting the fragment (7). If smaller screws are used, the surgeon must

Table 5.1. Screw Dimensions (in Millimeters)

Size of Screw	*Size of Glide Hole*	*Size of Thread (Pilot) Hole*	*Size of Tap*
4.5	4.5	3.2	4.5
3.5	3.5	2.7	3.5
2.7	2.7	2.5	2.7

become familiar with a different set of instrument dimensions, as outlined in Table 5.1.

One of the smaller diameter bone screws may be used in smaller, thinner slab fractures if the surgeon believes that the larger screw may split the bone (6). If the slab does split as the screw is tightened, the surgeon has no choice but to remove the slab of bone or to use two screws, one in each portion of the slab. A split slab usually requires considerable dissection of and trauma to the joint. Slab fractures of the third carpal bone also occur in combination with slab fractures of the radial carpal bone.

Multiple fractures of the carpal bones, such as a very large, displaced slab fracture of C3 with or without involvement of other bones (e.g., C4 and radial carpal bones), result in instability of the joint if unsupported. These injuries do require lag screw fixation of the affected bone(s) to prevent progressive collapse of the joint and a functionless limb. Lag screw fixation of multiple slab fractures greatly enhances the stability of the joint during the convalescence. Such an injury ends the horse's athletic career, but surgery is indicated to salvage the animal for breeding if it is sufficiently valuable.

Frequently a slab fracture requiring internal fixation occurs in a joint that has had a recent injection of corticosteroids. Certainly, a risk exists if an arthrotomy is performed, and it has been recommended that elective surgery, such as chip fracture removal, be delayed for 2 weeks (1). Radiographs should be taken and a clinical examination performed after the 2-week period to evaluate if infectious arthritis or progressive DJD has developed (1). With a slab fracture, a delay of 2 weeks before immobilization of the fragment can mean the end of the horse's career. During the delay there will be continued motion at the fracture site during normal weightbearing and damage to the affected bone (third carpal bone) and opposing carpal bone (radial carpal bone). Therefore, the owner should be told of the surgical risk (i.e., infection) and immediate screw fixation should be considered. Broad-spectrum antibiotics should be administered perioperatively.

REFERENCES

1. Bramlage LR. Surgical diseases of the carpus. Vet Clin North Am Large Animal Pract 1983;5:261.
2. Palmer SE. Lag screw fixation of a sagittal fracture of the third carpal bone in a horse. Vet Surg 1983;12:54.
3. Auer JA. Diseases of the carpus. Vet Clin North Am Large Animal Pract 1980;2:91.
4. Park RD, Morgan JP, O'Brien T. Chip fractures in the carpus of the horse: a radiographic study of their incidence and location. JAVMA 1970;157:1305.
5. Fackelman GE, Nunamaker DM. Manual of Internal Fixation in the Horse. New York: Springer-Verlag, 1982:37.
6. Vail GT, Wagner PC, Grant BD. Surgical repair of comminuted equine fourth carpal bone fractures. Equine Pract 1982;4:6.
7. Palmer SE, Adams FR. Repair of a slab fracture of the third carpal bone using ASIF small fragment technique: a case report. J. Equine Med Surg 1979;3:33.

Repair of Third Carpal Bone Slab Fracture Using Arthroscopic Surgery

Various forms of frontal and sagittal slab fractures occur in the carpal bones; the most common is a frontal slab fracture of the third carpal bone (1). The repair of such a fracture using arthrotomy has been described previously. Arthroscopic surgery to repair slab fractures has replaced arthrotomy in most practices and is described here. The technique uses the same principles of compression screw fixation as described under repair of fracture of the third carpal bone using arthrotomy. The difference is that the screw is placed through a stab hole and the positioning of the screw is ascertained using the combination of arthroscopic surgery to define the lateromedial width of the fracture and radiographs to define the positioning proximodistad. Details on the technique have also been described elsewhere (2–5). Small slab fractures also may be removed under arthroscopic visualization. The majority of fractures deemed appropriate for repair are fixed with 4.5-mm diameter cortical bone screws. The arthroscopic technique described here is used to treat all "routine" third carpal slab fractures (to distinguish from collapsing slab fractures, which may require an open reduction).

Anesthesia and Surgical Preparation

The surgical procedure is done with the horse under general anesthesia and the horse in dorsal recumbency. Before induction of anesthesia, the patient's limb is clipped from the midradius to the distal cannon area. The surgical site on the dorsal aspect of the joint is shaved immediately before or after anesthetic induction. Draping will include a plastic adhesive drape (Ioban, Ioban Orthopedics Products Division, 3M Center, St. Paul, MN) as well as an impervious draping system.

Additional Instrumentation

Appropriate arthroscopic instrumentation is required (see Appendix IV); ASIF instruments for lag screw fixation (see Appendix I) and a selection of ASIF cortical bone screws are also needed.

Surgical Technique

Arthroscopic surgery of the midcarpal joint is performed in the same fashion as previously described for a chip fracture of the distal aspect of the radial carpal bone. A lateral arthroscopic portal and a medial instrument portal are used, and a diagnostic examination of the joint is performed. The slab fracture is visualized and the fracture line debrided with a curet. It is usual to have a V-shaped section of bone come from the fracture line; this bone is removed. After debridement, the joint is irrigated. The carpus is then placed in maximal flexion (if it is not already in this position). Under arthroscopic visualization, two 18-gauge, 1.5-inch needles are placed into the midcarpal joint so that they are at either end (medial and lateral) of the fractured slab and are adjacent and parallel to the third carpal bone. The third needle is placed in the carpometacarpal joint (Fig. 5.3*A*) and a flexed lateral radiograph is taken. The needle placement as visualized in the joint determines the site of screw placement (halfway along the slab). The needle placement on the radiograph dictates the direction to ensure it is approximately midway proximal-distal and parallel within the third carpal bone. If a 4.5-mm cortical screw is to be placed, a stab incision with a no. 10 scalpel blade is made in the appropriate place and a 4.5-mm glide hole

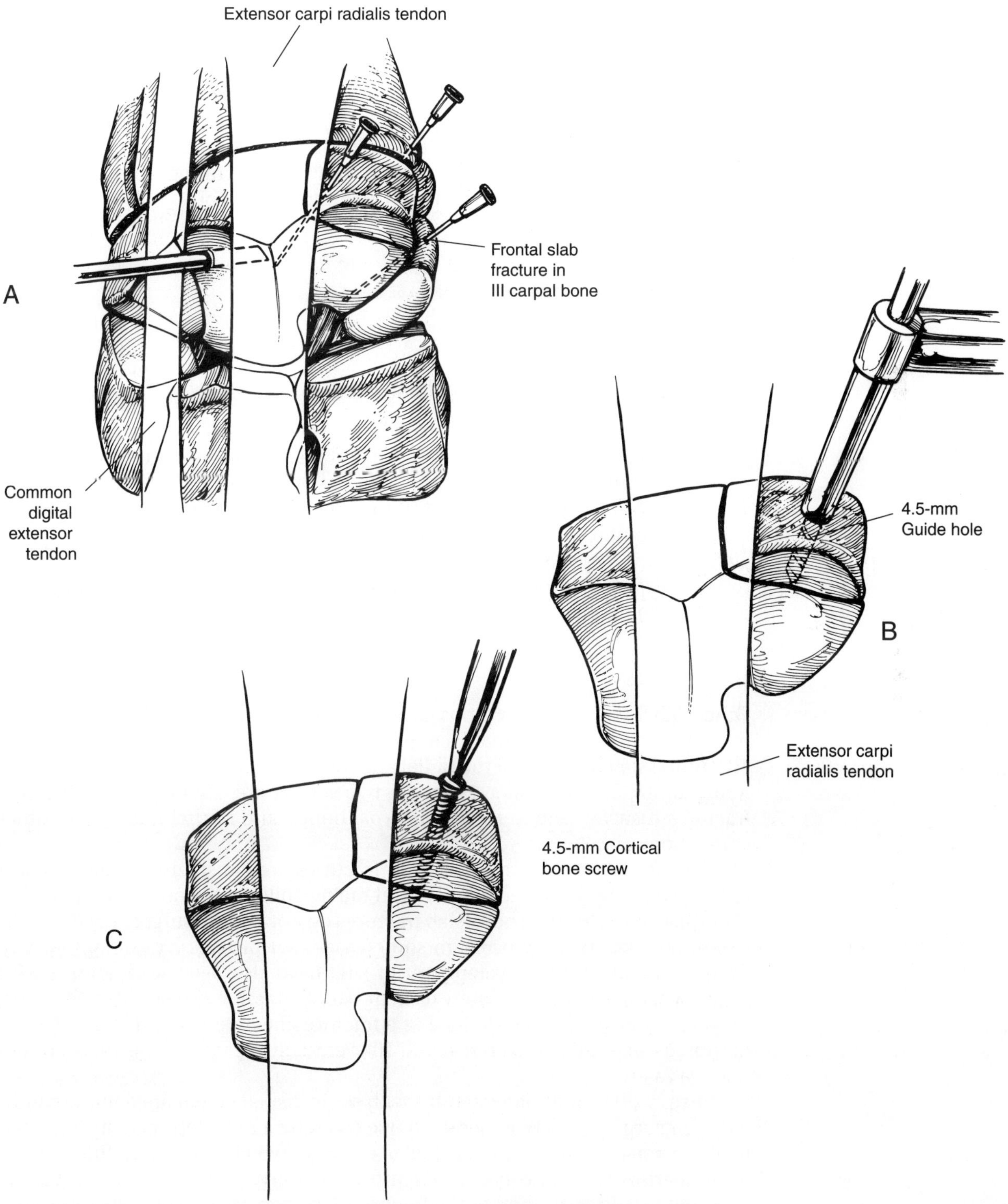

Figure 5.3, A–C. Lag screw fixation of slab fractures of the third carpal bone using arthroscopic surgery.

is drilled through to the fracture line (Fig. 5.3*B*). A 3.2-mm drill guide is inserted and a 3.2-mm hole is drilled in the third carpal bone. The hole is depth-gauged and tapped and a screw of appropriate length is selected. The screw is then placed to fix the fracture (Fig. 5.3*C*). The arthroscope is reintroduced to the joint to visualize the fracture reduction and to remove any additional debris. Sutures are placed in the skin incisions.

A 3.5-mm cortical screw can be used as an alternative (the author does so with smaller slab fractures). It has also been recommended as a routine measure (4). Third carpal slab fractures have also been repaired using the Herbert cannulated bone screw, which is a headless screw incorporating screw threads of two different pitches to create fracture compression, but failures have been observed.

Postoperative Management

While patients are recovering from anesthesia, a full-length padded bandage is applied to the operated limb to avoid trauma to the carpal joint. After recovery from anesthesia, smaller bandages utilizing a nonadhesive pad, sterile gauze (Kling, Johnson and Johnson Medical Inc, Arlington, TX), and elastic adhesive (Elastikon, Johnson and Johnson Medical Inc. Arlington, TX) may be applied. These bandages facilitate early exercise and passive flexion of the joint. Hand-walking is commenced 2 weeks after surgery (the sutures are removed at 10 to 12 days). Swimming may be used in the convalescent period any time after 3 weeks. In routine cases, stall confinement with an increasing regimen of hand-walking over 8 weeks is recommended. If radiographs obtained at that time reveal satisfactory progress in healing, the horse can be turned out. Another 3 months should pass before the horse returns to training at the track.

Comments

Other slab fractures of the carpus have been repaired arthroscopically, including frontal fractures of the radial facet of the third carpal bone (Schneider Type V) (1), frontal slab fractures of the radial and intermediate facets of the third carpal bone combined (Schneider Type VI—two screws are used here), sagittal slab fractures (usually seen in the third carpal bone), and frontal fractures of other carpal bones (6, 7).

All Thoroughbreds with carpal slab fractures are considered surgical candidates given appropriate economics and racing ability. Previous statements that undisplaced third carpal bone slab fractures do not require surgery need qualification (8). Healing may occur in some cases, but progressive osteoporosis of the slab fragment and development of DJD have also been seen. Horses with undisplaced slab fractures are excellent candidates for surgery. In one report in which undisplaced was defined as a fracture line of less than 1 mm, 12 Standardbreds were treated with rest and 10 eventually raced; 8 of the 10 raced well (9).

Horses with frontal slab fractures with some displacement are definite candidates for surgery (10). Whether the horse can return to athletic activity is related to the amount of associated articular damage, which influences the amount of osteoarthritis that develops. When fractures involve both facets, surgery is essential for restabilization of the fracture. Two papers have described the success rate of slab fracture after arthrotomy (9, 10). There has been one report of success rate with arthroscopic surgery (4). Horses with sagittal slab fractures (Schneider Type VIII) are also candidates for lag screw fixation. These fractures require a skyline radiographic demonstration. Arthroscopic examination has shown that they may be mobile. Conservative management of a series of 12 of these fractures resulted in a return of function in 7 (11), but the first author has treated horses that have not healed with conservative treatment and were later successfully treated with lag screw fixation.

REFERENCES

1. Schneider RK, Bramlage LR, Gabel AA, et al. Incidence, location and classification of 371 third carpal bone fractures in 313 horses. Equine Vet J 1988;6(Suppl):33–42.
2. Foerner JJ, McIlwraith CW. Orthopaedic surgery in the racehorse. Vet Clin North Am Large Animal Pract 1990;6:147–177.
3. McIlwraith CW. Diagnostic and Surgical Arthroscopy in the Horse. 2nd ed. Philadelphia: Lea & Febiger, 1990:76–83.
4. Richardson DW. Technique for arthroscopic repair of third carpal bone slab fractures in the horse. JAVMA 1986;188:288–291.
5. Bramlage LR. Surgical diseases of the carpus. Vet Clin North Am Large Animal Pract 1983;5:261–274.
6. Auer JA, Watkins JP, White NA, et al. Slab fractures of the fourth and intermediate carpal bones in five horses. JAVMA 1986;188:595–601.
7. McIlwraith CW. Fractures of the carpus. In: Nixon AJ, ed. Equine Fracture Repair. Philadelphia: WB Saunders, 1996:208–221.
8. Meagher DM. Joint surgery in the horse: selection of surgical cases and confirmation of the alternative. In: Proceedings of the 20th Annual Meeting of the AAEP, Las Vegas, NV, 1974:81–88.
9. Stephens PR, Richardson DW, Spencer PA. Slab fractures of the third carpal bone in Standardbreds and Thoroughbreds. JAVMA 1988;193:353–358.
10. Martin GS, Haynes PF, McClure JR. Effect of third carpal slab fracture and repair in racing performance in Thoroughbred horses: 31 cases (1977–1984). JAVMA 1988;193:107–110.
11. Fischer AT, Stover SM. Sagittal fractures in the third carpal bone in horses: 12 cases, 1977–1985. JAVMA 1987;191:106–108.

Repair of a Sagittal Fracture of the Proximal Phalanx (P1)

Longitudinal fractures of the proximal phalanx are seen in horses that perform strenuous activities such as racing, western performance events, trotting and pacing races, and jumping. These fractures can occur in a variety of configurations ranging from small hairline fissures in the fetlock joint to severely comminuted fractures with many pieces (1–4). Rarely are proximal phalangeal fractures open. All the different configurations of proximal phalangeal fractures seen in horses will not be discussed in this section. Instead, the authors will illustrate the steps required to repair a simple sagittal fracture of P1 that extends from the metacarpophalangeal joint to the junction of the middle and distal third of P1 (Fig. 5.4*A*). This is a relatively common configuration and would be a good case to try for a surgeon who has had relatively little experience with the ASIF technique. If there is any doubt, however, the surgeon should always practice screw placement on a cadaver limb.

The clinical signs of proximal phalangeal fractures vary. In severely comminuted fractures, severe lameness is present and crepitation will be evident. In some fractures, such as the longitudinal fissure commencing in the fetlock joint illustrated in Figure 5.4, the lameness can be subtle. Diagnostic nerve blocks or training when such fissures are present can result in complete dehiscence of the fracture and a marked decline in the prognosis for future athletic soundness. A small fissure may develop into a more complicated configuration under normal weightbearing (5).

For emergency transport to a facility where more elaborate treatment can be performed, the limb should be placed in a large, tight-fitting pressure bandage with support on the opposite limb. The animal will usually protect the limb because of extreme pain. If horses are to be shipped long distances with such a fracture or if the fracture is comminuted and unstable, the attending veterinarian may elect to place the limb in a fiberglass cast before transport. At least four radiographic views should be taken (AP, LM, and two obliques). There is often a duplication of the fracture line owing to the different course taken in the dorsal and palmar (plantar) cortices (Fig.5.4*A*). This may be mistaken for comminution or even sequestration. For fissures close to the articular surface, the x-ray beam should be directed at such an angle that it eliminates superimposition by the proximal sesamoid bones.

Horses with longitudinal fractures of the proximal phalanx should be considered candidates for rigid internal fixation because failure to reestablish the congruity of the joint surfaces (metacarpophalangeal and proximal interphalangeal) will result in degenerative disease of these joints (1–4, 6, 7). Some surgeons recommend that small fissures beginning at the proximal end of the proximal phalanx and not progressing any farther than 1 to 2 cm be handled conservatively. The fractures are presumed to be inherently stable and therefore stall rest could suffice. It can be argued, however, that fissures could continue farther distad at the microscopic level and could dehisce into a fracture with a poorer prognosis. The convalescent period is usually much shorter following internal fixation, and the total expense (including hospitalization) for treatment of the fracture may be less if handled surgically than if cast application is the sole method of therapy (2).

Periosteal proliferation resembling osselets on the proximal dorsal aspect of the proximal phalanx and demineralization along the fracture line are seen in fissures that have been handled conservatively. Such fractures should be given a guarded prognosis for athletic soundness (1, 5).

Internal fixation of proximal phalangeal fractures consists of insertion of one or more ASIF cortical bone screws using the lag screw principle (8). The authors

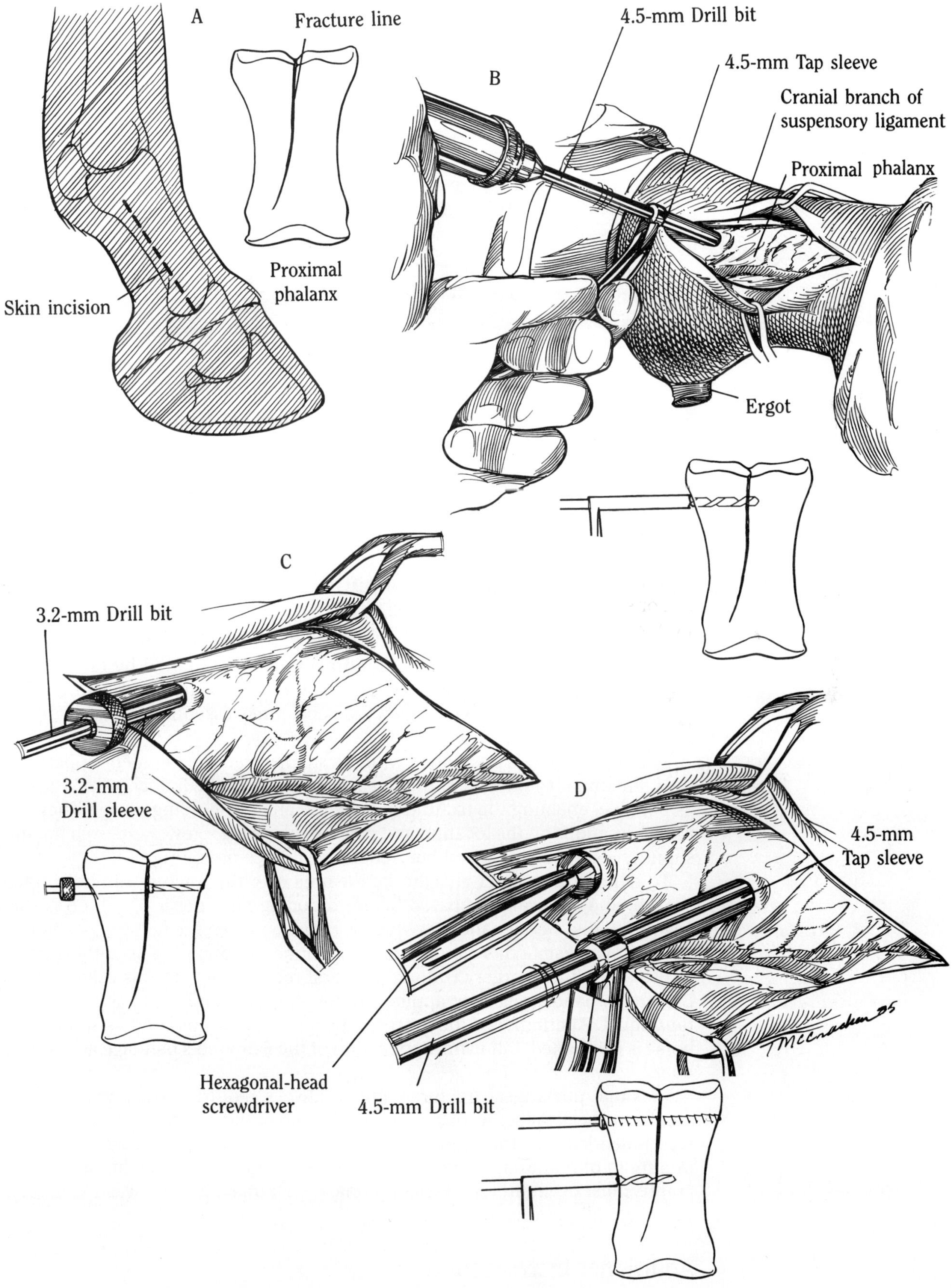

Figure 5.4, A–D. Steps in lag screw fixation of a sagittal fracture of the proximal phalanx.

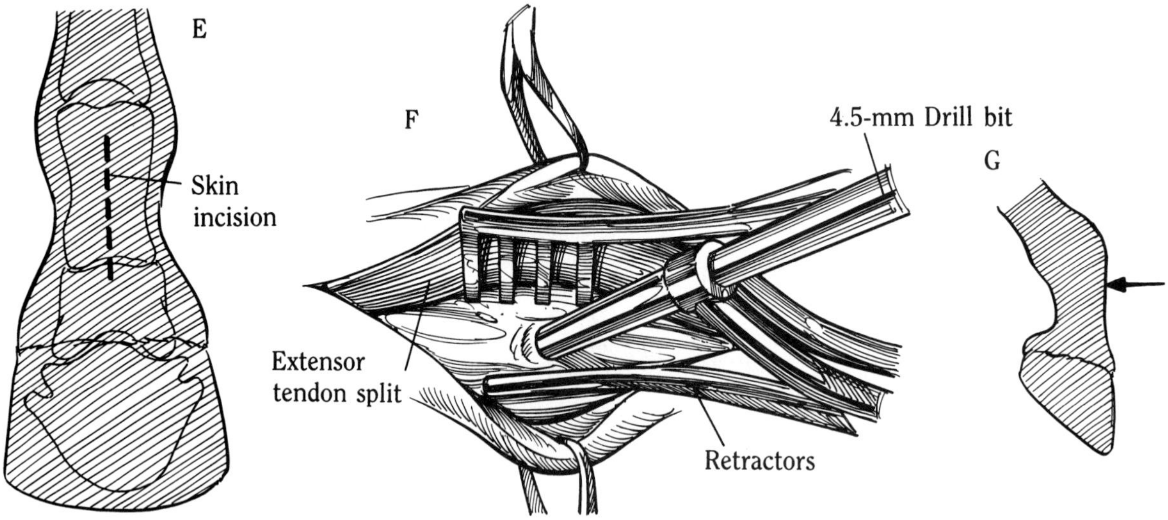

Figure 5.4, E–G. *(continued)* Steps in lag screw fixation of a frontal fracture of the proximal phalanx.

recommend that the introductory section on the lag screw principle be read now unless the reader has already done so.

Anesthesia and Surgical Preparation

The surgical procedure is done under general anesthesia with the horse in lateral recumbency. Before attempting screw fixation, the surgeon must be thoroughly familiar with the configuration of the fracture as determined by radiographs. Because the plane of the fracture frequently begins at the sagittal groove and spirals down the bone, oblique views are absolutely essential to "map out" the fracture lines.

The horse's limb is positioned with the smaller fracture fragment uppermost; thus, the threaded portion of the screw hole closer to the fetlock joint is as long as possible, enabling the fixation to have the greatest holding power. There are many variations on the location and position of the lag screws, and each fracture should be carefully assessed beforehand to reduce operating time.

To reduce time under anesthesia, the area over the fracture can be clipped, shaved, and surgically prepared before inducing anesthesia. The limb is then covered with a sterile bandage, which is removed when the horse is positioned. The use of an Esmarch's bandage and tourniquet is optional. The authors prefer to use both, if the surgery is done in lateral recumbency. In this case, a sterile Esmarch's bandage is now applied by the surgeon, and a nurse can apply a tourniquet. Alternatively, the limb can be shaved and prepared as soon as the horse is positioned, following application of the Esmarch's bandage and tourniquet.

Proximal phalangeal fractures almost always require intraoperative radiographs to check for screw placement and depth of the gliding hole. It is strongly recommended that the limb be positioned to facilitate this procedure with a minimum of redraping and chance to break aseptic surgical technique. Radiographs must be coordinated with technical staff to avoid time-wasting maneuvers that will prolong anesthesia.

Additional Instrumentation

This procedure requires instruments for lag screw fixation and an assortment of cortical and cancellous bone screws.

Surgical Technique

The surgical approach may be through stab incisions although, if more than two screws are to be inserted, the authors prefer a more extensive laterally or medially located incision (9) (Fig. 5.4, *B* and *C*). For fractures in a frontal plane whereby all the screws will be placed in a cranial to caudal direction, an I-shaped incision provides good visualization of the extensor tendon and corresponding branches of the suspensory ligament. Details of this approach are outlined in the section on pastern arthrodesis, although for lag screw fixation the position of the "I" must be moved proximad and the pastern joint should not be opened. If only one or two lag screws are to be placed in a cranial to caudal direction, a simple longitudinal incision will be adequate (2).

During initial experiences with lag screw fixation of these fractures, it was deemed necessary to place screws to ensure maximum resistance to shortening and maximal compression of the fracture by "inserting a screw along an imaginary line between a line perpendicular to the long axis of the bone and a line perpendicular to the fracture line" (1). However, with fractures close to a sagittal plane there is little tendency for slippage along the longitudinal plane of the fracture, and placement of screws at right angles to the fracture line or parallel to the metacarpophalangeal joint is technically easier than trying to bisect the angles between these two directions (10). Lag screws are inserted at the appropriate positions on the bone as dictated by the configuration of the fracture. Reduction of these fractures is generally not a problem because they usually align themselves as the fragments are compressed. The screw closest to the fetlock joint is usually inserted first, at the dorsal edge of the extensor branch of the suspensory ligament just distal to the palpable wing of P1 (5–8 mm distal to the distal extremity of the sagittal gravae on a densopalmar radiograph and control in a densopalmar direction on a lateromedial radiograph) (11) (Fig. 5.4*B*). Kirschner wires or 2.0-mm drill bits are used by some surgeons to estimate the anticipated positions of the lag screws.

In fissure fractures that are relatively undisplaced it is impossible to feel the 4.5-mm drill bit "arrive" at the fracture line (Fig. 5.4*B*). Since progression of this drill bit into the opposite cortex greatly reduces the holding power of the cortical screws, intraoperative monitoring of the drilling procedure with radiographs is necessary (2, 10). In addition, the distance to the fracture site should be measured preoperatively from radiographs. The authors prefer both methods even though they are more time-consuming. The configuration of the fracture will obviously dictate screw placement. Screws should not be placed beyond the radiographically visible fracture line because of the risk of entering a fracture plane (11).

When drilling the 3.2-mm holes that will eventually emerge from the opposite cortex (Fig. 5.4*C*), constant cleaning of the drill bit will ensure that small pieces of bone debris are not forced through the other side of the bone (2). The holes in the bone should be carefully countersunk to ensure that the heads of the screws will not bend on tightening (1). Care must be taken not to overcountersink, or the screw head will pull through the soft bone. If this occurs, a washer under the screw head may provide sufficient holding power to prevent the screw head from pulling through. When soft bone is encountered in young animals, ASIF partially threaded cancellous screws can be used. The threads of these screws should not cross the fracture line or the lag screw principle will be violated (8).

Following countersinking, the depth of the hole is measured carefully so as not to hook onto soft tissues (this will produce an excessively long implant). Tapping is done with a 4.5-mm tap sleeve to protect soft tissues. As soon as the tap emerges from the opposite cortex, it is removed.

The first screw is inserted and tightened partially but not completely. Subsequent screws are inserted as dictated by the configuration of the fracture (Fig. 5.4*D*). Tightening is completed. At this point a final series of intraoperative radiographs should be taken. Three radiographic views are recommended. For a simple sagittal fracture as shown in Figure 5.4*A*, these views would be one DP view and two oblique views that are approximately 15° from the DP view. They will show how well the fracture line is reduced and are the only accurate method to verify that the tips of the screws are not protruding beyond the bone (Fig. 5.4) (2).

The skin incisions are closed by standard methods using a suture material of the surgeon's choice. As mentioned previously, the screws may be placed through stab incisions.

For fractures that have a configuration that runs in a more frontal plane, a more dorsal approach is indicated whereby the extensor tendon is split longitudinally to gain access to the bone (Fig. 5.4, *E–G*). This approach can also supplement a more lateral approach if the fracture line spirals from a sagittal to a frontal plane.

Postoperative Management

Placement of the limb in a cast up to the top of the third metacarpus or metatarsus at least until recovery from anesthesia provides optimal safety. Heavy bandages or a plastic compression boot (Farley Compression Root, Equine Orthotics, Indian Harbour Beach, FL) are alternatives. A hand limb P1 fracture needs to be recovered in a cast or compression boot because of the high torsional forces. Undisplaced fractures that have been rigidly compressed by the lag screws as illustrated here can benefit from early motion, and, if used, the cast is removed after recovery. A more comminuted fracture does need a cast and may need as much as 2 to 3 months of casting. Radiographic evaluation will help monitor healing as well as the degree of DJD. The prognosis is generally good in fractures that are fresh and have no concurrent osteoarthritis (2–4, 6, 10), although decreased performance has been reported (5).

Return to exercise will vary depending on the individual horse. Hand-walking can usually commence in 4 weeks for simple fractures as illustrated here, and these horses can be turned out into a small paddock at 2 months. If radiographic healing is present at 3 months, training can be recommended.

REFERENCES

1. Fackelman GE. Sagittal fractures of the first phalanx (P1) in the horse. Vet Med Small Animal Clin 1973;68:622.
2. Gabel AA, Bukowiecki CF. Fractures of the phalanges. In: Symposium on Equine Orthopaedic Surgery. Philadelphia: WB Saunders, 1983.
3. Markel MD, Richardson DW. Noncomminuted fractures of the proximal phalanx in 69 horses. JAVMA 1985;186:573.
4. Markel MD, Martin BB, Richardson DW. Dorsal frontal fractures of the first phalanx in the horse. J Vet Surg 1985;14:36–40.
5. Tetens J, Ross MW, Lloyd JW. Comparison of racing performance before and after treatment of incomplete, midsag: Hal fractures of the proximal phalanx in Standardbreds: 49 cases (1986–1992). JAVMA 1997;210:82–86.
6. Ellis DR, Simpson DJ, Greenwood RES, et al. Observations and management of fractures of the principal phalanx in young Thoroughbreds. Equine Vet J 1987;19:43–49.
7. Fackelman GE, Nunamaker DM. Manual of Internal Fixation in the Horse. New York: Springer-Verlag, 1982.

8. Muller ME, Allgower M, Schneider R, et al. Manual of Internal Fixation. 2nd ed. New York: Springer-Verlag, 1979.
9. Milne DW, Turner AS. An Atlas of Surgical Approaches to the Bones of the Horse. Philadelphia: WB Saunders, 1979.
10. Turner AS. Large animal orthopaedics. In: Jennings PB, ed. The Practice of Large Animal Surgery. Philadelphia: WB Saunders, 1984;16:768–949.
11. Richardson DW. Fractures of the proximal phalanx. In: Nixon AJ, ed. Equine Fracture Repair. Philadelphia: WB Saunders, 1996:117–128.

Repair of Distal Condylar Fractures of the Third Metacarpal or Metatarsal Bones

Fractures of the condyles of the third metacarpal and metatarsal bones are seen predominantly in racing Thoroughbreds and Standardbreds. The configuration of the fracture covers a wide spectrum, ranging from a small fissure entering the fetlock joint to complete displacement and separation of the fragment from the parent cannon bone (1–4). The clinical signs can vary from mild lameness that is exacerbated by exercise in undisplaced fissure fractures to acute lameness with heat, pain, and swelling in displaced fractures. The fractures may involve the forelimbs or the hind limbs.

Radiographs of the affected fetlock joint should be taken to establish the diagnosis. At least five views should be taken: DP, lateral, two oblique views, and a 125° dorsopalmar (dorsoplantar) metacarpal (metatarsal) skyline view to evaluate the distal palmar (plantar) aspect of the metacarpus (metatarsus). Care should be taken to evaluate the radiographs for concomitant problems. The following conditions are sometimes seen with condylar fractures: (*a*) axial fractures of the proximal sesamoid bones; (*b*) apical fractures of the proximal sesamoid bones; (*c*) osteochondral fractures of the proximal aspect of the proximal phalanx; (*d*) distal palmar metacarpal subchondral disease or fracture fragments; (*e*) periarticular osteophytes indicative of DJD; and (*f*) suspensory desmitis (apparent clinically) (1–3). All other injuries associated with condylar fractures should be taken into account before surgery. Such injuries may have a significant bearing on the prognosis with respect to return to racing soundness. For example, at the fracture site the presence of undetected erosive (lytic) lesions on the palmar (plantar) region of the condyle and comminution with loose osteochondral fragments should be investigated (1, 5, 6) by taking a 125° dorsopalmar (dorsoplantar) metacarpal (metatarsal) skyline (125° DPMS) projection (1, 5, 6). When a fracture involves the medial condyle it will commonly travel a considerable distance up the bone to the nutrient foramen (3, 7). Multiple radiographic views are necessary to fully define the fracture planes (3, 7) because fractures of this configuration have a tendency to break catastrophically proximal to the region of the fracture site (7).

There are numerous types of fractures of the distal metacarpus or metatarsus. The most common fracture involves the lateral condyle and can be (*a*) incomplete; (*b*) complete-nondisplaced; (*c*) complete-displaced; or (*d*) an incomplete fracture originating on the distal palmar aspect of the third metacarpal condyle, requiring the special flexed dorsopalmar projection or a 125° dorsopalmar skyline projection to highlight the palmar aspect of the condylar fracture and diagnose the fracture (5, 8). Fractures also occur involving the medial condyle of the metacarpus or metatarsus. A more recent paper did not differentiate between undisplaced and displaced complete fractures as classified by Rick et al. (9) because they did not believe there was a certain radiographic means of determining whether there was dorsopalmar (dorsoplantar) displacement of the condylar fracture (10). This is a good point and could explain discrepancy between success rates of "displaced" fractures.

Lateral condylar fractures can be handled in a variety of ways, depending on the degree of separation of the fragments and the intended use of the animal. If the animal is to be retired for breeding purposes and there is minimum displacement of the fracture, pressure bandages or a plaster cast in combination with box stall rest for 8 weeks may suffice. An additional 8 weeks of stall confinement is required if there is considerable displacement of the fracture or the fragment. The convalescent period after a condylar fracture, much like that for fissure fractures of the proximal phalanx, is much shorter following internal fixation, and the total expense (including hospitalization) for treatment may be less if internal fixation is used. If the horse is intended for further athletic performance, the treatment of choice is lag screw fixation with two or more ASIF cortical bone screws (1–3, 7–10).

There are several aims of rigid internal fixation of such fractures: (*a*) to reestablish the congruity of the articular surface; (*b*) to minimize the gap that fibrocartilage has to bridge during the healing process; (*c*) to minimize movement at the junction of the articular cartilage and bone, reducing proliferative changes and subsequent joint stiffness (DJD); and (*d*) to ensure that the original fissure does not enlarge and become displaced to the point of complete dehiscence (1, 3, 4, 7, 12). Such fractures should be repaired as soon as the affected leg has "cooled out," which is generally 24 to 48 hours after the injury.

Anesthesia and Surgical Preparation

The horse may be positioned in lateral (with the affected leg uppermost) or dorsal recumbency. The author performs all these surgeries in dorsal recumbency, and a tourniquet is not necessary. The leg is prepared for surgery in a routine manner. To reduce anesthetic time, the limb can be clipped, shaved, and surgically prepared before inducing anesthesia. The limb is then covered with a sterile bandage that is removed when the horse is positioned. Alternatively, the limb can be shaved and prepared as soon as the horse is positioned.

Condylar fractures always require intraoperative radiographs to check for screw positioning and depth of the gliding hole. It is strongly recommended that the limb be positioned to facilitate this procedure (another advantage with dorsal recumbency) with a minimum of redraping and chance to break aseptic surgical technique. Radiographs must be coordinated with technical staff to avoid time-wasting maneuvers that will prolong anesthetic time.

Additional Instrumentation

This procedure requires instruments for lag screw fixation and an assortment of cortical bone screws. Arthroscopic technique is commonly used to assess the joint and thus arthroscopic equipment is also necessary.

Repair of a Displaced Fracture Using Arthrotomy

Minimally displaced fractures can be approached through stab incisions in the skin (discussed below), whereas displaced fractures are best approached through an incision extending from the lateral collateral ligaments of the fetlock joint to above the proximal exit point of the fracture. The latter, more extensive incision allows visualization of the proximal end of the fracture, thereby aiding alignment at the joint surface. It also gives better visualization of the configuration of the fracture, as these fractures sometimes spiral cranially or caudally. If the fracture is displaced, the more extensive incision will enable the surgeon to remove hematoma and bony debris from the fracture site. Some incisions (S-shaped) provide good exposure but may produce skin sloughs at the apices if they are too curved. The displaced fracture must be reduced before screw fixation. To evaluate reduction at the joint surface and remove loose osteochondral fragments at the palmar articular surface, an arthrotomy of the dorsal surface of the fetlock joint is usually performed (1, 3) but, more recently, reduction of displaced fractures has been done arthroscopically. The arthrotomy is done in the same location as would be used to remove an osteochondral fragment of the dorsal rim of P1 or hypertrophied synovial membrane (villonodular synovitis) and is described in this book. If the condylar fracture has a concurrent loose osteochondral fragment at the palmar articular surface, it is at this point in the procedure that the fragment must be removed. The metacarpophalangeal joint is slightly flexed, and periosteal elevators are used to distract the fractured condyle away from the metacarpus. The fracture site is cleaned of debris, and the typically triangular pieces of bone can be extracted from the palmar aspect of the joint.

To achieve reduction of a displaced fracture, large ASIF bone reduction forceps (Synthes Ltd., Wayne, PA) are used and are preferable to the c-clamp. When in position, the clamp should be tightened and a DP intraoperative radiograph taken (after placement of needles) to ensure that the drill will be directed parallel to the joint surface. When the surgeon is satisfied with the reduction of the fracture, the distal screw should be placed 1 to 2 cm proximal to the articular surface. To obtain adequate compression of the fracture site at the level of the articular surface, the more distal screw must be positioned carefully. Preferably, this screw should be placed proximad to the collateral ligament to minimize trauma to this structure. Conversely, in the management of smaller condylar fractures whose fracture lines do not extend very proximad, it may be necessary to place the most distal screw in the depression (fossa) of the most distal aspect of the bone.

Placement of the screw is begun by drilling the 4.5-mm gliding hole in the fracture fragment. Intraoperative radiographs are required to see that the 4.5-mm drill has crossed the fracture site when drilling this and subsequent gliding holes. The bone in this region is dense (Fig. 5.5, *A* and *B*).

The 3.2-mm sleeve is placed in the 4.5-mm glide hole, and the pilot hole is drilled without exiting the opposite cortex (Fig. 5.5*C*). Constant cleaning of the drill bit is essential during the drilling of these and subsequent holes in such dense bone. The depth gauge is used to determine the length of the cortical screw to be used, being careful not to catch the hook of the depth gauge on soft tissues if the pilot hole has been drilled completely through both cortices. It is difficult to measure the depth of the distal hole accurately, but a 52- or 54-mm long screw can usually be used. Tapping is performed after the depth is measured (Fig. 5.5, *D* and *E*). Using the countersink for the screw hole closest to the joint is not necessary and can be potentially injurious to the collateral ligament.

An ASIF cortical bone screw of appropriate length is inserted and tightened, but not excessively (Fig. 5.5*F*). An intraoperative radiograph is taken at this point to check fracture reduction and ensure that the threaded tip of the screw is not protruding into the opposite collateral ligament.

Once this screw is placed, the ASIF hexagonal-headed screwdriver can be left in place and the remaining screws inserted "freehand" in a sequence similar to the placement of the first screw. The 4.5-mm gliding hole must extend *beyond* the fracture line, and it may be necessary to take intraoperative radiographs to ensure this placement in undisplaced fractures. Screws that are placed more proximally should be countersunk to ensure even pressure on the screw head. Reduction of the fracture site can be monitored through the arthrotomy incision or with the arthroscope (Fig. 5.5*G*).

The arthrotomy incision is closed by a layer of simple interrupted absorbable sutures of synthetic absorbable or synthetic monofilament nonabsorbable material. The sutures should be preplaced in the joint capsule to facilitate accurate anatomic apposition and a tight seal. The subcutaneous fascia is closed with a simple continuous pattern using synthetic absorbable material, and the skin is closed with simple interrupted or vertical mattress sutures of monofilament nonabsorbable material. The wound through which the screws were placed is closed in two layers: subcutaneous fascia and skin. The tourniquet is then removed and a sterile dressing is placed over the incision.

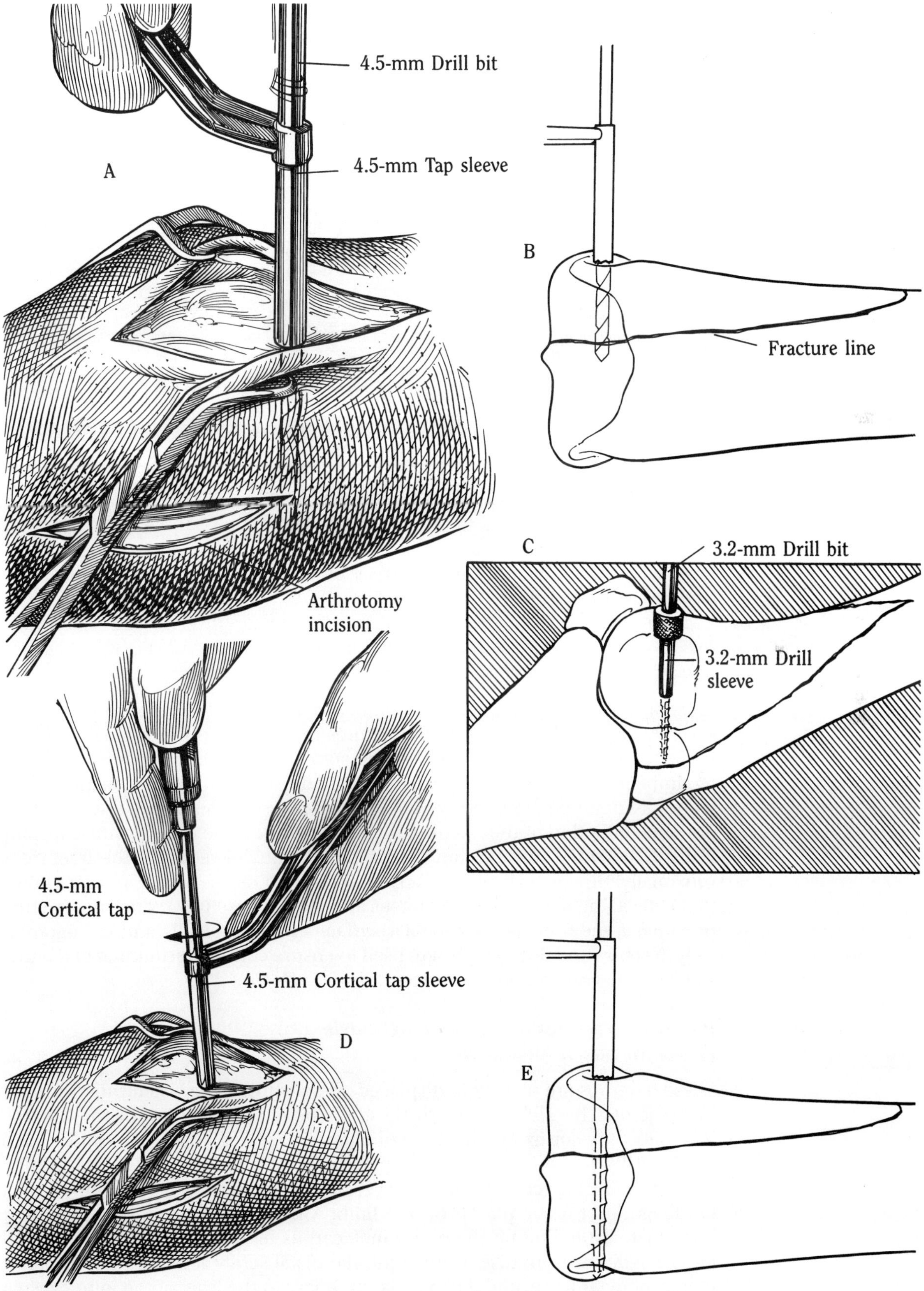

FIGURE 5.5, A–E. Steps in repair of a lateral distal condylar fracture in the metacarpus or metatarsus.

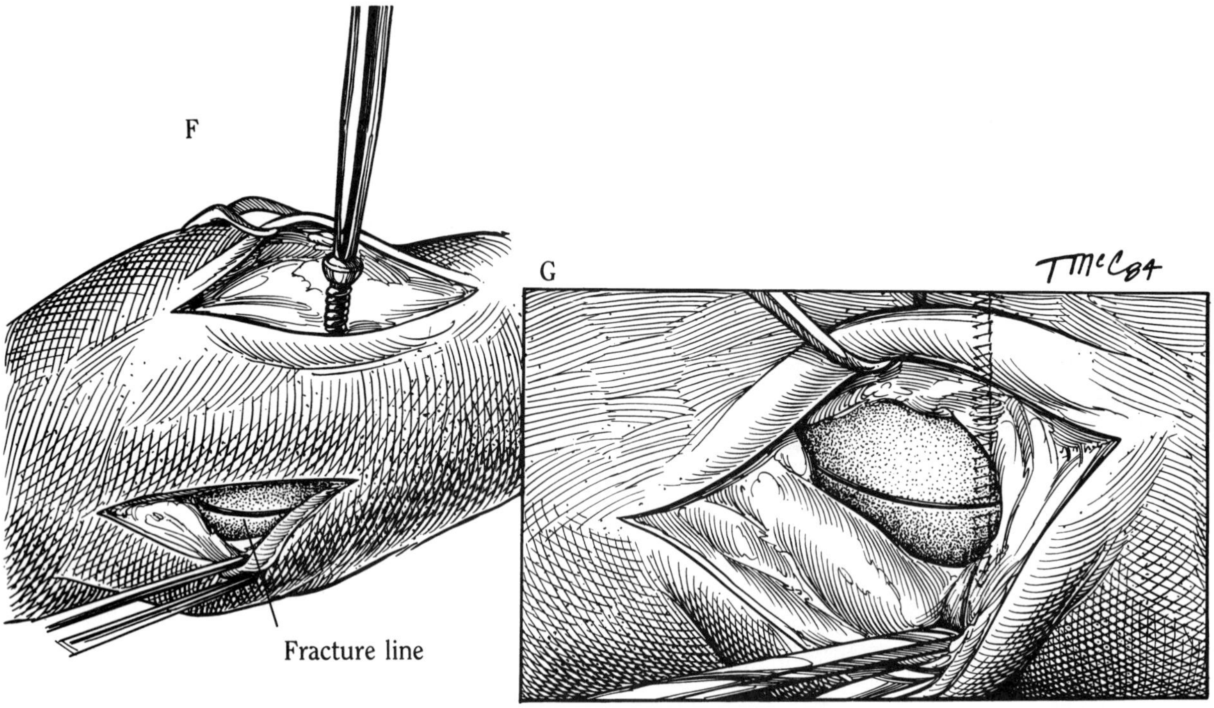

Figure 5.5, F–G. *(continued)* Steps in repair of a lateral distal condylar fracture in the metacarpus or metatarsus.

Repair Using Arthroscopic Visualization

This has become the first author's standard approach for the repair of all but severely displaced fractures. With fractures that are not obviously displaced on radiographs, the repair is done through stab incisions with the horse in dorsal recumbency. Diagnostic arthroscopy of the dorsal and palmar pouches of the fetlock is done concomitantly (both techniques are described elsewhere) to evaluate reduction of the fracture. Manipulations can be done arthroscopically if displacement is present, but the primary means of reducing the fracture is proximally, in which the open incision is used to clean out the fracture down to the distal metacarpus or metatarsus and then to carefully reduce the fracture proximally, monitoring the articular surface arthroscopically and radiographically. Needles and radiographs are used to ensure correct positioning of the first screw in the condylar fossa is made (Fig. 5.5, *H–J*).

Repair of Fractures of the Medial Condyle of Metacarpus or Metatarsus

These fractures are usually undisplaced, and arthroscopic visualization is used in the joint. The difference with these fractures is the failure of the fracture line to exit the cortex of the bone radiographically (Fig. 5.5*K*). Two options are available for treatment. One is the placement of multiple screws and putting two screws in lag screw fashion above the fracture line. This is followed by a full length cast being placed on the limb. A newer alternative is the use of a bone plate extending up the entire metacarpus or metatarsus (Fig. 5.5, *L* and *M*). To avoid compromise to the joint, the distal screw remains as a lag screw in the condylar fossa, and the plate commences at the level of the joint capsule insertion. The plate position may vary depending on the fracture. This is the preferred option in the first author's opinion for repair of medial condylar fractures.

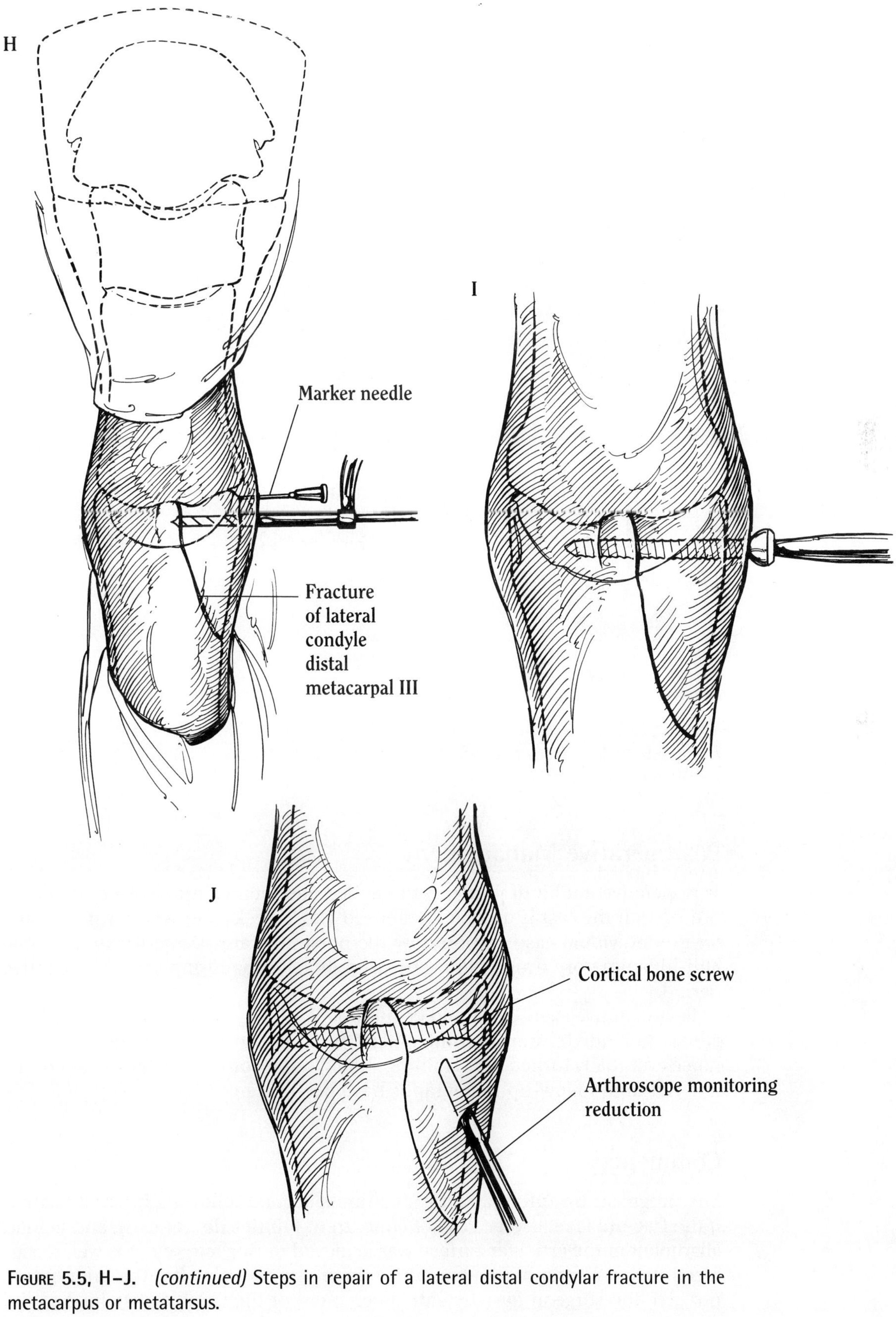

Figure 5.5, H–J. *(continued)* Steps in repair of a lateral distal condylar fracture in the metacarpus or metatarsus.

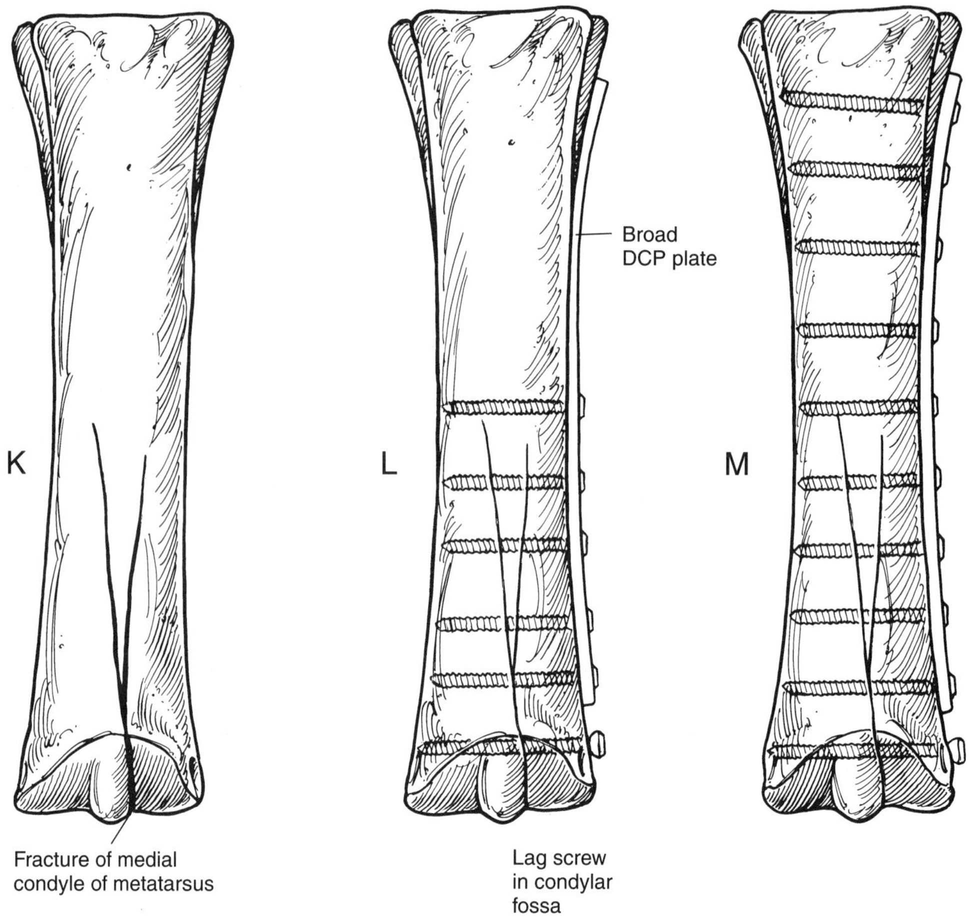

Figure 5.5, K–M. *(continued)* Steps in repair of a lateral distal condylar fracture in the metacarpus or metatarsus.

Postoperative Management

Perioperative antibiotics are recommended and tetanus prophylaxis should be provided. If the cast is used, it is removed 1 to 2 weeks after surgery depending on the individual case and on how the horse tolerates the cast. Nonsteroidal anti-inflammatory drugs should be used judiciously during the postoperative period.

Postoperative exercise should be minimal for the first 3 months. Box stall rest is recommended. After 3 months, hand-walking can be commenced and the horse eventually turned out. Training should not recommence for 4 to 8 months and not until follow-up radiographs have been taken.

Comments

The prognosis for future athletic soundness is good following internal fixation *if* the fracture is relatively fresh, if concurrent injuries do not exist, and if good alignment of the articular surface was achieved during surgery. It is well recognized that radiographic evaluation of the injury, shortly after the injury, does not give the surgeon an adequate assessment of the trauma sustained to the articular cartilage and joint capsule at the time of injury.

The presence of concurrent injuries appears to be a major factor in determining the future racing performance of the horse. The only way to be fully aware of these concurrent injuries is by performing a meticulous clinical and radiographic examination, including the 125° dorsopalmar metacarpal (metatarsal) skyline view.

For an undisplaced condylar fracture, with a concurrent osteochondral fragment in the palmar aspect of the fracture site, removal of this fragment is difficult without opening up the fracture site. Some patients, including those with large fragments, would benefit by leaving the fragment in place and not traumatizing the fracture further (1).

In the first follow-up study of condylar fractures in 71 Thoroughbreds, 4 Standardbreds, and 2 Grade horses (9), the fractures were classified as complete-displaced (46), complete-nondisplaced (6), and incomplete (21). Four horses had special incomplete (3) and complete (1) fractures of the third metatarsal bone extending from the medial condyle into the diaphysis. On follow-up, 12 of 38 horses with complete-displaced fractures continued racing after surgery and 0 of 6 continued racing with conservative treatment. The six horses with complete-nondisplaced fractures were operated on, and four continued to race after surgery. Eleven of twenty-one horses with incomplete fractures were operated on, and nine of eleven returned to racing. The other 10 were treated conservatively, and 9 of them returned to race. Winnings per race for the 35 Thoroughbreds analyzed were less than before the surgery when complete fractures or incomplete fractures were treated with surgery. However, nine Thoroughbreds with incomplete condylar fractures treated conservatively had higher earnings after treatment than before (9).

In a second study, the majority of the fractures were simple incomplete fractures (10). It was not considered practical to compare preinjury and postinjury racing performance because a large number of horses sustained their fractures in training before they raced. Medial and lateral condylar fractures showed similar percentages returning to racing and winning or being placed (however, some medial fractures suffered comminution and are not included in this follow-up). Of 69 nondisplaced lateral condylar fractures, 61% raced, 23.1% did not race, 10.1% were retired to stud, and 5.8% were euthanized. Of 39 medial condylar fractures, 61.5% raced, 15.4% did not race, 12.8% were retired to stud, and 10.3% were euthanized or died. Of 17 horses with complete and displaced lateral condylar fractures, only 17.6% raced. Two cases of medial metatarsal condylar spiral fractures sustained comminution 8 and 10 days after surgery. Another did so after 2 weeks of conservative treatment. They were euthanized. Three undisplaced condylar fractures recurred—two in the following year and one 2 years later. In another study, 6 of 15 cases of spiral medial condylar fracture suffered catastrophic comminution (7).

Typically, most surgeons leave the implants in place, but removing screws that cross dense bone cortices (more proximal) is logical. Some surgeons remove all screws (at approximately 4 months after insertion) (12).

The distal extremity of the fracture in the subchondral bone plate is the last to heal radiographically. The typical undisplaced condylar fracture will have healed proximally at 2 months, but the lucent line will still be visible beneath the articular surface. In the ideal case, the radiographically lucent line will have healed at 3 months, but it can often take more than 4 months.

REFERENCES

1. Adams SB, Turner TA, Blevins WE, et al. Surgical repair of metacarpal condylar fractures with palmar osteochondral comminution in two Thoroughbred horses. J Vet Surg 1985;14:32.
2. Barclay WP, Foerner JJ, Phillips TN. Axial sesamoid injuries associated with lateral condylar fractures in horses. JAVMA 1985;186:278.

3. Copelan RW, Bramlage LR. Surgery of the fetlock joint. Symposium on equine orthopaedics. Vet Clin North Am 1983;5:221.
4. Muller ME, Allgower M, Schneider R, et al. Manual of Internal Fixation. 2nd ed. New York: Springer-Verlag, 1979.
5. Pilsworth RC, Hopes R, Greet TRC. A flexed dorso-palmar projection of the equine fetlock in demonstrating lesions of the distal third metacarpus. Vet Rec 1988;122: 332–333.
6. Hornof WJ, O'Brien TR. Radiographic evaluation of the palmar aspect of the equine metacarpal condyles: a new projection. Vet Radiol 1980;21:161–167.
7. Richardson DW. Medial condylar fractures of the third metatarsal bone in horses. JAVMA 1984;185:761.
8. Kawcak CE, Bramlage LR, Embertson RM. Palmar condylar stress fractures of the distal metacarpus. In: Proceedings of the 38th Annual Meeting of the AAEP. 1992: 33–34.
9. Rick MC, O'Brien TR, Pool RR, et al. Condylar fractures of the third metacarpal bone and third metatarsal bone in 75 horses: radiographic features, treatments and outcome. JAVMA 1983;183:287.
10. Ellis DR. Some observations on condylar fractures of the third metacarpus and third metatarsus in young Thoroughbreds. Equine Vet J 1994;26:178–183.
11. Fackelman GE, Nunamaker DM. Manual of Internal Fixation in the Horse. New York: Springer-Verlag, 1982.
12. Ferraro GL. Lameness, diagnosis and treatment in the Thoroughbred racehorse. Vet Clin North Am Equine Pract 1990;6:63–84.

Internal Fixation of a Midbody Fracture of the Proximal Sesamoid Bone (With or Without Cancellous Bone Grafting)

Fractures of the proximal sesamoid bones occur in fast-gaited horses such as Thoroughbreds, Standardbreds, and racing Quarter horses (1–6). The injury also is seen in western performance horses, such as barrel racing and cutting horses, and occasionally in hunters, jumpers, and eventing horses. Fractures of one or both of the sesamoid bones can involve any level of the bone. Fractures of the apex of the bone are operated on by removal of the fragment using arthroscopic surgery (see pages 160–163) of the palmar or plantar recess of the fetlock joint.

A fracture of one proximal sesamoid bone in its midportion has been a dilemma for the equine surgeon with regard to surgical management. Treated conservatively, these fractures heal poorly because of poor blood supply and because the fragments are under continual tension of the suspensory apparatus. The resulting fibrous union lacks the strength to withstand strenuous exercise (1). Resection of the proximal fragment necessitates transection of considerable suspensory ligament attachment. It has been presumed that following such an operation, a fibrous tissue bridge would occur between the distal portion of the bone and the severed branch of the suspensory ligament. The end result would be of doubtful value to a fast-gaited horse. For this reason, alternative methods of management have been devised for the fracture of one sesamoid bone in its midportion.

Since the first edition of this text, the previously described autologous bone graft technique (7, 8), when used alone, has had poor results. The best method for treating these fractures is believed to be some form of internal fixation with or without an adjunctive bone graft. The first author generally does not use a bone graft along with compression and fixation for healing. However, other surgeons describe the use of bone graft in addition to screw fixation (4).

There are two options for internal fixation of midbody or large basilar fragments that have been described to provide continuity of an important component of the suspensory apparatus: lag screw fixation or repair with circumferential/transfixation wire. Such repair is recommended if return to racing is desired. The first author has the most experience with lag screw fixation in a proximal-distal direction. Alternatively, the screw has been placed in a distal-proximal direction by other authors. Circumferential wiring has more recently been described (5). Potential advantages of wiring over lag screw fixation include less soft tissue trauma, ease of implementation, and lack of need for specialized equipment. The disadvantages include the necessity of incisions into both the fetlock joint and deep digital flexor tendon and the possibility of wire breakage causing subsequent lameness. Both techniques are described here.

Anesthesia and Surgical Preparation

The surgical procedure is done with the horse under general anesthesia in lateral recumbency with the affected sesamoid bone uppermost. Before anesthetic induction, the limb is clipped from the coronet proximad to the proximal end of the cannon bone, around the limb's entire circumference. Following induction of the anesthetic, the area of the surgical incision is shaved. An Esmarch's bandage is applied to the limb, and a pneumatic tourniquet is applied just distal to the carpal joint. The surgical site is prepared for aseptic surgery in a routine manner.

If bone grafting is also being done, the tuber coxae or sternal area is clipped and prepared for harvesting an autogenous cancellous bone graft. The technique is described elsewhere in this book (pages 117–122).

Additional Instrumentation

Instrumentation for Lag Screw Fixation

Cancellous bone grafting requires bone curettes, a Weitlaner retractor, and casting material.

Surgical Technique

Lag Screw Fixation

A 4-cm incision is made between the branch of the suspensory ligament and the metacarpus, extending from the base of the sesamoid to immediately under the button of the splint bone (Fig. 5.6*A*). The incision is continued into the proximal palmar or plantar pouch of the fetlock joint to expose the apex of the sesamoid and the articular surface down to and including the fracture line (Fig. 5.6*B*). The limb is in flexion to facilitate reduction of the fracture, which is done while visualizing the fracture line. An ASIF reduction clamp may be used at this stage to maintain reduction of the fracture. A 1-cm stab incision is then made in the branch of the suspensory ligament in a position considered to provide the most bone fixation with the screw (Fig. 5.6*C*). A 4.5-mm glide hole is drilled down parallel to the articular surface until radiographs confirm it is through the fracture line (Fig. 5.6*C*). A 3.2-mm drill guide is then placed in the glide hole, and a 3.2-mm hole is drilled in the distal half of the sesamoid bone (Fig. 5.6*D*). After countersinking, depth gauging, and tapping, a 4.5-mm cortical bone screw is placed in lag screw fashion to stabilize the fracture (Fig. 5.6*E*).

Accurate placement of the screw is critical because there is insufficient bone for a second attempt. Recent innovations that could enhance the accuracy of placement include cannulated screws (Synthes or Herbert). If cancellous bone grafting is done, it is placed in the defect before final lag screw fixation (4).

Circumferential and Transfixation Wiring

In this technique, the same incision as described for lag screw fixation is done to expose the articular surface and apex of the sesamoid bone. A second incision is made into the digital tendon sheath through the anular ligament to expose the superficial and deep flexor tendons, the intersesamoidean ligament, and the palmar and plantar aspects of the fracture line (Fig. 5.6*F*). To place the wires, 16-gauge needles are placed in a frontal plane proximal and distal to the sesamoid bone. A 40-cm long strand of 18-gauge wire is initially threaded in an abaxial to axial direction through the distal needle and proximally along the axial margin of the bone. A 2-mm hole is drilled through the apex of the sesamoid, and the wire is inserted in an axial to abaxial direction through a needle placed in this hole. The distal free end is then tunneled over the abaxial surface of the sesamoid bone and brought out through the arthrotomy incision at the apex of the sesamoid bone. The ends are twisted to tighten and compress the fracture (Fig. 5.6, *G* and *H*). Again, bone grafting can be done to augment this repair, in which case the bone graft is placed into the fracture line before tightening of the wires.

The arthrotomy incision is closed with 0 synthetic absorbable suture in a continuous or interrupted pattern. The subcutaneous tissue is then apposed with a continuous suture of 2/0 absorbable suture, and the skin is closed with single interrupted sutures of nonabsorbable material. The anular ligament and tendon sheath are not apposed but the subcutaneous tissue over them is closed with a continuous suture of 0 polyglactin 910. The skin is closed with synthetic nonabsorbable sutures in a simple interrupted pattern. A sterile dressing is placed over the incision, and a fiberglass cast, extending to the proximal extremity of the metacarpus/metatarsus, is placed.

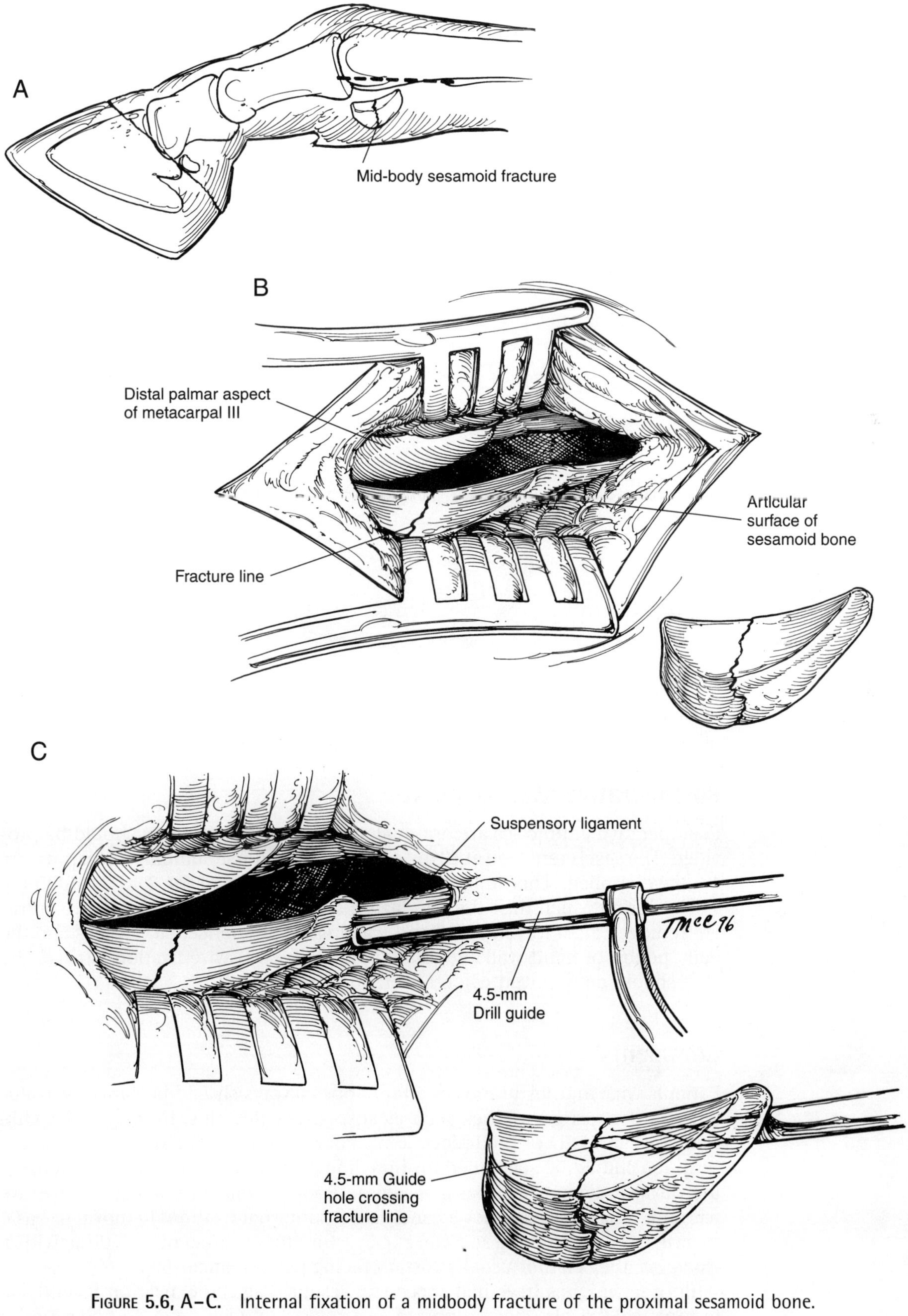

FIGURE 5.6, A–C. Internal fixation of a midbody fracture of the proximal sesamoid bone.

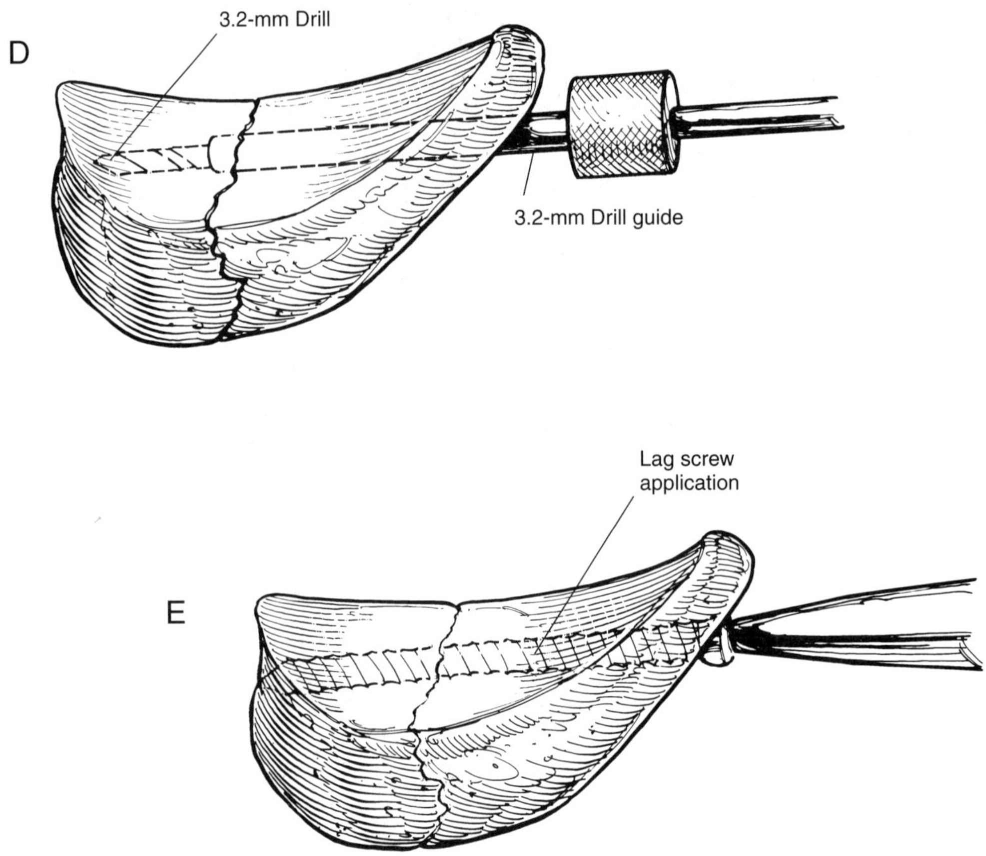

Figure 5.6, D–E. *(continued)* Internal fixation of a midbody fracture of the proximal sesamoid bone.

Postoperative Management

Postoperative antibiotics are optional, and tetanus prophylaxis should be provided. The cast is removed at 10 to 14 days with the horse standing and a pressure bandage applied. The limb should remained bandaged for 2 to 3 additional weeks during which time the bandage should be changed as required. Sutures are removed at 10 to 12 days. Hand-walking is commenced at 3 weeks and the daily period of hand-walking gradually increased. If wire fixation is used, the wire should be removed when healing occurs.

Comments

Patients with injuries to the sesamoid bones always should be carefully evaluated for concurrent injuries such as suspensory desmitis, intra-articular chip fractures, and DJD of the fetlock joint. Poor candidates for surgery of any description should be scheduled for breeding purposes if practical. Occasionally, the distal fragment of a basal sesamoid fracture will have a sagittal fracture within it; this fracture is not a candidate for internal fixation. Removal of basal fragments has been done and horses can return to a number of athletic activities. However, they cannot usually sustain racing performance.

Both techniques have had successful results. Lag screw fixation from distal to proximal has also been reported as a successful technique. In one series, 9 of 12 Standardbreds (75%) were able to race after surgery, and this number increased to 90% when two cases of septic arthritis were removed from the

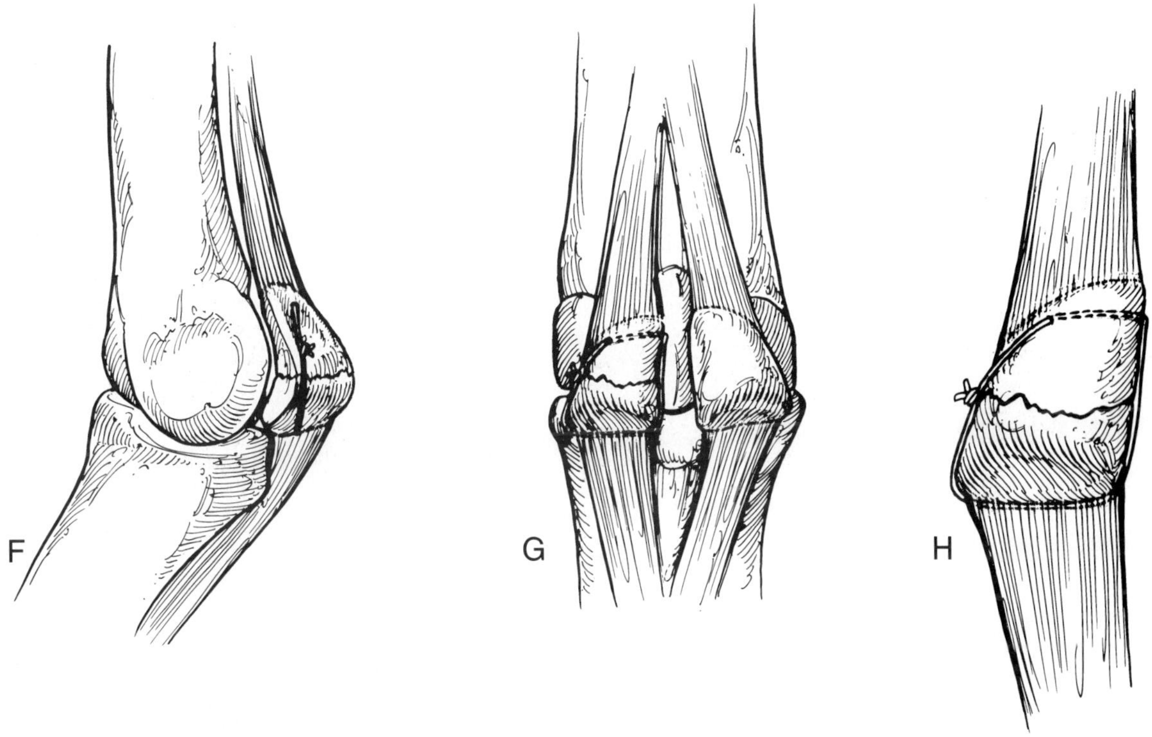

FIGURE 5.6, F–H. *(continued)* Internal fixation of a midbody fracture of the proximal sesamoid bone.

results. Five of eight Thoroughbreds (63%) were able to race, and one horse performed as a 3-day event horse after surgery. All Standardbreds and Thoroughbreds that had raced before injury had decreased earnings per race start after surgery, and all horses that had not raced before surgery were able to race after surgery (4).

In horses with midbody sesamoid fractures treated by wiring, 11 of 15 were able to resume athletic careers, with approximately 50% performing as well as or better than they had before injury (5). It could be said therefore that the prognosis for athletic use is reasonably good but the level of performance would be reduced. No comparable studies with conservative management or with cancellous bone grafting alone exist, but the prognosis is thought to be poor (1).

REFERENCES

1. Bukowiecki CF, Bramlage LR, Gabel AA. Proximal sesamoid bone fractures in the horse. A review, current treatments and prognosis. Compend Cont Edu Pract Vet 1985; 7:S684.
2. Fackelman GE. Compression screw fixation of proximal sesamoid fracture. J Equine Med Surg 1978;2:32–39.
3. Fretz PB, Barber SM, Bailey JV, et al. Management of proximal sesamoid bone fractures in the horse. JAVMA 1984;185:282–284.
4. Henninger RW, Bramlage LR, Schneider RK, et al. Lag screw and cancellous bone graft fixation of transverse proximal sesamoid bone fractures in horses: 25 cases (1983–1989). JAVMA 1991;199:606–612.
5. Martin BB, Nunamaker DM, Evans LH, et al. Circumferential wiring of mid-body and large basilar fractures of the proximal sesamoid bone in 15 horses. Vet Surg 1991;20: 9–14.

6. McIlwraith CW. Diagnostic and surgical arthroscopy of the metacarpophalangeal and metatarsophalangeal joints. In: McIlwraith CW, ed. Diagnostic and Surgical Arthroscopy of the Horse. Philadelphia: Lea & Febiger, 1990:93–95.
7. Medina L, Morgan LE, Wheat JD, et al. Treatment of basal fractures of the proximal sesamoid bones in the horse using an autogenous bone graft. In: Proceedings of the 26th Annual Convention of the AAEP, New Orleans, LA, 1981:345.
8. McIlwraith CW, Turner AS. Equine Surgery: Advanced Techniques. Philadelphia: Lea & Febiger, 1987.

Compression Plating of Simple and Comminuted Fractures of the Third Metacarpal or Metatarsal (Cannon) Bones

Fractures of the cannon bones are common in horses because of their vulnerability. They are also common in foals, especially during halter-breaking accidents or when a mare stands on the foal. Because of the poor soft tissue covering, they are frequently open. When the horse is being transported to a facility for further evaluation, radiographic assessment, and possible repair, the injured leg should be in a well-applied splint, a Robert Jones bandage, or a fiberglass cast. If not, the fracture will certainly become open if it is not already, and the fracture ends will soon become abraded and smoothed off.

The question whether to repair the fracture with internal fixation or external coaptation alone will depend on the configuration of the fracture, the size of the subject, economics, and the skill of the surgeon. The following section of this chapter is not meant to be a complete treatise on compression plating in horses. The authors are assuming that the surgeon about to attempt repair of such a fracture has been to one of the recognized AO-ASIF courses on internal fixation of fractures. This chapter should be regarded as a "refresher" that can remind the surgeon of some of the many details that must be attended to if such a repair is undertaken.

A good radiographic study of the entire bone, including the joint above (i.e., carpometacarpal) and the joint below (i.e., metacarpophalangeal joint) the fracture, is mandatory. This should include oblique views or any other views that may more accurately define the configuration of the fracture. Hairline fissure fractures that extend proximad or distad may be present and will markedly affect the method of repair, location of plate(s) and lag screws, as well as the prognosis. An open fracture should not discourage the surgeon from internal fixation with plates and screws. In fact, it should be a greater indication for internal fixation (1, 2). One exception to this rule is an open fracture that enters the nutrient foramen of the third metacarpal. This has an extremely poor prognosis and should not be attempted. It has been well demonstrated experimentally in laboratory animals and clinically in man and the horse that bone will heal in the face of infection if the right biomechanical situation exists, namely, *stability at the fracture site.*

Although the subject of case selection is important and should not be underestimated, it will not be discussed in great detail here. Obviously, a young animal of lighter body weight is going to heal more rapidly than a mature or aged horse greater than 400 kg in body weight.

Anesthesia and Surgical Preparation

The horse (foal) should be started on broad-spectrum antibiotics immediately before surgery. This will ensure the presence of the antibiotic in the hematoma at the time of surgery. Antibiotic coverage should continue for 24 hours after suction drains are removed (see "Repair of a Comminuted Fracture").

Safe general anesthesia is essential. The animal is positioned and suitably padded with the affected limb uppermost. Shortly after induction, two holes are drilled into the hoof wall, and baling wire is looped through the holes and twisted back on itself and held by an assistant. A large-diameter soft rope is threaded around the sternum or groin of the foal and secured to counteract traction that may be exerted on the distal limb. Steady continuous traction is commenced as soon as a suitable plane of general anesthesia has been reached. Surgical preparation must include the entire circumference of the fractured bone and extend from proximal radius to the coronet. After clipping the limb, the surgical site is shaved and the entire limb prepared for aseptic surgery.

Draping of cannon bone fractures must be done thoroughly; a full complement of drapes should be available. The draping should create a sterile field and must maintain such a field despite the handling and manipulation that inevitably occurs during the repair. The drapes should never become dislodged. A sterile adhesive plastic drape should be applied in such a manner that the limb is as free as possible and the surgeon has a constant view of the surrounding anatomy.

The location of the plate to repair a diaphyseal fracture of a cannon bone will depend on the configuration of the fracture. Strain gauge measurements have shown that the third metacarpal bone is axially loaded and the dorsolateral aspect of the third metatarsal bone is under tension during normal weightbearing (3, 4). With the fractures shown in Figure 5.7, *A–D,* the plate could be placed virtually anywhere except the caudal aspect of the bone. Because soft tissue coverage is critical to the outcome of internal fixation of the cannon bones, an approach that splits the lateral digital extensor tendon has been recommended (5), and it is this approach that is presented here.

Additional Instrumentation

This procedure requires instruments for bone plate application and a complete inventory of ASIF dynamic compression plates (DCPs) of various sizes (see Appendix II). Also required are a suction drain and material for fiberglass cast application.

Surgical Technique

The skin incision is made directly over the lateral digital extensor tendon as shown in Figure 5.7*E* (5, 6). As soon as the skin incision has been made, sterile towels are sewn or stapled to the wound edges, incorporating the plastic adhesive drape in the sutures or staples. Stapling the skin towels to the wound edge is advantageous because the application time is shorter than that for suturing the drapes to the limb (7). The fibers of the tendon are split, dividing the tendon longitudinally along most of its length into two equal portions. The periosteum is also incised down to the bone, and the periosteum is reflected in preparation for application of the bone plate (Figure 5.7*F*).

When the surgical site has been exposed, hematoma and tissue debris are removed by suction. Small bony fragments that will not be incorporated in the repair are removed with forceps. Throughout the procedure, tissues should be kept moist but not allowed to become completely waterlogged because of excess flushing.

Repair of a Simple Fracture

The fracture is reduced carefully by manipulating the fracture ends as steady judicious traction is applied with the aid of the baling wire held by a non-scrubbed assistant. The fracture must be reduced carefully without damaging the bone ends; otherwise, good anatomic interdigitation of the fracture will not occur. Reduction should be such that limb alignment (rotation, angulation) is good. Once the fracture has been reduced, it can be temporarily secured with a lag screw. Inserting the screw is easiest if there is some obliquity to the fracture line, as shown in Figure 5.7*G,* but may be impossible if the fracture is a transverse one. This lag screw will provide additional compression at the fracture site. The screw should be a 4.5-mm bone screw of appropriate length. Because the hole

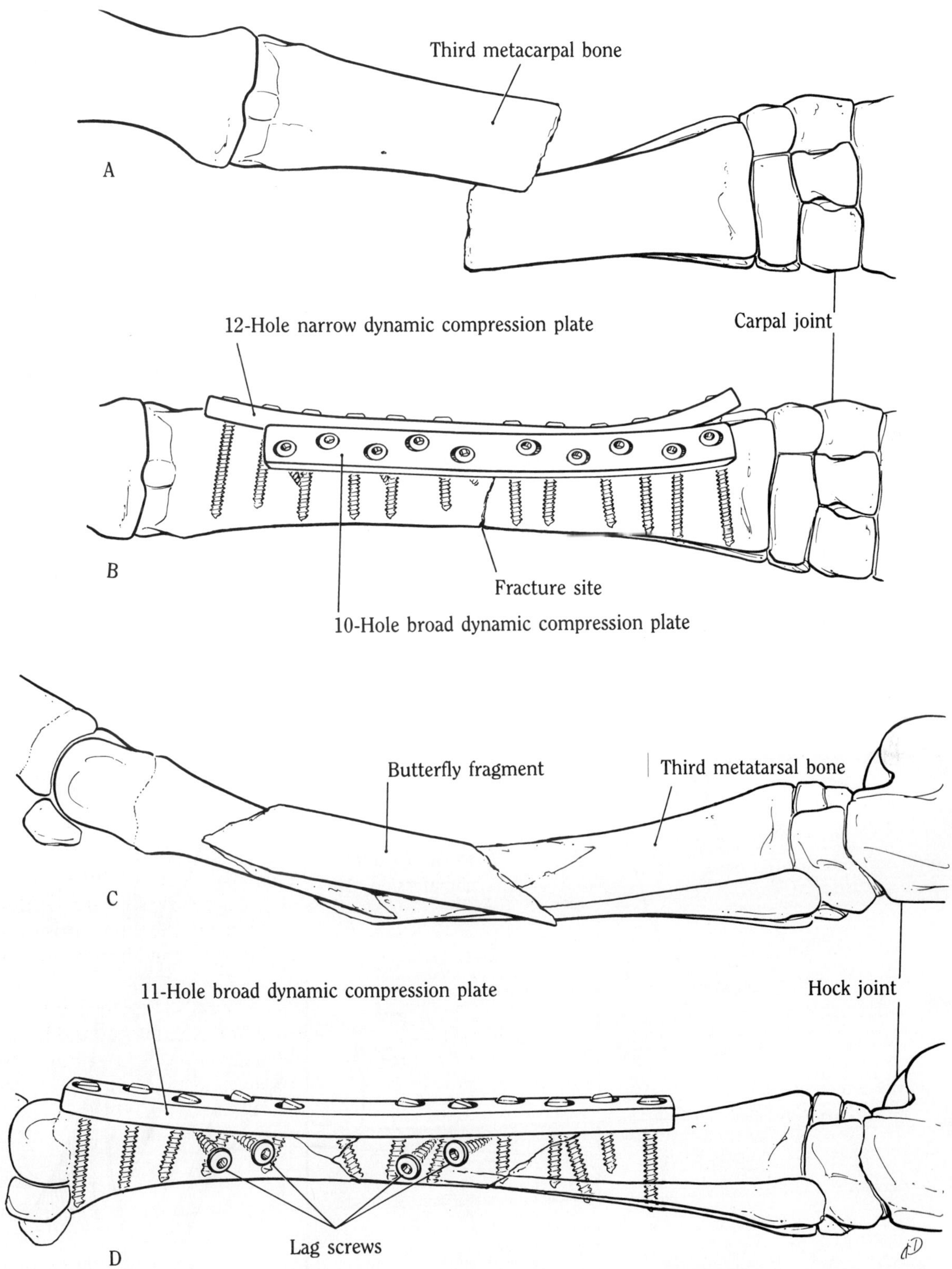

Figure 5.7. **A.** Line drawing (from radiographs) of a simple fracture of the third metacarpus (adult). **B.** Completed repair of the simple third metacarpal fracture in Figure 5.5*A*. Two bone plates were required to complete the repair. **C.** Line drawing (from radiographs) of a comminuted fracture of the third metatarsus (foal). **D.** Completed repair of the fracture in Figure 5.5*C*. One bone plate and four lag screws were required to complete the repair.

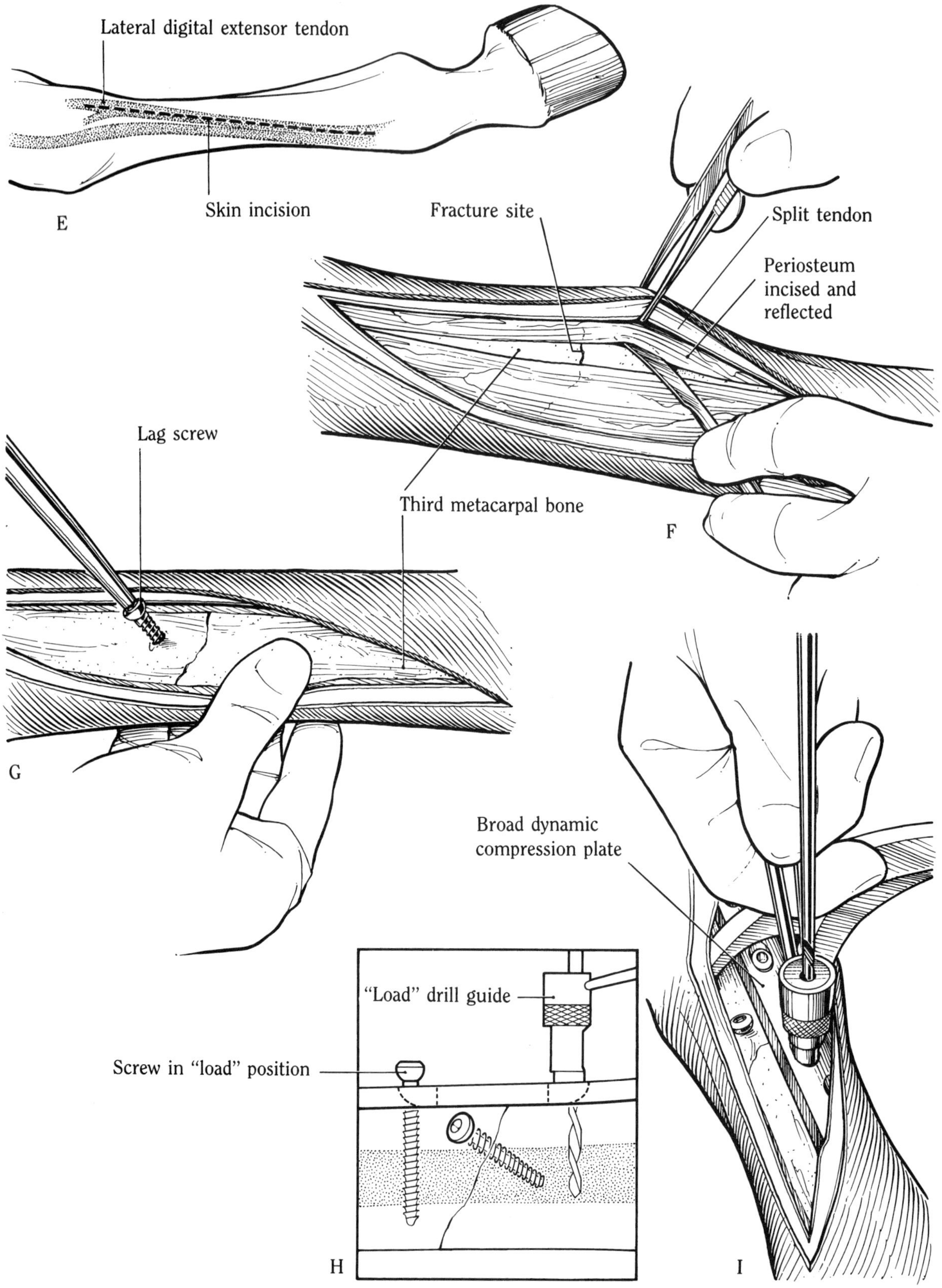

Figure 5.7, E–I. *(continued)* Steps in repair of a simple fracture of the third metacarpus or metatarsus.

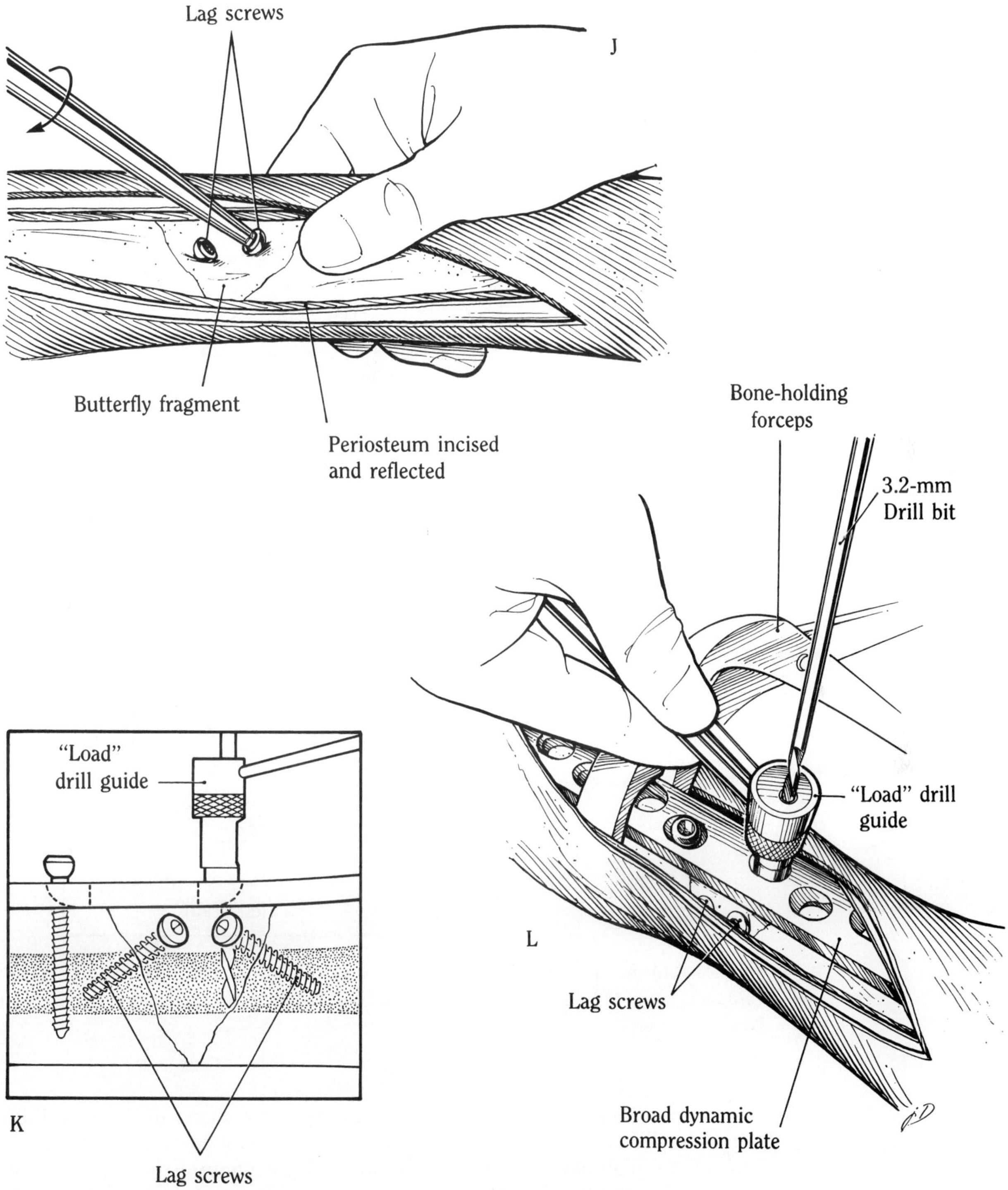

FIGURE 5.7, J–L. *(continued)* Steps in repair of a comminuted fracture of the third metacarpus or metatarsus.

is drilled in an oblique direction, it should be adequately countersunk to prevent plastic deformation of the head of the screw.

A compression plate of suitable length is selected. Aluminum templates are useful to help select the correct size of the plate and to contour it. The plate should span the bone from one metaphysis to the next. The most suitable implant currently available for long bone fracture repair is the broad DCP. The

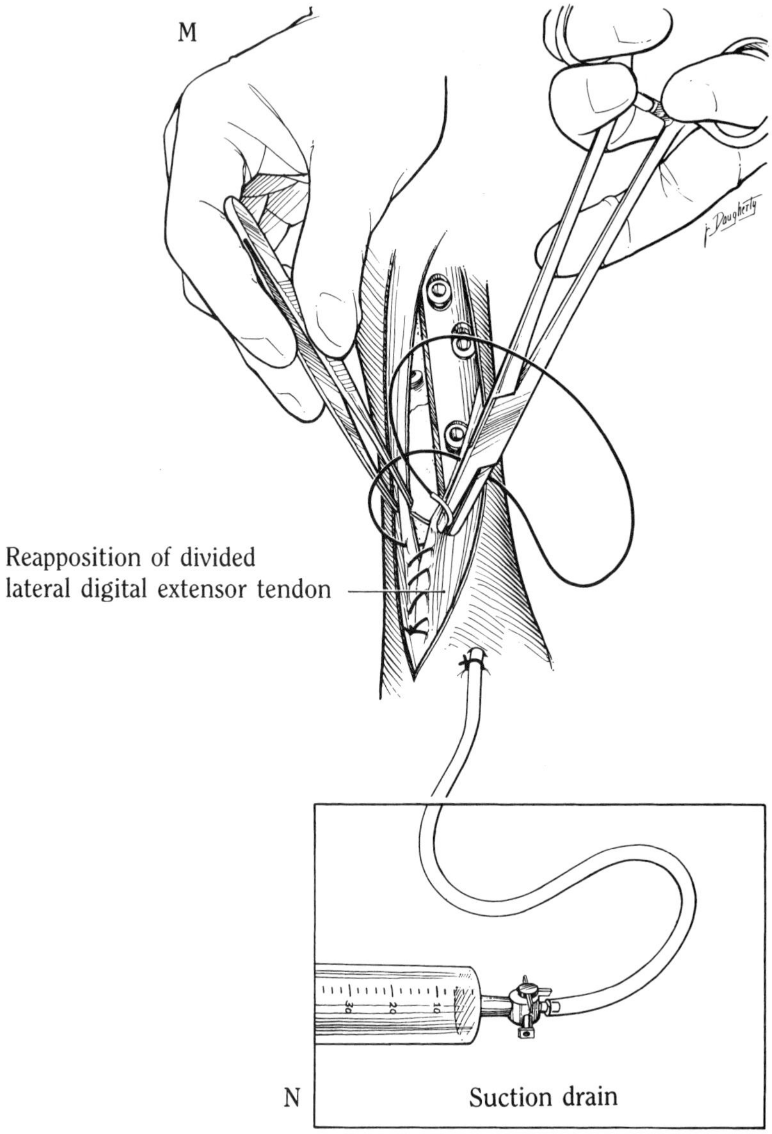

Figure 5.7, M–N. *(continued)* Closure of the wound following plate application, showing re-apposition of the lateral digital extensor tendon, with use of a suction drain to evacuate blood or serum.

plate is contoured (bent and twisted) to match the shape of the aluminum template. For the fracture shown in Figure 5.7*A*, a small amount of "pre-bending" of the plate will help provide more uniform compression opposite the fracture site. This is achieved by providing a 2-mm gap under the plate at the fracture site (8).

Slight twisting of the plate will be required. The authors find it easier to do this by holding the plate in the bending press and using *one* of the bending irons to achieve the twist. The surgeon should try to contour the plate as perfectly as possible without excessively prolonging the operating time.

The plate is attached to the bone by inserting the first screw through the plate approximately 1 cm from the fracture site. The screw is not tightened completely. The plate is then displaced toward the fracture site to bring the shaft of the screw up against the displaced edge of the screw hole. The screw on the other side of the fracture is inserted through the plate using the yellow "load" drill guide. Both screws should engage both cortices of the bone (Fig. 5.7, *H* and *I*). When the tap is passed through the plate, it should pass through the 4.5-mm tap sleeve with the plate protector positioned at its end.

The two screws are situated at either side of the fracture site, located eccentrically in the holes in the plate (i.e., in the "load" position). As the two screws are alternately tightened, compression will be observed at the fracture site. The remaining screws are placed in the neutral position using the corresponding neutral or "green" drill guide. As an alternative to placing a lag screw across the fracture before fixation, a lag screw can be placed through the plate and across the fracture to provide interfragmentary compression.

The remaining screws should engage in both cortices of the bone and should be angled to cross the bone at its greatest diameter wherever they are located. Cortical bone screws, either 4.5 or 5.5 mm in diameter, can be used for the remaining screws.

If the bone is very soft, such as may be encountered in the metaphysis of newborn foals, either 5.5-mm or 6.5-mm cancellous screws can be used. These larger screws are also useful if the surgeon inadvertently strips the threads of one of the cortical screws.

In certain-sized individuals (e.g., > 250 kg), an additional plate (broad or narrow compression plate) will be required. This should be situated at 90° to the first plate, with all the screws placed in the "neutral" position. If a second plate is applied, the original lag screw should be removed and, if possible, used as one of the screws in the plate (Fig. 5.7*B*). Every step of the repair should be aimed at achieving maximum stability at the fracture site.

Repair of a Comminuted Fracture

The fracture illustrated in Figure 5.7*C* is comminuted and has a small "butterfly" fragment. It is in three parts and can be converted into a two-part fracture by reattaching the fragment to the parent bone with a lag screw. At this point the fracture is reduced with another lag screw (Fig. 5.7*J*). The fracture is then repaired as described above for repair of a simple fracture. The fragment should be positioned *under* the plate, as shown in Figure 5.7*K*. Additional compression could be achieved at the fracture line by placing lag screws through the appropriate holes in the plate and directing them across the fracture plane (Fig. 5.7*L*).

All holes in the plate should be filled. If a fracture line appears directly under one of the holes in the plate, instead of leaving it void, it should be filled. A glide hole is drilled through the fracture site until the medullary cavity is reached. The 3.2-mm drill sleeve is placed in the hole, a 3.2-mm hole is drilled and tapped, and a 4.5-mm cortical screw of appropriate length is inserted (Fig. 5.7*D*).

Placement of a suction drain is advisable to evacuate the hematoma at the surgical site (an ideal medium for bacteria). The drain should be placed along the entire length of the incision and then tunneled by means of a trocar through several centimeters of soft tissues. The tube should be under constant vacuum (Fig. 5.7, *M* and *N*).

The incision is closed by first apposing the divided lateral digital extensor tendon and using a synthetic absorbable suture material in a simple continuous pattern (Fig. 5.7*M*). The subcutaneous tissue and skin are closed by the pattern and materials of the surgeon's choice. For adults and yearlings, the limb should now be placed in a full-limb fiberglass cast that extends to the proximal end of the radius or tibia, whichever is appropriate. For foals, rather than apply a cast, a well-applied Robert Jones bandage will sometimes suffice in a well-stabilized fracture by rigid internal fixation. The suction drain is brought out through the cast. The reservoir (bellows apparatus) should be attended to every hour for the first 12 hours so that as much hematoma as possible is removed. The reservoir should never be allowed to back flow, and solutions of any description should not be flushed up the tubing. Antibiotics should be continued until at least 24 hours after removal of the drain. The drain is removed when the collection of fluid is diminished, usually after a clot of blood, fibrin, and tissue debris has formed within the lumen. The cast can be removed anytime after 24 hours in young foals and can coincide with drain removal. Older animals require periods of extended immobilization.

The animal is confined to a box stall. Because foals are likely to be the most appropriate candidates, a box stall large enough to accommodate the mare and foal should be available. Shavings or a light bedding of straw is also recommended to enable the foal to ambulate without becoming trapped by deep bedding.

Comments

The surgical approach described for cannon bone fractures provides a maximum amount of soft tissue over the implant should breakdown of the skin incision occur (5). If the fracture configuration dictates that a more dorsal (cranial) approach is required, the common (or long) digital extensor tendon can be split in a similar fashion.

Subperiosteal dissection creates the least amount of trauma to the soft tissues and provides the best postoperative blood supply to the healing bone (9). In addition, removal of the periosteal layer allows the plate to have more intimate contact with the bone, thereby increasing bone-to-plate friction. For similar reasons, the plate should be contoured with as much precision as time permits. One method to improve friction between the plate and the bone is a technique called plate luting. The fracture is repaired as described; when the repair is complete, all screws passing through the plate are loosened to permit the plate to be lifted off the bone slightly. Polymethylmethacrylate (PMMA) is mixed into the dough stage and then applied to the ventral surface of the plate. The plate is now attached firmly to the bone. The PMMA will form a thin layer between the plate and bone. As the plate is tightened, most of the PMMA will be forced to the sides. This excess is removed.

Pre-bending is another important maneuver to achieve more uniform compression across the fracture site. It would not be possible for a comminuted fracture such as the fracture shown in Figure 5.7*C* or for a very oblique fracture line, but it is suitable for the fracture shown in Figure 5.7*A*.

If comminution does exist, the comminuted region should be placed under the plate and consideration be given to the insertion of a cancellous bone graft. Comminuted fractures repaired with internal fixation must be supplemented with external coaptation, even though both methods are frowned on in human orthopaedics.

Screws with large diameters (5.5-mm cortical) have been recommended to achieve greater holding power (10, 11). One advantage of the larger screws is that they have the same pull-out strength as the partially threaded cancellous screws. A fully threaded screw is preferable to a partially threaded screw, especially if removal of the implants is anticipated when the fracture has healed.

The biggest obstacle to overcome in the surgical repair of cannon bone fractures is preservation of the viability of the soft tissues covering the implants. The energy that caused the fracture has in part been displaced into the soft tissues and overlying skin, making them vulnerable to the additional insult of surgery. On occasion, the insult of surgery is too much and the skin sloughs over the implants. This sloughing admits infection so that implants eventually loosen and the fracture becomes unstable.

The AO-ASIF DCP, with its uniquely designed screw holes, should be used. The DCP is more versatile than previously used older plates, and the screws can be angled without creating excessive stress on the screw heads. Plate removal is an additional procedure with additional expense involved. It is not routinely recommended unless a specific indication exists. Common indications include drainage and fistula formation, usually resulting from infection around the implants. If the animal is destined to be used for some form of athletic performance, then implant removal *is* usually necessary because screws placed from the dorsal cortex to the palmar cortex in a sagittal plane in (cranial to caudal) have an "anchoring" effect, not allowing normal flexion of the bone during maximal loading. This results in pain and soreness until the implants are removed.

REFERENCES

1. Turner AS. Large animal orthopaedics. In: Jennings PB, ed. Practice of Large Animal Surgery. Philadelphia: WB Saunders, 1984:816.
2. Schneider RK, Jackman BR. Fractures of the third metacarpus and metatarsus. In: Nixon AJ, ed. Equine Fracture Repair. Philadelphia: WB Saunders, 1996:179–194.
3. Brewener AA, Thomason J, Goodship A, et al. Bone stress in the horse forelimb during locomotion at different gaits. A comparison of two experimental methods. J Biomechanics 1983;16:565
4. Turner AS, Mills EJ, Gabel AA. In vivo measurement of bone strain in the horse. Am J Vet Res 1975;36:1573.
5. Bramlage LR. Fractures of the third metacarpal and metatarsal bones. Paper presented at the 16th Annual Course on Internal Fixation of Fractures and Non-Unions. Columbus, Ohio, 1985.
6. Milne DW, Turner AS. An Atlas of Surgical Approaches of the Bones of the Horse. Philadelphia: WB Saunders, 1979.
7. Morris DM. The use of skin staples to secure skin towels in areas difficult to drape. Surg Gynecol Obstet 1984;159:387.
8. Fackelman GE, Nunamaker DM. Manual of Internal Fixation in the Horse. New York: Springer-Verlag, 1982.
9. Bramlage LR. Long bone fractures. Symposium on Equine Orthopaedics. Vet Clin North Am 1983;5:285.
10. Yovich JV, Turner AS, Smith FW. Holding power of orthopaedic screws in equine third metacarpal and metatarsal bones: I. Foal bone. J Vet Surg 1985;14:221.
11. Yovich JV, Turner AS, Smith FW. Holding power of orthopaedic screws in equine third metacarpal and metatarsal bones: II. Adult horses. J Vet Surg 1985;14:230.

Plate Fixation of a Simple Fracture of the Olecranon

Fractures of the olecranon are relatively common, especially in younger horses. A kick from another horse, a sudden fall, and avulsion of a part of the bone by the pull of the triceps brachii muscle are the usual causes of such fractures (1–11). A simple olecranon fracture generally responds well to internal fixation if certain principles are followed, and for this reason the authors believe it is appropriate to describe the method of repair of such a fracture.

A horse with a fracture of the olecranon will bear a variable amount of weight on the limb, depending on the location of the fracture and the degree of disruption of the triceps-olecranon apparatus. The typical stance of an animal with an olecranon fracture resembles the dropped elbow stance of radial paralysis. Swelling and crepitation may be evident on palpation, but the amount will depend on the location of the fracture and the degree of comminution and instability.

The diagnosis of a fracture of the olecranon is confirmed with radiographs (craniocaudal and medial-to-lateral views). The lateral view usually shows the fracture configuration most clearly and is best taken with the x-ray beam directed in a medial-to-lateral direction across the cranial aspect of the chest. Olecranon fractures can assume a variety of configurations. Most commonly, the fracture occurs through the semilunar notch of the elbow joint, although other configurations may be seen that range from an avulsion of the epiphysis of foals to severe comminution of the ulna with luxation of the radius craniad (Monteggia fracture) (7). Distraction of the proximal fragments is sometimes severe, owing to the pull of the triceps brachii muscle. If the surgeon is new or inexperienced at ASIF compression plating techniques, it would be unwise to attempt one of the complicated fractures of the olecranon. These cases are best referred to surgeons with more experience.

Olecranon fractures have been managed by surgical or nonsurgical methods in different situations. The configuration of the fracture will often determine which method will be chosen. For minimally displaced fissure fractures, treatment with absolute stall rest for 6 to 8 weeks, prevention of "contracted" flexor tendons of the affected limb, and support of the contralateral limb may suffice. Cross-tying is sometimes indicated to prevent the animal from lying down and displacing the fracture on rising. The affected limb should be radiographed periodically to check for distraction or displacement of the fragments, in which case internal fixation is indicated. In extremely comminuted fractures, nonoperative management may be the only alternative because of the large number of fragments. Economics may also be a deciding factor in the method of repair. Nonoperative treatment, however, should not be regarded as a "conservative" approach because, in the authors' opinion, it has a higher chance of failure than does operative treatment. Surgical treatment, when applicable, results in restoration of normal elbow joint mechanics and possible return to athletic soundness. In the authors' experience, this is rarely the case after nonsurgical treatment (11).

If nonsurgical management is elected, a number of complications can arise, including (*a*) "contraction" of the flexor tendons of the affected limb with stiffness of joints; (*b*) severe atrophy of the triceps brachii muscle; (*c*) failure of fracture union, resulting from excessive distraction of fragments; (*d*) permanent pain and stiffness of the elbow joint, resulting from secondary DJD; (*e*) angular limb deformities (in young animals) such as valgus or varus deformities of the carpus of the contralateral limb, resulting from excessive compensatory weightbearing; and (*f*) laminitis in adult horses, resulting from compensatory overload of the uninjured limb (11).

The main goal of surgical intervention in olecranon fractures is to offset the distracting forces of the triceps brachii muscle and to reestablish continuity of the articular surface of the elbow joint (1–11).

The most satisfactory technique for repair of a fractured equine olecranon is rigid stabilization, using dynamic compression plating along the caudal aspect of the bone, and this method is described. Fortunately, the tension surface of the bone is its caudal aspect because of the pull of the triceps brachii muscle. Pinning and tension-band wiring techniques, which are successful in olecranon fractures in small animals and man, have limited application in the horse, owing to the greater body weight of the patient (11). Because the stability is less with pinning and wiring devices, convalescence is frequently prolonged, and weightbearing is delayed (6). One exception to the preference for plate fixation is the very proximal avulsion fracture of the olecranon process that is impossible to plate because of the lack of bone within the proximal fragment.

Because the plate is subjected to tensile forces, which it resists extremely well, fracture repair is generally not fraught with the problems of implant failure that occur in the other tubular long bones of adult horses. Most olecranon fractures respond dramatically postoperatively because early weightbearing and pain-free ambulation occur soon after rigid internal fixation.

Anesthesia and Surgical Preparation

The surgical procedure is done under general anesthesia with the horse placed in lateral recumbency with the affected limb uppermost.

Before induction of anesthesia, the entire elbow region is clipped, including a portion of the lateral thorax and forelimb. By clipping the limb before surgery, the anesthetic time can be reduced.

Additional Instrumentation

Compression plating of the olecranon requires a full complement of long bone plating instruments and an assortment of cortical and cancellous screws (see Appendix I).

Surgical Technique

The limb is draped, using sterile plastic adherent drapes for the immediate surgical site. A curvilinear skin incision is made as illustrated in Figure 5.8*A*. Using a muscle separation technique, the bone is approached between the ulnaris lateralis muscle and the humeral head of the deep digital flexor muscle (12). The ulnaris lateralis muscle is reflected craniad and the humeral and ulnar heads of the deep digital flexor muscle caudad, exposing the caudal aspect of the ulna (Fig. 5.6*B*).

Olecranon fractures are usually easy to reduce (11). Bone reduction forceps with points are useful in reduction of fractures that are being treated some time after the original injury. In chronic cases, fibrous tissue may be interposed between the fracture fragments, making perfect reconstruction of the fracture impossible. In such cases, the bone plate should be applied without extensive debridement because once the fracture is stabilized, ossification usually proceeds rapidly (13).

The compression plate should be contoured to fit the caudal aspect of the bone (Fig. 5.8*C*). Some twisting of the plate may be required. A technique has been described in which the distal parent fragment of the olecranon is "shaved" with an osteotome or chisel to aid in seating the plate on the rounded caudal

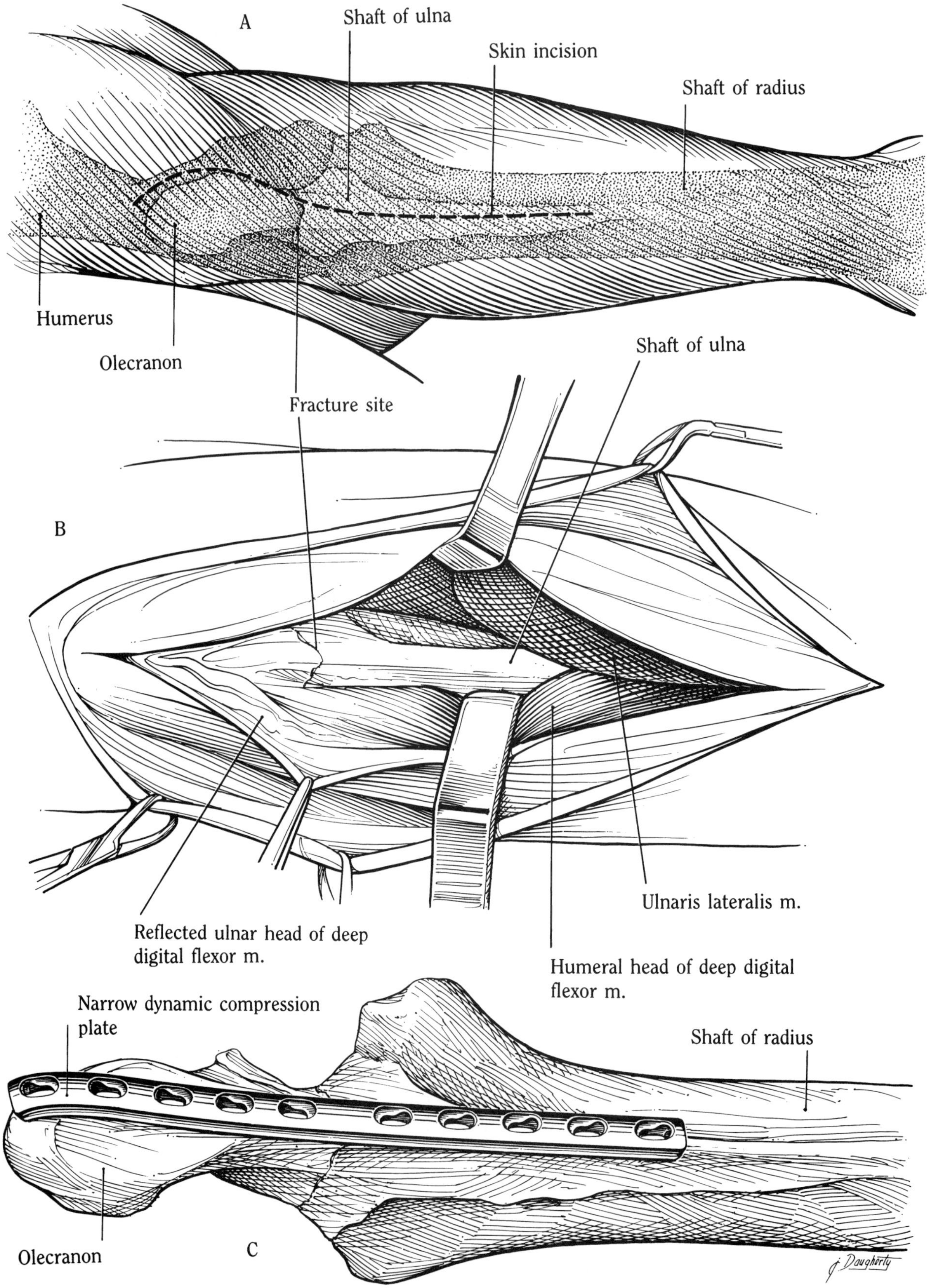

Figure 5.8, A–C. Compression plating of simple fracture of the olecranon.

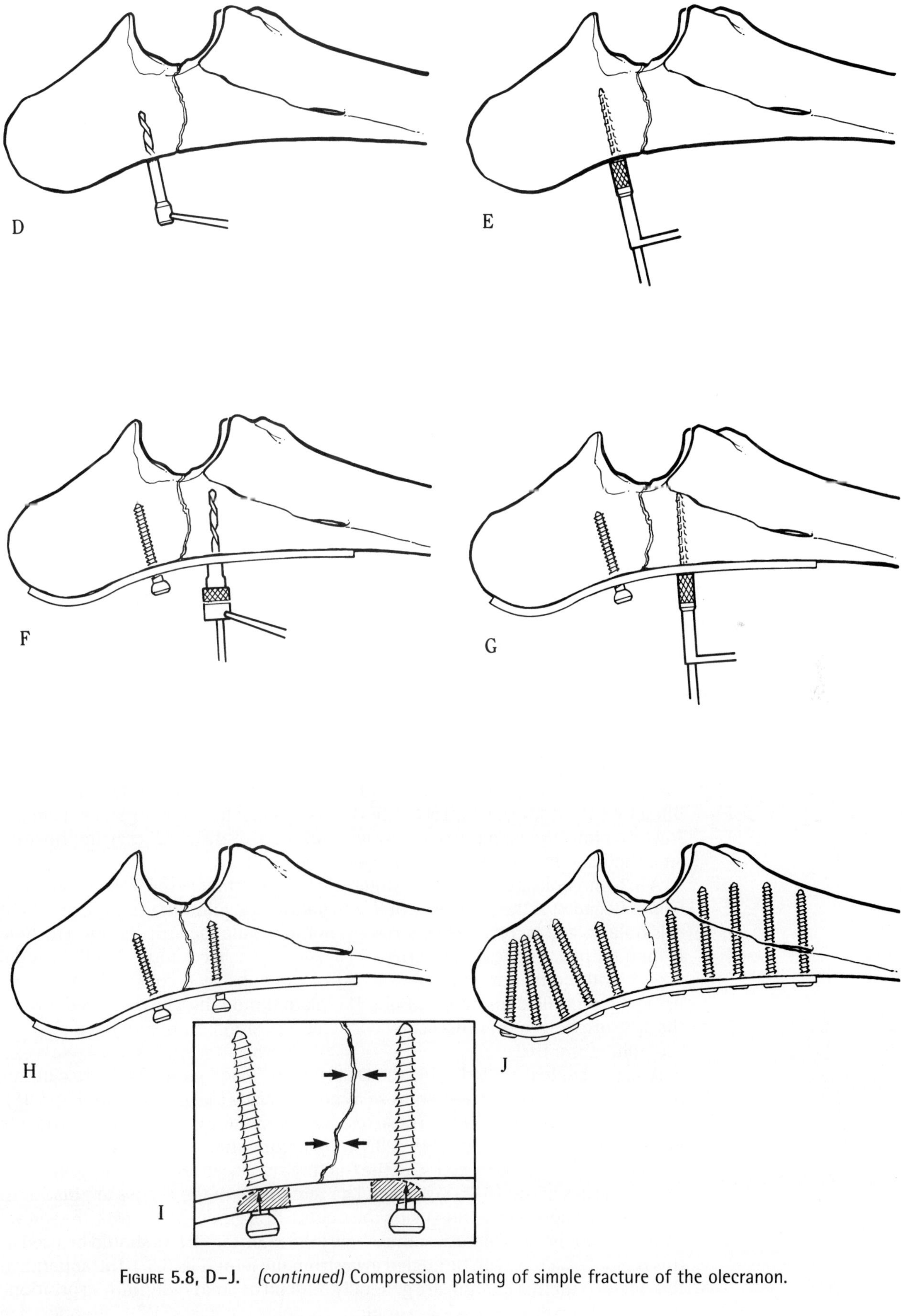

FIGURE 5.8, D–J. *(continued)* Compression plating of simple fracture of the olecranon.

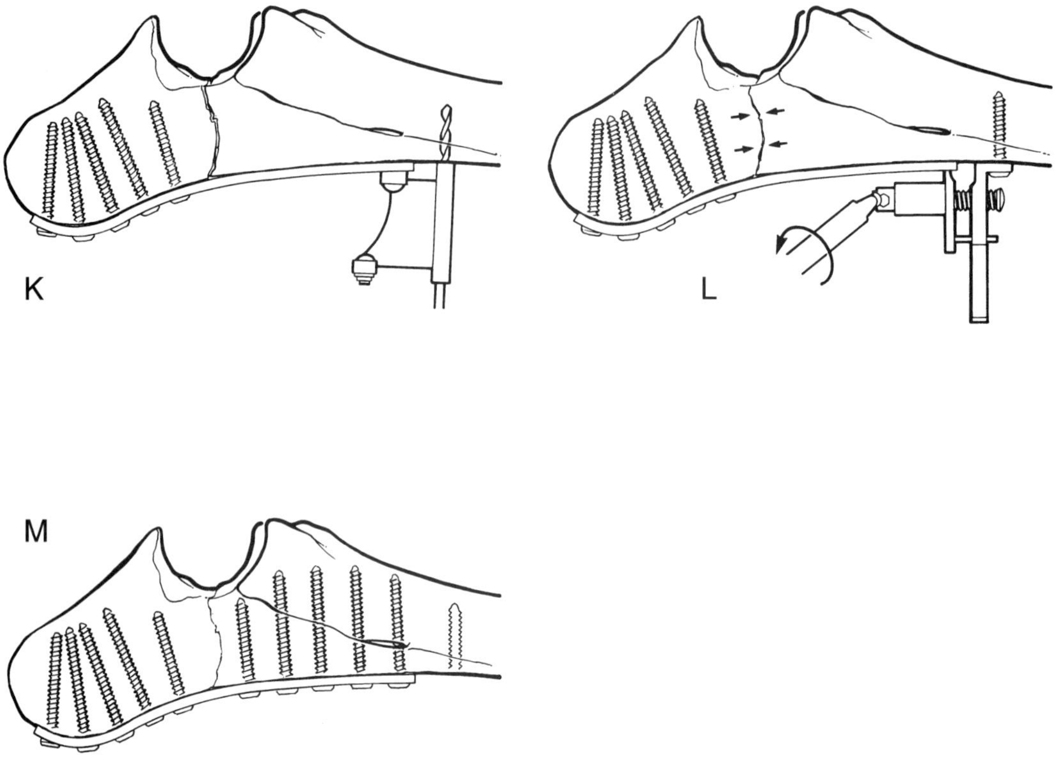

Figure 5.8, K–M. *(continued)* Compression plating of simple fracture of the olecranon.

aspect of the bone (5). This technique is useful for some fresh fractures and may be essential for long-standing injuries when callus and fibrous tissue have produced an irregular surface to the bone.

Application of the Plate

The plate of appropriate length is applied by the techniques and methods outlined by ASIF (13, 14). A narrow ASIF DCP is suitable for most horses. For simple fractures into the semilunar notch without a lot of distraction at the fracture site, the plate is applied in the following sequence.

A 3.2-mm hole is drilled approximately 1 cm proximal to the fracture site (Fig. 5.8*D*). Because of the proximity of the radiohumeral joint, the screw inserted in this hole should be relatively short so as not to invade the articulation. The hole is then tapped (Fig. 5.8*E*). A narrow DCP is accurately contoured to the caudal aspect of the ulna and loosely attached to the bone by a cortical bone screw, using the predrilled, pretapped hole. The plate should then be displaced toward the fracture line so that this screw occupies a position on the inclined slope of the hole of the DCP.

A second hole is drilled using the DCP yellow "load" guide. The screw in this hole should also be relatively short so as not to invade the articulation (Fig. 5.8*F*). The hole is tapped (Fig. 5.8*G*). These two screws are now positioned eccentrically away from the fracture site (Fig. 5.8*H*). Tightening the screws reduces the fracture and produces compression of the fracture site because of the self-compressing properties of the DCP (Fig. 5.8*I*). The remainder of the screws are placed in the so-called neutral position using the neutral drill guide. At all costs, the screws should avoid the articulation of the elbow joint. Shorter screws should be used in this region, or screws can be angled away from the joint (Fig. 5.8*J*). Intraoperative radiographs for this fracture are generally difficult as far as determining positioning, and the risk of breaking aseptic technique increases. With preoperative planning and knowledge of where the elbow joint is in relationship to the fracture site, the surgeon can complete the operation without such an interruption. Because of the density of the bone in the proximal radius, the distal screws need only engage the caudal radial cortex (Fig. 5.8*J*). The blood vessels in the interosseous foramen should be avoided (14). Cortical bone screws are used throughout the repair except when the bone of the proximal ulna is soft, as may occur in foals or yearlings.

If a larger fracture gap exists, the tension device can be readily used because additional distal exposure is easily obtained (12). With this device, a relatively large fracture gap can be closed and compressed. All the screws proximal to the fracture site are first inserted. The special drill guide for the compression device is secured to the plate and a 3.2-mm hole is drilled (Fig. 5.8*K*). The removable tension device is attached to the plate and secured to the bone with a 4.5-mm cortical bone screw. A socket wrench is used to slightly tighten the tension device and simultaneously provisionally reduce the fracture (Fig. 5.8*L*). The tension device is then tightened to produce compression at the fracture site. The distal screws are now inserted and the compression device is removed (Fig. 5.8*M*).

The judicious use of power tapping and of the power screwdriver attachment will greatly speed up the operation and reduce the time the animal is anesthetized and the wound exposed to room air. Reducing the pressure of the compressed nitrogen source to diminish the torque generated by the drill decreases the chances of instrument breakage.

In very young animals, the ulna should not be attached to the radius with screws because this procedure will cause abnormal development of the elbow joint as the proximal radial physis continues to grow. In such cases, the screws should be inserted *only* through the ulna if at all possible. If the ulna is so thin that screw fixation of the ulna alone would jeopardize the repair, the screws will have to be placed in the caudal cortex of the radius, but the plate must be removed before elbow dysplasia develops.

Suction drains should be used if excessive hematoma at the fracture site is anticipated. Pressure bandaging is difficult with the incision this far up the limb. Another option is to suture a stent bandage directly over the incision.

Postoperative Management

The postoperative management of olecranon fractures should consist of pressure bandaging while the animal is confined to a box stall. Casting or splinting is not only impossible but is probably detrimental because of placing unwanted forces on the fracture site.

If the fracture can be adequately stabilized at surgery, the prognosis for future soundness is generally good to excellent. Postoperatively, horses with olecranon fractures begin almost immediate weightbearing. Failure to bear weight within 7 to 10 days of surgery is usually indicative of continued instability at the fracture site or infection of the fixation.

Whether the plates should be removed from olecranon fractures in mature horses is still undetermined. The authors' tendency is to leave them in place unless there is a loose screw that could potentially migrate or there is infection around the implants. If infection is present, the implants must not be removed until the fracture has healed. In young animals (less than 5 months) that still may have continued growth of the proximal radial physis, plate removal is necessary to avoid elbow dysplasia and subsequent lameness.

REFERENCES

1. Brown MP, Norrie RD. Surgical repair of olecranon fractures in young horses. J Equine Med Surg 1978;2:545.

2. Clem M, De Bowes R, Douglass J, et al. The effects of fraction of the ulna to the radius in young foals. Vet Surg 1988;17:338–345.
3. Colahan PT, Meagher DM. Repair of comminuted fractures of the proximal ulna and olecranon in young horses using tension band plating. Vet Surg 1979;8:105.
4. Denny HR, Barr A, Waterman A. Surgical treatment of fractures of the olecranon in the horse: a comparative review of 25 cases. Equine Vet J 1987;19:319–325.
5. Fackelman GE, Nunamaker DM. Manual of Internal Fixation in the Horse. New York: Springer-Verlag, 1982.
6. Fretz PB. Fractured ulna in the horse. Can Vet J 1973;14:50.
7. Kopf N, Rettenbacher G. Die Zuggurtung der Olekranofractur Beim Pferd. Pract Tierarzt 1981;7:598.
8. Levine SB, Meagher DM. Repair of an ulnar fracture with radial luxation in a horse. Vet Surg 1980;9:58.
9. Milne DW, Turner AS. Atlas of Surgical Approaches to the Bones of the Horse. Philadelphia: WB Saunders, 1979.
10. Muller ME, Allgower M, Schneider R, et al. Manual of Internal Fixation. 3rd ed. New York: Springer-Verlag, 1979.
11. Nixon AJ. Fractures of the ulna. In: Nixon AJ, ed. Equine Fracture Repair. Philadelphia: WB Saunders, 1976:231–241.
12. McGill CA, Hilbert BJ, Jacobs KV. Internal fixation of fractures of the ulna in the horse. Aust Vet J 1982.58:101.
13. Monin T. Repair of physeal fractures of the tuber olecranon in the horse using a tension band method. JAVMA 1978;172:287.
14. Denny HR. The surgical treatment of fractures of the olecranon in the horse. Equine Vet J 1976;8:20.

Application of Fiberglass Cast

A cast is commonly an essential part of treatment of fractures and luxations. Frequently, a cast is used to "protect" a fracture that has been repaired with plates and/or screws, especially during the recovery period from anesthesia when excessive forces may disrupt the repair. Casts are also useful for temporary immobilization of fractures distal to the distal third of the radius and tibia. Fractures proximal to this level are temporarily immobilized with a Robert Jones bandage with a lateral splint to prevent abduction of the limb (1). Casting is also used as a sole method of treating certain fractures that are too comminuted for repair by internal fixation with plates and/or screws (2–4). Transfixation casting incorporating transversely placed pins that are then incorporated into the cast has been useful in the management of comminuted fractures. The pins may be directly incorporated into a fiberglass cast, or, alternatively (as advocated by some surgeons), pins are incorporated within the cast using a U-bar (5). In vitro testing has shown, however, no advantage to incorporating a U-bar into the construct when fiberglass cast material is used (6, 7).

Another frequent indication for cast application at Colorado State University Veterinary Teaching Hospital is distal limb lacerations, especially those involving the bulbs of the heels and coronet. Despite an initial higher expense, a cast provides superior immobilization of the wound edges to pressure bandaging alone. Pressure bandaging is sometimes useful in the initial stages of management when there is extensive suppuration or contamination, but a cast placed on the limb at the earliest opportunity is the best method to achieve rapid wound healing. Casts are also a vital adjunct to tendon lacerations in horses because of the inability of most commercially available suture materials to withstand the enormous tensile forces subjected to the repair by large animals. Certain cases of so-called contracted tendons or flexural deformities in foals require casts either as a sole method of treatment or as an adjunct to surgery.

One variation in the casting method is the so-called tube or sleeve cast. This cast extends from the proximal end of the radius to just below the fetlock joint, the foot being exposed. In foals, the most common indication for a tube cast is the condition referred to as "hypoplasia" or delayed ossification of the carpal bones. The authors have also used the tube cast as a support to the repair of comminuted fractures of the carpus.

The greatest advantage of the tube cast is that normal weightbearing can occur and the flexor tendons are under normal physiologic tension while the axial alignment of the limb is maintained. The limb will not adopt the hyperextension conformation because of tendon flaccidity seen if the entire limb, including the foot, is placed in the cast. The animal also has better footing while in the cast.

Casting is by no means a benign procedure, and it does take experience and some practice to become confident in the technique. It is hoped that this section will aid the reader in becoming confident in the technique. Once perfected, fiberglass casting will become a useful method of therapy that will yield rewarding results.

Additional Instrumentation

Many different materials for cast application in horses have been available over the years. With recent advances in the fiberglass and plastic industry, strong lightweight materials are now in routine use. The fiberglass products have essentially replaced the use of plaster. A variety of knitted fiberglass fabrics, impregnated with a polyurethane resin that is activated on exposure to water, are now

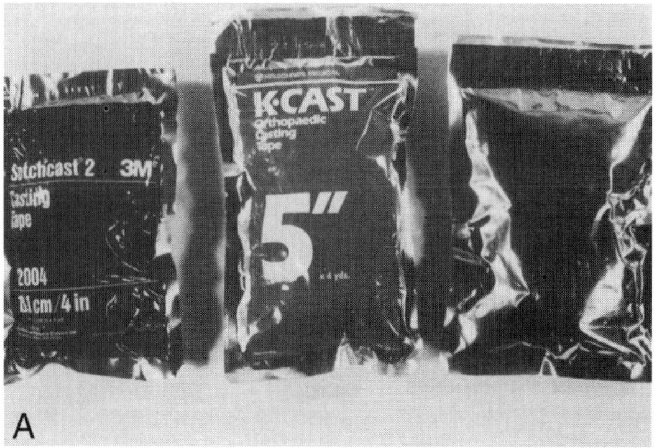

Figure 5.9, A. Types of fiberglass cast material available for large animals: *left*, Scotchcast (3M Company, 3M Animal Care Products, St. Paul, MN); *center*, K-Cast (Kirschner Medical, Timonium, MD); *right*, Delta Lite (Johnson and Johnson, Medical Inc, Arlington, TX).

used for cast application on large animals (Fig. 5.9*A*). The material is lightweight and therefore ideal for use in foals, unlike the heavier plaster-based products that were previously used. The material is also durable and water resistant and water permeable. Most materials available rapidly harden to maximum strength, enabling the horse to stand and bear weight after approximately 20 minutes of curing.

The fiberglass products are relatively radiotransparent, enabling fracture healing to be evaluated. It is possible, however, to check *fracture alignment* with reasonable accuracy after the cast has been applied (4).

The fiberglass products are more expensive than the traditional plaster- and resin-impregnated plaster products. However, *less* material will be used, and with the greater durability of the fiberglass products the cost is virtually the same. All fiberglass casting products have an expiration date stamped on the package, which should be observed. The rolls are stored in sealed foil pouches that, if punctured, result in premature hardening. The pouches should be kept in a cool, dry atmosphere and the stock rotated. The pouches should remain in the original shipping boxes to avoid excess handling and the possibility of puncturing. Refrigeration will increase shelf life. During the actual casting procedure, one pouch should be opened at a time to minimize exposure to air. The roll of fiberglass tape and its resin should feel soft and pliable. If curing has occurred within the pouch, the roll will feel firm and be difficult or impossible to unravel. Disposable gloves should be worn during the casting procedure because the resin will adhere to the skin, and allergic skin reactions are a possibility. Various fiberglass products have been compared, with no significant differences; however, their strength is superior to that of plaster (8, 9).

One of the disadvantages of the fiberglass products currently available is the relative difficulty in shaping the product to the contours of the limb, compared with plaster. This seems especially true in foals whereby sharper corners have to be turned during the application process. It is less of a problems than before but an alternative is the use of "combination" casts, which consist of a very thin layer of resin-impregnated plaster, and then apply fiberglass over the plaster or the use of special cast padding.

Veterinarians have been frequently confused regarding *how much* padding to use under a cast. A good rule to follow, stated simply, is "as little as possible." Through years of trial and error, it has become customary to use no more than two layers of orthopaedic stockinette. Some stockinette products are made of waterproof synthetic fiber, enabling hydrotherapy to be carried out *while the cast is on.* This is not a common method of therapy, and the authors do not

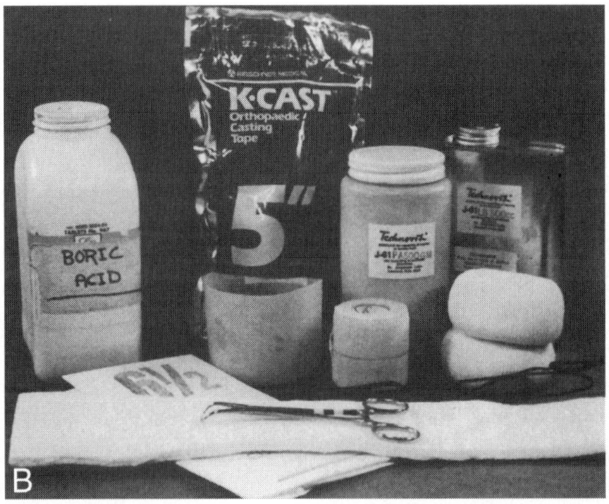

Figure 5.9, B. Equipment necessary for cast application (see Appendix I).

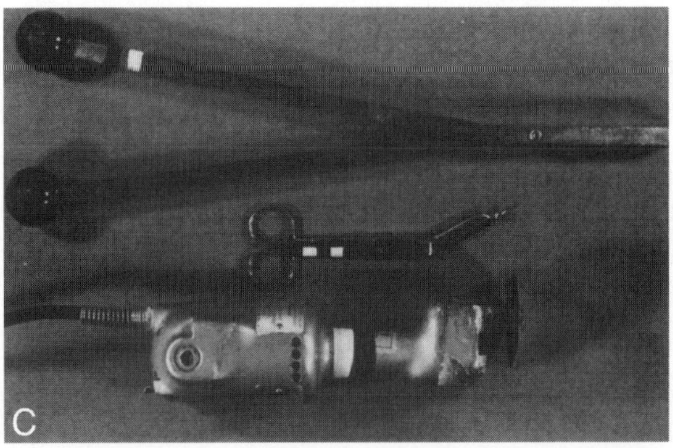

Figure 5.9, C. Equipment necessary for cast removal (see Appendix I).

insist that the stockinette be waterproof. The only bit of padding other than stockinette that is "permitted" is a strip of orthopaedic felt placed at the top of the cast or an anulus or ring of felt to protect the prominence over the accessory carpal bone if the cast extends above the carpal joint.

One final word of advice before cast application: the operator should always assemble *all* the equipment needed to apply the cast and attend to the wound *before general anesthesia is induced.*

The equipment necessary to apply the cast is listed in Appendix III and illustrated in Figure 5.9, *B* and *C.*

Technique of Cast Application

Method of Restraint

Cast application is difficult in the standing horse but can be done on a temporary basis using fiberglass material. An optimal job requires the animal to be motionless and relaxed. Nevertheless, cast application is occasionally indicated in standing horses for various reasons. Fractures of the long bones in yearlings and adults of such a size that physical restraint is out of the question are a real dilemma to manage on an emergency basis. Temporary immobilization is an important adjunct to treatment if the animal is to be transported to a facility where further treatment is undertaken. If the attending veterinarian is confident with intravenous anesthesia techniques, then a temporary bandage is applied, anesthesia is induced, and a cast is applied. However, a fiberglass cast is much easier to use in the standing horse than a plaster cast and is appropriate in many situations. Some fractures will be better handled using a Robert Jones dressing, with a lateral splint to prevent abduction, if the fracture is in the proximal two thirds of the radius or tibia (1).

The horse should be positioned in lateral recumbency with the limb to be cast uppermost. The limb should be in a "natural" position that will permit normal ambulation. Very slight flexion of the carpal joint will reduce the torsional forces at the fracture site (3). Because of the reciprocal apparatus, the hind limb will be more difficult to work with. Some slight flexion is desirable; but extension in the hind limb will make the limb considerably longer than the opposite member, and the horse will tend to drag it as this leg attempts to ambulate.

With the exception of tube casts, the cast should encase the *entire* foot and end proximally at one of four points: the proximal end of the radius/axillary region and the proximal end of the tibia/tibial crest region or immediately distal to the carpus or tarsus, where cannon bones start to flare. A cast should never end in the midmetacarpus (midmetatarsus) because it causes intense stress and severe rub sores. Ending the cast in the midtibia, midradius region will result in a loose cast when the animal stands and the muscles are under tension. This will be accentuated when muscle atrophy occurs if cast immobilization is prolonged.

The golden rule for fracture treatment stating "the joint above the fracture and the joint below the fracture must be immobilized" is, for the most part, applicable to the horse. The notable exception to this would be management of a *very* distal fracture of the tibia or radius. A full-limb cast does provide *some* immobilization of fractures in this region despite the inability to extend the cast above the elbow or stifle joint. Some of these fractures would obviously be supplemented with internal fixation.

Traction on the limb in some form or another is desirable in various instances. Traction will aid in positioning the limb as well as reducing and aligning the fracture fragments, especially comminuted fractures of the proximal and middle phalanges, and the cannon bones. The ideal method to provide traction is to drill holes in the hoof wall at the same angle as one would drive a horseshoe nail. Through these holes is looped a length of bailing wire, twisted on itself and wrapped around some sort of object that will allow an assistant to provide steady sustained traction during the casting procedure (Fig. 5.9*D*). A strong, well-trained assistant is indispensable during cast application in both foals and

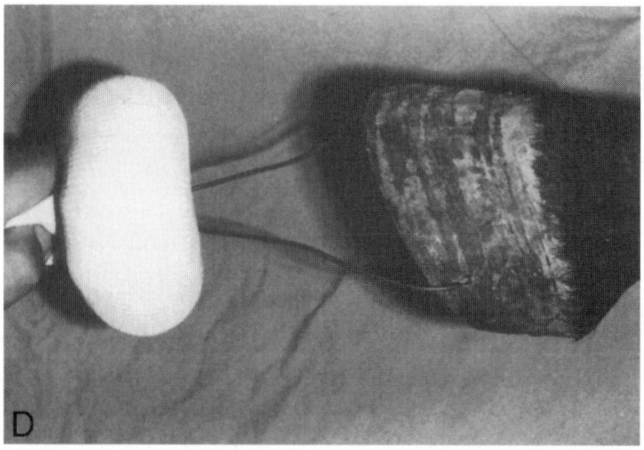

Figure 5.9, D. Baling wire used to provide traction. The stockinette is threaded over the wire in preparation to be rolled up the limb.

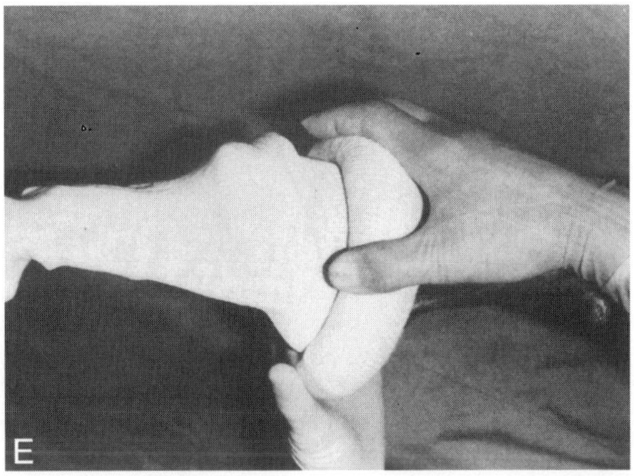

FIGURE 5.9, E. Stockinette being rolled up the limb without disrupting dressings or disturbing the flattened hair.

adult horses. Another assistant must diligently maintain alignment during the curing process. It is not uncommon for assistants to become so involved in the application of the cast that they neglect the posture of the limb. A common end result is a bow in the limb because of inadequate support under the carpus or tarsus. The assistant must support these areas with a *flattened* hand, so as not to indent the curing cast with the fingers.

PREPARATION OF THE LIMB

The wound or surgical site must be appropriately dressed and covered before application of the stockinette. This may entail clipping, shaving, debriding, and suturing, or any combination of these procedures. A nonadhering dressing held in position with some cotton gauze (e.g., Kling) is now applied. If a cast is being applied to reduce formation of granulation tissue, it is prudent to trim the granulation tissue *before* the cast is applied, preferably the day before casting. The authors prefer to trim granulation tissue as generously as possible, apply a pressure bandage to the wound to allow for hemostasis, and *then* apply the cast the following day. The skin under the cast should be dry and the hair flat.

APPLICATION OF STOCKINETTE AND FELT

One or two layers of stockinette are now rolled up the limb, rather than pulled, which would disrupt any dressings and disturb the flattened hair (Fig. 5.9*E*). The size of the stockinette is important. Excessively large stockinettes will not conform to the limb and will be "baggy," especially below the carpus and tarsus. Excessively small stockinettes will be impossible to stretch over the hoof or impossible to roll up over the more muscular parts of the limb in the case of a full-limb cast.

After the stockinette is in place, a strip of felt is positioned at the top of the cast and secured with a towel clamp (Fig. 5.9*F*). This felt and the stockinette are the *only* padding used in virtually all our casts, with one or two exceptions. For full-limb casts above the carpus, an anulus or "doughnut" of felt must be positioned and secured over the accessory carpal bone region (Fig. 5.9*G*). Some surgeons will apply a thin strip of felt around the coronet to protect this region from the oscillating saw during cast removal. With a tube cast, an additional strip of felt is necessary at the distal end of the cast.

APPLICATION OF FIBERGLASS TAPE

If available, a thin layer of resin-impregnated (or rapid-setting) plaster should be applied to the limb. This is an important step, especially in foals.

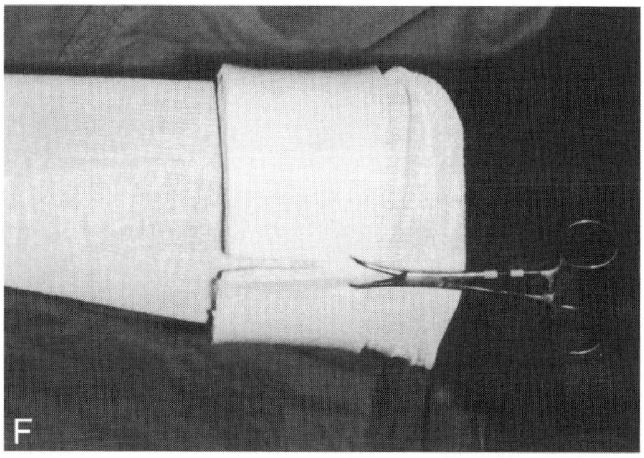

Figure 5.9, F. A strip of felt secured at the top of the limb by a towel clamp.

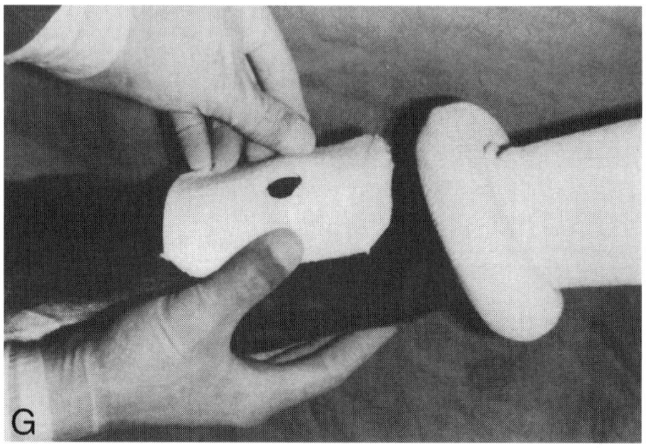

Figure 5.9, G. Positioning a specially shaped piece of felt over the accessory carpal bone region.

The fiberglass tape is available in various widths; 4-, 5-, and 6-inch widths are suitable for all sizes of horse. The authors prefer to begin the cast with a few layers of the narrower tape (e.g., 4 inches) because it seems easier to conform it to the contours of the limb and then use wider tape for succeeding layers (e.g., 5 or 6 inches) to expedite the procedure. In a comparison of 2-, 3-, 4-, and 5-inch width casting material, 5-inch material produced the strongest casts (10).

The tape is removed from its foil pouch and immersed in water for 10 to 15 seconds. The recommended temperature for curing is 70 to 75°F (room temperature), but this can be varied accordingly to alter the speed of curing. Warmer temperatures will decrease the curing time and are recommended only when the operator has become familiar with the product and has had experience with the casting technique. The tape should not be wrung out.

The tape is applied in a spiral fashion, first encircling the felt at the top of the cast and proceeding distad (Fig. 5.9*H*). If plaster has already been applied, the fiberglass can be applied directly over the plaster. The tape should overlap the previous turn by approximately one-half to one-third the width of the tape. Slightly more tension should be applied than the operator is used to with plaster products (Fig. 5.9*I*).

Exactly *how much* fiberglass to apply without compromising strength yet avoiding a cumbersome overweight cast is a matter of judgment, and certainly there is no substitute for experience. At least 3 to 4 layers are required for foals and 4 to 6 layers for adults. For the beginner, the first few casts may be a little heavier than desired, but subsequent ones can be made lighter when the properties of the fiberglass are discovered. A broken cast is not only expensive (time and materials) but can spell disaster if intended to protect internal fixation of a fracture during recovery from anesthesia. A broken cast will mean immediate anesthesia and re-application of a new and stronger cast.

To produce a smooth cast, the tape must be folded, twisted, or pleated. Small pleats are advisable in the more contoured areas such as the articulations over the fetlock (Fig. 5.9*J*).

Longitudinal splints of casting material used in plaster casts are not usually necessary with fiberglass because of its inherent strength, but splints may increase the strength of the cast (10). Nevertheless, the cast should be reinforced around and immediately below the carpal and tarsal joints, which are regions where full-limb casts frequently fail.

As the cast is constructed, it will become obvious that eventually the traction device must be removed. If the device was necessary for fracture reduction and alignment, it is advisable to wait 10 minutes until some curing has occurred so that fracture reduction is not compromised. Excess stockinette is then removed (Fig. 5.9*K*), followed by removal of the traction device by cutting the baling wire (Fig. 5.9*L*). The stockinette is folded up over the toe and an additional roll of fiberglass tape is used to encase the entire toe (Fig. 5.9*M*). An important step at this point is the construction of some form of heel block to reduce the fulcrum

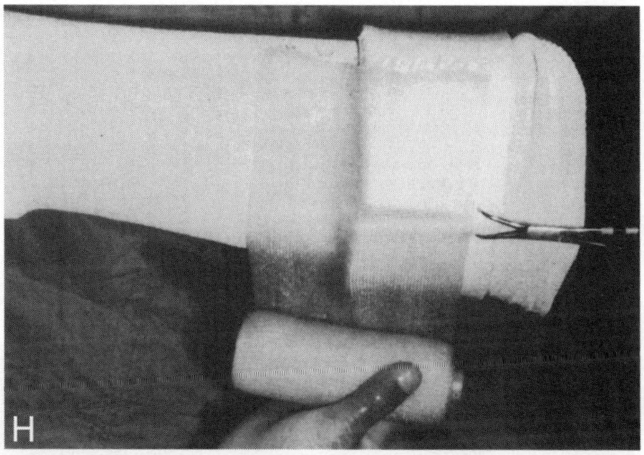

Figure 5.9, H. Application of the fiberglass tape, beginning at the top of the limb and proceeding distad.

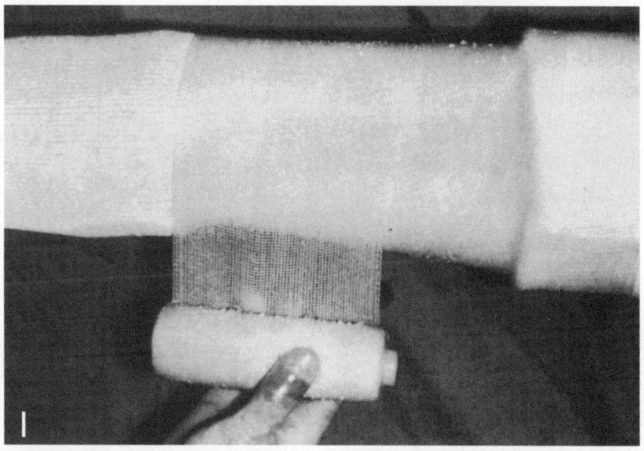

Figure 5.9, I. The tape should spiral distad, overlapping the previous turn by approximately one-half to one-third.

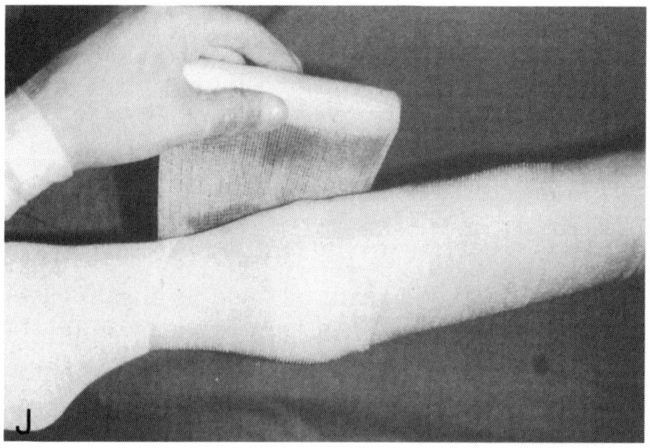

Figure 5.9, J. Folding or twisting tape in the more contoured areas such as the fetlock joint.

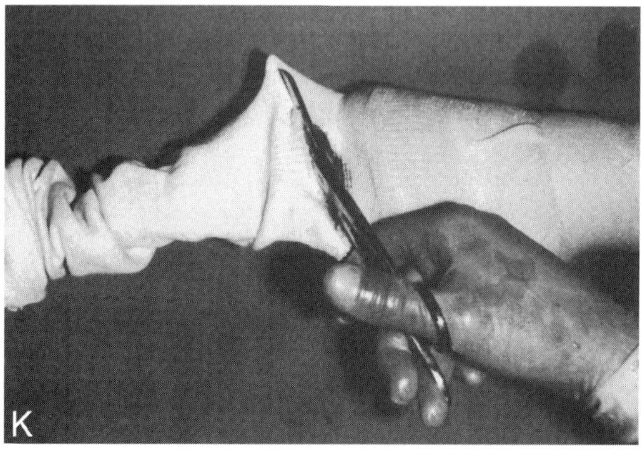

Figure 5.9, K. Removal of excess stockinette.

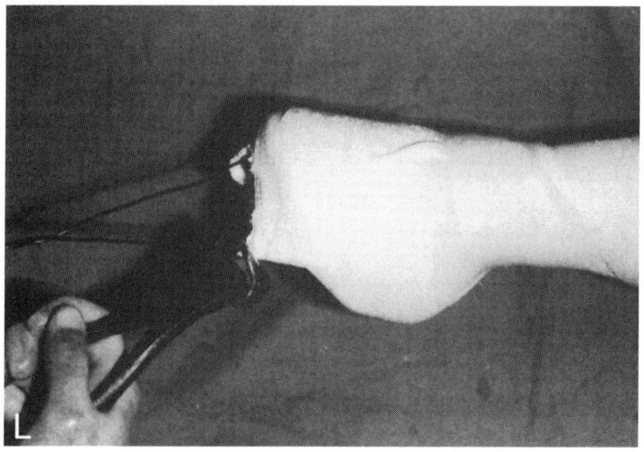

Figure 5.9, L. Removal of traction device.

effect that will occur if the horse bears weight purely on the toe and not the heel. The most expensive method is to place a roll of casting tape under the heel and secure this roll into position with the same roll of tape used to cover the toe (Fig. 5.9*N*). A cheaper method is to take a previously shaped block of wood that can be positioned and taped into place. At this point in the procedure an assistant should commence mixing the acrylic (optional) that will be used as a toe cap. An acrylic cap will reduce a lot of wear on the toe of the cast (Fig. 5.9*O*). The authors have found that fiberglass tape is easily abraded on rough surfaces as the horse walks. Once the toe has been exposed, reduction in the immobilizing effect of the cast is immediate, and movement will produce rubbing sores on the coronet and heel bulbs. Sufficient stockinette and cast

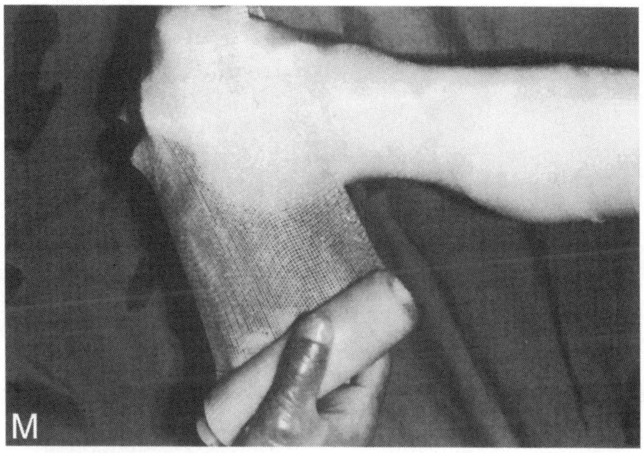

FIGURE 5.9, M. Encasing the entire foot with the cast.

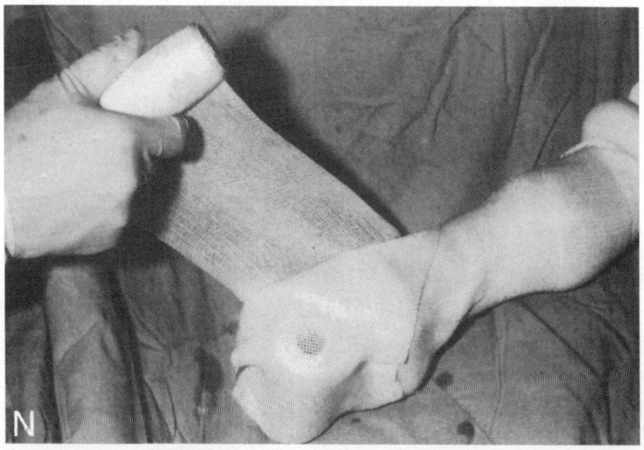

FIGURE 5.9, N. Roll of casting tape placed under the heel and secured in position with additional tape.

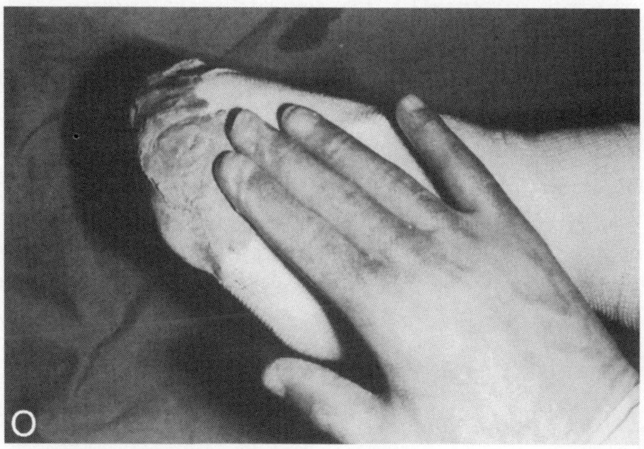

FIGURE 5.9, O. Acrylic cap placed on the toe to reduce excessive wear on the toe of the cast.

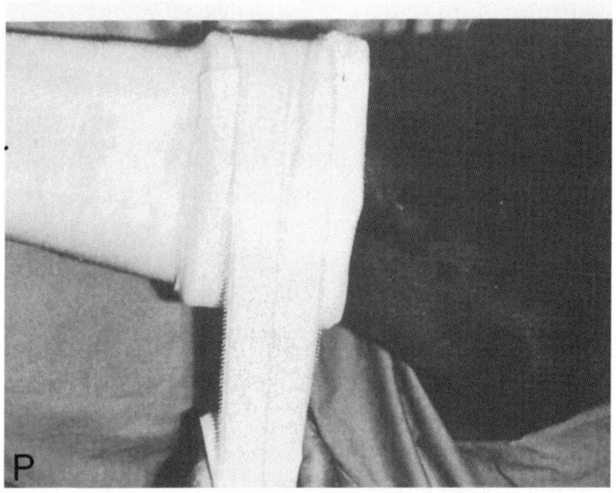

Figure 5.9, P. Elastic adhesive bandage applied to top of cast.

tape must be used to protect the toe from the exothermic reaction of the acrylic, but modern fiberglass tapes have a minimal exothermic reaction.

When the cast is complete and the toe cap (in the case of casts encasing the toe region) in place, silicone handcream is applied to the operator's gloved hands and then used to smooth out any sharp edges that may be remaining on the surface of the cast. The handcream should never be used until completion of the cast because it will interfere with adherence of succeeding layers of casting tape.

Adhesive dressing such as Elastikon is applied to the top of the cast to secure the stockinette (Fig. 5.9*P*). It can be spiraled onto the bare limb to "seal" the top of the cast, preventing hay and debris from entering the cast.

The currently quoted time required for the cast to harden to permit weightbearing in adult horses is 20 minutes. Certainly, it is unwise to take shortcuts at this point just to expedite the procedure. As mentioned, a broken cast because of inadequate time to cure is not only costly in time and materials but could potentially mean the demise of the horse.

Tube or Sleeve Cast

A sleeve cast is used primarily for orthopaedic conditions of the forelimb, such as collapsed or hypoplastic carpal bones in foals, and for this reason the description to follow will apply to the forelimb. The same principles apply to the hind limb, as this cast is also used in early cases of collapsed tarsal bones. A sleeve cast extends from the proximal end of the radius to slightly distal to the fetlock joint. The stockinette is applied to the limb and the orthopaedic felt is applied at the top of the cast in an identical fashion to that for the preceding cast. An additional piece of orthopaedic felt approximately 6 cm in width is then applied to the fetlock joint (Fig. 5.9*Q*).

The fiberglass tape is applied in a spiral fashion but ends at the fetlock joint articulation or slightly distal to it. Shortly into the curing process, the stockinette is cut at the tip of the toe and folded back on itself and taped onto the cast itself. This will cause the felt to curve around and produce a rounded edge of fiberglass tape that will be less likely to form a potentially dangerous sharp edge of fiberglass (Fig. 5.9*R*).

Convalescence

The equine patient with a limb in a cast must have diligent aftercare to ensure that minor problems do not develop into more serious ones. The patient should

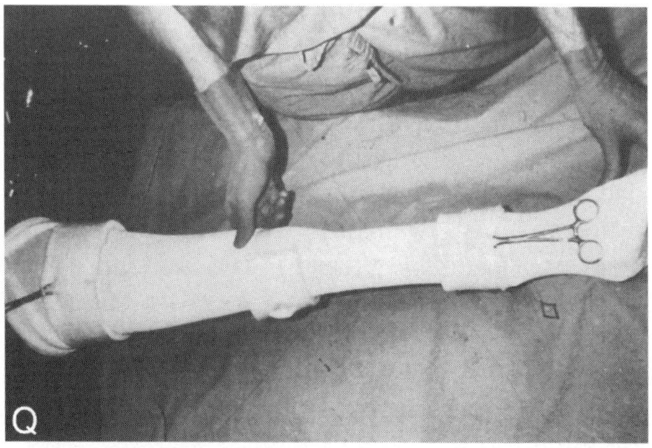

FIGURE 5.9, Q. Positioning of orthopaedic felt for a tube or sleeve cast. Note additional piece of orthopaedic felt at fetlock joint.

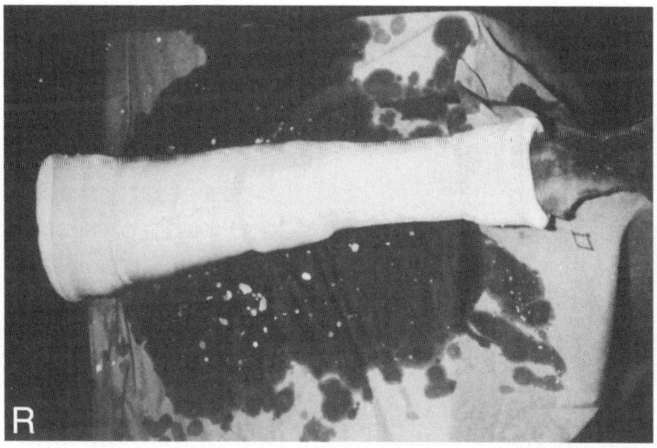

FIGURE 5.9, R. Completed tube or sleeve cast.

be hospitalized in a confined area with light bedding. The authors prefer straw. The bedding must be kept clean and dry. The cast should be closely inspected to see that it has not cracked. Frequently, cracks are not obvious and may be nothing more than hairline fissures that will open up when the animal places an excessive amount of weight on the limb. If a cast breaks, its immobilizing effect is lost. Casts seem to break in certain areas, such as the proximal extremities of the cannon bones just distal to the carpus or tarsus, or in the pastern region.

A patient with a cracked cast should be scheduled for general anesthesia and replacement of the cast at the earliest opportunity. If the cast has become completely separated into two units, it should be "patched up" with two or three rolls of fresh fiberglass tape immediately. If only a small hairline fissure has developed, it should be patched but the horse should be taken off feed and scheduled for general anesthesia and cast change the next day. No hard and fast rules can be established regarding the urgency of replacing a damaged cast; each case has to be evaluated individually.

The value of daily grooming, adequate nutrition, and general tender loving care for orthopaedic patients should never be underestimated (11).

Pressure sores and rubbing sores should not be regarded as "occupational hazards" of casting the limbs of horses. All attempts must be made to minimize them, but occasionally they occur no matter how meticulously the cast is applied. The thin, fine skin in foals is particularly susceptible to pressure and rubbing sores. The most consistent sign of serious problems developing under a cast *is increased reluctance to use the limb.* The authors encourage that, at least daily, the horse be walked just a few paces out of its box stall and then returned to the stall so that the amount of weightbearing can be monitored from one day to the next. If the horse appears less agile and more reluctant to step out on the cast, it should alert the clinician to a potential problem. When evaluating the use of the cast, one should always take into account if the horse is on analgesics such as nonsteroidal anti-inflammatory drugs. It is possible that such drugs are masking a serious problem under the cast. Swelling above the cast is cause for alarm and, in most cases, warrants a cast change to investigate the problem. If the cast has been used for an extensive soft tissue injury, swelling above the cast can be anticipated and remedied by pressure bandaging above the cast. If there is no apparent explanation for the swelling, a cast change should be scheduled as early as practical.

Pressure sores under a cast occur more frequently in certain sites, such as the accessory carpal bone, abaxial surface of the proximal sesamoid bones, and the proximal dorsal metacarpus/metatarsus in horses with casts that end in this region. Many pressure sores and rubbing sores will resolve merely by applying another cast. The next cast will often provide subtle alterations in fit that will allow the sores to resolve spontaneously. Rubbing and pressure sores should be cleaned of exudate and a nonadherent dressing applied and held in position with cotton gauze (e.g., Kling). Tetanus prophylaxis should be provided unless it was done previously.

Cast loosening is more likely to occur with the larger full-length casts that end in the muscular regions of the proximal parts of the forearm and crus. This is caused by muscle atrophy as a result of disuse and sometimes swelling reduction as a result of the immobilizing effect of the cast. If the limb is severely swollen as a result of soft tissue injuries or cellulitis, an attempt should be made to reduce the swelling with pressure bandaging, hydrotherapy, and anti-inflammatory drugs before the cast is applied.

Localized osteoporosis is a loss of mineral content of the bones that are immobilized within the cast. The problem is most severe in growing animals because of the rapid bone turnover and is most noticeable in the proximal sesamoid bones and phalanges (3). The process is reversible when the animal is free of the cast and some weightbearing is resumed. Despite its regular appearance, it is extremely rare for an animal with localized osteoporosis as a result of immobilization to sustain a pathologic fracture. The osteopenic effects of casting in the equine forelimb have been assessed using the noninvasive techniques of ultrasound velocity, single photon absorptiometry, and radiographic photodensitometry (12). The general trend was for the measures of bone quality in the limb in the cast to be reduced compared with the control. These values tended to recover after cast removal, particularly when full mobility was possible by returning the horse to a paddock 4 weeks after cast removal. The reduction in the bone parameters while the limb was in a cast was small. There were changes in the limb opposite the cast, implying the changes could be the result of operations associated with confinement. The small changes observed may be associated with the fact that the horses were still bearing weight on the immobilized limb. The authors considered that an 8-week period of immobilization would cause a greater degree of osteopenia than was demonstrated in this experiment.

A more insidious problem associated with immobilization of the limbs is atrophy of articular cartilage. Immobilization impairs the diffusion of nutrients into the articular cartilage from the synovium because of the absence of the intermittent loading of the joint. Joint stiffness, a problem that haunts human orthopaedic surgeons, does not seem a problem in horses unless the joint itself has been injured (3). Intra-articular fractures with accompanying joint capsule tearing are prone to this.

Joint laxity and flaccidity of the flexor tendons are also seen following cast

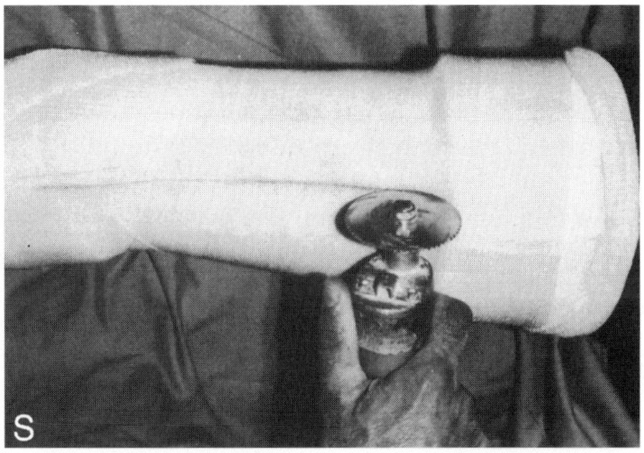

FIGURE 5.9, S. Cuts on the medial and lateral surfaces of the cast.

application, especially in foals. Shoes with heel extensions are required if the condition is severe.

Cast Removal

In adult horses, the cast can be left in place for 3 to 5 weeks unless complications develop. Casts on the limbs of foals should be changed at least every 14 days because of limb growth within the cast. Casts used to immobilize extensive soft tissue injuries may require changing every 10 to 14 days, depending on the amount of wound drainage and suppuration.

To remove a cast, an electric oscillating saw is the recommended instrument (Fig. 5.9*C*). Unfortunately, they are noisy, and sedation is often necessary. These saws will cut skin if they are not used with care. Cuts are made on the medial and lateral surfaces of the cast, as well as under the hoof (Fig. 5.9*S*). Because of its strength, it is essential that complete full thickness cuts be made when removing a fiberglass cast. It is virtually impossible to remove a cast by cutting one side and merely scoring the other side in the hope it will fracture down the scored side.

It is usual to cut the last cast off with the horse standing so that anesthesia can be avoided. If anesthesia is necessary, the resultant two halves of the cast can be reapplied to the limb to protect the injury while the horse is recovering from anesthesia and then removed with the horse standing.

Following removal of the cast, a "rebound" edema of the limb is common. Therefore, one should always anticipate pressure bandaging the limb for several weeks after cast application.

REFERENCES

1. Bramlage LR. Current concepts of emergency first aid treatment and transportation of equine fracture patients. Comp Contin Edu 1983;5:564.
2. Edwards GB, Clayton-Jones DG. Use of Hexcelite for the immobilization of the limbs of large animals. Vet Rec 1978;102:397.
3. Fessler JF, Turner AS. Methods of external coaptation. Symposium on Equine Orthopaedics. Vet Clin North Am Large Animal Pract 1983;5:311.
4. Horney FD, Dingwall J. The clinical use of light cast. Can Vet J 1975;16:201.
5. Nemeth F, Back W. The use of the walking cast to repair fractures in horses and ponies. Equine Vet J 1991;23:32–36.
6. McClure SR, Watkins JP, Bronson DG, et al. In vitro comparison of the standard

short limb cast and three configurations of short limb transfixation casts in equine forelimbs. Am J Vet Res 1994;155:1831–1834.
7. Parente EJ, Nunamaker DM. Stress protection afforded by a cast on plate fixation of the distal forelimb in the horse in vitro. Vet Surg 1995;24:49–54.
8. Bartels KE, Penwick RC, Freeman LJ, et al. Mechanical testing and evaluation of eight synthetic casting materials. Vet Surg 1985;14:310–318.
9. Houlton JEF, Breorley MJ. A comparison of some casting materials. Vet Rec 1985; 117:55–58.
10. Wilson DG, Vanderby R. An evaluation of fiberglass cast application techniques. Vet Surg 1995;24:118–121.
11. Dingwall JS, Horney FD, McDonnel W, et. al. A comparison of breaking strengths of various casting materials. Can Vet J 1973;14:62.
12. Buckingham SHW, Jeffcott LB. Osteopenic effects of forelimb immobilization in homes. Vet Rec 1991;128:370–373.

Harvesting of Cancellous Bone Graft

Autogenous cancellous bone grafting is an important adjunctive procedure in the treatment of certain orthopaedic problems in the horse. Cancellous bone grafting is used in the horse (*a*) as an aid in the ossification of defects accompanying primary internal fixation of fractures; (*b*) in the treatment of delayed union or nonunions; (*c*) in the treatment of osteomyelitis; (*d*) in the promotion of surgical arthrodesis; (*e*) in the healing of midbody and basal sesamoid fractures; and (*f*) to promote healing in the treatment of subchondral cystic lesions. Cancellous bone is the usual form of bone graft used in the horse because of its excellent osteogenic and osteoinductive properties, as well as its ready availability (1).

The fate of autogenous cancellous bone grafting following transplantation has been the subject of many studies. It is generally believed that few cells survive the transplantation procedure, although both donor and recipient cells should be considered as contributing to the new cell population. More importantly, the graft stimulates the formation of new bone by osteoinduction (properly attributed to bone morphogenic protein [BMP]) and other growth factors) (2) and also provides a scaffold for ingrowth of blood vessels and multipotential mesenchymal cells (osteoconduction) (3). It is well recognized that autogenous cancellous bone revascularizes more quickly than homogenous cancellous bone with an earlier and greater production of new bone. In addition, autogenous cancellous bone is immunologically more desirable (4). Note that a cancellous graft should be placed, ideally, in a region of rich blood supply.

Harvesting of cancellous bone graft is generally performed while surgery is being done on another part of the body (e.g., internal fixation of a long bone fracture or surgical exposure of a sesamoid fracture). To minimize operating time, the use of two surgical teams is appropriate. If surgery time is delayed, the graft will suffer unnecessary exposure, thereby decreasing survival of graft cells (5). The exposure of the cancellous bone is timed so that graft material can be transferred immediately from the donor site to the surgical region.

Harvesting of cancellous bone from the tuber coxae and sternum is described (5–7). The proximal tibia is an alternative, and this procedure has been reported to be safe despite previous questions on the potential for pathologic fractures (4).

Anesthesia and Surgical Preparation

Harvesting of bone from the tuber coxae is done with the horse under general anesthesia and in lateral recumbency. Generally, the tuber coxae that will be up when the horse is under surgery for the primary problem will be selected. A large area over the tuber coxae should be clipped before induction of anesthesia. Immediately before or after induction, the immediate area of the tuber coxae is shaved and surgical preparation is then made. The plastic adhesive drape is used.

Harvesting of cancellous bone from the sternum is done with the horse under general anesthesia and in dorsal recumbency. A large area of sternum is clipped and the skin shaved from the manubrium to the xiphoid and extends 15 cm to each side. The area is surgically prepared and a plastic adhesive drape used.

Additional Instrumentation

It is convenient to have two sets of instruments, one for the primary procedure and the other for the bone graft, because the surgeons are usually working on opposite sides of the horse.

Surgical Technique

Tuber Coxae

There are two different approaches to the tuber coxae. The technique depicted uses a skin incision that passes in a perpendicular fashion over the tuber coxae as illustrated in Figure 5.10*A*. The length of the incision will vary according to the amount of bone graft needed (from 10 to 25 cm). If a small amount of graft is required, as with sesamoid bone grafting, a small incision is sufficient. If a major amount of cancellous bone will be removed, as with an involved fracture, the incision must be larger to allow greater exposure of the tuber coxae. An alternative approach is to make a curvilinear incision over the caudal aspect of the tuber coxae and reflect the skin craniad. The subcutaneous tissue and fascia are incised in the same plane as the skin to expose the tuber coxae (Fig. 5.10*B*). An incision is then made in the periosteum that outlines the area of the cortical window that will be made to expose the cancellous bone beneath (Fig. 5.8*B*). This incision passes through the lateral cortex of the tuber coxae and will be 5 × 2.5 cm if a large amount of bone is to be removed. An osteotome is used to cut a window through the bone (Fig. 5.10*C*). If a small amount of bone is required, a quarter-inch drill hole through the cortex is often sufficient. Once the osteotome has incised through the cortex into the cancellous bone space, the segment of corticocancellous bone is removed and discarded. Cancellous bone within the tuber coxae is then removed with a curette as required (Fig. 5.10*C*). Following completion of graft harvesting, the area is flushed with saline solution to remove all debris. The cortical bone is not replaced and only the soft tissue is closed. The fascia and subcutaneous tissue are closed with interrupted sutures of 2/0 synthetic absorbable material. The skin is closed with a row of simple interrupted or vertical mattress sutures using nonabsorbable monofilament material supported by vertical mattress tension sutures (Fig. 5.10*D*). A stent bandage using a roll of gauze (Kling) is sewn over the surgical site.

In young animals, a thick layer of cartilage will be found over the end of the tuber coxae. The bone is soft enough that a curette can usually be used to create the window.

Harvesting of Bone from the Sternum

This technique uses a midline skin incision extending from a point approximately 20 cm cranial to the xiphoid and extending 10 cm caudad (6). The incision is continued through the subcutaneous tissue and pectoral musculature until the ventral aspect of the caudal sternum is exposed (Fig. 5.10*E*). The pectoral muscle is then elevated from the sternum on either side of midline using a periosteal elevator (Fig. 5.10*F*). Cartilage that forms the ventral border of the sternum is then removed with rongeurs until cancellous bone is exposed (Fig. 5.10*G*). If 1 to 2 cm of cartilage is removed without identifying cancellous bone, the procedure should be repeated 2 cm cranial or caudal to this site. However, the occurrence of this problem is usually obviated by using the caudal sternebrae, not the cranial sternebra. The caudal sternebrae have less muscle and less cartilage covering the cancellous bone. In addition, the cranial aspect of the sternum has a large keel of cartilage for the attachment of the pectoral muscles, and the caudal sternebrae are closer to each other. After exposure of the cancellous bone, a large curette is used to remove as much cancellous bone as possible (Fig. 5.10, *H* and *I*). The cancellous bone is easily distinguished from cartilage. The presence of cartilage on the curette signifies removal of all cancellous bone within a particular sternebra. After completion of graft harvesting, the area is flushed with sterile solution to remove all debris. The muscle and subcutaneous tissues are apposed in two layers with simple interrupted sutures of 0 synthetic absorbable material. The skin is closed with a row of simple interrupted or

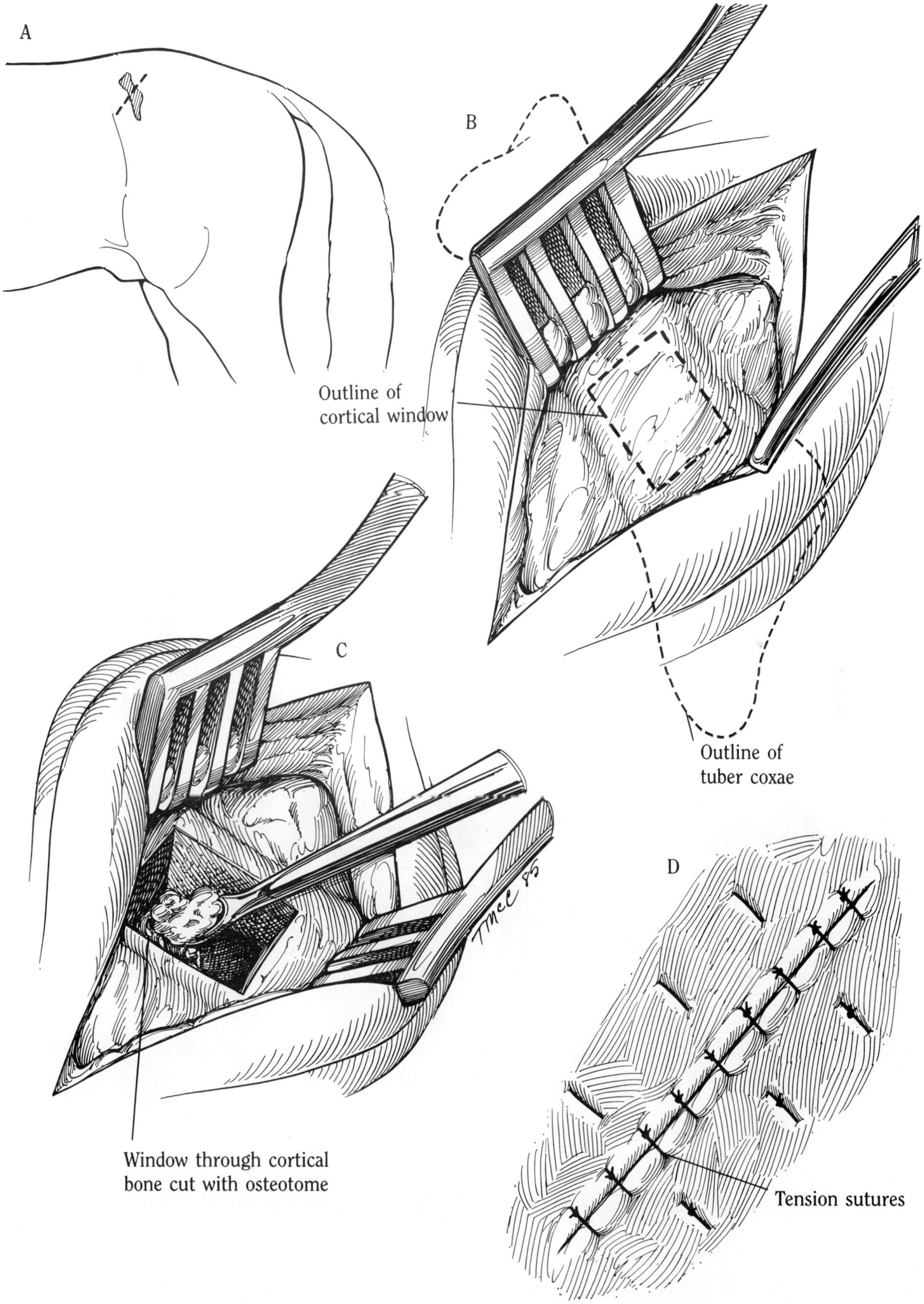

FIGURE 5.10, A–D. Harvesting of cancellous bone.

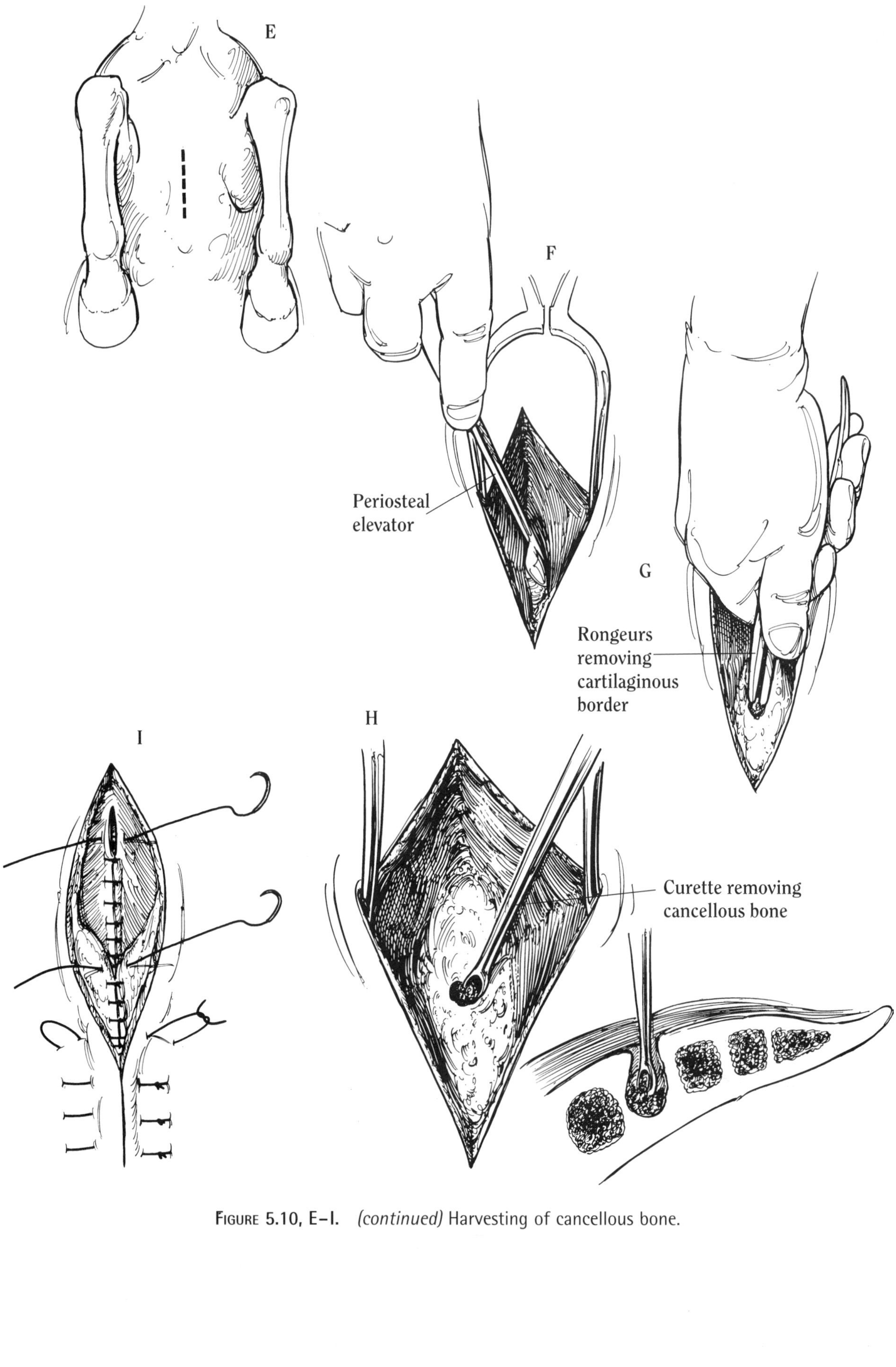

Figure 5.10, E–I. *(continued)* Harvesting of cancellous bone.

vertical mattress sutures using nonabsorbable monofilament material. A stent bandage using a roll of gauze (Kling) is then sewn over the surgical site.

Postoperative Management

Phenylbutazone is administered postoperatively because pain from the graft site can be severe. Antibiotics are not necessary for the graft harvesting itself, but they may be used depending on the other, primary surgical procedure being performed. If the graft is removed before the recipient site has been prepared, it should be placed on a sponge moistened with blood. The stent bandage is removed in 1 week, the tension sutures in 10 days, and the skin sutures closing the incision are removed in 14 days.

Comments

Alternative approaches to the tuber coxae, including the use of curvilinear incisions away from the prominence of the tuber coxae and a window in the gluteal cortex of the ileum, have been described. However, the technique described here is simpler, and the authors have not experienced complications with it. It is important that the only cortex removed is from the end of the ilium, as damage to cortex on the sides could promote postoperative fracture.

The experience gained from experimental and clinical cases indicates that the sternum is a suitable site for collection of cancellous bone and is readily accessible when the horse is in dorsal recumbency (6). The main advantages of this site are the absence of tension in the skin, the dependent location of the site, and ease of access in dorsal recumbency. The most common complication reported is peri-incisional edema and serum drainage, but most incisions heal without problems. It has been shown that the defect in the sternebra heals by second intention. Although the amount of bone healing has not been defined, there appears to be no problems with instability or pathologic fractures of the sternum (6). Other alternatives to autogenous cancellous bone grafting have been evaluated and include ceramics composed of calcium phosphate salts with a calcium:phosphorus ratio close to that of bone, demineralized bone matrix (which contains BMP), or pure forms of BMP (8). At present it is thought that from a practical and economic point of view, autogenous bone tends to be the "gold standard" in promoting bone formation in defects in the horse. The use of the ceramic material β-tricalcium phosphate was evaluated in surgically created subchondral bone defects in horses with no advantage shown when compared with control defects (9).

REFERENCES

1. DeVries WJ, Runyon CL, Martinez SA. Effect of volume variations on osteogenic capabilities of autogenous cancellous bone graft in dogs. Am J Vet Res 1996;57:1501–1505.
2. Heiple KG, Goldberg VM, Powell AE, et al. Biology of cancellous bone grafts. Orthop Clin North Am 1987;18:179–185.
3. Turner AS. Large animal orthopaedics. In: Jennings PB, ed. Practice of Large Animal Surgery. Philadelphia: WB Saunders, 1984.
4. Boero MJ, Schneider JE, Mosier JE, et al. Evaluation of the tibia as a source of autogenous cancellous bone in the horse. Vet Surg 1989;18:322–327.
5. Stashak TS, Adams OR. Collection of bone grafts from the tuber coxae of the horse. JAVMA 1975;167:397.
6. Richardson GL, Pool RR, Pascoe JR, et al. Autogenous cancellous bone grafts from the

sternum in horses. Comparison with other donor sites and results of use in orthopaedic surgery. Vet Surg 1986;1:9–15.
7. Slocum B, Chalman JA. Cancellous bone graft from the wing of the equine ilium: the surgical approach. Arch Am Coll Vet Surg 1975;4:39.
8. Burchardt H, Enneking WF. Transplantation of bone. Surg Clin North Am 1978;58: 403.
9. Rose PL, Auer JA, Hulse D, et al. Effect of β-tricalcium phosphate in surgically created subchondral bone defects in male horses. Am J Vet Res 1988;49:417–424.

Transphyseal Bridging With Screws and Wire

Angular limb deformities in foals are frequently caused by an imbalance of physeal growth. For various reasons, endochondral ossification is proceeding faster on one side of the growth plate than the other. The clinical appearance is a valgus or varus deformity. A *valgus* deformity is defined as a deviation of the line away from the midline distal to the joint in which the deviation originates (1). A *varus* deformity is a deviation of the limb toward the midline distal to the joint in which the deviation originates. The most common location of angular limb deformities is the carpal joint, where valgus deformities predominate (2–4). In the authors' experience, the next most common location is the fetlock varus deformity, with carpus varus and tarsus valgus being less common. Other deformities (e.g., tarsus varus) are extremely rare.

Conservative therapy is adequate for the management of most angular limb deformities seen in equine clinical practice. This would include trimming of the hooves to remove the fulcrum effect caused by a long toe and confinement to reduce concussive forces that would occur if unrestricted exercise were permitted.

As part of the clinical examination of a foal with an angular limb deformity, a radiograph of the affected joint is indicated. This is particularly important in the carpal joint, where the radiograph may reveal abnormalities within the bones of the carpus or at the level of the proximal ends of the metacarpal bones. If these abnormalities are severe, surgery is not indicated because it will not be directed at the primary abnormality. Such foals may be candidates for other methods of therapy, such as "tube" casting (4).

Before attempting surgery that relies on active growth of a physis, it is vital that the surgeon realize how much *growth potential* remains in that physis. Although it is useful to know from radiographs when a growth plate has closed, it is of greater importance to the surgeon to know when the physis has completed most of its growth. For example, although radiographic evidence of closure of the distal metacarpal and metatarsal physes is seen at approximately 9 months, it is well known by surgeons who have attempted to correct angular deformities of the fetlock joint that most of the growth in this region is complete by 3 months of age. Therefore, it is the authors' belief that deformities of the fetlock joint should be operated on as soon as they are noticed, instead of adopting a wait-and-see policy that may work in certain deformities of the carpus and tarsus. Certain angular deformities of the distal metacarpus and metatarsus, as well as diaphyseal angular deformities, can be corrected only by a wedge osteotomy and internal fixation using compression plating techniques (5, 6). These techniques are beyond the scope of this book; the reader is encouraged to consult the bibliography.

Although the radiographic closure of the distal radial physis occurs between 24 and 30 months, most of the longitudinal growth has occurred by 9 to 10 months. Surgery is not advocated at this late stage either because continual asymmetric loading of the carpal or tarsal joints for this condition can lead to osteoarthritic changes. For this reason, surgery on the carpal and tarsal joints should be done when the foal is between 6 weeks and 4 months of age. One other factor that is operational in making such a decision is the severity of the deviation. If a relatively mild deformity has been steadily correcting itself following hoof trimming and confinement, the surgeon may elect to delay surgery for a few weeks. This approach is not applicable to the fetlock joint.

Metallic implants to cause temporary physeal arrest have been used to correct certain angular limb deformities in man and animals. The aim of such surgical procedures is to temporarily bridge the metaphysis to the epiphysis, causing retardation of maturation and calcification of endochondral ossification on the metaphyseal side of the growth plate that will decrease longitudinal bone growth on that side. Metal staples have been used to bridge physes in both foals and children. The technique was modified in 1972 and now utilizes an ASIF bone screw placed on each side of the physis, with two figure-8 wires connecting the heads (7). This is, in the authors' opinion, the preferred method because the implants are easier to remove and the screws can be inserted independently at convenient sites on either side of the physis. In addition, it is believed that immediate compression is applied across the growth plate, thereby hastening correction, and the implants are stronger than staples (2, 3). Even though they are placed extraperiosteally, less soft tissue blemish is associated with the use of screws and wire than with staples (2).

The procedure can be done alone or in combination with the technique of hemicircumferential transection of the periosteum and periosteal stripping for certain deformities, particularly in the fetlock joint, and is described in the next section of this book. The procedure of transphyseal bridging using screws and wire also has been done in calves and llamas (8, 9).

Anesthesia and Surgical Preparation

The surgery is done under general anesthesia. Inhalation anesthesia such as halothane is preferable. In most foals that are candidates for this surgery, anesthesia can be induced by administration of the gas by mask. Anesthesia in older foals can be induced by intravenous techniques and maintained by an inhalation anesthetic. The foal is then placed in lateral recumbency with the side of the metaphysis/epiphysis to be bridged uppermost.

If the screws and wire are to be combined with the periosteal stripping procedure, the screws and wire should be inserted first because the risk of wound infection is higher and demand for asepsis greater when implants such as these are used. If both procedures are being done on the same growth plate, both surgical sites must be clipped, shaved, and prepared for surgery in a routine manner. A sterile plastic adhesive drape is applied to the limb so that it is tightly adherent to both surgical sites and stuck to itself in a seam at the cranial or caudal surface of the limb.

Additional Instrumentation

Transphyseal bridging requires a 3.2-mm drill bit (if ASIF cortical bone screws are to be used) or a 3.6-mm drill bit (if ASIF cancellous bone screws are to be used). An assortment of cortical or fully threaded cancellous bone screws, ranging from 32 to 40 mm in length, is required. Also needed are the corresponding 4.5-mm or 6.5-mm cancellous bone tap, 4.5- or 6.5-mm ASIF tap sleeves, a power or hand-held drill, 18-gauge (1–2 mm) stainless steel wire, a wire twister of the surgeon's preference, and wire cutters. Equipment for taking intraoperative radiographs (without compromising sterile technique) is necessary. This includes a portable x-ray machine, sterile cassette covers, and cassettes.

Surgical Technique

Distal End of the Radius (Carpus Valgus Deformity)

An 8- to 9-cm semi-elliptical incision is made with the apex facing caudally, centered over the medial radial epicondyle. The incision should end distally, at the level of the antebrachiocarpal joint (Fig. 5.11*A*). The skin and subcutaneous flap that has been created is reflected craniad, and its apex is grasped carefully with a Backhaus towel clamp. The distal radial physis is then located by probing the most prominent area in the surgical field with an 18- or 20-gauge sterile disposable hypodermic needle. Probing is best done by "walking" the needle along the metaphysis distad toward the epiphysis, exerting firm pressure by the index finger placed over the hub of the needle (Fig. 5.11*B*). Small hematomas may result from this procedure but are of no consequence. If the surgeon is unsure of where the needle is located, then an intraoperative radiograph is indicated at this point. As an additional aid, another needle can be placed in the antebrachiocarpal joint and a radiograph then taken.

To facilitate placement of the screw in the distal radial epiphysis, a small stab incision is made in the collateral ligament that invests the epiphysis of the distal extremity of the radius. A 3.6-mm or 3.2-mm hole is drilled to a depth of approximately 40 mm in the distal radial epiphysis, attempting to go parallel to the plane of the growth plate and antebrachiocarpal (radiocarpal) joint space. If a cortical bone screw is to be used, then a 3.2-mm drill bit will be used; if a cancellous bone screw is being used, either a 3.6-mm or a 3.2-mm drill can be used. If the operation is being performed by the surgeon for the first time, the authors recommend that the surgeon take an intraoperative radiograph at this point to check if the drill, and subsequently the screw, is likely to endanger the physis or, more importantly, to invade the antebrachiocarpal joint. The soft tissues should be protected during drilling (and tapping) of these holes by using the appropriate tap sleeve. Once the surgeon is confident with this operation, insertion of the first screw hole can be done "freehand" without intraoperative radiographs. The hole is then tapped, using the 4.5mm tap (cortical screws) or 6.5-mm tap (cancellous screws) and protecting the soft tissue with the appropriate tap sleeve (Fig. 5.11*B*). Tapping is an optional step, and it has been recommended that the screw in the epiphysis be placed in a self-tapping manner because the bone is relatively soft (10).

A 4.5-mm cortical or 6.5-mm fully threaded cancellous bone screw of 32 to 38 mm in length is inserted. The screw should not be tightened to a point that the head disappears below the level of the collateral ligament. After this step, the authors advise obtaining an intraoperative radiograph regardless of the surgeon's experience because placement of this screw is one of the most critical steps of the whole operation. While the radiograph is being developed, the second remaining screw can be inserted in the metaphyseal region in a similar manner to the first. The hole should be placed in one cortex only. Because the bone is denser in this region, threads should be cut in the hole using the appropriate tap. The location of this screw is much less critical than the one located in the distal radial epiphysis; however, it must be located so that neither it nor the wire lies directly under the skin incision. If this occurs, infection may enter through the skin incision and establish itself around the implants during the convalescence. A chronically draining wound or even localized osteomyelitis and screw loosening may occur. The screw should not be seated so deeply that the head is buried in the bone.

Two independently placed figure-8 wires should be placed around the heads of the screws. The wire should be twisted to produce a symmetrically even twist in the wire (Fig. 5.11*C*). The wire is then cut and the protruding twisted piece of wire bent down so that it lies alongside the figure-8 wire. A second, similarly placed piece of wire is applied directly over the first, and the twisted ends are folded down beside the wire loops pointing distally so that no sharp pieces of wire protrude from the surgical site (Fig. 5.11*C*). This is also important to facilitate removal. Any sharp protruding pieces of wire may cause pressure necrosis of the skin during the convalescence.

There are numerous ways to join or twist wire to prevent it from loosening.

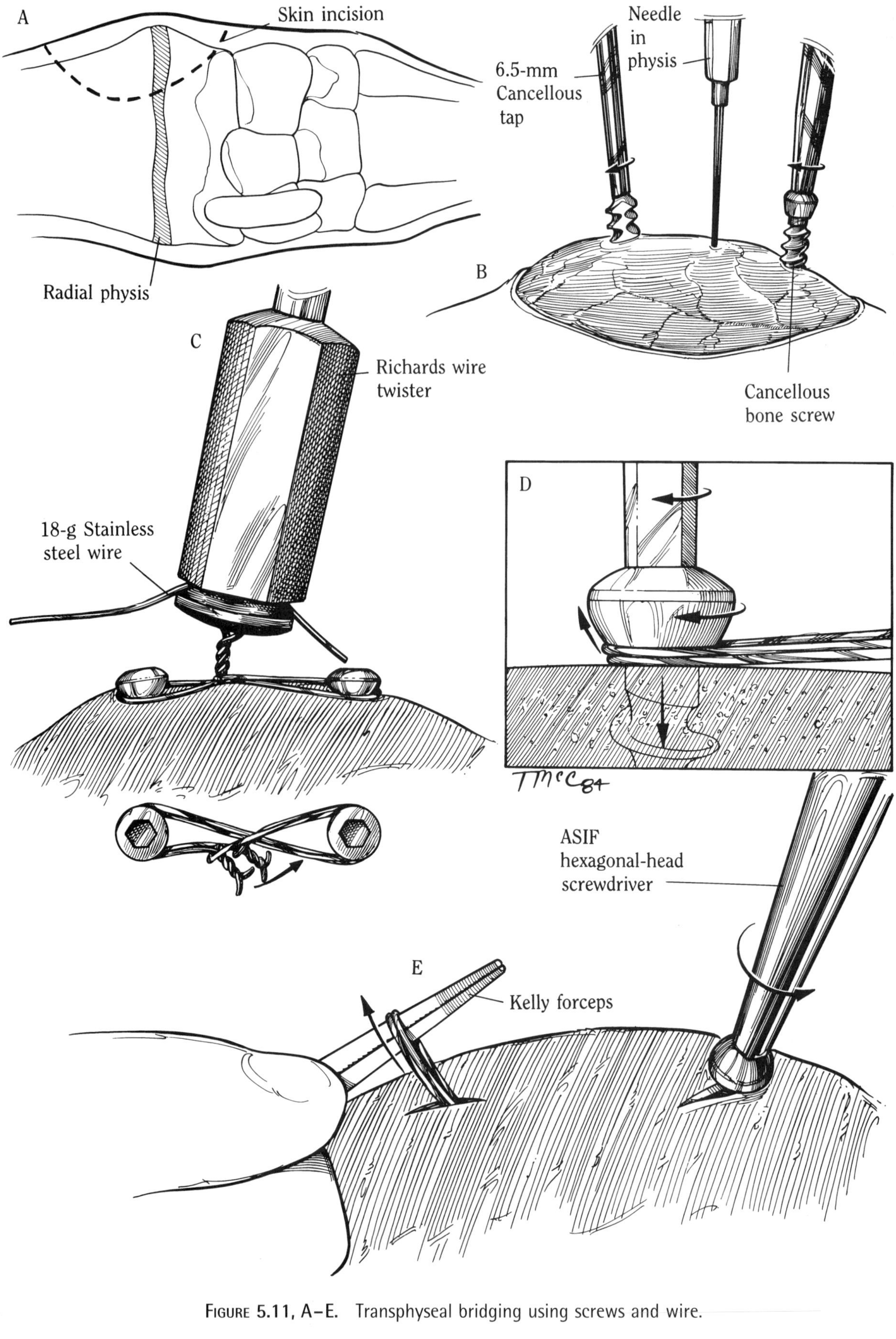

Figure 5.11, A–E. Transphyseal bridging using screws and wire.

Some texts advocate the ASIF cerclage wire tightener, which uses a hook-in-eye configuration to hold the wire (10). Specially prepared ASIF 1.2-mm cerclage wire with a loop twisted on the end by the manufacturer is required. The authors prefer the wire twister manufactured by Richards (Richards Manufacturing Company, Memphis, TN) but believe that surgeons should use whatever they are comfortable with. When the surgeon is satisfied with the security of both wires, additional tension is then brought about in the wires by alternately tightening the screws. The wire will slide along the inclined plane of the spherical screw heads (Fig. 5.11*D*). The screws should not be tightened so much that they disappear from sight or that the wire slips off the heads (10). The surgeon should palpate the implants with the index finger to check that they are not protruding excessively.

The subcutaneous tissues are very thin in this area, but the authors strongly recommend that they be apposed over the implants during closure. A simple continuous suture of synthetic absorbable suture material should be used. Catgut is not recommended in this region because of its inflammatory properties. The skin edges are apposed using a simple interrupted pattern with the appropriate synthetic monofilament suture material. At this point, an intraoperative radiograph is taken to check for correct placement of implants and for documentation in case postoperative problems arise.

Distal Ends of the Third Metacarpal and Metatarsal Bones

Angular limb deformities resulting from an imbalance of growth of the distal metacarpal or metatarsal physis are not as common as those occurring in the carpus. Because the distal metacarpal and metatarsal growth plates close much sooner, surgery for angular limb deformities of this region should be attempted as soon as the deformity is noticed, provided the foal is less than 2½ months of age. The authors also recommend that these deformities be treated by hemicircumferential transection of the periosteum and periosteal stripping on the opposite metaphysis of that bone, *as well* as the transphyseal bridging described here.

Varus deformities in this region are the usual situation. In this case, transphyseal bridging is done on the lateral aspect of the physeal region, and the periosteal stripping is done on the medial side. The surgical procedure is essentially the same as described for bridging of the distal radial physis. A semi-elliptical skin incision is made, making sure to stay dorsal to the palmar (plantar) vein artery and nerve in the region of the fetlock joint and at the same time ensuring there is no potential for implants to be situated directly under the skin incision. Because the epiphysis of these bones is relatively larger compared with the distal radial or tibial epiphyses, there is a little more room for error during the placement of the distal bone screw. Nevertheless, an intraoperative radiograph is indicated to be absolutely sure the metacarpophalangeal joint space or the physis has not been invaded and relocation of the screw is not indicated. Closure of the skin and subcutaneous layers should be performed meticulously in this area.

Distal End of the Tibia

Deformities caused by an imbalance of growth of the distal tibial physis are less common. Screw and wire insertion can be performed, but it requires meticulous placement of the distal bone screw because of the irregular shape of the distal tibial epiphysis. Intraoperative radiographs are mandatory for this surgery because it is relatively easy to inadvertently place the screw into the tarsocrural joint space. The screw in the epiphysis must therefore be angled upward to prevent this. The authors recommend taking an intraoperative radiograph following the placement of a sterile disposable hypodermic needle in both the physes and the tarsocrural joint. Another intraoperative radiograph is recommended to check the direction of the drill bit. Placement of the screw in the metaphysis is relatively straightforward. The end result will be two screws placed in different directions, something that cannot be achieved readily with staples.

Postoperative Management

A sterile nonadhesive dressing is placed over the incision, and then the affected joint is bandaged with materials of the surgeon's choice. A full-limb bandage using cotton may be indicated, but the authors believe that a light gauze and elastic adhesive bandage covering only the affected joint may be all that is required if carefully applied.

The authors believe perioperative antibiotics are indicated because implants such as screws have been shown to increase the likelihood of infection (6). Nonsteroidal anti-inflammatory drugs are not generally indicated. If the foal becomes lame during the convalescence, the causes of the lameness should be identified quickly and treated aggressively.

The foal should be confined during the convalescence to reduce concussion on the growth plates. The hooves should receive the appropriate trimming. Frequently, foals are fed mineral supplements or given injections of various vitamins. The authors believe these are unnecessary in most situations unless a true deficiency can be identified. Certainly, older animals undergoing this surgery (e.g., weanlings) should be fed a ration that has the appropriate calcium: phosphorus ratio. Analysis of the diet of older foals frequently reveals a mineral imbalance. The status of other trace minerals as an adjunct to the treatment of angular limb deformities in foals should also be determined; for example, a zinc excess or copper deficiency may exist in individual instances.

Implant Removal

When the axis of the limb is straight, the implants must be removed to prevent *overcorrection* of the deformity. Owners must be alerted to this, and good client education and communication are essential in this regard.

Removal of the screws and wire with the foal standing and under local anesthesia (around the screw heads) should not be considered because an uncooperative foal can easily cause a break in aseptic technique, especially if difficulty arises in locating the distal screw.

To remove the screws, a stab incision is made over the more readily palpable proximal (metaphyseal) screw head. Subcutaneous tissues are parted, using a mosquito hemostat, and then the hexagonally shaped "well" in the head of the screw is located. The hexagonal-tipped screw driver is carefully manipulated into the head of the screw to remove the screw (Fig. 5.11*E*). A second stab incision is made in the vicinity of the head of the distal screw, and the hexagonal well in the screw head is located. Typically, more fibrous tissue will be covering the screw head of the distal screw. This screw is now removed (Fig. 5.11*E*). A pair of curved Kelly forceps is used to retrieve the two pieces of wire that formed a loop around the proximal screw head by hooking the tip of the forceps through this loop and bending the two bits of wire out the proximal stab incision. When the forceps are securely anchored through both pieces of wire, the wire is pulled out the *proximal* incision with a sharp tug. An assistant will be required to hold the limb during this maneuver (Fig. 5.11*E*).

One or two simple interrupted skin sutures are placed in each stab incision, and a light pressure bandage is applied to the affected joint for 7 to 10 days. Skin sutures are removed in 10 days.

REFERENCES

1. Fretz PB, Pharr JW, McIlwraith CW, et al. Varus vs. valgus. [Letter] JAVMA 1982;181: 636.
2. Fretz PB, Turner AS, Pharr J. Retrospective comparison of two surgical techniques for correction of angular limb deformities in foals. JAVMA 1975;172:281.
3. Leitch M. Angular limb deformities arising in the carpal region in foals. Compend Cont Edu Pract Vet 1979;1:539.
4. Leitch M. Musculoskeletal disorders in neonatal foals. Symposium on neonatal equine disease. Vet Clin North Am Equine Pract 1985;1:189.
5. Fretz PB, McIlwraith CW. Wedge osteotomy for angular limb deformities in foals. JAVMA 1983;182:245.
6. Petty W, Spanier S, Shuster JJ, et al. The influence of skeletal implants on incidence of infection. J Bone Joint Surg 1985;67A:1236.
7. Fackelman GE, Frolich D. The current status of ASIF technique in large animals. In: Proceedings of the 18th Annual Meeting of the AAEP, San Francisco, CA, 1972:325.
8. Adams SB, Amstutz HE. Surgical correction of angular limb deformity of the forelimbs of a 7-month-old calf. Vet Surg 1983;12:58.
9. Fowler ME. Angular limb deformities in young llamas. JAVMA 1982;181:1338.
10. Fackelman GE, Nunamaker DM. Manual of Internal Fixation in the Horse. Berlin: Springer-Verlag, 1982:91.

Hemicircumferential Transection and Periosteal Stripping

The technique of horizontal transection of the periosteum and periosteal stripping has been used to achieve physiologic leg lengthening in man (1–3). Two mechanisms explain this phenomenon. Earlier theories hypothesized that the periosteal stripping induced local vascular changes that subsequently affected bone growth. More recently, experiments have shown that periosteal transection allows a *mechanical release* of fibroelastic periosteal tension (4). The technique of hemicircumferential transection of the periosteum and periosteal stripping (hereafter called simply periosteal stripping) was first successfully applied to correct angular limb deformities in foals by Auer et al. in 1982 (5).

The authors currently use periosteal stripping as the primary surgical technique for angular limb deformities caused by imbalance of physeal growth of the distal radius metacarpus (metatarsus) and tibia. For angular limb deformities of the fetlock joint (usually a varus deformity) the authors sometimes use periosteal stripping in combination with transphyseal bridging with screws and wire (discussed in the preceding section).

Because periosteal stripping is a "stimulation" procedure, i.e., it increases bone growth, it should be obvious to the reader that the procedure is performed on the opposite site of the metaphysis from that for the retardation procedure of transphyseal bridging. For a valgus deformity of the carpus (6), therefore, the periosteum is transected on the lateral aspect of the distal radial metaphysis (5, 7, 8).

Anesthesia and Surgical Preparation

The surgical procedures must be done under general anesthesia with the side of the bone to be operated on uppermost. Alternatively, if both sides are to be operated on, the foal can be placed in lateral recumbency to avoid having to change position. If both periosteal stripping and transphyseal bridging are to be performed (e.g., on the distal metacarpal or metatarsal physis), then the procedure involving the implants (screws and wire) would logically be done first. When implants are being used, the risk of wound infection is greater because of the "foreign body effect" of the implants; therefore, the demand for asepsis during surgery is more critical.

Once the screws and wire have been inserted and the wound closed (see "Surgical Technique"), the animal can be rolled over and the periosteal stripping performed on the opposite metaphysis. Care must be taken not to break aseptic technique as the foal is rolled over. Consequently, if both procedures are contemplated, both surgical sites must be clipped, shaved, and prepared for surgery in a routine manner. A sterile plastic adhesive drape is applied to the limb so that it adheres tightly over both surgical sites and is stuck to itself in a seam at the cranial or caudal surface of the limb.

Additional Instrumentation

Periosteal stripping requires a periosteal elevator and a no. 12 Bard-Parker scalpel blade and a periosteal elevator.

Surgical Technique

The technique described herein is slightly modified from the one first described by Auer et al. (5). A 6-cm vertical straight skin incision is made on the most lateral (or medial) aspect of the metaphysis of the affected bone. The skin incision should extend distad to about the middle of the adjacent epiphysis (Fig. 5.12*A*). The subcutaneous tissue and areolar tissue also are incised carefully. Care must be taken to avoid nearby tendons and their tendon sheaths. In the carpus valgus deformity, there is a natural depression between the common and lateral digital extensor tendons. The incision is located in this depression. In a varus deformity of the carpus, the medial aspect of the distal end of the radius is relatively free of such structures. The approach for the lateral aspect of the distal tibial metaphysis is slightly different because of the lateral location of the lateral digital extensor tendon. Two vertical incisions through the skin and subcutaneous tissues (cranial and caudal to the lateral digital extensor tendon) are made to enable sufficient exposure of the metaphysis.

With the skin edges carefully held apart with two Backhaus towel clamps placed on the skin edges, an 18- or 20-gauge sterile disposable needle is used to locate the physis. The distal radial physis is located close to the most prominent part of the bone in the surgical field. It can be found by "walking" the needle along the metaphysis distad toward the epiphysis, exerting firm pressure by the index finger placed over the hub of the needle (Fig. 5.12*B*). Small hematomas may result from this procedure, but they are of no consequence. An inverted T-shaped incision is made in the periosteum, using a bold stroke of a no. 20 scalpel blade (Fig. 5.12*C*). The horizontal component of the T should be approximately 1 cm proximal to the growth plate; however, the exact distance is apparently not critical (Fig. 5.12*C*). To ensure that the maximum amount of hemicircumference is transected, the surgeon can use the "hooked" blade of a no. 12 scalpel blade. The inverted T incision through the periosteum creates two triangular flaps that will be stripped from the underlying metaphysis (Fig. 5.12*D*). The authors have found that elevation of the periosteum by a periosteal elevator before using the no. 12 scalpel blade will facilitate further transection of the periosteum. The tendon sheaths of the extensor tendons are occasionally entered during this maneuver, but the authors have seen no untoward effects if this happens, and suturing should not be attempted. The periosteum is allowed to lie in its slightly retracted position and is not sutured.

In foals with valgus deformities of the carpus, as discussed, periosteal transection will be made laterally. An adjunctive surgical procedure that the authors recommend is to palpate and transect the remnant of the distal extremity of the ulna with a no. 11 scalpel blade or a rongeur forceps. This will eliminate any restraining (tethering) effect this bone may have on the lateral side of the bone (7) (Fig. 5.12*E*).

The subcutaneous tissues are apposed with a simple continuous pattern using a coated synthetic absorbable suture (e.g., 2/0 polyglactin 910 or polyglycolic acid) (Fig. 5.12*F*). Before finishing this layer of closure, the authors have found it useful to squeeze out any remaining hematoma, using several cotton gauzes rolled in a cylindrical shape. Skin edges are apposed using a nonabsorbable monofilament suture such as nylon or polypropylene (Fig. 5.12*F*). The hematoma can again be removed by squeezing it out one end of the incision with gauze, just before placing the last two or three remaining skin sutures.

Postoperative Management

The skin incision is covered with a nonadhesive dressing and held in place with a gauze bandage. A light elastic bandage is then applied over the entire joint so that it adheres to the bare skin, thereby minimizing the chance of its slipping.

Preoperative antibiotics are administered only if the periosteal stripping procedure is combined with insertion of implants on the other side of the bone or in another location in the horse. They are not used for a routine uncomplicated case wherein periosteal stripping is the sole procedure.

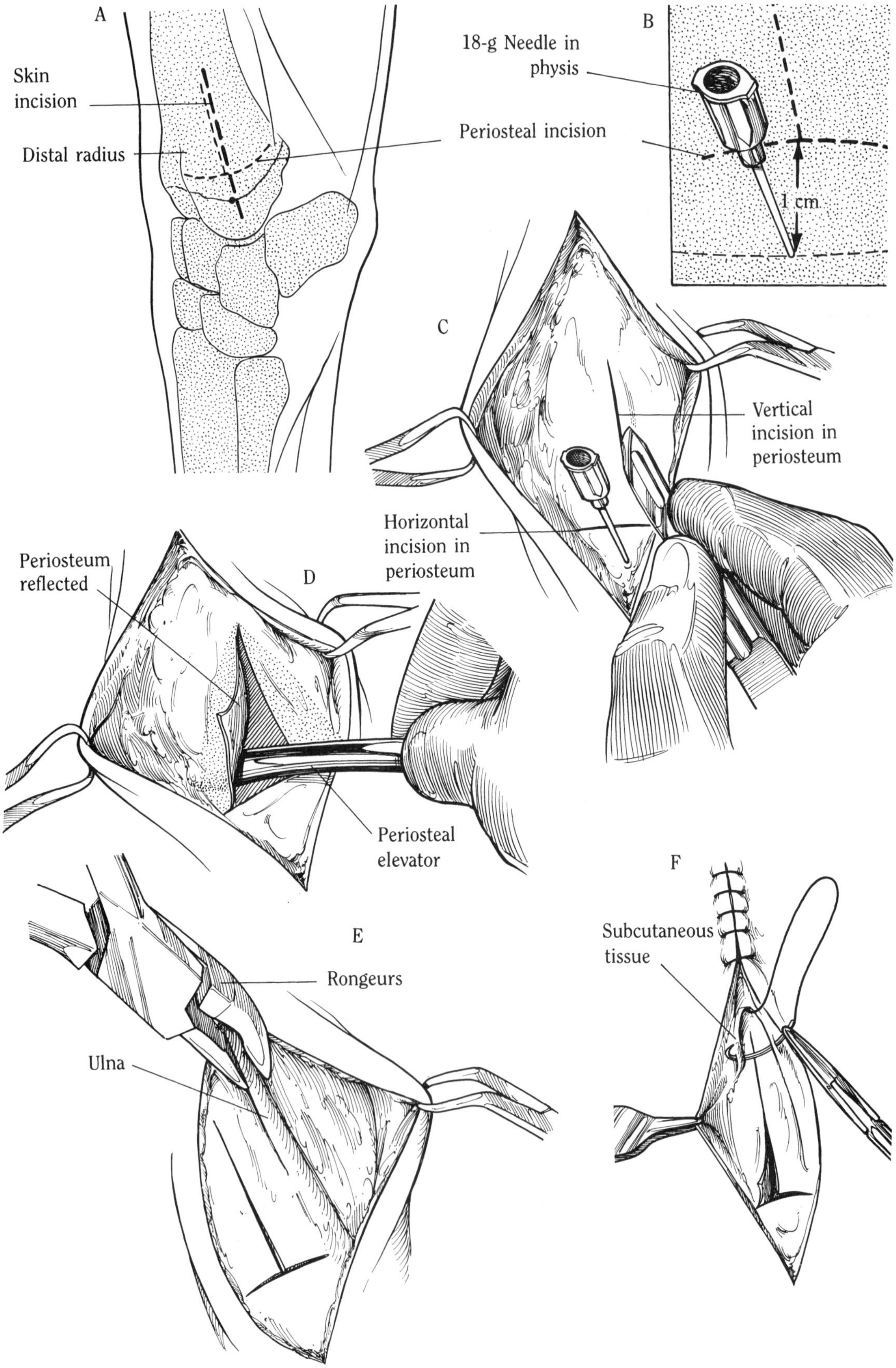

Figure 5.12, A–F. Steps in correction of carpal valgus deformity by hemicircumferential transection of the periosteum and periosteal stripping.

The wound is kept under a sterile wrap for at least 10 days to minimize swelling at the surgical site. The authors change a bandage at day 3 to 5, with the second bandage being identical to the first. Skin sutures are removed at 10 to 14 days. Nonsteroidal anti-inflammatory drugs are not necessary.

During the convalescence while the limb straightens, the foal must remain relatively confined to minimize concussion of the growth plate that would be caused by excessive activity. Although complete confinement of the mare and her foal to a box stall is desirable and recommended, this often meets with resistance from the owners. They frequently prefer the mare to be out in sunlight to help induce regular ovulation. As a compromise, the authors recommend that they both be placed in a stall that has a small run attached to it. Under no circumstances, however, should the foal be running free with the mare in a large pasture.

Comments

The advantages of periosteal stripping are that it is a relatively straightforward procedure, it does not require implants, and it does not require the mandatory second operation in transphyseal bridging for removal of screws and wire. Hospitalization is considerably shorter, and the overall operation is therefore cheaper for the client. It is also cosmetically appealing, and the procedure can be repeated if further correction is needed (5). Interestingly, the technique, if used as a sole procedure, has not in the authors' experience resulted in overcorrection of an angular limb deformity (7).

Failure to correct the angular limb deformity seems to be the only complication and occurs in only a small percentage of cases (5, 7). If it happens, the surgeon is faced with a decision to either repeat the periosteal stripping or perform the more complicated and expensive transphyseal bridging on the opposite side of the metaphysis.

REFERENCES

1. Chan KP, Hodgson AR. Physiologic leg lengthening. Clin Orthop 1970;68:55.
2. Crilly GR. Longitudinal overgrowth of chicken radius. J Anat 1972;112:11.
3. Jenkins DHR, Cheng DHF, Hodgson AR. Stimulations of bone by periosteal stripping. J Bone Joint Surg 1975;57B:482.
4. Houghton GR, Dekel S. The periosteal control of long bone growth. Acta Orthop Scand 1979;50:635.
5. Auer JA, Martens RJ, Williams EH. Periosteal transection for correction of angular limb deformities in foals. JAVMA 1982;181:459.
6. Fretz PB, Pharr JW, McIlwraith CW, et al. Varus vs valgus. [Letter] JAVMA 1982;181:636.
7. Bertone AL, Turner AS, Park RD. Further observations of the use of periosteal transection and stripping for the treatment of angular limb deformities in foals. JAVMA 1985;187:145.
8. Leitch M. Musculoskeletal disorders in neonatal foals. Equine practice symposium on neonatal equine disease. Vet Clin North Am 1985;1:189.

Arthrotomy of the Dorsal Aspect of the Fetlock Joint

In the past, the indications for dorsal arthrotomy of the fetlock joint included removal of osteochondral chip fragments from the dorsal proximal aspect of the proximal (first) phalanx, removal of osteochondritis dissecans (OCD) fragments from the sagittal ridge of the distal articular surface of the third metacarpal bone, and removal of chronic proliferative synovitis (villonodular synovitis) masses from the dorsal aspect of the fetlock joint (1–5). Arthrotomy is now considered obsolete for the treatment of proximal phalangeal chips, OCD fragmentation from the distal metacarpus, and most cases of villonodular synovitis (5, 6). It is recognized, however, that removal of large fragments through arthrotomy may be indicated in a practice situation when arthroscopic surgery is not available. Arthrotomy still may be indicated for the removal of large masses of chronic proliferative synovitis (3, 4), as these are not always amenable to arthroscopic surgery (6). Arthrotomy is also used for the enucleation of subchondral cystic lesions from the distal metacarpus (where the arthroscopic technique is more difficult).

Anesthesia and Surgical Preparation

Dorsal arthrotomy is done with the horse under general anesthesia and, depending on the surgeon's preference, in lateral or dorsal recumbency. With dorsal recumbency and the limb suspended, natural hemostasis is achieved. If the procedure is done in lateral recumbency, an Esmarch's bandage and a pneumatic tourniquet are generally used. Before induction of anesthesia, the patient's limb is clipped from the hoof to just below the carpus all the way around the limb.

Following anesthetic induction, the area of the surgical incision is shaved and a routine surgical preparation performed. Draping should include the use of a plastic adhesive drape. Some surgeons do the surgical preparation before induction of anesthesia. Radiographs should always include oblique views to ascertain the exact location of the lesion. Depending on the location of the lesion, the approach may be medial or lateral to the common digital extensor tendon.

Surgical Technique

A skin incision approximately 5 cm long is made 1 cm medial or lateral to the common digital extensor tendon over the fetlock joint. Figure 5.13*A* illustrates a medial approach to the metacarpophalangeal joint for removal of a fragment of the proximal phalanx. The subcutaneous fascia is incised along the same line as the skin incision. The incision is continued through the fibrous joint capsule (Fig. 5.13*B*). The dorsal branch of the palmar metacarpal artery and dorsal branch of the artery of the proximal phalanx are ligated or cauterized, if encountered. The incision is completed through the synovial membrane.

With villonodular (chronic proliferative) synovitis, the arthrotomy incision is centered over the synovial reflection of the distal metacarpus. The mass is removed after grasping it with Allis forceps and severing the base with a scalpel (Fig. 5.13*C*). With large lesions, the mass can extend across the entire side of the joint; in some situations, two arthrotomy incisions, one on each side of the common digital extensor tendon, may be necessary. Sagittal sectioning of the mass before severing the base may also facilitate removal.

When operating on subchondral cystic lesions of the distal aspect of the meta-

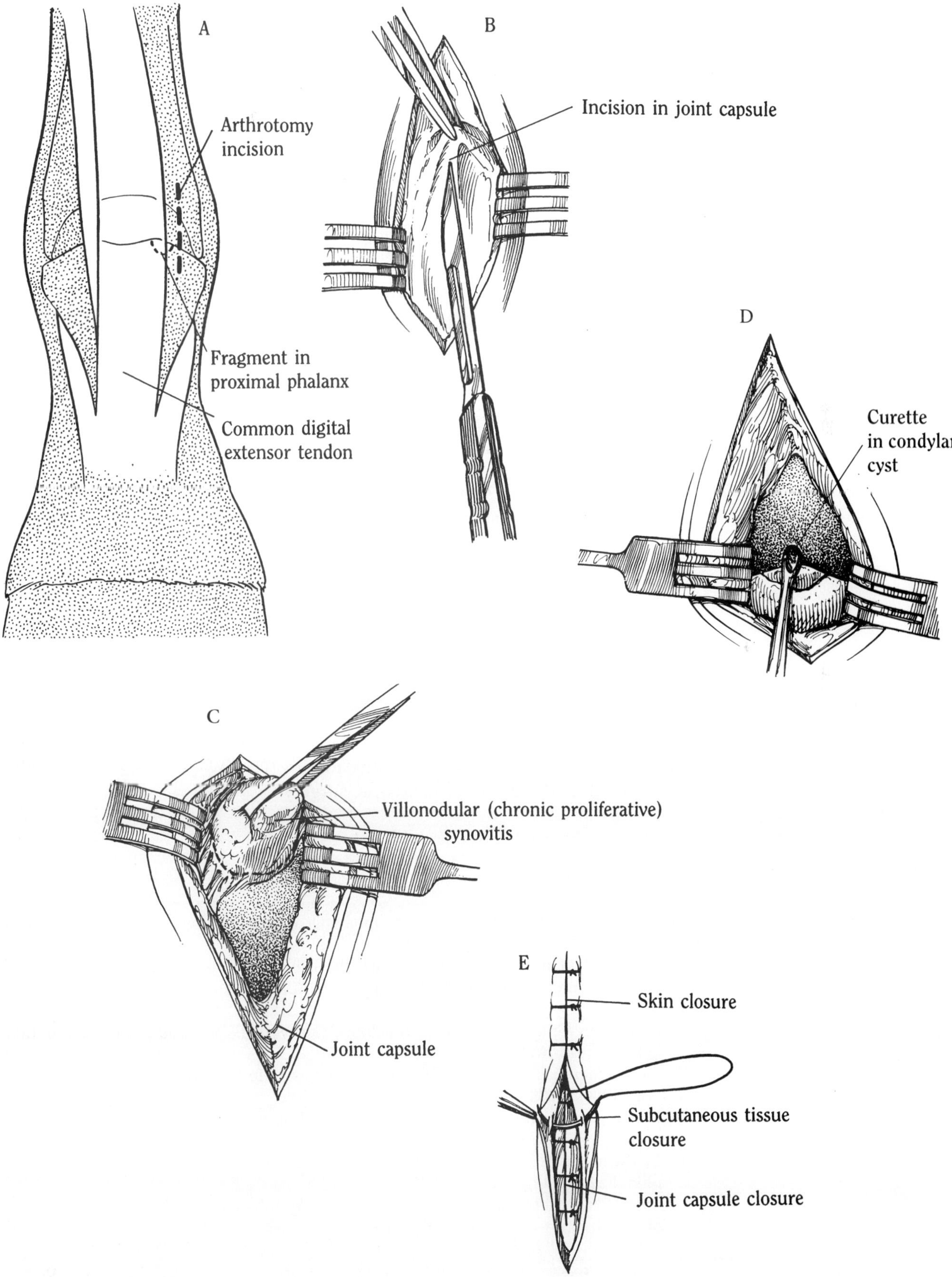

Figure 5.13, A–E. Dorsal arthrotomy of the fetlock joint.

carpus, the joint is flexed after the arthrotomy is completed. Flexion is continued until the opening of the cystic lesion is visible (Fig. 5.13*D*). A curette is then used to enucleate the contents of the lesion (Fig. 5.13*D*). When all affected tissue is removed and there is healthy bone in the cavity, the articular defect is trimmed and the joint flushed before closure of the arthrotomy.

Following any procedure in the joint, it is flushed with saline solution or balanced electrolyte solution, and suction is used to remove fluid. The fibrous joint capsule is closed, using interrupted sutures of 2/0 synthetic nonabsorbable or absorbable material. The sutures in the joint capsule do not penetrate synovial membrane, and preplacement of the sutures in the joint capsule ensures that penetration does not occur and that there is ideal approximation of the incision edges (Fig. 5.12*E*). The subcutaneous fascia is closed in a continuous pattern using 2/0 synthetic absorbable suture material. (Fig. 5.12*E*). The skin is closed in an interrupted pattern using 2/0 nonabsorbable monofilament suture material (Fig. 5.12*E*). The tourniquet is removed (if one has been used), a sterile dressing is placed over the incision, and a firm pressure bandage is placed immediately on the leg from just below the carpal joint to the foot.

Postoperative Management

The use of antibiotics is optional. The skin sutures are removed in 10 to 12 days, but the bandage is maintained on the limb for another 10 days. Postoperative radiographs are taken within 24 hours of surgery; these films are of value for comparative purposes when follow-up progressive radiographs are made at a later date. The horse is stall-rested with hand-walking for 6 weeks, and can then be turned out in a small area. At least 4 months' rest before training is recommended.

Comments

Calcification of the joint capsule has been reported as a complication of tunnel arthrotomy in the metacarpophalangeal joint (7). This potential complication is obviated by the use of arthroscopic surgery.

REFERENCES

1. Haynes PF. Disease of the metacarpophalangeal joint and metacarpus. Vet Clin North Am Large Animal Pract 1980;2:49.
2. Meagher DM. Joint surgery in the horse: the selection of surgical cases and the consideration of alternatives. In: Proceedings of the Annual Meeting of the AAEP, Las Vegas, NV, 1974:81.
3. Nichols FA, Grant BD, Lincoln SD. Villonodular synovitis of the equine metacarpophalangeal joint. JAVMA 1976;168:1043.
4. Van Veenendaal JC, Moffatt RE. Soft tissue masses in the fetlock joint of horses. Aust Vet J 1980;56:533.
5. Yovich JV, McIlwraith CW, Stashak TS. Osteochondritis dissecans of the sagittal ridge of the third metacarpal and metatarsal bones in horses. JAVMA 1985;186:1186.
6. McIlwraith CW. Diagnostic and Surgical Arthroscopy in the Horse. 2nd ed. Philadelphia: Lea & Febiger, 1990.
7. Raker CW. Calcification of the equine metacarpophalangeal joint following removal of chip fractures. Arch Am Coll Vet Surg 1975;4:66.

Arthrotomy of the Tarsocrural (Tibiotarsal) Joint

Arthrotomy of the tarsocrural joint is indicated for the surgical treatment of OCD lesions and removal of fragments associated with trauma when the alternative technique of arthroscopic surgery is not available (1). Such lesions occur in the distal intermediate ridge and malleoli of the tibia and in the trochlear ridges of the talus (1). Arthroscopic surgery is the preferred technique for the treatment of such lesions (2), but arthrotomy may still be used in occasional cases when a large fragment off the distal aspect of the lateral trochlear ridge of the talus is embedded in the soft tissue. In addition, fragments from the lateral malleolus are seldom operable by arthroscopic techniques. Traumatic fragments off the lateral malleolus of the tibia should be removed with an arthrotomy that extends proximal from the joint cavity.

The exact location and extent of the lesions should be ascertained with preoperative radiographs. Lesions of the distal intermediate ridge of the tibia, lateral trochlear ridge of the talus, and lateral malleolus of the tibia are operated on through a dorsolateral arthrotomy approach. This technique is presented sequentially below. The indications for a dorsomedial arthrotomy approach are fewer but include lesions on the medial trochlear ridge of the talus and the medial malleolus of the tibia.

Anesthesia and Surgical Preparation

The dorsolateral arthrotomy is done under general anesthesia either with the horse placed in lateral recumbency with the affected limb up or in dorsal recumbency with the limb extended. Before induction of anesthesia, the patient's limb is clipped from the middle of the crus to the fetlock joint all the way around the leg. Following induction of anesthesia, the immediate surgical area is shaved and the limb prepared. The use of a tourniquet is optional.

Additional Instrumentation

The procedure requires retractors, curettes, periosteal elevators, and a bulb syringe.

Surgical Technique

The limb is draped with a draping system of the surgeon's choice, which should include plastic adherent drapes. A 3-cm vertical skin incision is made lateral to the long digital extensor tendon from the lateral malleolus distad to the level of the middle extensor retinaculum (Fig. 5.14*A*). The incision is continued through the subcutaneous tissue, avoiding the cranial tibial artery and deep peroneal nerve that lie plantar to the long digital extensor tendon. Synovial distension of the joint, which is usually present in these cases, facilitates identification of the dorsolateral pouch of the tarsocrural joint. If synovial distension is not obvious, the joint pouch can be made more obvious by intra-articular injection of fluid. The joint capsule is incised in the center of this pouch (Fig. 5.14*B*). Hand-held retractors will facilitate exposure of the lesion, particularly those of the intermediate ridge of the tibia proximally (Fig. 5.14*C*).

Lesions of the distal intermediate ridge of the tibia are operated on by retracting the incision proximad and reaching over the lateral trochlear ridge to the lesion. The fragments may be loose (and can be simply lifted out), or separation of the fragment from the parent bone with an elevator or osteotome may

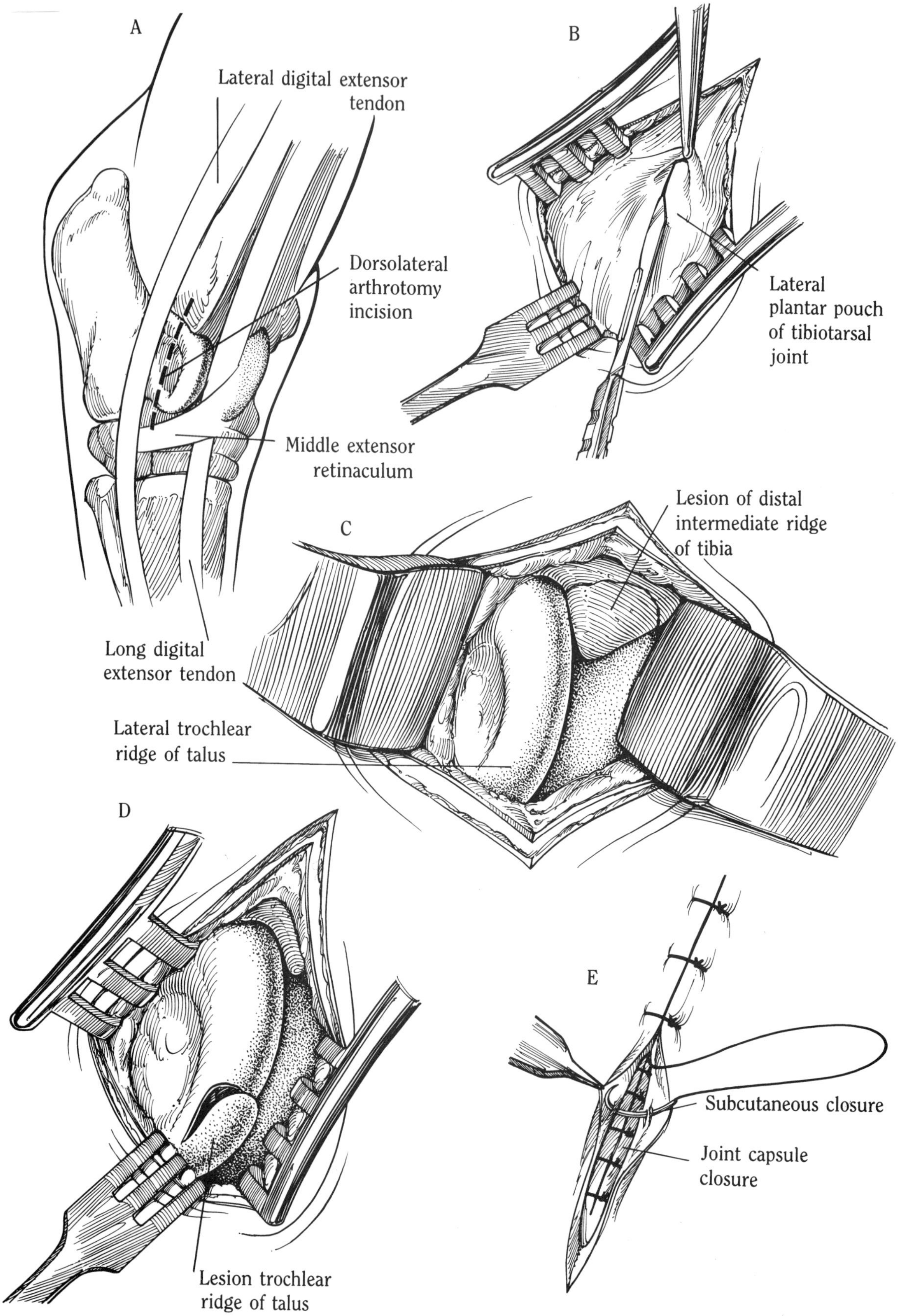

Figure 5.14, A–E. Arthrotomy of the tarsocrural joint.

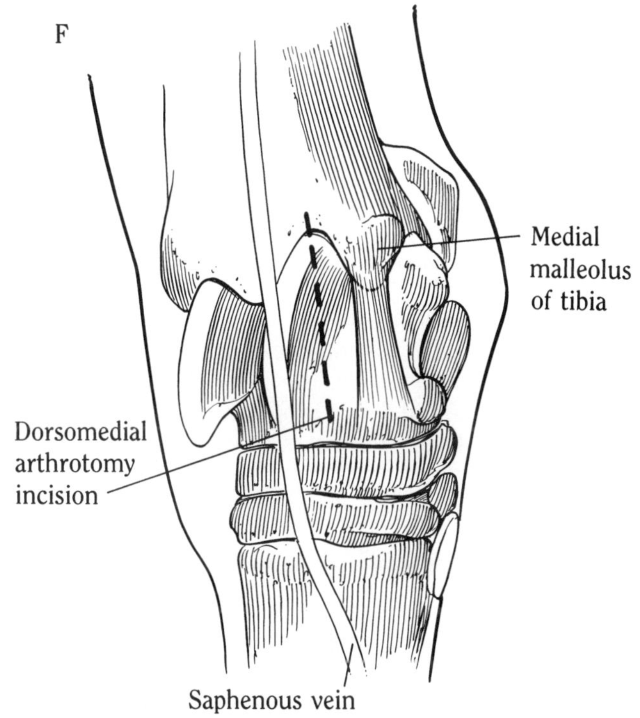

Figure 5.14. F. *(continued)* Arthrotomy of the tarsocrural joint.

be required. Following removal of the fragment, any loose tags of bone and cartilage are removed.

With lesions of the lateral trochlear ridge of the talus, a flap is generally present, and this is elevated and removed (Fig. 5.14*D*). In some instances, a large osteochondral fragment requiring dissection from the joint capsule is present. Any loose or undermined articular cartilage is removed, and the subchondral bone in the base of the defect is curetted. Some surgeons will also elect to drill holes in the healthy subchondral bone to facilitate vascularization and subsequent healing of the defect (forage) (3). In some cases of lateral trochlear ridge OCD, an osteochondral fragment will have already completely separated from the defect and be located in the dorsomedial joint pouch. It may be possible to grasp this lesion through the dorsolateral arthrotomy, but in some situations an additional dorsomedial arthrotomy may be necessary. The removal of these loose bodies is important because these separated fragments continue "to grow" and may become very large.

A lesion of the lateral malleolus will require some additional dissection of the fragment from the fibrous capsule (most of these should not be operated on).

Once all intra-articular lesions have been attended to, the joint is flushed and the arthrotomy is closed. The fibrous joint capsule and retinaculum are closed with simple interrupted sutures of absorbable synthetic material or monofilament nonabsorbable material (Fig. 5.14*E*). The sutures should not penetrate the synovial membrane. Preplacement of the sutures in the joint capsule and retinaculum ensures accurate apposition and a tight seal. The subcutaneous tissue is closed with a simple continuous suture of absorbable synthetic material, and the skin is closed with interrupted sutures using monofilament nonabsorbable material (Fig. 5.14*E*). The immediate surgical site is covered with a nonadherent pad and gauze bandage, and the limb is wrapped with a tight pressure bandage up to the middle of the crus.

If dorsomedial arthrotomy is necessary, it also is done through the large dorsomedial joint pouch, with care being taken to avoid the cranial branch of the medial saphenous vein (Fig. 5.14*F*).

Some cases of OCD necessitate two arthrotomies to manage both the original defect and the loose body or bodies. If arthroscopic surgery is available, double arthrotomies are not necessary.

Postoperative Management

The limb is maintained in a firm pressure bandage for 2 weeks, during which time the bandage is changed on several occasions. Skin sutures are removed at 10 to 12 days. During convalescence, the horse is kept in a stall and hand-walked. Training is not resumed for at least 4 months after surgery.

REFERENCES

1. McIlwraith CW. Surgery of the hock, stifle and shoulder. Symposium on Equine Orthopaedics. Vet Clin North Am 1983;5:333.
2. McIlwraith CW. Diagnostic and Surgical Arthroscopy in the Horse. 2nd ed. Philadelphia: Lea & Febiger, 1990.
3. Ficat RP, Ficat C, Gedeon P, et al. Spongialization: a new treatment for diseased patellae. Clin Orthop 1979;144:74.

Arthrotomy of the Femorotibial Joint

Arthrotomy of the femorotibial joint has essentially been replaced by arthroscopic surgery. It has been primarily used in the past for the surgical treatment of subchondral cystic lesions of the medial condyle of the femur (1–3). This technique was initially developed because results with conservative management of femoral cystic lesions have been poor at Colorado State University, despite some reports of a reasonable return to clinical soundness with conservative treatment (4, 5). Horses with cystic lesions may perform well up to a certain level and then become lame with harder work. Some horses can perform satisfactorily within a certain range of work. With more athletic pursuits, problems may be anticipated.

Surgical techniques that have been investigated include an extra-articular approach to the cyst with curetting and packing of the defect with a cancellous bone graft (McIlwraith CW, unpublished data, 1981), open curettage of the cyst through a femorotibial arthrotomy with (6) or without (2, 3) cancellous bone grafting, or replacement of the defect with a polymer carbon fiber and fluorocarbon (Proplast, Dow Corning Corp., Midland, MI) (7). The first technique has been abandoned because of poor results, and curettage of the cyst without cancellous bone grafting is the method of choice (now usually done arthroscopically).

Anesthesia and Surgical Preparation

The arthrotomy is done under general anesthesia with the horse placed in dorsal recumbency and the stifle joint flexed. Before induction of anesthesia the patient's limb is clipped in the area of the stifle, and the immediate surgical site is shaved directly after induction of anesthesia and positioning of the patient.

Additional Instrumentation

This arthrotomy procedure requires retractors and curettes, as well as a flushing and vacuuming system.

Surgical Technique

Following surgical preparation, the site is draped. With the limb in a flexed position, the femorotibial joint can be directly approached between the middle and medial patellar ligaments (Fig. 5.15*A*). A 5-cm vertical skin incision is made from below the patella distad to the tibial tuberosity, over the medial condyle that can be palpated. The incision is extended through superficial and deep stifle fascial layers into the femoropatellar fat pad (Fig. 5.1*B*), and the femoropatellar fat pad is dissected away at this location to expose the femorotibial joint capsule. This latter dissection should be conducted with care in the more proximal part of the incision to avoid penetration of the femoropatellar joint capsule. Using this approach, the femorotibial joint is reached and is identified by palpating the medial femoral condyle beneath it. After the joint capsule has been cleared of fat and elevated away from the condyle with forceps, a 2-cm incision is made through the joint capsule (Fig. 5.15*C*). With the aid of hand-held retractors and limb manipulation (slight flexion or extension), the articular component of the lesion can be exposed (Fig. 5.15*D*).

The articular defect serves as identification for the deeper cystic lesion. It will vary from a small dimple or crack to a more widely eroded area. The latter situation tends to occur in horses that have been worked while under anti-inflammatory medication because of lameness. The opening is then penetrated

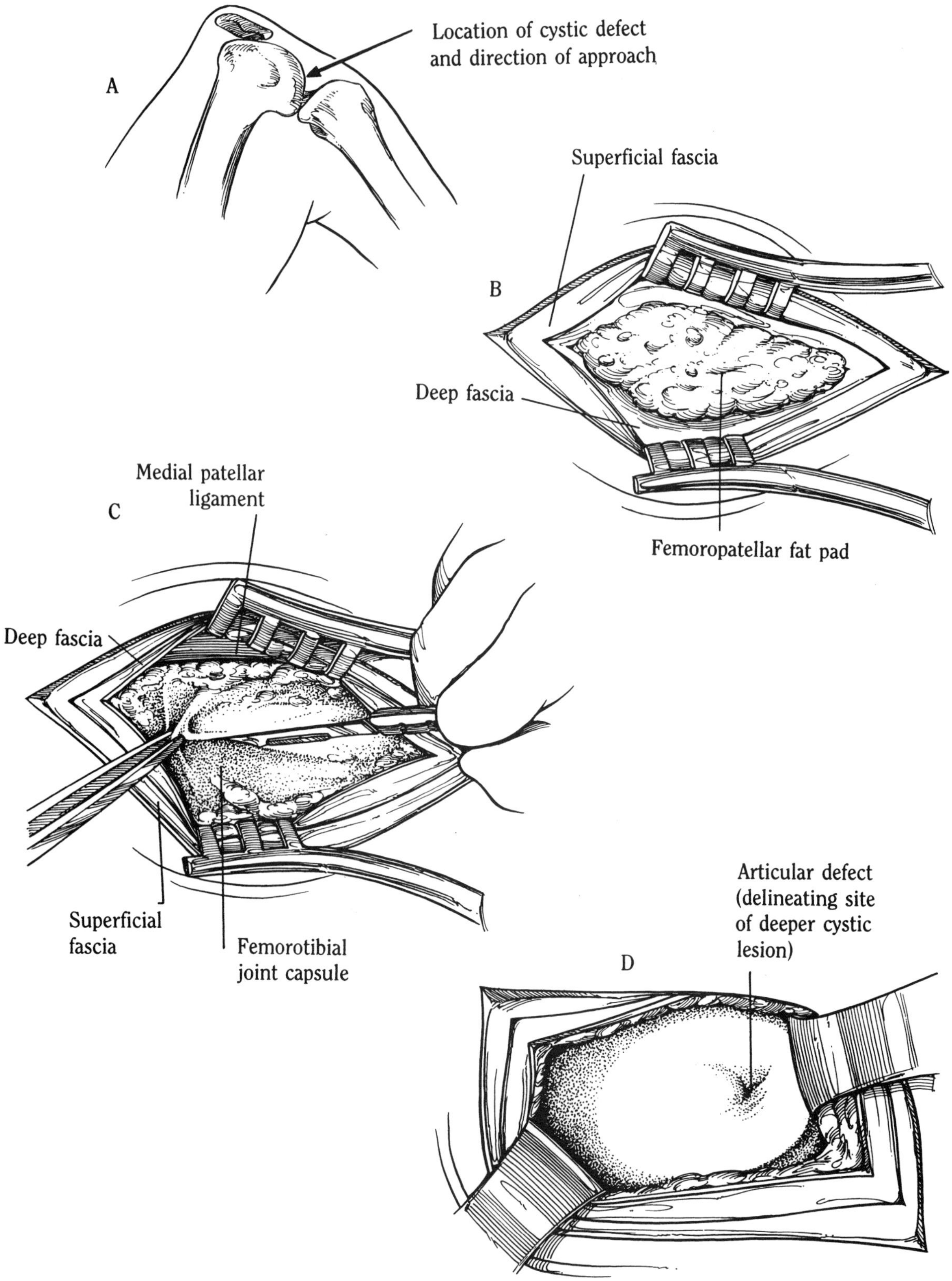

Figure 5.15, A–D. Arthrotomy of the femorotibial joint.

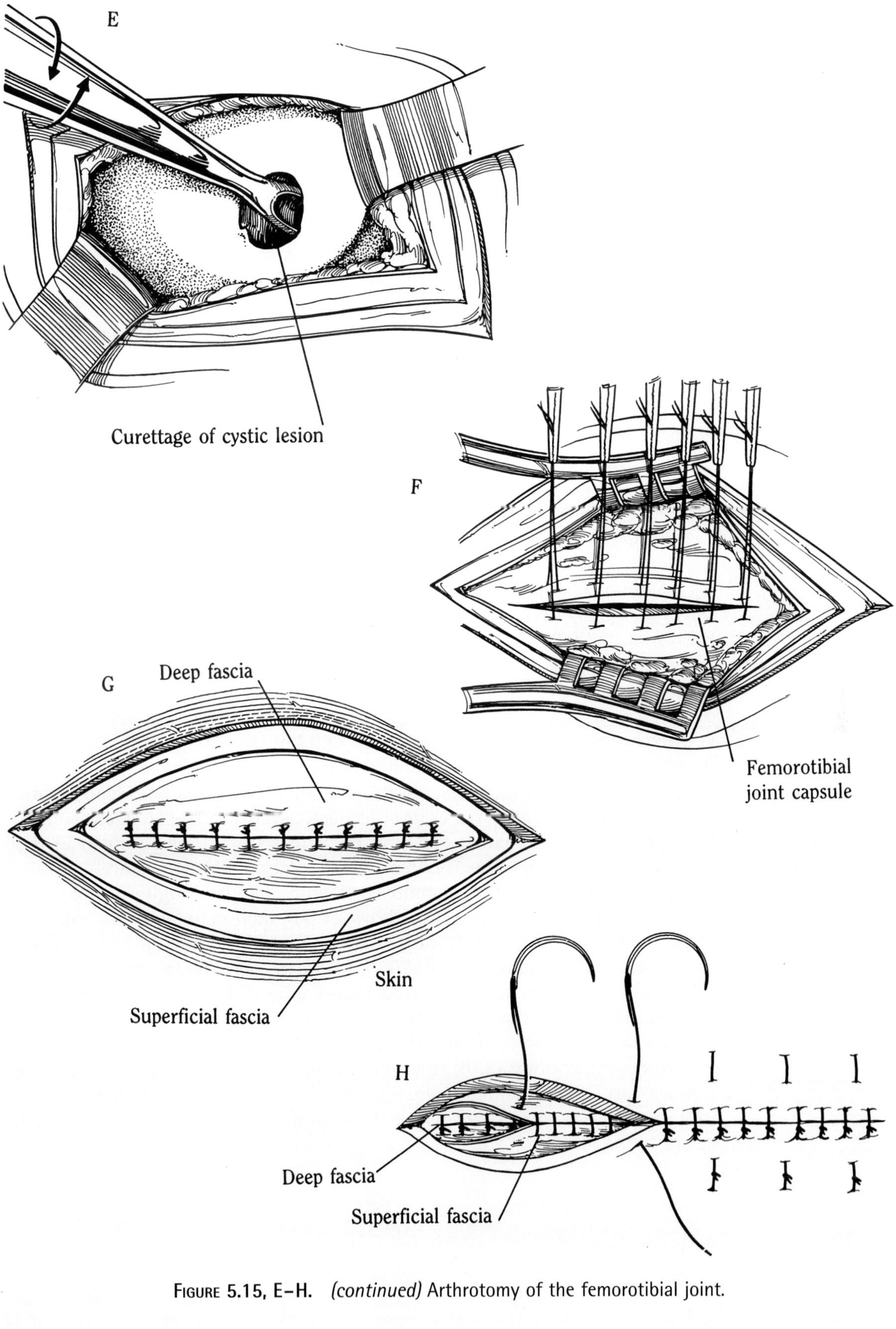

FIGURE 5.15, E–H. *(continued)* Arthrotomy of the femorotibial joint.

to enter the cyst for curettage (Fig. 5.15*E*). Curettage of the cystic lesion should be thorough, with careful debriding of the entire wall of the cyst and elimination of sclerotic bone, which is commonly present at the periphery.

Before closure, the femorotibial joint is irrigated thoroughly. The femorotibial joint capsule is closed with simple interrupted sutures of 2/0 synthetic absorbable suture material (Fig. 5.15*F*). The deep fascia is closed with simple interrupted sutures of 0 or 1 synthetic absorbable material (Fig. 5.15*G*), and the superficial fascia and subcutaneous tissues are closed with a continuous suture using 0 synthetic absorbable suture material. The skin incision is closed with simple interrupted sutures using 2/0 nonabsorbable monofilament material, supported by vertical mattress tension sutures of 0 nonabsorbable monofilament material (Fig. 5.15, *G* and *H*). The incision is covered with a stent bandage.

Postoperative Management

Skin sutures are removed at 2 weeks. The horse is maintained standing, using an overhead wire, for 3 weeks. The horse is maintained in a stall for another 6 weeks (with daily hand-walking) and then can be turned out into a small area. The horse is not put into training for 6 months, and then is brought back into training gradually.

Postoperative radiographs will show variable degrees of osseous healing of the defect. However, continued lucence of the cystic defect is not incompatible with functional soundness (3). It is suggested that the degenerate tissue within the cystic lesion is replaced with fibrous tissue. Lack of osseous healing has also been reported following adjunctive cancellous bone grafting (6).

Femorotibial arthrotomy through an approach between the medial patellar ligament and the medial femorotibial (collateral) ligament has worked well for other surgeons (1, 3). Based on personal experience, the authors believe the approach described is more convenient and has worked well. In one study of 51 horses with unilateral or bilateral femorotibial arthrotomy for the treatment of medial condylar bone cysts, a total of 60 cysts were treated. Treated horses responded to the surgery 3 to 12 months postoperatively. In 42 horses, lameness was reduced or eliminated, enabling them to return to and remain in their intended function. Of these 41 horses, 35 were sound, 4 had not started training, and 7 showed partial improvement (2 of which had no long-term follow-up). Of the remaining nine horses, two showed no reduction in lameness and seven were not followed up. Arthrotomy was successful in reducing or eliminating lameness in 82% of all horses and 95% of those where follow-up was possible. Lameness was eliminated in 35 of 51 horses originally operated on, which is a 69% success rate. Although cancellous bone grafting is a logical adjunct, the authors do not perform it because their results have been the same as those reported with grafting (3, 6), thereby making the second surgical procedure unnecessary. Also, the authors are apprehensive about maintaining the cancellous bone in situ when there is an open communication distad from the cystic cavity to the joint.

REFERENCES

1. Kold SE, Hickman J. Use of an autogenous cancellous bone graft in the treatment of subchondral bone cysts in the medial femoral condyle of the horse. Equine Vet J 1983; 15:312.

2. McIlwraith CW. Surgery of the hock, stifle and shoulder. Vet Clin North Am Large Animal Pract 1983;5:333.
3. White NA, McIlwraith CW, Allen D. Curettage of subchondral bone cysts in medial femoral condyles of the horse. Equine Vet J 1988;(Suppl 6):120–124.
4. Jeffcott LB, Kold SE. Clinical and radiological aspects of stifle bone cysts in the horse. Equine Vet J 1982;14:40.
5. Stewart B, Reid CF. Osseous cyst-like lesions of the medial femoral condyle of the horse. J Am Vet Med Soc 1982;180:254.
6. Kold SE, Hickman J. Results of treatment of subchondral bone cysts in the medial condyle of the femur with an autogenous bone graft. Equine Vet J 1984;16:414.
7. Valdez H. The use of carbon bio materials in repairing osteochondrotic lesions in the horse. In: Proceedings of the 27th Annual Meeting of the AAEP, New Orleans, LA, 1981:239–242.

Arthrotomy of the Shoulder Joint

Arthrotomy of the shoulder joint is indicated for the treatment of OCD and subchondral cystic lesions of the glenoid (1–5). There are few reports in the literature of surgically treating OCD in this joint, probably because of the difficulty in adequately exposing the humeral and glenoid surfaces of the shoulder joint and the knowledge that DJD commonly occurs in association with OCD in the equine shoulder (6).

Follow-up on operations for OCD using the technique about to be described is encouraging (4). Not only was it possible to return horses to athletic soundness, but also it was possible to markedly improve function where extensive degenerative change was present. The surgical approach described is modified from one described for the dog (7). Arthroscopic surgery is the method preferred for treating OCD at the shoulder but it is difficult and limited to young patients. The arthroscopic technique is described elsewhere.

Anesthesia and Surgical Preparation

Accurate identification of the problem before the operation is important. Intra-articular analgesia is usually induced to localize the lameness problem to the shoulder joint, and radiographs are made under general anesthesia. Radiographs with the horse standing are often inadequate and may not demonstrate lesions. An arthrogram can be done by introducing 7 mL of diatrizoate methylglucamine (Renografin, E.R. Squibb & Sons, Inc., Princeton, NJ) into the affected joint, but the authors do not consider this to be necessary routinely.

The shoulder is clipped before surgery, and the horse is placed on a regimen of perioperative antibiotics and given tetanus toxoid. Phenylbutazone is also administered perioperatively.

Surgical Technique

After draping, a 20-cm skin incision is made, beginning 2.5 cm caudal to the spine of the scapula and curving over the shoulder joint caudal to the infraspinatus tendon (which can be palpated) (Fig. 5.16*A*). The deep fascia is incised to expose the caudal border of the brachiocephalicus muscle. This is elevated and retracted craniad to expose the underlying aponeurosis of the deltoideus muscle, which is located over the infraspinatus muscle. The dense aponeurotic portion at the cranial aspect of the deltoid muscle is severed, and the deltoideus muscle retracted caudad to reveal the teres minor muscle below (Fig. 5.16*B*). This exposure is also facilitated by cranial retraction of the infraspinatus muscle (Fig. 5.16*B*). The insertion of the teres minor on the humerus is transected, leaving enough of the attachment to be sutured, and the muscle belly is retracted caudad, using Gelpi retractors to expose the joint capsule beneath. Care must be taken to avoid the caudal circumflex humeral artery and vein and axillary nerve, which are positioned caudad to the surgical region. The joint capsule may sometimes be distended. The joint capsule is incised parallel to the palpable rim of the glenoid cavity (Fig. 5.16*C*).

Accessibility to lesions will vary, with access tending to be easier when bone remodeling is extensive. In other situations, the careful insertion of a curved instrument into the glenoid notch to distract the humeral head from the glenoid cavity is important. Extreme adduction of the distal limb will expose additional portions of the caudal humeral head, and this maneuver needs to be done forcibly. As with other cases of OCD, detached or loose cartilage flaps are removed and the subchondral bone is debrided of all abnormal tissue with a curette. The use of a fiberoptic lighting source to expose deeper regions of the joint is also

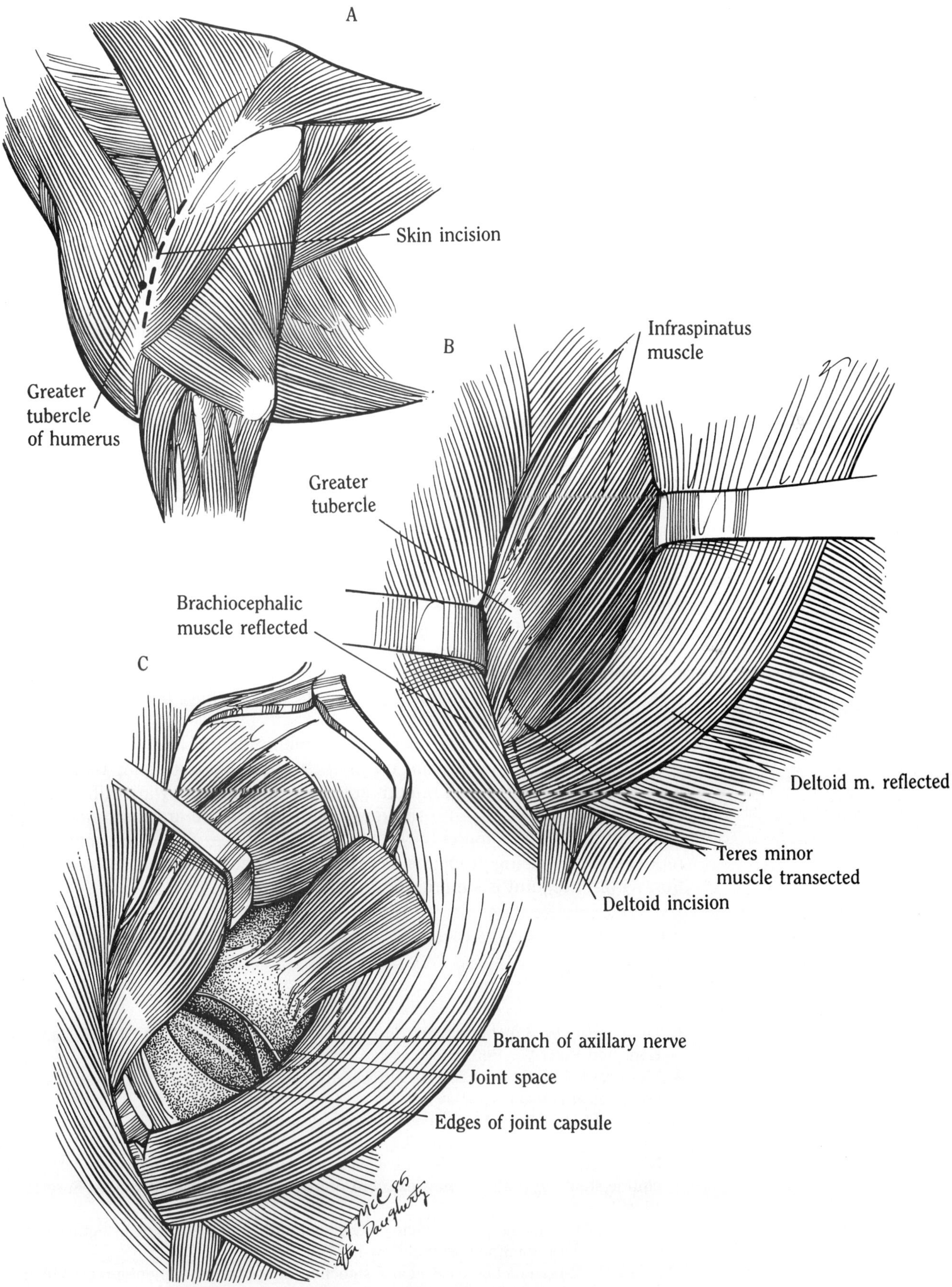

Figure 5.16, A–C. Muscle-separating approach to the shoulder joint of the horse.

advantageous. Cystic lesions in the glenoid cavity are identified by cartilaginous dimpling or cracking and curetted. An angled curette is useful. After debridement and removal of fragments, the joint is flushed thoroughly to remove loose pieces of bone and cartilage.

The joint capsule is closed with interrupted sutures of 2/0 polyglactin 910. The teres minor muscle is reattached to the humerus with simple interrupted sutures of 1 polyglactin 910, and the severed aponeurotic origin of the deltoid muscle is similarly sutured. The free caudal border of the brachiocephalic muscle is replaced over the deltoid muscle and sutured with a simple continuous pattern using 1 polyglactin 910. The subcutaneous tissue is also apposed using a simple continuous suture of 0 polyglactin 910, and the skin is apposed with simple interrupted sutures of monofilament nonabsorbable suture material, or with skin staples. A stent bandage is secured over the wound.

Postoperative Management

Antibiotics and phenylbutazone are administered for 5 days following surgery. The horse is stall-rested with hand-walking for 1 month and then can be turned out into a small area with a gradual increase in exercise. A total of 6 months' rest is allowed before resuming training.

Comments

This surgical approach to the shoulder joint differs from two previous techniques for arthrotomy in the horse that have involved longitudinal or transverse tenotomy of the infraspinatus tendon (5, 8). The approach described maintains the stability of the joint afforded by the infraspinatus tendon and allows better exposure of the caudal humeral head than the authors have been able to achieve by longitudinal tenotomy.

Adequate surgical access does require manipulation and traction. Arthroscopic techniques have now been developed that allow superior visualization to the shoulder (9). Surgical manipulations with arthroscopy are difficult, however, and do not yet fit into the description of routine arthroscopic surgery. Arthrotomy does not require the specialized experience of the arthroscopic technique, and no healing problems have been observed. Conversely, the visualization within the joint is superior with arthroscopy.

REFERENCES

1. McIlwraith CW. Subchondral cystic lesions (osteochondrosis) in the horse. Compend Cont Edu Pract Vet 1982;4:394.
2. McIlwraith CW. Diagnostic and Surgical Arthroscopy in the Horse. 2nd ed. Philadelphia: Lea & Febiger, 1990.
3. Mason TA, MacLean AA. Osteochondrosis dissecans of the head of the humerus in two foals. Equine Vet J 1977;9:189.
4. Nixon AN, Stashak TS, McIlwraith CW, et al. A muscle-separating approach to the equine shoulder joint for the treatment of osteochondritis dissecans. Vet Surg 1984; 13:247.
5. Schmidt GR, Dueland DR, Vaughan JT. Osteochondrosis dissecans of the equine shoulder joint. Vet Med Small Animal Clin 1975;70:542.
6. Nyack B, Morgan JP, Poole RR, et al. Osteochondritis of the shoulder joint of the horse. Cornell Vet 1981;71:149
7. Birkeland R. Osteochondritis dissecans in the humeral head of the dog: comparison

of results achieved with conservative and surgical treatment. Nord Vet Med 1967;19: 294.

8. De Bowes RM, Wagner PC, Grant BD. Surgical approach to the equine scapulohumeral joint through a longitudinal infraspinatus tenotomy. Vet Surg 1982;11:125.
9. Bertone AL, McIlwraith CW. Arthroscopic approaches and intra-articular anatomy of the equine shoulder joint and approaches for the surgical treatment of osteochondrosis. Vet Surg 1987;16:312–317.

Arthroscopic Surgery of the Carpal Joints

Arthroscopic surgery in the carpal joints is indicated for the removal of osteochondral chip fractures, debridement of degenerative subchondral lesions, treatment of third carpal slab fractures, and diagnosis and treatment of tearing of the medial palmar intercarpal ligament (1–5). The advantages of arthroscopic surgery over conventional arthrotomy for the treatment of these problems have been documented (1, 2, 6, 7). It is the authors' opinion that these advantages are sufficient to make the use of arthrotomy for the removal of such fragments obsolete. The equine carpal joints have been the most frequently operated on by arthroscopic surgery and have served somewhat as the showpiece for the procedure. Basic principles of arthroscopic surgery for the removal of small fragments will be described. For more details, the reader is referred to another textbook (1).

The authors also use arthroscopic surgery to operate on carpal slab fractures, and it is described on page 62–65.

Anesthesia and Surgical Preparation

This surgical procedure is done with the horse under general anesthesia. The horse may be placed in lateral or dorsal recumbency, but the authors prefer dorsal recumbency with the limb suspended. This position facilitates operation on the horse from both sides (this is commonly necessary when multiple fragments are present).

Before induction of anesthesia, the patient's limb is clipped from the midradius to the distal cannon area. The immediate surgical site on the dorsal aspect of the joint is shaved immediately before or after induction of the anesthesia. Draping will include a plastic adhesive drape as well as a special impervious drape (General Econopak Inc., Philadelphia, PA).

Additional Instrumentation

Appropriate arthroscopic instrumentation is required (see Appendix IV) (1).

Surgical Technique

Arthroscopic surgery uses the principle of triangulation. Preoperative radiographs will have ascertained the site of the chip fractures or subchondral bone disease but arthroscopic examination frequently finds additional pathologic change that was not identified on the radiographs. As a general principle, the arthroscope is inserted on the side opposite the lesion, and surgical instruments are inserted over the lesion. When lesions are present on both sides, the positions of instrument and arthroscope will be reversed appropriately.

A chip fracture off the distal aspect of the radial carpal bone will be used as an example. Two skin incisions are made before distension of the joint. The incision for the arthroscope is placed laterally, between the extensor carpi radialis and the common digital extensor tendons. The portal for the instrument is located medially, medial to the extensor carpi radialis tendon. These incisions are made before joint distension so that the surgeon can be sure they are located away from the tendon sheaths. The intercarpal (midcarpal) joint is then distended with saline or polyionic electrolyte solution, and the arthroscopic cannula is inserted through the joint capsule using the sharp trocar. The sharp trocar is then exchanged for a blunt obturator to complete placement of the arthroscopic sheath within the joint. The arthroscope is then inserted, and the ingress fluid line and light cable are attached. The joint can then be examined.

The pathologic changes at various sites within the joint are ascertained. This examination is facilitated by the placement of an egress cannula through the site of the instrument portal (Fig. 5.17*A*). The egress cannula is used to allow flushing of fluid through the joint to clear it of any debris or blood. When the view is clear, the stopcock on the egress cannula is closed and the egress cannula can be used as a palpating instrument to ascertain the mobility of chips and the size and nature of other lesions. Once the diagnostic arthroscopy is completed, the chip can be removed.

An instrument portal through the joint capsule is then made, using a trocar or no. 11 scalpel blade (Fig. 5.17*B*). Carpal chips can be divided into four categories, and the techniques for their removal vary accordingly. If the chip is fresh and mobile, forceps are inserted through the instrument portal and the chip is removed. When there are strong fibrous attachments at the fracture line or to the fibrous joint capsule, the fragment is loosened with a periosteal elevator inserted through the instrument portal (Fig. 5.17*C*). When bony reattachment is developing or has occurred, an osteotome is used to free the fragment from the parent bone. The osteotome is held in correct position by the surgeon who is visualizing its position, and an assistant taps the osteotome on command. When there is extensive bony reattachment, a motorized burr can be used to remove the protruding lesion.

After removal of the separated chip fragment using forceps (Fig. 5.17, *D* and *E*), the defect is then debrided with a curette (Fig. 5.17, *F* and *G*). (The selection of forceps to remove fragments depends on both the preference of the surgeon and the size of the fragment.) Debridement of the defect includes the removal of defective bone as well as elevated, fragmented, or loose articular cartilage. Partial thickness defects of articular cartilage (where there is firm attachment of the remaining cartilage to the bone) are not debrided. These principles are based partly on knowledge of cartilage healing in the horse and partly on subjective feeling (1). When debridement of the defect is completed, the joint is irrigated using a large-bore (4.5-mm) egress cannula.

Chip fragments at different locations vary in their ease of removal, on the degree of associated joint damage, and also on the prognosis. Chip fractures off the distal intermediate carpal bone are removed using a medial arthroscopic approach and a lateral instrument approach (the actual site of these lateral and medial portals is always the same with any chip in the carpal joint). Chip fragments off the proximal aspect of the third carpal bone are removed with a lateral arthroscopic approach and a medial instrument approach. Generally, lesions in the radiocarpal (antebrachiocarpal) joint are more difficult to operate on because the joint capsule is drawn more tightly against the dorsal surface of the bones in this joint, thus allowing less room for manipulation of the instruments. Surgery in this joint is facilitated if the limb being operated on is in approximately 30 degrees of flexion, in contrast to 90 degrees of flexion in the intercarpal joint. With lesions of the proximal radial and proximal intermediate carpal bone, the forceps have to approach the lesion end on, and the distance from the synovial membrane to the lesion is small. For lesions of the proximal radiocarpal bone, the arthroscope is placed through the lateral portal and the instrument through the medial portal. These positions are switched for operating on the proximal aspect of the intermediate carpal bone. Fractures off the distal lateral aspect of the radius are operated on with the arthroscope placed medially and the instrument placed laterally. These fragments are generally of a larger size. Similarly, fragments off the medial aspect of the distal radius are operated on with the arthroscope placed laterally and the instrument placed medially. Further detail on surgery at each of these locations is presented elsewhere (1).

Carpal fragments of all sizes are amenable to arthroscopic surgery, and suturing of portals in the joint capsule is unnecessary even with large fragments.

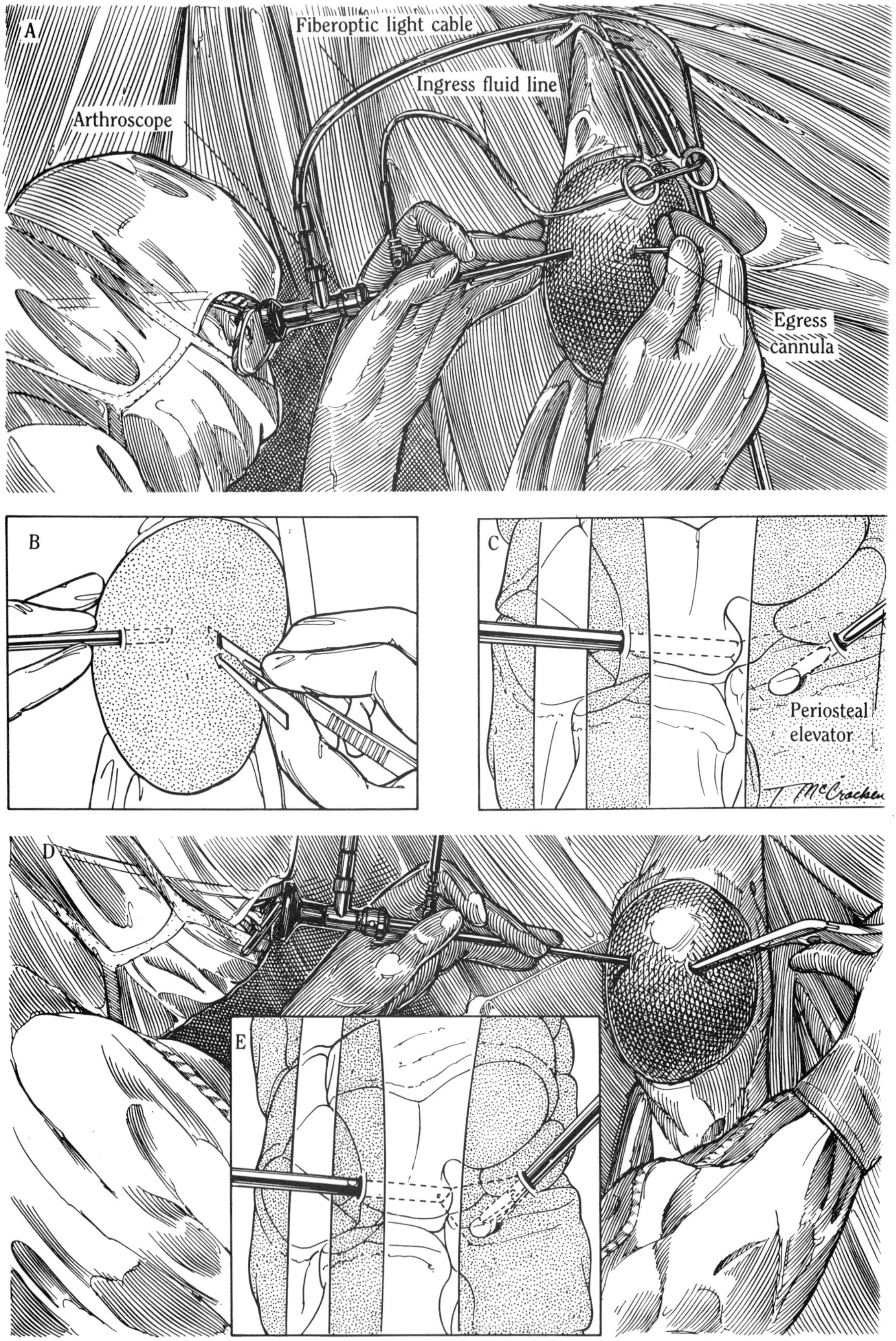

Figure 5.17, A–E. Arthroscopic surgery of the carpal joint.

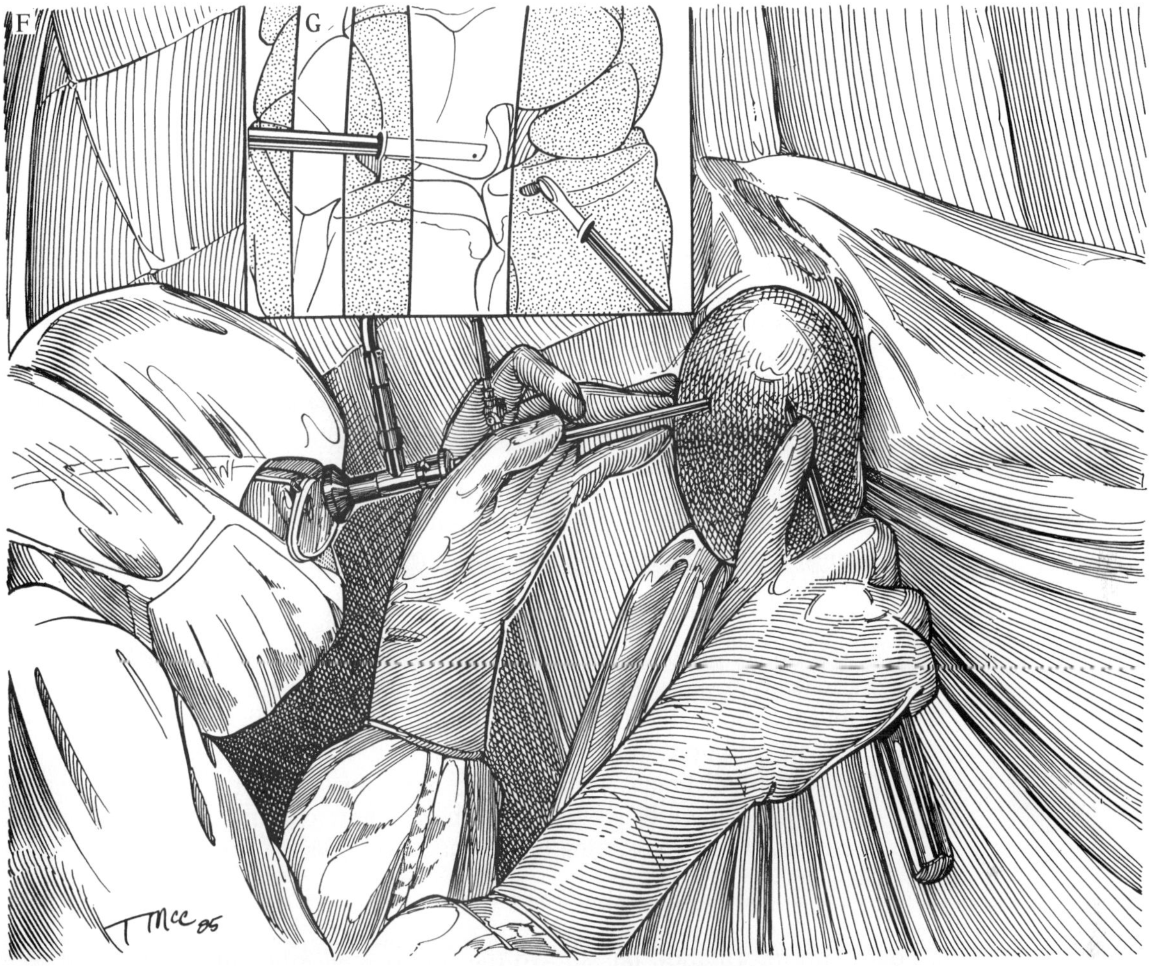

Figure 5.17, F–G. *(continued)* Arthroscopic surgery of the carpal joint.

Multiple fragments in multiple joints can be conveniently operated on with arthroscopic surgery, whereas multiple arthrotomies in such situations would not be appropriate. Spurs or osteophyte are removed only if they are broken off or if their interposition into the joint makes them likely candidates for later fracture or if they will preclude normal joint closure. Most spurs visible on preoperative radiographs are *not* candidates for removal, and the best example of these are ones that commonly occur on the proximal aspect of the intermediate carpal bone.

Intraoperative and/or postoperative radiographs are important to ensure that no fragments are left within the joint. While the arthroscopic surgeon must be careful to ensure that all interarticular fragments are removed, at the same time it is important that the surgeon realize that osseous densities within the joint capsule are not candidates for removal.

Postoperative Management

While patients are recovering from anesthesia, full-length padded bandages are applied to the operated limbs to avoid trauma to the carpal joints. After recovery from anesthesia, small bandages consisting of a nonadhesive pad, a sterile gauze (Kling), and an elastic adhesive (Elastikon) are applied. These bandages facilitate early exercise and passive flexion of the joint. Hand-walking is commenced at

7 to 10 days. Swimming is commonly used during the convalescent period for many horses. With simple fractures, horses can be put into training at 6 weeks, and some horses are started considerably earlier without any problems. Horses with associated cartilage and bone damage have appropriately longer periods of convalescence.

Comments

The advantages of arthroscopic surgery can be listed as follows (1–5):

1. Less trauma to the soft tissues with resultant benefits both in the cosmetic appearance of the carpus and in decreased functional compromise.
2. Better visualization of lesions.
3. Earlier return to racing or other athletic activity. This advantage is considered to be related to maintenance of normal joint function, particularly in the soft tissues, not to differences in cartilage healing.
4. Improved racing performance after surgery (2).
5. Treatment of more cases possible (multiple lesions).
6. Correction of the problem instead of treatment with medication. Many trainers who were not satisfied with the results from arthrotomy and therefore would rely on rest, retirement, or continued work with medication now request arthroscopic surgery.
7. Considerably decreased convalescent costs for arthroscopy compared with arthrotomy. Not only is the time from surgery to commencement of training decreased, but also training time is decreased because of less loss of fitness (7).

Follow-up information has shown that the overall functional ability and cosmetic appearance of the limbs are excellent. Postsurgical follow-up information has been reported for 445 racehorses. After surgery, 303 (68.1%) raced at a level equal to or better than preinjury level, 49 (11%) had decreased performance or still had problems referable to the carpus, 23 (5.2%) were retired without returning to training, 28 (6.3%) sustained another fracture, 32 (7.2%) developed other problems, and 10 (2.2%) sustained collapsing slab fractures while racing. Comparing the results of arthroscopic surgery in this series with the results of arthrotomy is difficult because of the variable methods used in the past to assess success. However, earlier reports on arthrotomy considered return to competition or starting in one race as a success; using such criteria, the success rate in the arthroscopic follow-up study would be 88.6% for Thoroughbreds and 88.8% for Quarter horses.

When horses were separated into four categories of articular damage, the performance in the two most severely affected groups was significantly inferior. A total of 133 of 187 horses with grade 1 damage (71.1%), 108 of 144 horses with grade 2 damage (75%), 41 of 77 horses with grade 3 damage (53.2%), and 20 of 37 horses with grade 4 damage (54.1%) returned to racing, as well as or better than before injury. The success rate among cases with grade 1 and 2 lesions was significantly greater than that among cases with grade 3 and 4 lesions ($P < 0.01$). Refragmentation in grade 3 and 4 cases is common, as is osteophytosis and enthesitis on the dorsal surface of the carpal bones.

Although arthroscopic surgery is the technique that should be used for operated problems of the carpal joints, recognize that the technique requires skill and experience and careful learning. Without these qualifications the advantages of arthroscopic surgery are quickly lost.

REFERENCES

1. McIlwraith CW. Diagnostic and surgical arthroscopy in the horse. Philadelphia: Lea & Febiger, 1990.
2. McIlwraith CW, Yovich JV, Martin GS. Arthroscopic surgery for the treatment of osteochondral chip fractures in the equine carpus. JAVMA 1987;191:531–540.
3. Richardson DW. Technique for arthroscopic repair of third carpal bone slab fractures in the horse. JAVMA 1986;188:288–291.
4. McIlwraith CW. Tearing of the medial palmar intercarpal ligament. Equine Vet J 1992; 24:367–371.
5. McIlwraith CW. Fractures of the carpus. In: Nixon AJ, ed. Equine Fractures. Philadelphia: WB Saunders, 1995:208–221.
6. McIlwraith CW. Experiences in diagnostic and surgical arthroscopy in the horse. Equine Vet J 1984;16:11.
7. McIlwraith CW. Arthroscopy in retrospect. In: Proceedings of the 30th Annual Convention of the American Association of Equine Practitioners, Dallas, TX, 1984:57–66.

Arthroscopic Surgery of the Dorsal Aspect of the Fetlock Joint

Arthroscopic surgery of the dorsal aspect of the fetlock joint is indicated for the following conditions:

1. Proximal dorsal chip fractures of the proximal phalanx (1–3).
2. Villonodular (chronic proliferative synovitis) synovitis of appropriate size (2, 4, 5).
3. OCD of the sagittal ridge of the distal metacarpus or metatarsus (2, 6).
4. Subchondral cystic lesions of the distal metacarpus.

The removal of osteochondral chip fragments from the proximal dorsal aspect of the proximal phalanx is the most common indication for arthroscopic surgery in this joint (2). The use of arthrotomy in such conditions is now generally considered inappropriate unless there are special circumstances. The technique for removing these chip fractures will be illustrated. Arthroscopic surgery for the removal of avulsion fragments of the proximal palmar or proximal plantar rim of the proximal phalanx is more difficult, but a technique has been developed and is described next.

Arthrotomy may still be used for large fractures of the proximal lateral or proximal medial eminence (7). Arthroscopic surgery is appropriate for less extensive villonodular synovitis cases, but arthrotomy may still be necessary when large masses fill the entire dorsal joint space (previously described). With OCD of the distal sagittal ridge of the distal articular surface of the third metacarpal or metatarsal bone, arthroscopic surgery is recommended (2).

Villonodular synovitis or chronic proliferative synovitis is a slowly developing intra-articular mass arising from the normal flatlike synovial projection at the proximodorsal attachment of the fetlock joint. It most commonly occurs in the metacarpophalangeal joints and is considered to arise as a sequel to trauma, probably a combination of concussion and severe hyperextension. Histologically, the mass contains dense fibrous connective tissue, arguing against comparisons with pigmented villonodular synovitis in humans (5). These cases can be operated on using an arthroscopic approach to the dorsal aspect of the fetlock joint (2).

Anesthesia and Surgical Preparation

For arthroscopic surgery in the dorsal aspect of the fetlock joint, the horse is placed under general anesthesia in dorsal recumbency. The limb is suspended for surgical preparation, and it may be suspended or rested on the horse's forearm during the operation. The limb is clipped before surgery from below the carpus to the foot and shaved immediately before or after induction of anesthesia.

Additional Instrumentation

These arthroscopic procedures require arthroscopic instrumentation (see Appendix IV).

Surgical Technique

A chip fracture off the medial aspect of the proximal phalanx within the fetlock joint will be used as an example. The joint is distended with saline or electrolyte solution before making any incisions (Fig. 5.18*A*). The general principles of triangulation and arthroscopic surgery have been previously described in the section on carpal arthroscopy. The skin incision for the arthroscopic portal is made over the bulge lateral to the common digital extensor tendon created by joint distension. The arthroscopic sleeve is inserted using the sharp trocar, and after passing through the joint capsule, it is angled proximad to avoid creating iatrogenic damage to the sagittal ridge of the distal metacarpus. After placement of the arthroscopic sheath, the arthroscope is inserted and the fluid line and light cable are attached.

For surgical procedure on a chip fracture off the medial proximal aspect of the proximal phalanx, the instrument portal is made in the lower half of the medial bulge created by joint distension. The portal through the joint capsule is made with a trocar or scalpel blade as previously described in the procedure on carpal arthroscopic surgery. If there is a question regarding the correct site for placement of the instrument portal, it can be ascertained by inserting an 18-gauge needle through the proposed site to check for positioning. The external and internal positioning of the arthroscope and instrument is illustrated in Figure 5.18, *B* and *C*. As in the carpus, fragments can be removed with forceps if they are loose or they may require separation with a periosteal elevator. Following removal of the fragment, loose tags are removed from the defect, but debridement is kept to a minimum in an attempt to avoid any potential periosteal proliferation at the surgical site caused by capsular trauma (8), The joint is irrigated with polyionic solution and the skin incisions are closed.

For surgery on villonodular synovitis, the arthroscope is placed in the same position as described above, although some surgeons prefer it more distal. The instrument portal is made after ascertaining the best location with the needle, and the villonodular mass is resected directly with sharp severance of the base and removal with Ferris Smith rongeurs (Fig. 5.18*D*). An option is to use two instrument portals, one above the other, and having one to hold the lesion and the more proximal one to sever the mass. The mass can also be resected with motorized equipment. If the lateral mass cannot be removed with the lateral arthroscopic and medial instrument approach, the instrument and arthroscope are changed in position. Further details can be obtained elsewhere.

For OCD, the same lateral arthroscopic portal is used as previously described. The best position for the instrument portal is ascertained using a needle and an instrument portal created with a no. 11 blade on the medial side (Fig. 5.18*E*). Flaps are elevated and removed with Ferris Smith rongeurs and the defect debrided with a curet.

Arthroscopic surgery may also be used for debridement of a subchondral cystic lesion of the distal metacarpus. The technique is more difficult because flexion of the joint is required to expose the cystic lesion, and this makes arthroscopic manipulation more difficult. The arthroscope is placed in the same position as previously described but the instrument portal needs to be on the same side. Its position is distal to the arthroscopic portal and the ideal position is ascertained by the prior use of a needle.

Postoperative Management

A sterile dressing is placed over the incisions, and a firm leg bandage is applied to the lower leg. This wrap is maintained with changes for 10 days, at which time the sutures are removed and no further bandaging is necessary. Handwalking is begun 7 to 10 days after surgery. Swimming is used during the convalescence of some of these patients. For horses with uncomplicated chip fractures of the proximal dorsal aspect of the proximal phalanx, training can be resumed 2 months after surgery (2, 3). A longer lay-up time of 4 months is recommended

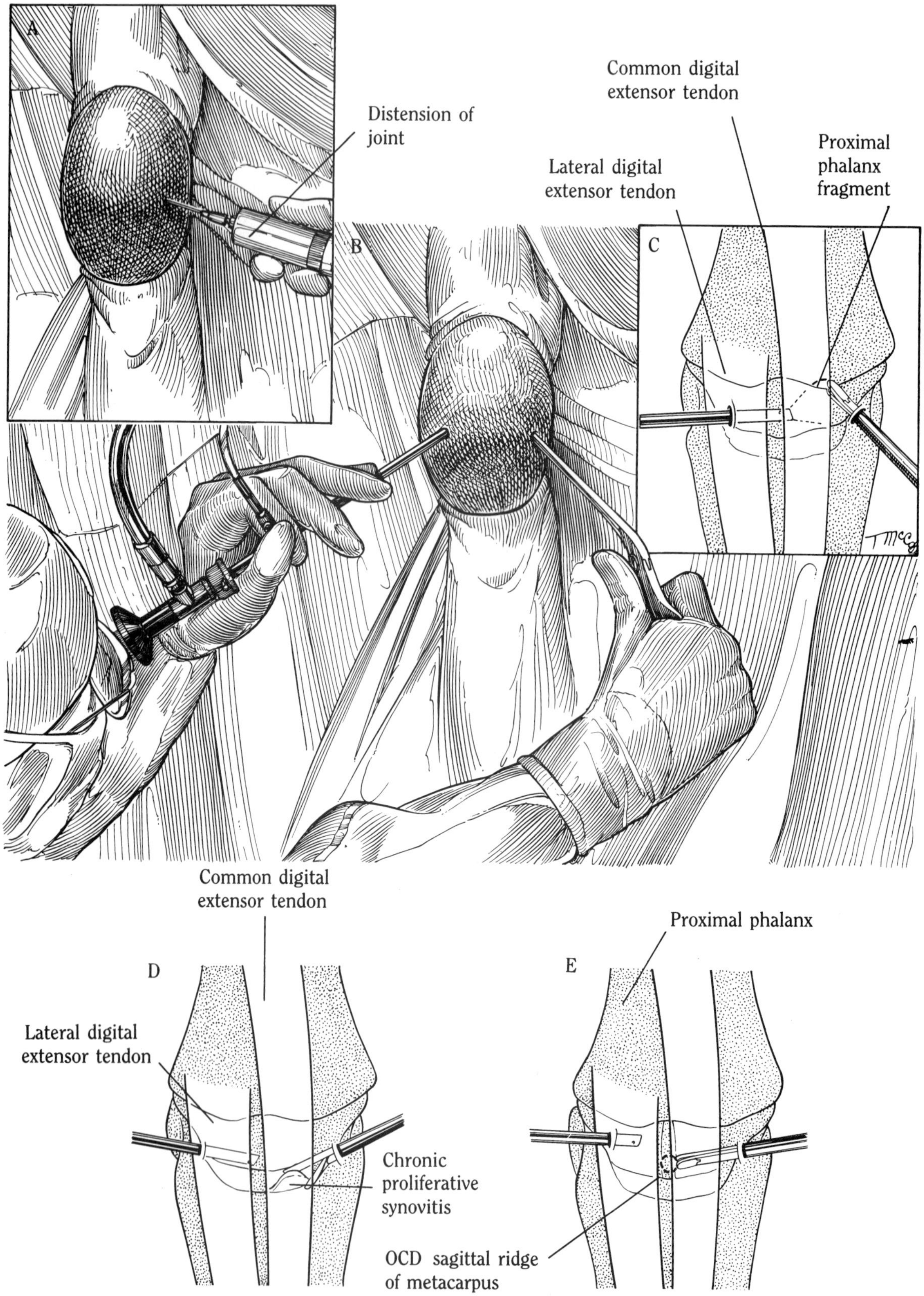

FIGURE 5.18, A–E. Arthroscopic surgery for the dorsal aspect of the fetlock joint.

for horses with chronic proliferative synovitis and larger fractures off the proximal aspect of the proximal phalanx.

Comments

The advantages of arthroscopic surgery over arthrotomy have been described elsewhere in this textbook and are well documented in the literature (2, 3, 9). As mentioned before, caution is needed in that these advantages apply only when sufficient skill and experience in the technique have been developed.

The results of arthroscopic surgery for proximodorsal P1 chip fragments are excellent and have been reported in 336 horses (3). When a proximodorsal P1 chip fragment is the solitary lesion, 92.0% of Thoroughbred racehorses return to racing and 71.4% return at the same level. This figure is lowered to 72.4% and 52.6%, respectively, when there are concomitant lesions such as wear lines and erosions on the distal metacarpus.

With OCD, the prognosis varies depending on time of surgery relative to first appearance of clinical signs, hind limb versus forelimb, and the presence of secondary osteoarthritis.

Excellent results with arthroscopic surgery have been reported for villonodular synovitis (4). The average rest period was 3 months. In uncomplicated cases of chronic proliferative synovitis, of 13 horses in which follow-up information was available between 6 and 30 months postsurgery, 12 returned to their previous level of training, and the owner or trainer reported no recurrence of lameness. Of these 12 horses, they all raced and 6 of them won a race. One horse that did not recover satisfactorily was an eventing horse that had severe osteoarthritis at the time of arthroscopic surgery.

REFERENCES

1. Yovich JV, McIlwraith CW. Arthroscopic surgery for removal of chip fragments of the first phalanx. JAVMA 1986;188:273.
2. McIlwraith CW. Diagnostic and Surgical Arthroscopy in the Horse. 2nd ed. Philadelphia: Lea & Febiger, 1990 KS. Veterinary Medicine Publishing Company, 1984.
3. Kawcak CE, McIlwraith CW. Proximal dorsal first phalanx osteochondral chip fragmentation in 336 horses. Equine Vet J 1994;26:329–396.
4. Kannegieter NJ. Chronic proliferative synovitis of the equine metacarpophalangeal joint. Vet Rec 1990;127:8–10.
5. van Veenendaal JC, Moffatt RE. Soft tissue masses in the fetlock joint of horses. Aust Vet J 1980;56:533–536.
6. Yovich JV, McIlwraith CW, Stashak TS. Osteochondritis dissecans of the sagittal ridge of the third metacarpal and metatarsal bones in horses. JAVMA 1985;186:1186.
7. Petterson H, Ryden G. Avulsion fractures of the caudoproximal extremity of the first phalanx. Equine Vet J 1982;14:333.
8. Raker CW. Calcification of the equine metacarpophalangeal joint following removal of chip fractures. Arch Am Coll Vet Surg 1975;4:66.
9. McIlwraith CW. Fetlock fractures and luxations. In: Nixon AJ, ed. Equine Fracture Repair. Philadelphia: WB Saunders, 1996:153–162.

Arthroscopic Surgery of the Palmar (Plantar) Aspect of the Fetlock Joint

Arthroscopic surgery of the palmar (plantar) aspect of the metacarpophalangeal (tarsophalangeal) joint is indicated for (*a*) removal of palmar (plantar) (type I) osteochondral fragments; (*b*) apical fragmentation of the sesamoid bones; (*c*) abaxial fragmentation of the sesamoid bones; (*d*) selected basilar fragmentation of the sesamoid bones; and (*e*) diagnostic arthroscopy during reduction of distal metacarpal or metatarsal condylar fractures (1–3).

Two types of fragments of the palmar or plantar part of the metacarpophalangeal and metatarsophalangeal joints have been described: type I, osteochondral fragments of the palmar or plantar aspect (also called bony fragments of the palmar or plantar part of the metacarpophalangeal and metatarsophalangeal joint) (4–7); type II, osteochondral fragments of the palmar or plantar aspect of the fetlock joints or ununited proximoplantar tuberosity of the proximal phalanx (4–6). Surgery is rarely indicated with type II osteochondral fragments. However, type I osteochondral fragments are articular and frequently cause clinical signs. Type I fragments originate from the plantar aspect of the proximal phalanx just medial or lateral to the sagittal groove. Type II fragments arise from the plantar eminence of the proximal phalanx. Lameness is often only evident at high speeds for advanced work.

The etiopathogenesis of proximal plantar osteochondral fragmentation is uncertain. Some investigators consider them to be traumatic fractures and others consider them manifestations of OCD. The origin of the pain is uncertain (8). Because there was no evidence of recent fracture or bone to bone contact, the fragments themselves are probably not the origin. Soft tissue damage or tearing around the fragment may occur at the limits of joint motion, particularly during extension of the joint associated with high-speed gaits. Examination of metatarsophalangeal joints with fragments at necropsy showed a partial subluxation of the proximal sesamoid above the fragment during flexion and a dorsal protrusion of the fragment into the joint during extension. Such mechanical factors may be involved when one considers that synovial membrane overlies the fragment.

Techniques for the removal of apical, abaxial, and basilar sesamoid fragments have been described elsewhere (3). These cases are diagnosed with conventional radiographs.

Anesthesia and Surgical Preparation

The surgical procedure is done with the horse under general anesthesia in dorsal recumbency. The fetlock is slightly flexed. Before anesthetic induction, the limb is clipped from the coronet proximal to the proximal end of the cannon bone, around the limb's entire circumference. After induction of the anesthetic, the area of the surgical incision is shaved and the surgical area is prepared.

Additional Instrumentation

Arthroscopic instrumentation must include a flat sesamoid knife (Sontec) as well as a curved Foerner elevator.

Surgical Technique

The joint is distended with fluid and an 8-mm skin incision made at the proximal central area of the distended palmar (plantar) pouch. A no. 11 blade is used to

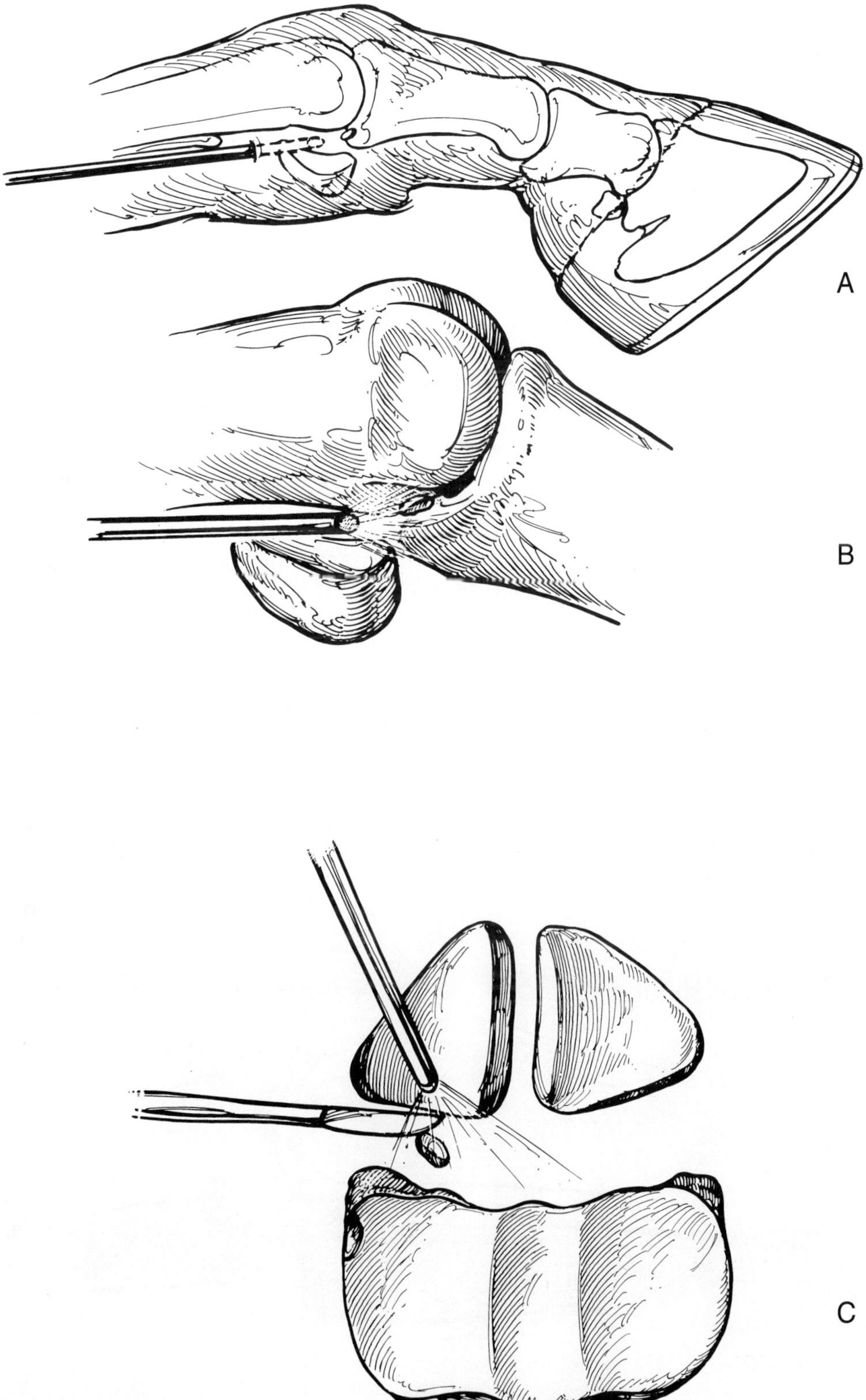

Figure 5.19, A–C. Arthroscopic surgery of the palmar (plantar) aspect of the fetlock joint.

continue the incision into the joint and an arthroscopic sleeve inserted using the conical obturator. After removal of the conical obturator, the arthroscope is placed and examination of the joint carried out. After diagnostic arthroscopy, the arthroscope is focused on the area of the fragment (Fig. 5.19, *A* and *B*). A needle is used to ascertain the best location for the instrument above the proximal plantar eminence of the first phalanx. The instrument should come in parallel to the base of the sesamoid, and a no. 11 blade is used to make the portal in this direction. A probe is then placed through the portal to evaluate the fragment, which is palpable through the synovial membrane (and usually visible). A flat sesamoid knife is then used to incise the proximal attachment of the fragment (Fig. 5.19*C*). This incision is continued around under the fragment and the curved knife is then used to sever the axial attachments. The fragment is then removed with 4 × 10-mm Ferris Smith cup rongeurs (Fig. 5.19*D*). After removal of the fragment, the soft tissue in the defect is trimmed and the joint lavaged. The portals are closed with skin sutures using 2/0 monofilament nylon.

The same approach is used for surgery for apical sesamoid fractures, abaxial sesamoid fractures, and basilar sesamoid fractures. The instrument approach depends on the location of the fragment but is always ascertained with placement of a needle. For apical fragments, the portal is distad to the arthroscope and opposite the fracture line. The instrument can then be inserted in the fracture line, as well as giving good positioning for severing the suspensory and intersesamoidean ligament attachments. After elevation of the fragment, a flat sesamoid knife is used to sever the suspensory attachments. A curved Foerner elevator is then used to sever the intersesamoidean ligament attachments and ensure severance of all attachments around the abaxial side. The fragment is then removed with Ferris Smith rongeurs. Further details are available elsewhere (8).

The technique for removing abaxial sesamoid fragments is the same, but only suspensory ligament attachments need to be removed. The basilar fragments are also removed using the same instrument approach as for palmar (plantar) first phalanx fragments. The distal soft tissue attachments of the fragment are

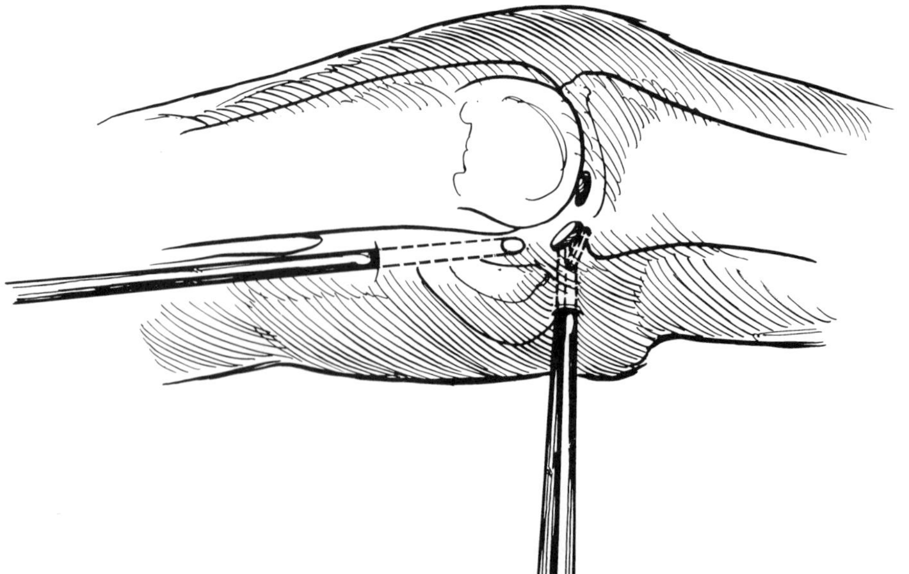

Figure 5.19, D. *(continued)* Arthroscopic surgery of the palmar (plantar) aspect of the fetlock joint.

severed and the fragment elevated. The fragment is then removed with Ferris Smith intervertebral disk rongeurs.

Comments

Results of arthroscopic surgery have been published on a series of 119 horses; Standardbred racehorses represent 109 (92%) of those affected (8). In 55 of 87 (63%) racehorses and in 100% of the 9 nonracehorses, performance returned to preoperative levels after surgery. Abnormal surgical findings consisting of articular cartilage fibrillation and synovial proliferation were significantly ($P <$ 0.0001) associated with adverse outcomes; these findings were documented in 31% of the 32 horses without successful outcome and in only 2% of the 55 horses with successful outcomes.

REFERENCES

1. McIlwraith CW. Fetlock fractures and luxations. In: Nixon AJ, ed. Fractures in the Horse. Philadelphia: WB Saunders, 1996:153–162.
2. McIlwraith CW, Foerner JJ. Removal of osteochondral fragments from the proximal or plantar aspect of the first phalanx. In: McIlwraith CW, ed. Diagnostic and Surgical Arthroscopy. 2nd ed. Philadelphia: Lea & Febiger, 1989:105–108.
3. McIlwraith CW. Diagnostic and Surgical Arthroscopy in the Horse. 2nd ed. Philadelphia: Lea & Febiger, 1990.
4. Barclay WP, Foerner JJ, Phillips TN. Lameness attributable to osteochondral fragmentation of the plantar aspect of the proximal phalanx in horses: 19 cases (1981–1985). JAVMA 1987;1991:855–857.
5. Grondahl AM. The incidence of bony fragments and osteochondrosis in the metacarpo- and metatarsophalangeal joints of Standardbred Trotters: a radiographic study. J Equine Vet Sci 1992;12:81–85.
6. Grondahl AM. Incidence and development of ununited proximoplantar tuberosity of the proximal phalanx in Standardbred Trotters. Vet Radiol Ultrasound 1992;33:18–21.
7. Nixon AJ, Pool RR. Histologic appearance of axial osteochondral fragments from their proximoplantar/proximopalmar aspect of the proximal phalanx in horses. JAVMA 1995;207:1076–1080.
8. Fortier LA, Foerner JJ, Nixon AJ. Arthroscopic removal of axial osteochondral fragments of the plantar/palmar proximal aspect of the proximal phalanx in horses: 119 cases (1988–1992). JAVMA 1995;206:71–74.

Arthroscopic Surgery of the Tarsocrural (Tibiotarsal) Joint

Arthroscopic surgery is the preferred method of treatment for cases of OCD or traumatically created fragments involving the tarsocrural joint (1, 2). The sites of such lesions include the distal intermediate ridge and medial malleolus of the tibia and the trochlear ridges of the talus. Arthroscopic surgery is also used for the treatment of traumatically induced chip fragments of the tarsocrural joint as well as diagnostic arthroscopy of this joint. Traumatically induced fragments off the lateral malleolus generally require arthrotomy if they are considered suitable for surgical treatment.

The exact location of the lesions should be ascertained as well as possible with preoperative radiographs. Experience with arthroscopy has taught us, however, that the surgeon must be prepared to find lesions that were not demonstrable on preoperative radiographs. In addition to decreasing the trauma associated with removal of these fragments, compared with arthrotomy, arthroscopic surgery has improved the surgeon's diagnostic capabilities in this joint and the ability to identify "new" lesions.

Anesthesia and Surgical Preparation

The surgical procedure is done under general anesthesia with the horse in dorsal recumbency. Frequently, bilateral lesions are present, and both joints are operated at the same time. Before induction of anesthesia, the patient's limb(s) is(are) clipped from the middle of the crus to the middle of the metatarsus. Following induction of anesthesia, the areas over the dorsolateral and dorsomedial pouches of the tarsocrural joint are shaved, and a routine surgical preparation of the hock is done.

Additional Instrumentation

This procedure requires arthroscopic instrumentation (see Appendix IV).

Surgical Technique

An impervious draping system is used, as well as sterile plastic adherent drapes in the immediate area. (The general technique of arthroscope and instrument insertion and triangulation was discussed earlier.) One difference with the tarsocrural joint is that the joint is distended with sterile fluid before making any skin incisions. This joint distension is effected through the dorsomedial pouch, and 50 to 100 mL of fluid is injected. This distension enables identification of both the dorsolateral and the dorsomedial outpouching of the tarsocrural joint. To operate on lesions of the distal intermediate ridge of the tibia, or the lateral trochlear ridge of the talus, a medial approach with the arthroscope is made. The lateral approach with the arthroscope is made if the primary area of concern includes the medial trochlear ridge of the talus. For lesions of the medial malleolus of the tibia, lateral and medial arthroscopic approaches have been used.

To insert the arthroscope through the medial pouch, an 8-mm skin incision is made slightly dorsal to the center of the outpouching but lateral to the cranial branch of the medial saphenous vein. This incision will be approximately 1 cm lateral to the complex of extensor tendons over the dorsal aspect of the joint. The arthroscopic sheath and sharp trocar are then pushed through the subcutaneous tissue and joint capsule with the limb maintained in extension. When the bone on the medial nonarticular portion of the talus is contacted, the sharp trocar is replaced with the blunt obturator, and the limb is flexed to enable passage of the arthroscopic sheath across the joint. The arthroscope, the fiberoptic cable, and the ingress fluid system are then connected and visualization can begin.

If the arthroscope is to be placed from the lateral side, it is inserted through the dorsolateral pouch. The skin incision is made in the center of the dorsolateral pouch with the limb in extension. Flexion is again used to facilitate passage of the sheath and obturator over the dorsal aspect of the trochlear ridges of the talus.

The placement of the instrument and arthroscope to operate on a lesion off the distal intermediate ridge of the tibia is illustrated in Figure 5.20*A*. The instrument is placed through the distal part of the bulge of the dorsolateral pouch. Such a placement is necessary to enable passage of the instrument over the lateral trochlear ridge and onto the intermediate ridge lesion. This approach is also represented diagrammatically in Figure 5.20*B*. The technique for operating on a lesion on the lateral trochlear ridge is illustrated in Figure 5.20*C*. Alternatively, the arthroscope may also be placed laterally. Lesions of the medial malleolus are operated on using a triangulating approach from the same side or the opposite side, depending on the surgeon's preference. Unless fragments of the lateral malleolus are small, their embedment in other soft tissues of the joint is too extensive for arthroscopic surgery to be carried out conveniently. Further details on the arthroscopic techniques in the tarsocrural joint are available elsewhere (1, 2).

Fragments and flaps are separated with an elevator or osteotome followed by removal with forceps. The area of the lesions is debrided with a curette. The joint is then flushed, and the arthroscope and sheath are removed from the joint. Each skin incision is closed with one or two simple interrupted sutures of nonabsorbable material. The tarsus is bandaged using a nonadhesive pad, gauze bandage, and elastic adhesive bandage. A full pressure wrap is not considered necessary.

Postoperative Management

The bandage is maintained with changes for 10 days, at which time the sutures are removed and bandaging is no longer necessary. The horse is maintained in a stall for 1 month and can then be turned out into a small area. Athletic training (if the age of the animal is appropriate) can be resumed in 6 to 8 weeks.

The technique and results of arthroscopic surgery for the treatment of OCD in 318 tarsocrural joints in 225 horses has been reported (2). Arthroscopic surgery was an effective technique for treating OCD, and the overall functional ability and cosmetic appearance of the limbs were excellent. Postsurgical follow-up information was obtained for 183 horses, of which 140 (76.5%) raced successfully or performed their intended use after surgery. Of the remaining 43, 11 were considered to still have a tarsocrural joint problem, 19 developed other problems precluding successful performance, 8 were considered poor racehorses without any lameness problems identified, 3 were euthanized because of septic arthritis, and 2 died of other causes. There was no significant effect of age, sex, or limb involvement on the outcome. The size of the intermediate ridge lesions had no effect on prognosis, but the presence of degenerative or erosive changes in the articular cartilage significantly decreased the prognosis. The synovial effusion resolved in 117 of 131 racehorse joints (89.3%) and 64 of 86 nonracehorse joints (74.4%) with follow-up. The outcome for synovial fluid resolution was inferior for lesions of the lateral trochlear ridge of the talus or medial malleolus of the tibia, compared with distal intermediate ridge lesions. There was no significant relationship between resolution of effusion and successful performance outcome.

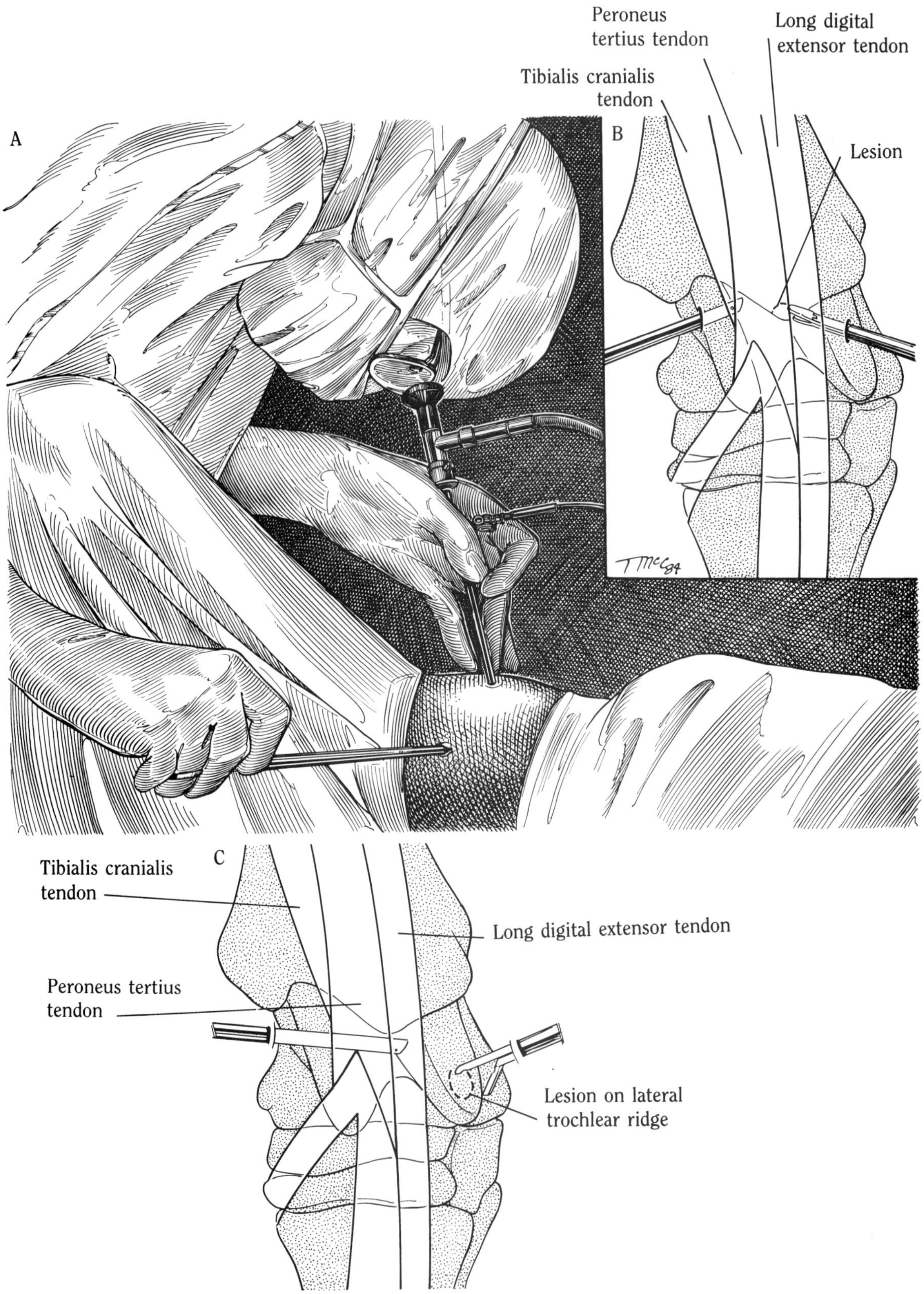

Figure 5.20, A–C. Arthroscopic surgery of the tarsocrural joint.

REFERENCES

1. McIlwraith CW. Diagnostic and Surgical Arthroscopy in the Horse. 2nd ed. Philadelphia: Lea & Febiger, 1990.
2. McIlwraith CW, Foerner JJ, Davis DM. Osteochondritis dissecans of the tarso neural joint: results of treatment with arthroscopic surgery. Equine Vet J 1991;23:155–162.

Arthroscopic Surgery of the Femoropatellar Joint

Arthroscopic surgery of the femoropatellar joint is the preferred method of surgically treating OCD of the lateral trochlear ridge, the medial trochlear ridge, or the patella. The advantages include decreased tissue trauma, a less complicated convalescence, and good results in terms of return to athletic function (1–4). There is rapid resolution of both synovial effusion and lameness following the surgery. Contraindications to surgery include marked loss of articular cartilage and bone on the trochlear ridges, lateral luxation of the patella, or remodeling change of the patella seen on radiographs. The use of arthroscopy has improved our diagnostic capabilities in this joint, as well as offering an improved method of surgical treatment.

The technique is also used for the treatment of fragmentation of the distal aspect of the patella and selected fractures of the proximal aspect of the patella (2, 5).

Anesthesia and Surgical Preparation

The surgical procedure is done with the horse under general anesthesia and in dorsal recumbency. The limbs are maintained in extension during surgical procedures, but the opposite limb is flexed when not being operated on to minimize the risk of postoperative femoral nerve paresis. Before induction of anesthesia, the area of the stifle is clipped and the immediate surgical site is shaved either before or after anesthetic induction. An impervious draping system is used.

Additional Instrumentation

Arthroscopic instrumentation including motorized abrading equipment is necessary (see Appendix IV).

Surgical Technique

Both limbs may be operated on at once. The affected limb is maintained in an extended position during surgical procedures while the other limb is kept in a flexed position. Prior distension of the femoropatellar joint is not usually necessary. An 8-mm skin incision is made midway between the distal border of the patella and the tibial crest between the lateral and middle patellar ligaments. This incision is continued through the superficial and deep fascia into the femoropatellar fat pad. The arthroscopic sleeve, containing a blunt obturator, is then inserted through this incision and directed at an angle of 45° up under the patella. With pressure, the sheath and obturator will pass through the thin femoropatellar capsule and up the trochlear groove. If resistance is encountered, the sheath is moved lateral to pass up the gap between the patella and lateral trochlear ridge into the suprapatellar pouch. When the arthroscopic sleeve is inserted up into the suprapatellar pouch, the examination is begun in this position. Sequential examination of the femoropatellar joint is continued by withdrawing the scope down the trochlear groove and alternatively examining the lengths of the medial and lateral trochlear ridges. The entire examination of the joint can be completed with the arthroscope placed through this single portal.

The site of instrument portals will vary depending on the location of the lesion. The same principles of triangulation as described in the carpus are used,

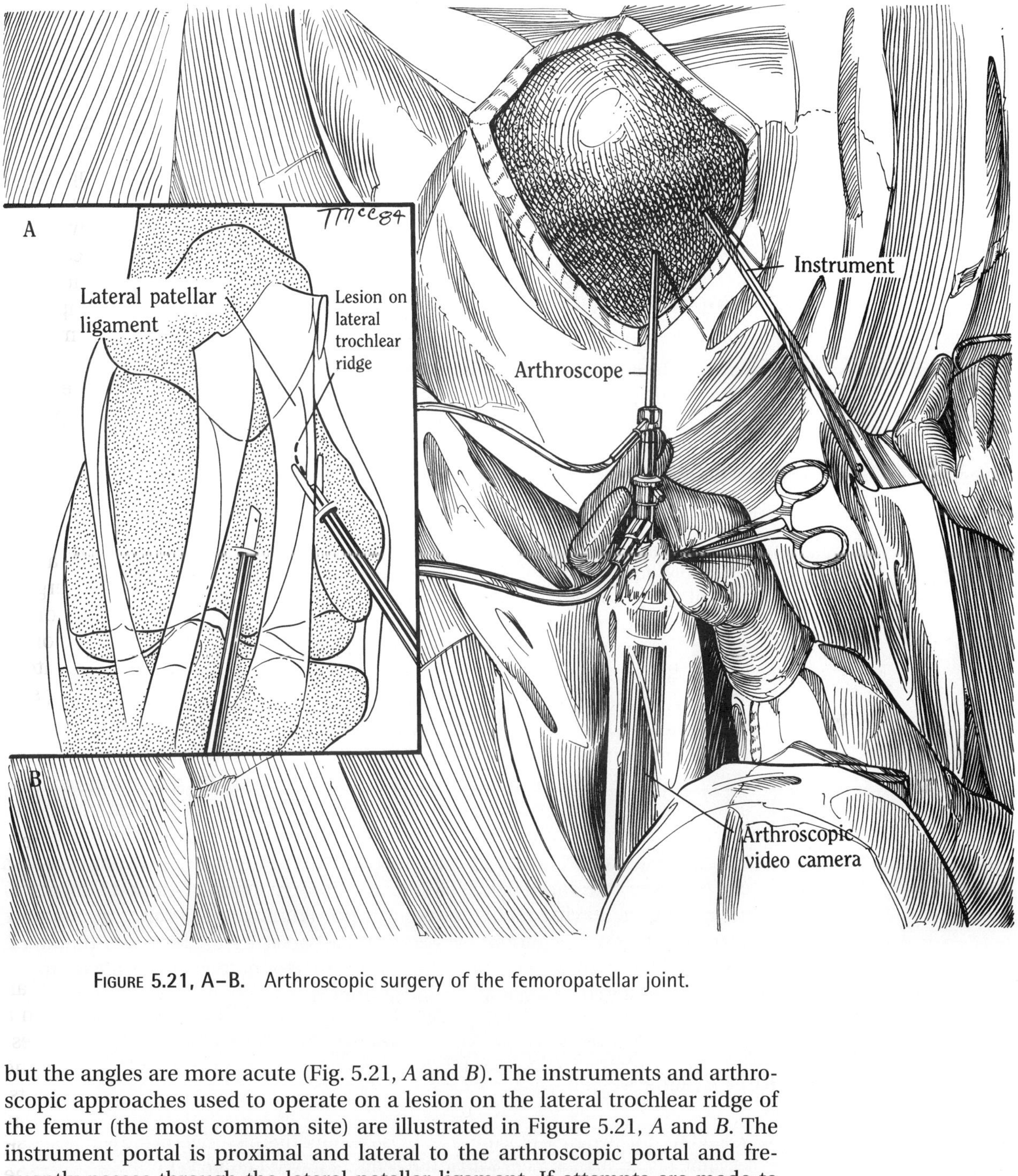

FIGURE 5.21, A–B. Arthroscopic surgery of the femoropatellar joint.

but the angles are more acute (Fig. 5.21, *A* and *B*). The instruments and arthroscopic approaches used to operate on a lesion on the lateral trochlear ridge of the femur (the most common site) are illustrated in Figure 5.21, *A* and *B*. The instrument portal is proximal and lateral to the arthroscopic portal and frequently passes through the lateral patellar ligament. If attempts are made to make the portal more lateral than the lateral patellar ligament, it is difficult to manipulate the instrument to operate effectively on lesions on the lateral trochlear ridge. Making an instrument portal through the lateral patellar ligament does not seem to be of any consequence. Lesions are operated on by elevating the flaps or fragments and removing them with forceps. Loose bodies are similarly removed with forceps. The lesions are debrided with a combination of basket forceps, curettes, and mechanical abrading equipment. These maneuvers are presented in more detail elsewhere (1, 2).

For the lesions in less frequent locations, different instrument portals are necessary. A more distal portal is required for lesions of the distal lateral trochlear ridge. Similarly, proximal and distal portals between the middle and medial patellar ligament are used to operate on the medial trochlear ridge of the femur. If lesions are on the underside of the patella, a distal portal medial or lateral to the middle patellar ligament is necessary for the instrument to be effectively passed proximad under the patella and manipulated on the articular surface of the patella.

Following debridement of lesions, the joint is flushed and the skin incisions are closed with nonabsorbable suture material. No bandaging is necessary.

For lesions on the patella, the instrument portal is usually approximately 2 cm lateral to the arthroscopic portal. The ideal position is ascertained.

Postoperative Management

The use of antibiotics is optional, but the horses are placed on phenylbutazone for 5 days following surgery. Skin sutures are removed in 12 to 14 days. The horse is maintained in a stall for 1 month and can then be turned out into a small area. Training exercise can be resumed 3 months after the arthroscopic surgery. Synovial effusion generally resolves within 1 month of surgery.

Comments

The results of arthroscopic surgery for the treatment of OCD on 252 femoropatellar joints in 161 horses has been reported. In the study were 82 Thoroughbreds, 39 Quarter horses, 16 Arabians, 9 Warmbloods, and 15 of various breeds. Twenty-two horses were under 1 year of age at the time of surgery, 68 were yearlings, 36 were 2-year-olds, 21 were 3-year-olds, and 14 were 4 years of age or older. Ninety-one had bilateral lesions and 70 had unilateral lesions. Follow-up information was obtained on 134 horses: 86 (64%) of these 134 horses returned to their intended use or achieved their intended use, 9 (7%) were in training, 21 (16%) were unsuccessful, and 18 (13%) were unsuccessful because of other reasons. Horses with grade 1 lesions (< 2 cm in length) had a significantly higher success rate (78%) than did horses with grade 2 (2–4 cm) or grade 3 (> 4 cm) lesions (63% and 54% success rates, respectively). The overall success rate of 64% was compared with a 68% success rate in terms of named Thoroughbred yearlings achieving racing. There was no significant difference in outcome as it related to sex, racehorse versus nonracehorse, lesion location, unilateral versus bilateral involvement, presence or absence of patella or trochlear groove lesions, or presence or absence of loose bodies.

REFERENCES

1. Foland JW, McIlwraith CW, Trotter GW. Osteochondritis dissecans of the femoropatellar joint: results of treatment with arthroscopic surgery. Equine Vet J 1992;24:419–423.
2. McIlwraith CW. Diagnostic and Surgical Arthroscopic Surgery in the Horse. 2nd ed. Philadelphia: Lea & Febiger, 1990; KS, Veterinary Medicine Publishing Company, 1984.
3. McIlwraith CW, Martin GS. Arthroscopic surgery for the treatment of osteochondritis dissecans in the equine femoropatellar joint. Vet Surg 1985;14:105.
4. Martin GS, McIlwraith CW. Arthroscopic anatomy of the equine femoropatellar joint and approaches for treatment of osteochondritis dissecans. Vet Surg 1985;14:99.
5. McIlwraith CW. Osteochondral fragmentation of the distal aspect of the patellar in hanaes. Equine Vet J 1990;22:157–163.

Arthroscopic Surgery of the Femorotibial Joint

Arthroscopic surgery of the medial or lateral femorotibial joint (usually medial) is indicated for (*a*) subchondral cystic lesions of the medial condyle of the femur; (*b*) tearing of the medial or lateral meniscus or cranial ligaments of the meniscus; (*c*) tearing of the cruciate ligaments; and (*d*) diagnostic evaluation for any other damage or disease. Early papers were restricted to diagnostic examination of the femorotibial joints (1–3). Use of arthroscopic surgery to treat cystic lesions of the medial condyle of the femur was first described by Lewis (4). The most common indication in the past has been for the treatment of subchondral cystic lesions of the medial condyle of the femur, but the ability of femorotibial arthroscopy to diagnose conditions undetectable by other means has increased greatly in recent years (1, 5).

Anesthesia and Surgical Preparation

The surgical procedure is done with the horse under general anesthesia in dorsal recumbency. The stifles are flexed at 90°. The areas of the stifle are clipped before anesthesia. Shaving is usually done on the table. The surgical area is prepared.

Additional Instrumentation

Arthroscopic instrumentation should include motorized equipment for synovial resection and bone debridement.

Surgical Technique

Two approaches are used for diagnostic arthroscopy of the medial femorotibial joint: cranial (2) and lateral (4). The lateral arthroscopic approach is always used for subchondral cystic lesions and is recommended as the initial approach for other diagnostic arthroscopy.

The joint is not distended. For the lateral approach, the site of the arthroscopic portal is caudal to the lateral patellar ligament, cranial to the long digital extensor tendon, and approximately 2 cm proximal to the tibia. An incision is made in the skin and fascia of the stifle. The arthroscopic cannula with the cannula obturator is then directed medially and slightly caudad to penetrate the synovial membrane in the lateral aspect of the medial femorotibial joint. The obturator can be flipped through the synovial membrane on the axial side of the medial condyle. The obturator is removed and the arthroscope inserted. Details of the examination of diagnostic arthroscopy have been described elsewhere (1).

The intercondylar eminence of the tibia and the axial side of the medial condyle of the femur are used as initial reference points. The cranial ligament of the medial meniscus and the cranial portion of the medial meniscus are visible by moving the arthroscope medially along the distal aspect of the medial condyle. With advancement of the arthroscope, the condyle and cranial aspect of the meniscus are visible up to close to the area of the medial collateral ligament. The arthroscope is then retracted to the center of the joint and rotated upward to visualize the central weightbearing area of the medial condyle of the femur. Further retraction allows visualization of the proximal axial portion of the medial condyle, the cranial cruciate ligament, and the caudal cruciate ligament.

If further visualization in the caudal area of the intercondylar fossa is required, the arthroscope is placed through a cranial portal. This portal has usually been made by prior placement of a spinal needle and an incision with a no. 11 blade. The cranial approach with the arthroscope is also the first part of entering the lateral femorotibial joint. Once the arthroscope has been placed in the dorsal pouch, its end is placed against the septum near the axial edge of the lateral condyle. The arthroscope is then replaced with a conical obturator and the sheath and obturator inserted through the synovial membrane into the lateral femorotibial joint.

Examination of the lateral femorotibial joint is similar to the medial, with initial recognition of the cranial ligament of the lateral meniscus, the lateral condyle of the femur, and lateral meniscus. The long digital and popliteal tendons are also recognized.

For arthroscopic surgery of a subchondral cystic lesion, the lateral arthroscopic portal is used. Examination reveals the dimple in the cartilage (sometimes a clear hole) demarcating the location of the cystic lesion. A spinal needle is used to determine the optimal cranial instrument portal to enucleate the cystic lesion. This instrument portal is then made with a no. 11 blade and the cystic lesion explored with a probe (Fig. 5.22*A*). The contents of the cystic lesion are removed with a curet and/or motorized abrader. Undermined cartilage at the surface is removed with a curet. When all defective tissue is removed, the joint is lavaged. Debris tends to accumulate in the intercondylar area close to the attachment of the cranial cruciate ligament. A large egress cannula is used for this purpose. Arthroscope and instrument portals are closed with skin sutures.

For treatment of traumatic injuries of the medial femorotibial joint, the lateral arthroscopic portal is usually used. Partial tears to the cranial and caudal cruciate ligament are debrided using a cranial instrument portal and a motorized resector. Although only the cranial-axial area of the medial meniscus is visible in a joint where the cruciate ligaments are intact, a number of tears regularly occur in this visible portion. The torn portion of the meniscus is debrided using a combination of hand instruments and motorized resection (Fig. 5.22*B*). At the completion of all procedures, the joint is lavaged.

Comments

Results of arthroscopic surgery for the treatment of subchondral cystic lesions of the medial femoral condyle in horses have been published (4, 6). In the most recent study, where more sensitive analyses of the results were done, 23 of 31 (74%) horses had a successful result and 8 of 31 (26%) had an unsuccessful result (6). Within this group of horses, the prognosis for successful results after arthroscopic surgery was not associated with age, sex, size of lesion, unilateral versus bilateral lesions, whether the lesion was drilled, the presence of osteochondritis associated with the subchondral cystic lesions, or whether the lesion enlarged after surgery. Follow-up radiographs were available for 14 horses, and in 9 of these, the subchondral cystic lesion enlarged after surgery. Postoperative cystic enlargement was associated significantly with drilling of the lesion bed at the time of surgery (6). Because of these findings, drilling of the lesion bed is not now recommended. Also, in an effort to decrease cystic enlargement, intra-articular corticosteroids are also used and have resulted in a decreased incidence of cystic enlargement.

A small series of meniscal tears treated with arthroscopic surgery has been published (3). The first author's experiences are consistent with this data.

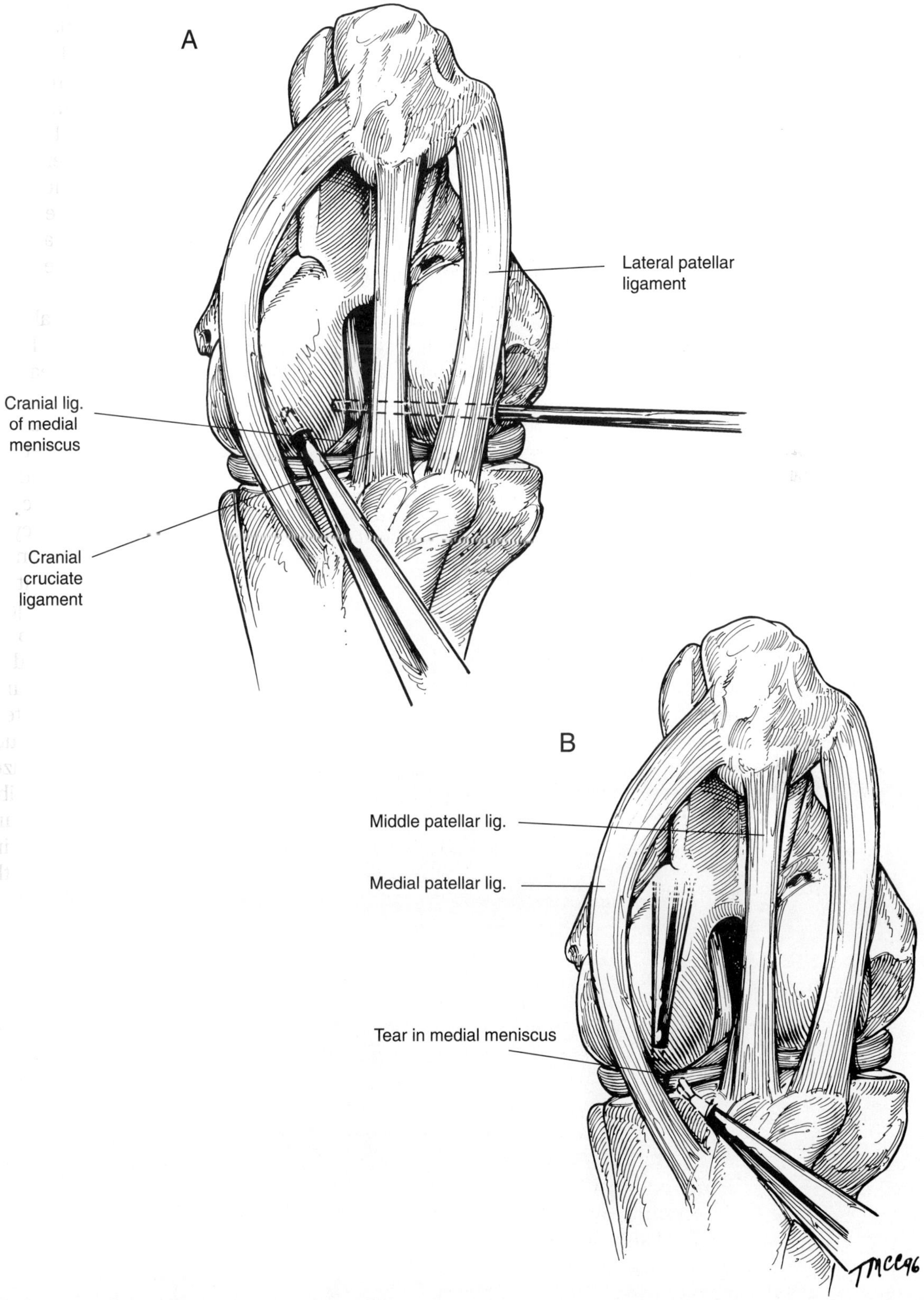

Figure 5.22, A–B. Arthroscopic surgery of the femorotibial joint.

REFERENCES

1. McIlwraith CW. Diagnostic and Surgical Arthroscopy in the Horse. 2nd ed. Philadelphia: Lea & Febiger, 1990.
2. Moustafa MAI, Boero JJ, Baker GJ. Arthroscopic examination of the femorotibial joints of horses. Vet Surg 1987;16:352–357.
3. Nickels FA, Sande R. Radiographic and arthroscopic findings in the equine stifle. JAVMA 1982;181:918–924.
4. Lewis RD. A retrospective study of diagnostic and surgical arthroscopy of the equine femorotibial joint. In: Proceedings of the American Association of Equine Practitioners, New Orleans, LA, 1987:887–893.
5. Walmsley JP. Vertical tears of the cranial horn of the meniscus and its cranial ligament in the equine femorotibial joint: 7 cases and their treatment by arthroscopic surgery. Equine Vet J 1995;27:20–25.
6. Howard RD, McIlwraith CW, Trotter GW. Arthroscopic surgery for subchondral cystic lesions of the medial femoral condyle in horses: 41 cases (1988–1991). JAVMA 1995; 206:842–850.

Surgical Treatment of Infective (Septic) Arthritis

In addition to antibiotic therapy, the institution of some form of joint drainage and irrigation is usually appropriate in the treatment of infective arthritis (1). The presence of a purulent effusion retards the action of many antibiotics by decreasing the metabolic rate of the bacteria. In addition, pH values drop in septic effusions, and the activity of aminoglycosides is reduced significantly with a decrease in pH (2). The primary indication for joint drainage, however, is the removal of substances potentially deleterious (metalloproteinases, E group prostaglandins, free radicals, and cytokines) to the articular cartilage.

Methods of joint drainage include needle aspiration, through-and-through lavage, distension irrigation, and arthrotomy with or without synovectomy. The selection of a particular technique depends on the individual case as well the preference of the clinician. Techniques have been adapted from the human medical literature, but controlled data in the horse are necessary to assess relative efficacy of the different methods. Recent experiments have attempted to elucidate the situation (3). It should not be implied that the use of any of these techniques will lead consistently to a successful result. In the authors' experience, there is still no panacea for the condition, and there is marked variation in success.

Two drainage techniques will be described. In early cases of infective arthritis, through-and-through lavage of the joint is appropriate. When the inflammatory process becomes chronic, lavage and distension irrigation lose their effectiveness because fibrin clots become too large or too organized for aspiration. In these instances, arthrotomy and joint debridement are indicated. In studies with induced septic arthritis in rabbits, it was found that by 7 days postinfection, the exudate had organized to the extent that surgical debridement was the only means of effective removal (4). More recent work in the human clinical literature emphasized that arthrotomy needs to be done at an early stage, not as a last resort (5). In analysis of results in the treatment of 28 cases of septic arthritis of the human wrist, of the 10 wrists with good or excellent results, all had had the arthrotomy within 10 hours of diagnosis. Of the 13 with a fair or poor result, surgery had been delayed for 16 hours or longer (5). The long-term results deteriorated in direct proportion to increasing time until treatment and the number of procedures performed (5). The current tendency of the authors with cases of equine septic arthritis is for earlier intervention or earlier arthrotomy.

The degree of increased surgical aggressiveness proposed for the treatment of equine septic arthritis and the timing are still a little uncertain. Recent work with an experimental model did document that arthrotomy more effectively removed fibrin from the joint than any one of three lavage regimes (3). However, when horses were euthanized and the joints examined, most parameters were not significantly different. It is considered that the advantages of aggressive surgical debridement differ among clinical cases of diverse pathogenesis.

Through-and-Through Lavage

Through-and-through lavage is generally done by placing two needles or catheters on opposite sides of the joint (Fig. 5.23*A*). One serves as an inflow tract and the other as an outflow tract, and periodic distension of the joint is achieved by occluding the outflow tract and applying pressure to the ingress line. This procedure is ideally done under general anesthesia and aseptic conditions, but in some instances lavage while the horse is standing is appropriate. Three to six liters of fluid are flushed through joint. A balanced polyionic electrolyte solution is preferred, as this will more closely approximate the pH of normal synovial

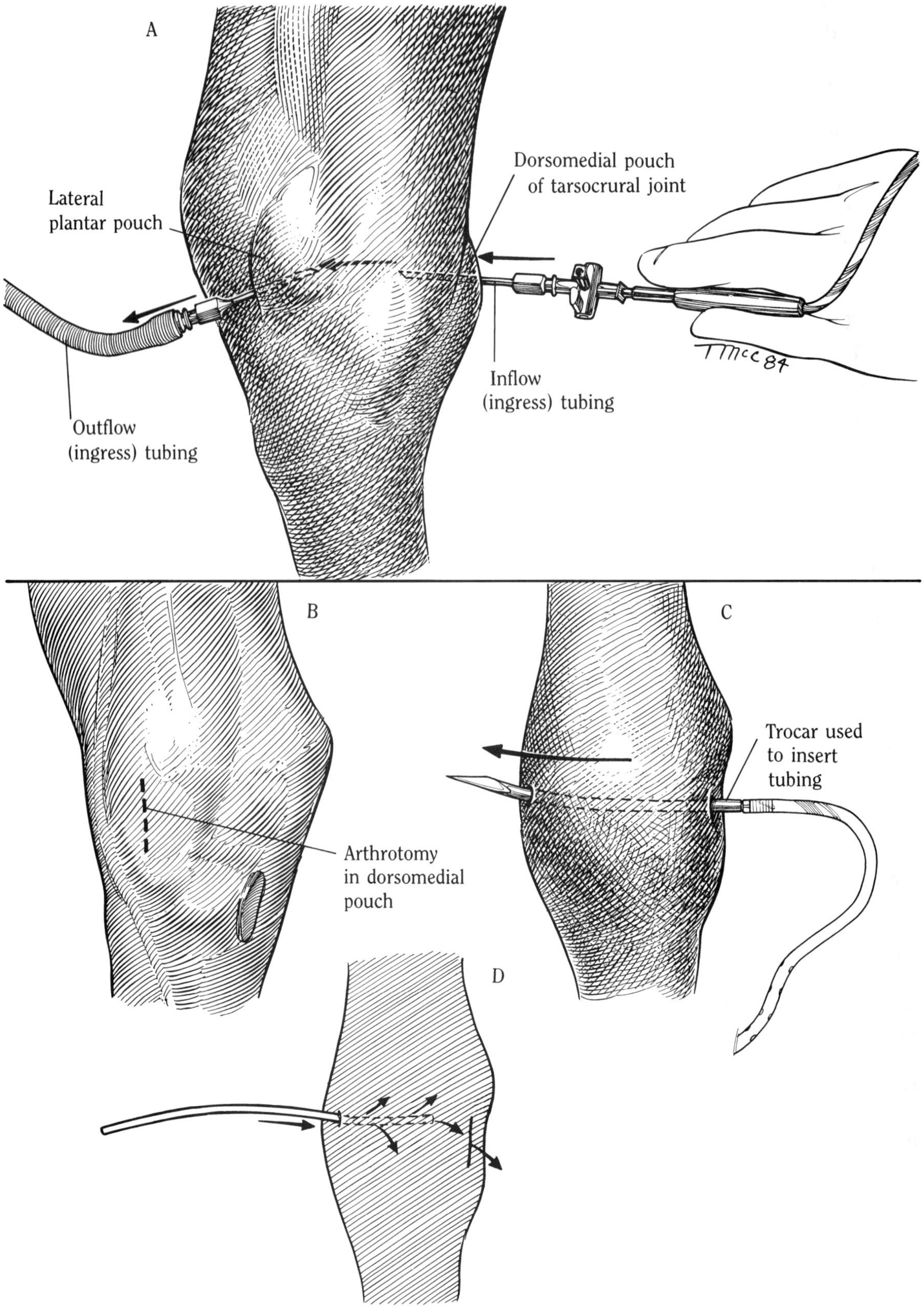

Figure 5.23, A–D. Surgical treatment of infectious arthritis.

fluid. The addition of antibiotics to the irrigating solution is optional, but the authors do not do it. Some clinicians add povidone-iodine solution (Betadine) to the irrigating solution. However, recent experimental work has shown that too concentrated a solution is deleterious to the joint. It has been shown that if the concentration of povidone-iodine in solution is 0.2% or less, no deleterious effects are experienced (6). Conversely, addition of chlorhexidine-surfactant (Novalsan) solution is definitely contraindicated (6). Opinions among clinicians also vary on the timing for irrigation or lavage. Experimental work at Colorado State University did not show significant differences between one-, two-, and three-lavage regimes.

Arthrotomy with Implantation of an Ingress Flushing System

The site of the arthrotomy incision is usually the same as for an elective arthrotomy in the respective joint. Identification of landmarks will be more difficult, however, because of the periarticular swelling generally associated with septic arthritis. The technique is a simple one and is illustrated in Figure 5.23, *B–D*, using the tarsocrural joint as an example. In this case an arthrotomy incision is made through the dorsomedial pouch of the tarsocrural joint (Fig. 5.23*B*). After the skin incision is made distal to the medial malleolus of the tibia, a careful inspection is made to ensure that the cranial branch of the medial saphenous vein is not within the area. Because of the capsular and subcutaneous swelling, the location of the vein may be difficult to ascertain before making the skin incision. The incision is then continued through the subcutaneous tissue and fibrous joint capsule. Gray, hyperplastic synovial membrane will usually be encountered at this stage and it is similarly incised.

This arthrotomy will be left open to heal on its own. With resolution of infection, the synovial membrane will close over the defect and second intention healing will occur. Once arthrotomy has been performed, a quarter-inch fenestrated drain (Orthopaedic Equipment, Bourbon, IN) is inserted through the dorsolateral pouch using a trocar as illustrated in Fig. 5.23*C*. Care must be taken to ensure the fenestrations are within the joint and not in the subcutaneous tissue (Fig. 5.23*D*). A three-way stopcock is connected to the drain, the drain is sutured in an appropriate position, and the limb is bandaged. This technique is always done under general anesthesia with aseptic conditions. At the time of surgery, the joint is flushed thoroughly and flushing is continued on a twice-daily basis for 7 to 10 days. The length of the fenestrated portion and the number of fenestrations on the drain are recorded (a case of part of the drain being pinched off and left in the joint has been recorded [3]).

During arthrotomy, as much pathologic synovial membrane as possible is removed. Fibrin is also debrided from the joint. However, synovectomy is difficult because chronically affected joints have extensive thickening of the fibrous joint capsule, and multiple arthrotomy incisions will be required to remove the entire synovial membrane. Suction drains and closure of the arthrotomy are unsatisfactory because of clogging of the drain and rapid cessation of effective drainage. The Penrose drain is an alternative, but retrograde contamination of the joint is a risk. The leaving of an open arthrotomy has not been associated with untoward complications.

Postoperative Management

The joint is flushed twice daily through the ingress system and the bandage is changed daily. Broad-spectrum antibiotics are maintained systematically throughout the period of treatment. When the joint has closed, analysis of synovial fluid is one of the methods of gauging the effectiveness of treatment. Sequential follow-up radiographs are also recommended.

Other ancillary follow-up medications have been proposed. The use of systematic nonsteroidal anti-inflammatory agents is logical both for comfort of the patient and to decrease prostaglandin levels within the inflamed joint. Although the use of intra-articular corticosteroids has been proposed, once the actual sepsis is apparently resolved, the authors believe it is a hazardous practice. Although acknowledging that they aid circulation and plasma membrane integrity, prevent intracellular water sequestration, inhibit capillary and fibroblast proliferation, prevent kinin release, complement activation and prostaglandin synthesis, and have specific effects against metalloproteinases and cytokines, the reader must recognize that the authors' experimental work has shown that 50% of joints still cultured positive after apparent clinical resolution of the problem (3). Sodium hyaluronate has been used by some clinicians with reportedly good results.

REFERENCES

1. McIlwraith CW. Treatment of infectious arthritis. Vet Clin North Am Large Animal Pract 1983;5:363.
2. Ward TT, Steigbigel RT. Acidosis of synovial fluid correlates with synovial fluid leukocytosis. Am J Med 1978;64:933.
3. Bertone A, McIlwraith CW, Jones RL, et al. Comparison of treatments for experimentally induced equine infectious arthritis. Am J Vet Res 1987;48:519–529.
4. Daniel D, Akeson W, Amiel D, et al. Lavage of septic joints in rabbits: effects of chondrolysis. J Bone Joint Surg Am 1976;58–A:393.
5. Rashkoff EV. Septic arthritis of the wrist. J Bone Joint Surg 1983;65–A:824.
6. Bertone A, McIlwraith CW, Powers B, et al. The effect and comparison of four antimicrobial joint lavage solutions on synovial membrane and articular cartilage in the horse. Vet Surg 1986;15:305.

Surgical Relief of Carpal Canal Syndrome

A condition somewhat related to anular ligament constriction of the fetlock occurs in the carpal canal of the horse (1, 2). It is also a well-recognized condition in the wrist joint of man known as carpal tunnel syndrome (1, 5). Through the carpal canal of the horse run the deep and superficial flexor tendons as well as the medial palmar artery and vein, the lateral palmar artery and vein, and the medial palmar nerve (4) (Fig. 5.24*A*). The accessory carpal bone and the palmar carpal canal anular ligament contribute to the relatively nondistendible carpal canal. The carpal synovial sheath invests the tendons in this area.

Any enlargement of the contents of or narrowing of the carpal canal can cause pain and lameness in a fashion similar to that seen in the palmar or plantar tendon sheath of the fetlock joint. Infection and trauma in the region are also potential causes of the condition (5). Pressure on the medial palmar nerve may also contribute to the lameness (1). Any thickening of the flexor tendons, such as would occur in a case of very proximally located tendinitis of either the deep or superficial flexor tendon, can cause the condition. Carpal canal syndrome in the horse has been associated with a fracture of the accessory carpal bone (1, 2, 6). This fracture is more common in jumping and steeplechase horses, although all breeds are potentially susceptible. Following fracture, swelling at the fracture site with subsequent fibrosis and callus formation results in a relative narrowing of the canal with pressure on the flexor tendons, nerves, and blood vessels.

Carpal canal syndrome is manifested by a bulging of the carpal sheath adjacent to the digital extensor and ulnaris lateralis muscles. There may be reduced arterial pulse distal to the lesion (4). There is pain on flexion or extension of the limb (1). Radiographs may reveal a healing fracture of the accessory carpal bone. Nerve conduction studies used in man have not been done in horses but would be of interest in this condition. The surgical technique is similar to that described previously (1).

Distension of the carpal sheath may also be seen as a manifestation of osteochondroma of the distal radius. The latter can be confirmed by radiographs and/or ultrasonography and has been treated successfully by the first author using an arthroscopic technique.

Anesthesia and Surgical Preparation

The operation is done with the patient under general anesthesia in lateral recumbency with the affected limb down. The caudal aspect of the carpus is prepared for aseptic surgery in a routine manner.

Surgical Technique

A 15-cm-long incision is made longitudinally from 3 cm above to 5 cm below the accessory carpal bone, parallel and caudal to the common digital vein (Fig. 5.24*B*). A longitudinal strip of the volar anular ligament up to 1-cm wide is removed parallel to the axis of the limb (Fig. 5.24*C*). Care must be taken not to lacerate the lateral palmar vein, which is close to the retinaculum (6) (Fig. 5.24*A*). The length of the strip should be a little greater than the zone of thickening, but rarely does it include the entire longitudinal length of the anular ligament (Fig. 5.24*D*).

The subcutaneous tissues are closed using either continuous or simple interrupted sutures of synthetic absorbable material. These sutures should provide a good watertight seal to prevent the formation of synovial fistula. The skin is closed with nonabsorbable sutures in a suture pattern of the surgeon's choice.

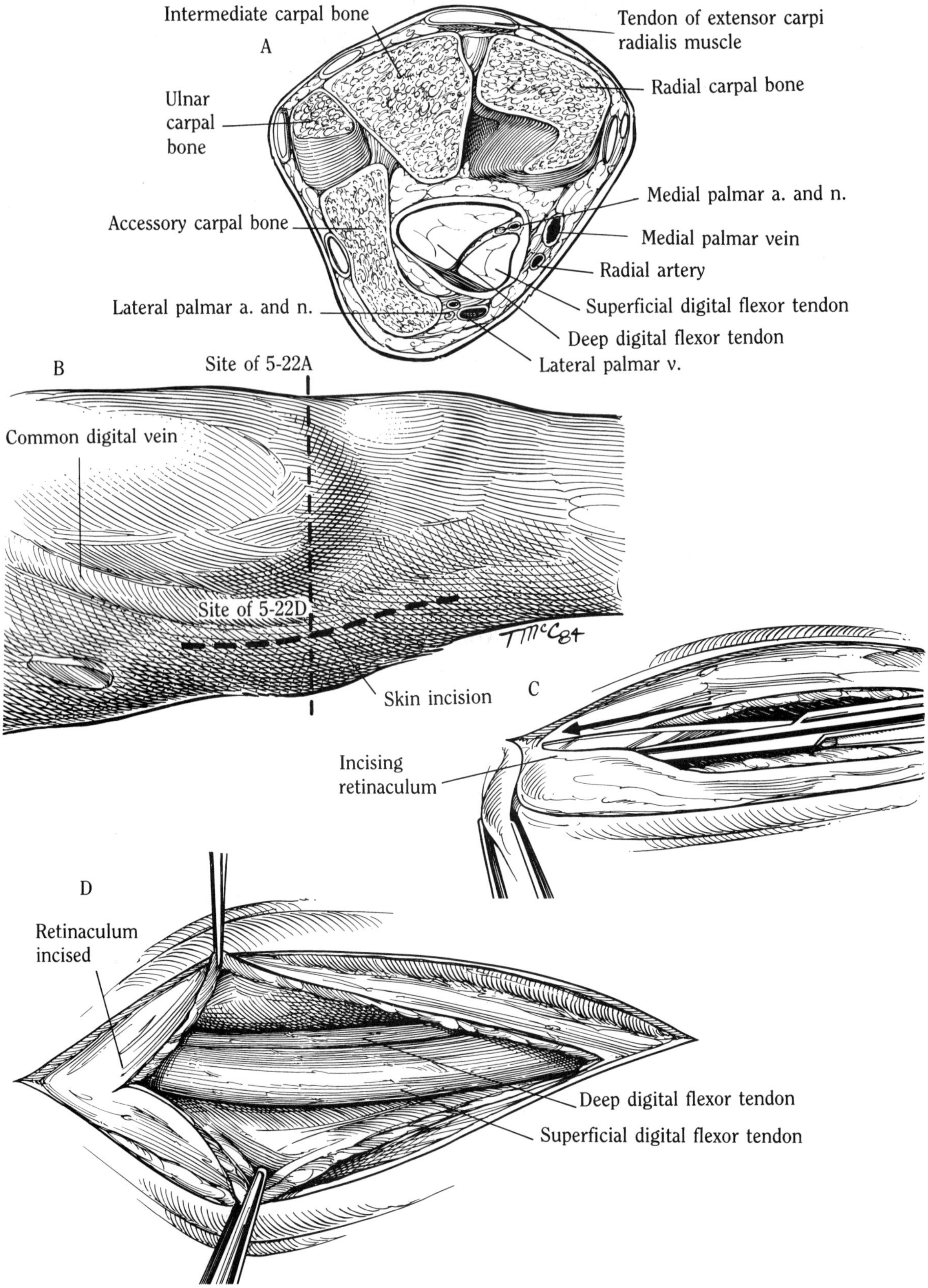

FIGURE 5.24, A–D. Surgical relief of carpal canal syndrome.

Postoperative Management

A sterile dressing is placed over the incision, and the entire limb is placed in a protective bandage. Care must be taken to avoid a pressure sore over the prominence of the accessory carpal bone when a bandage is applied to this area. In the authors' experience, they have observed an early favorable response following surgery in a limited number of cases.

Phenylbutazone is administered intravenously to reduce postoperative pain and facilitate early return of use of the limb. Antibiotics are not administered routinely. Sutures are removed at 12 to 14 days, and bandaging may be discontinued 3 to 4 days later.

Comments

Case selection is important in this condition. Ideally, a surgical candidate should be free of chip fractures within the carpus or associated DJD. These conditions would affect the prognosis adversely. The most difficult decision that faces the surgeon is whether the cause of the lameness is instability at the fracture site of the accessory carpal bone or the carpal tunnel syndrome itself. Injecting local anesthesia into the carpal sheath may aid in the localization of the lameness. The dramatic response to surgery seen in selected cases is similar following treatment of carpal tunnel syndrome in human patients (5).

REFERENCES

1. MacKay-Smith MP, Cushing LS, Leslie JA. "Carpal canal" syndrome in horses. JAVMA 1972;160:993.
2. Turner AS. Large animal orthopaedic surgery. In: Jennings PB, ed. Textbook of Large Animal Surgery. Philadelphia: WB Saunders, 1984:934.
3. Lieberman JS. Neuromuscular electrodiagnosis. In: Joumans JR, ed. Neurological Surgery, Vol. 1. Philadelphia: WB Saunders, 1982:630.
4. Getty R. Heart and arteries. In: Getty R, ed. Sisson and Grossman's The Anatomy of the Domestic Animal. 5th ed. Philadelphia: WB Saunders, 1975:592.
5. Milford L. The hand. In: Edmonson AS, Crenshaw AH, eds. Campbell's Operative Orthopaedics. 6th ed. St. Louis: CV Mosby, 1980:361.
6. Radue P. Carpal tunnel syndrome due to fracture of the accessory carpal bone. Equine Pract 1981;3:8.

Superior Check Ligament Desmotomy (After Bramlage)

Superior check ligament (accessory ligament of the superficial digital flexor [SDF]) desmotomy was initially described as a surgical treatment for metacarpophalangeal flexural deformities in young horses. Reported results vary (1–3), however, and it is now recognized that the SDF tendon is not necessarily the primary unit in metacarpophalangeal flexural deformities (4). In cases in which the SDF appears to be the most involved structure, superior check ligament desmotomy may be indicated.

More recently, superior check ligament desmotomy has been reported as a treatment for SDF tendonitis in racehorses (5–7). The rationale for the surgery is that is interrupts the transfer of the weightbearing load on the tendon to the distal radius, bringing the muscle and tendon proximal to the superior check ligaments (and therefore enhanced elasticity to the functional unit) into use during weightbearing (5). In a study of cadaver limbs, superior check desmotomy (SCD) did cause elongation of the muscle belly when load was applied to the limb, but strain in the SDF tendon increased rather than decreased as expected; however, it is uncertain how relevant this data is to the in vivo situation (8).

Anesthesia and Surgical Preparation

Surgery is done with the patient under general anesthesia and either in lateral recumbency with the affected leg down or in dorsal recumbency with the leg suspended. The latter position is preferable in terms of hemostasis. The leg will have been clipped previously from midradius to midmetacarpus. The medial side of the antebrachium is surgically prepared.

Surgical Technique

A 10-cm skin incision is made between the cephalic vein and the caudal border of the radius, over the flexor carpi radialis tendon and extending from the level of the central chestnut proximad to the medial malleolus of the radius (Fig. 5.25*A*). The incision is continued through the subcutaneous tissue and antebrachial fascia. A transverse branch of the cephalic vein may or may not require ligation (the incision can often be continued under it). The cephalic vein is retracted caudal, exposing the lateral wall of the flexor carpi radialis tendon sheath. The facial sheath of the flexor carpi radialis is incised (Fig. 5.25*B*) along its medial wall to expose the flexor carpi radialis tendon. Gelpi retractors are placed to retract the tendon caudal and expose the medial wall of the sheath, which adheres to the superior check ligament (Fig. 5.25*C*). The fibers of the superior check ligament are now visible (Fig. 5.25*D*). There are two lamellae in the superior check ligament. The major group is the transverse group of fibers that lie closer to the surgeon, and the more oblique lamellae are oriented from proximocaudal on the radius and inserting craniodistad into the SDF tendon. The transverse lamellae are incised first; once they are incised, the more oblique lamella comes into view. The oblique fibers are less taut than the transverse fibers and are more difficult to transect. An incision is made into the middle of the oblique lamella and a Kelly forceps passed through the lamellae to lift the fibers up and facilitate their incision. Using the Kelly forceps also protects the flexor carpi rete vasculature beneath the proximal aspect of the superior check ligament. As the incision is continued proximad, care is taken to identify the nutrient artery for the SDF tendon in the proximal border (Fig. 5.25*E*). The artery is isolated and transection of the ligament completed (Fig. 5.25*F*). Transection

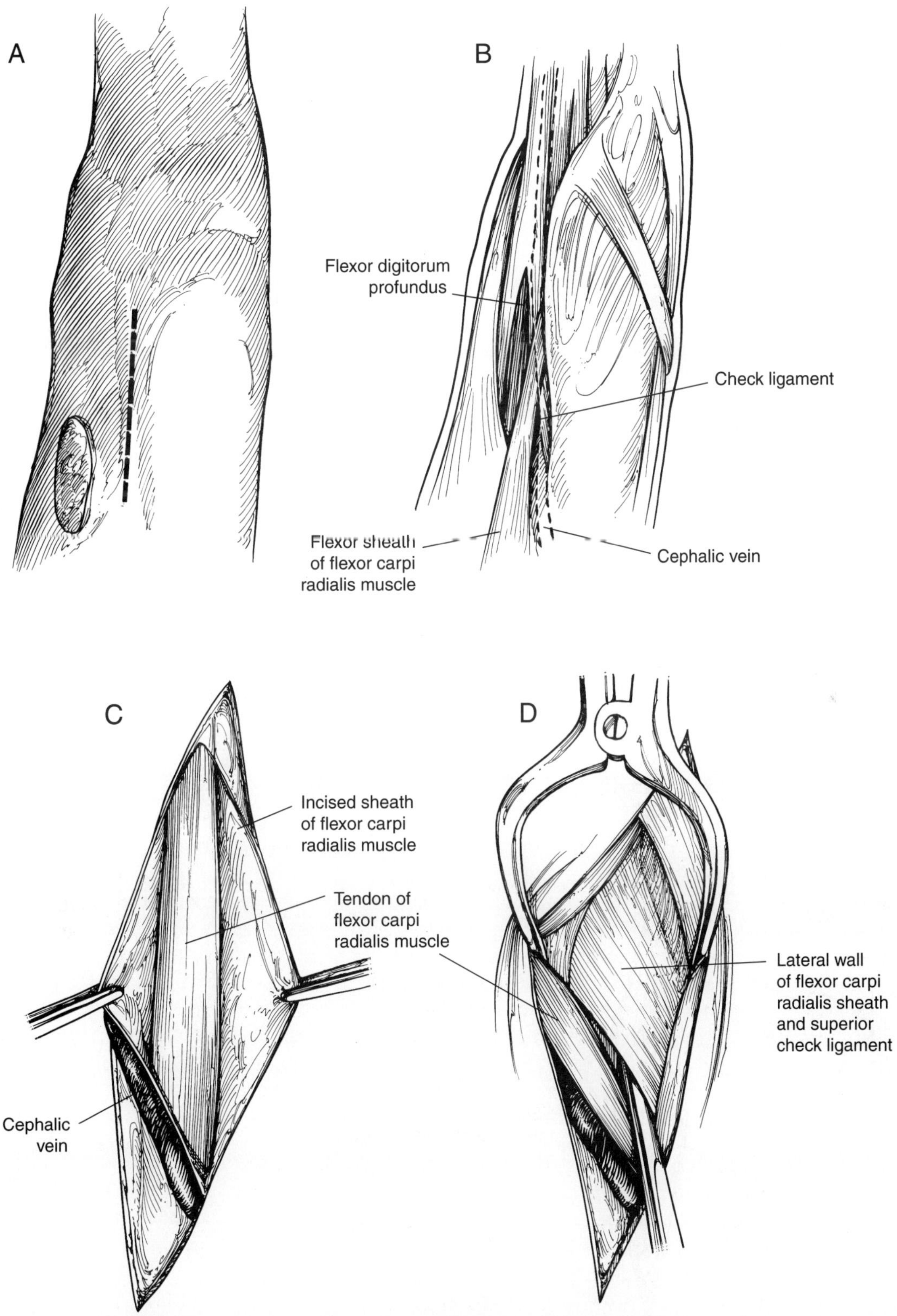

FIGURE 5.25, A–D. Superior check ligament desmotomy (after Bramlage).

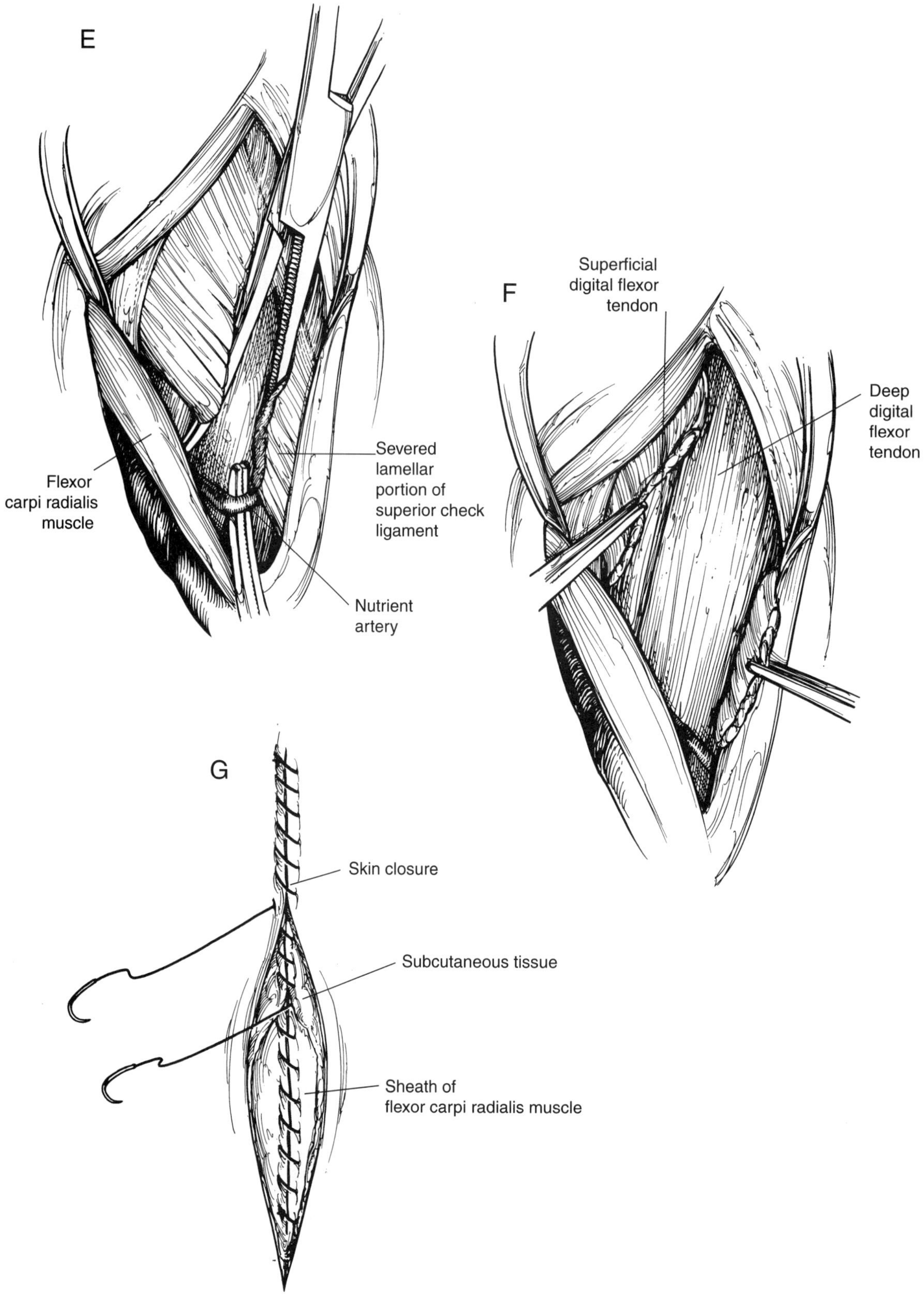

Figure 5.25, E–G. *(continued)* Superior check ligament desmotomy (after Bramlage).

of the ligament is then completed distad. Complete transection distally usually causes entry into the carpal tendon sheath, which is immediately axial to the distal aspect of the check ligament. This is not a problem.

When the ligament is thoroughly divided, palpation will reveal that there is no attachment between the superior check ligament and the radius except for the nutrient artery mentioned previously. The radial head of the deep flexor tendon is seen within the central and proximal areas of the incision (Fig. 5.25*F*).

The incision in the flexor carpi radialis sheath is closed with simple interrupted sutures of 2/0 synthetic absorbable material. The antebrachial fascia and subcutaneous tissue is closed with a continuous suture of 2/0 synthetic absorbable material (Fig. 5.25*G*), and the skin is closed with interrupted sutures of 2/0 nonabsorbable material.

Postoperative Management

A sterile dressing is placed over the incision and a pressure bandage is applied. The latter is critical to help eliminate accumulation of serum at the surgery site and obviate postoperative healing problems. Sutures are removed at 12 to 14 days and bandaging may be discontinued 3 to 4 days later. Routine aftercare involves 2 weeks of stall rest, 2 weeks of hand-walking, and 1 month of paddock exercise followed by three-times weekly exercise at a trot for 2 months to stretch the tendon. Ultrasound examination is done at 120 days to determine if the horse is ready to increase exercise (7).

Comments

The technique described is a modification of that initially described (2). The approach is more caudal and the limits of the superior check ligament are more easily defined. In addition, the closure of the medial wall of the flexor carpi radialis sheath facilitates elimination of dead space and minimizes the potential for hematoma formation and adhesions.

The most common complication is seroma, and the incidence of this varies. In one study, it occurred in 2 of 40 horses (9); in another study, it was associated with 23 (64%) incisions between day 2 and day 14 postsurgery (10).

The first report on the use of superior check desmotomy in the treatment of SDF tendinitis was in 1986 in Thoroughbreds, in which 19 of 24 horses (79%) that completed the trial were able to complete two races without recurrence of the tendonitis (5). Five horses became lame again as a result of recurrence, for a total of 19 of 36 (53%) being able to return to competition without injury. This was considered significantly better than the expected rate of return without treatment. In a later paper on Thoroughbreds, the race records before and after surgery of 51 Thoroughbred racehorses were obtained (6). Thirty of the 36 horses had no recurrence of tendonitis. When the highest postinjury class of race was compared with the class of the last two races before surgery, 25 of the 32 horses that started after surgery completed at or above their preinjury class. Seven horses competed in a lower class. Subsequent work in 61 Standardbred racehorses showed that 82% of all horses raced after surgery and 69% completed five or more starts (11). These studies suggested that superior check desmotomy allows Standardbred horses with SDF tendinitis to race and earn money without recurrence of tendinous injuries. Horses that have not raced before injury may be expected to earn less money and record slower lifetime race marks after surgery than horses that are racing at a time of injury.

Other papers subsequently have confirmed the suggested value of superior check desmotomy in Standardbreds (33 of 38 horses completed five or more races after surgery, with recurrence of tendinitis in 6 and an overall success rate of 27 of 38) (9). In an Australian study, 13 of 25 (52%) Thoroughbreds raced on five or more occasions and 10 of 15 Standardbreds (66%) raced on five or more occasions (12). When compared with the subjective impression that 20 to 30% of horses with SDF tendinitis can return to racing after a prolonged rest, the results suggest that bilateral superior check ligament desmotomy improved the prognosis for a horse returning to racing after injury to the SDF tendon. Superior check ligament desmotomy may also be used in conjunction with surgical tendon splitting. It has been suggested that tendon splitting provides more rapid improvement in the ultrasonographic appearance of core lesions, and it is appropriate to drain grade III or IV lesions, in which the fluid is most often a hematoma or seroma as a result of the hemorrhage that accompanies the initial tendon injury (13).

REFERENCES

1. Fackelman GE. Flexure deformity of the metacarpophalangeal joints in growing horses. Compend Cont Edu Pract Vet 1979;9:51.
2. Jann HW, Beroza GA, Fackleman GE. Surgical anatomy for desmotomy of the accessory ligament of the superficial flexor tendon (proximal check ligament) in horses. Vet Surg 1986;15:278.
3. Wagner PC, Shires GMH, Watrous BJ et al. Management of acquired flexural deformities in the metacarpophalangeal joint in equidae. JAVMA 1985;187:915.
4. McIlwraith CW. Diseases of joints, tendons, ligaments and related structures. In: Stashak TS, ed. Lameness in Horses. 4th ed. Philadelphia: Lea & Febiger, 1987:339.
5. Bramlage LR. Superior check ligament desmotomy as a treatment for superficial digital flexor tendinitis: initial report. In: Proceedings of the 32nd Annual Convention of the American Association of Equine Practitioners. 1986:365–369.
6. Bramlage LR, Rantanen NW, Genovese RL, et al. Long-term effects of surgical treatment of superficial digital flexor tendinitis by superior check desmotomy. In: Proceedings of the 34th Annual Meeting of the AAEP. 1988:655–656.
7. Bramlage LR. Surgical management of tendinitis and desmitis. Proc Dubai Conference, 375–378, March 27–30, 1996.
8. Shoemaker RŞ, Bertone AL, Mohammad LN, et al. Desmotomy of the accessory ligament of the superficial digital flexor muscle in equine cadaver limbs. Vet Surg 1991; 4:245–252.
9. Hawkins JF, Ross MW. Transection of the accessory ligament of the superficial digital flexor muscle for the treatment of superficial digital flexor tendinitis in Standardbreds: 40 cases (1988–1992). JAVMA 1995;206:674–678.
10. Cote N, Marcoux M, Lepage OM. Complications of desmotomy of the accessory ligament of the superficial digital flexor tendon. A retrospective study of 19 cases (1986–1989). Pract Vet Equine 1994;26:103–107.
11. Hogan PA, Bramlage LR. Transection of the accessory ligament of the superficial digital flexor tendon for treatment of tendinitis: long-term results in 61 Standardbred racehorses (1985–1992). Equine Vet J 1995;27:221–226.
12. Fulton IC, MacLean AA, O'Really JL, et al. Superior check ligament desmotomy for treatment of superficial digital flexor tendinitis in Thoroughbreds and Standardbred horses. Aust Vet J 1994;71:233–235.
13. Henninger R, Bramlage L, Schneider R. Short-term effect of superior check ligament desmotomy and percutaneous tendon splitting as treatment for acute tendinitis. In: Proceedings of the 36th Annual Meeting of the AAEP, Lexington, Kentucky, 1990: 539–540.

Arthrodesis of the Proximal Interphalangeal Joint

Arthrodesis of the proximal interphalangeal joint is used in treating DJD of the pastern joint, luxations of the pastern joint, and fractures involving the pastern joint. The proximal interphalangeal (pastern) joint is a common site for DJD in horses (1–3). It can occur as a sequela to a severe sprain of the pastern or a deep wire cut in the pastern region.

In young horses, high ringbone is occasionally seen in the hind limbs, secondary to subchondral cystic lesions (2, 4). These cysts are possible manifestations of osteochondrosis. The exact cause of the subchondral cyst is uncertain, but it appears to be unrelated to the smaller subchondral cysts seen in humans secondary to DJD. The pastern joint of the opposite hind limb should also be radiographed. There may be lesions in the opposite pastern joint as well as in other joints that are predisposed to the syndrome of OCD and subchondral bone cyst formation (2).

Arthrodesis is also indicated for certain fractures of the middle phalanx (P2) that do not involve the distal interphalangeal joint (2, 5–9). It has been the authors' experience that, if such fractures are allowed to heal by external coaptation alone, the resulting callus enlarges the pastern area and may interfere with tendon function. Such fractures are usually so unstable that not only is healing protracted but also the proximal phalanx becomes driven into the fracture site to produce severe hyperextension of that joint and a limb that may be even nonfunctional for pasture soundness (5). Various techniques of arthrodesis of the equine pastern joint have been documented (9). Earlier techniques used a joint drilling procedure that removed as much of the articular cartilage as possible. Other methods employ a more radical approach to the joint, using a variably shaped skin incision and a transection of the dorsal joint capsule of the pastern joint. With these methods, a more thorough curettage of the joint surface is possible.

Arthrodesis for high ringbone usually entails removal of a variable amount of periosteal new bone from the dorsal region of the joint, which forms in response to the original disease. To gain access to the joint, some collateral ligament transection is necessary, although the authors recommend that these ligaments be preserved as much as possible because they contribute to the final stability of the joint. The use of internal fixation as part of the surgical procedure aids in the horse's convalescence. The method described here is a modification of the lag screw fixation as described by Schneider and co-workers (1). The convalescent time and cost of hospitalization can be reduced because the cast can be removed earlier, since the lag screws make the joint inherently more stable (1, 9). This finding has also been substantiated by others (2).

Clipping of the entire limb up to the level of the proximal end of the metatarsus or metacarpus is best done before induction of anesthesia to reduce the time under anesthesia.

Anesthesia and Surgical Preparation

The surgical procedure is done with the horse under general anesthesia with the affected limb uppermost. The limb is positioned on a leg stand so that placement of a cassette for intraoperative radiographs will be possible without having to move the horse and risk a break in aseptic technique. The authors prefer to have the limb supported just below the hock or carpus with the rest of the limb free, approximately half a meter above the table surface.

The dorsal aspect of the affected pastern joint is shaved; an Esmarch bandage and a pneumatic tourniquet are then applied just below the carpal or tarsal joint as appropriate. The area of the surgical incision is prepared for aseptic surgery in a routine manner.

The use of a plastic adhesive drape is recommended. Because the foot region will be fairly close to the surgical site, it is advisable to place a separate plastic drape and a pair of sterile rubber surgical gloves over the foot before applying the drape over the surgical site.

Additional Instrumentation

ASIF equipment for lag screw fixation with 4.5-mm cortical bone screws (see Appendix I), includes curettes, chisel (1–2 cm wide), mallet, strong periosteal elevator, and equipment for intraoperative radiographs.

Surgical Technique

To obtain adequate exposure of the pastern joint, thereby ensuring a more thorough removal of articular cartilage, the joint must be exposed through its dorsal aspect. An I-shaped incision is made over the dorsal surface of the proximal and middle phalanges. The proximal part of the incision extends across the middle of the proximal phalanx, and the distal part of the incision is placed approximately 0.5 cm above the coronet (Fig. 5.26*A*). The two incisions are connected by a sagittal incision down the dorsal aspect of the proximal and middle phalanges. The skin is reflected, exposing the common (or long) digital extensor tendon and the two branches of the interosseous (suspensory) ligaments. A Z-plasty is performed in the common (or long) extensor tendon and, if necessary, the branches of the suspensory ligament (Fig. 5.26*B*). The extensor tendon is carefully dissected away from the joint capsule of the pastern joint, and the pastern joint is identified by probing with sterile disposable hypodermic needles. Following identification of the joint, the joint capsule is transversely incised using sharp dissection. The collateral ligaments can be completely severed to allow exposure of the joint surfaces. In the authors' experience, partial severance is usually adequate. If arthrodesis is done for a proximal middle phalangeal fracture, there is usually enough instability of the joint that even less collateral ligament need be severed to permit adequate exposure. However, in arthrodesis for the treatment of ringbone, severing a certain amount of collateral ligament is necessary.

Following the arthrotomy, a suitable instrument such as a heavy-duty periosteal elevator is used to pry the joint surfaces apart so that as much hyaline cartilage as possible can be visualized. A curette is then used to denude as much cartilage from the ends of the bone as possible. Access to the caudal aspects of the proximal and middle phalanges for curettage is facilitated by an assistant forcefully flexing the joint (1, 2) (5.26*C*).

Following removal of the articular cartilage, a shelf is made approximately 2.5 cm proximal to the joint and on the middle of the proximal phalanx. This shelf is used to seat the heads of the screws. Two or three lag screws (depending on the size of the horse) are placed across the pastern joint, engaging as much of the middle phalanx as possible (Fig. 5.26, *D–F*). Usually, 4.5-mm cortical bone screws are used, but 5.5-mm screws are sometimes used in large horses. Care must be taken not to drill the 3.2-mm pilot hole too far and damage the navicular bone when the drill emerges from the caudal cortex of the middle phalanx. A roughly parallel configuration of the lag screws is recommended (5) (Fig. 5.26, *G* and *H*). With the avulsion fractures of the middle phalanx, care must be taken not to direct the screws into the fracture site (4). Intraoperative radiographs are an essential part of this surgical procedure. The authors believe the best time to take one is following the placement of the first lag screw. Only

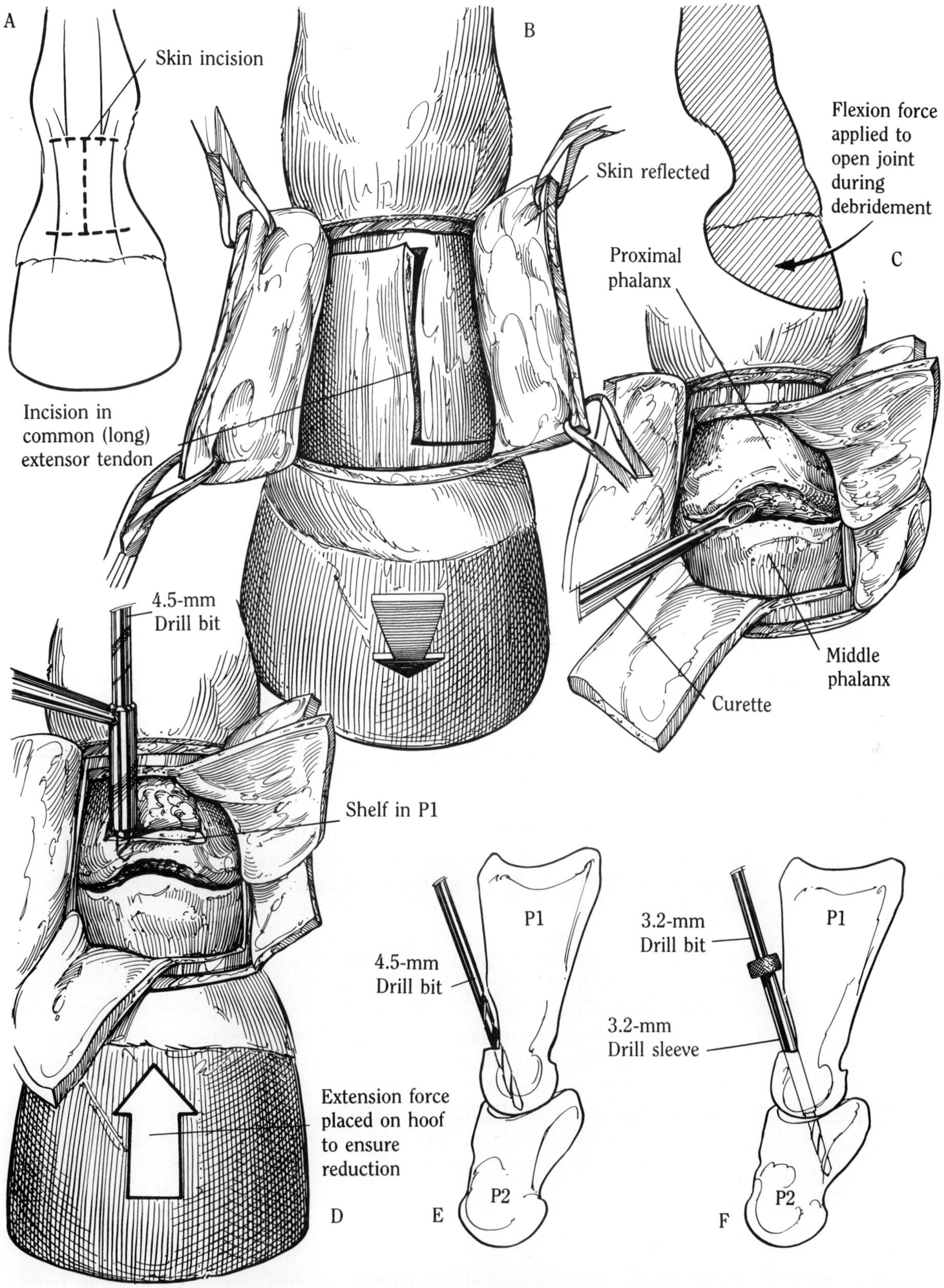

Figure 5.26, A–F. Arthrodesis of the pastern joint using lag screws.

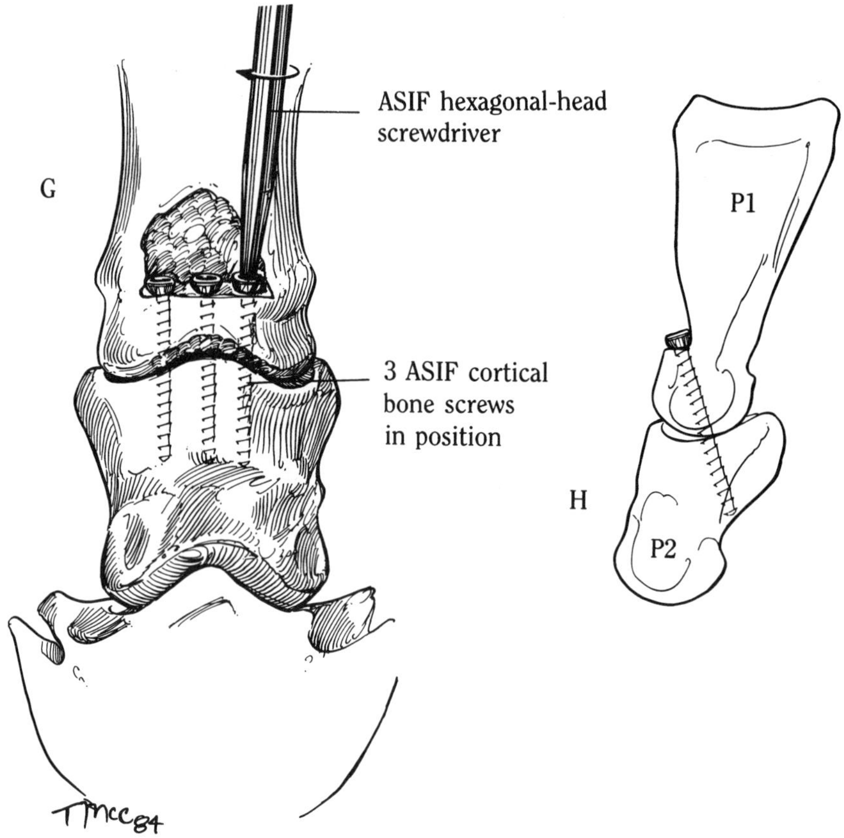

Figure 5.26, G–H. *(continued)* Arthrodesis of the pastern joint using lag screws.

a true lateral view need be taken. From the radiograph the surgeon will be able to note if the screw is in the correct direction and engaging as much of P2 as possible and if it is of the correct length. The screw must not protrude beyond the palmar cortex of P2 and endanger the navicular bone; yet, at the same time, it should engage this cortex to ensure maximum holding power. Following placement of the first screw, the remaining two or three screws are placed on either side of this screw, making the necessary adjustments in screw direction and length for them. A lateral and dorsopalmar (dorsoplantar) radiograph is then taken as a final record of the arthrodesis.

The authors have found that it is virtually impossible to include any subcutaneous layer in the closure. For that reason, the authors proceed directly to closure of the skin when the joint capsule and extensor tendons have been apposed. Following closure of the wound and removal of the adhesive drapes, nonadherent dressings are applied and maintained in position with cotton gauze such as Kling. The tourniquet is released and a fiberglass/plastic combination cast is applied to the top of the proximal extremity of the metatarsus or metacarpus.

Postoperative Management

Prophylactic antibiotics are administered for 3 to 5 days. Horses usually require analgesics such as phenylbutazone for several days and sometimes for as long as 10 days. Preoperative administration of phenylbutazone is also recommended. The dose of phenylbutazone can be reduced gradually over the period of administration. If the horse begins to use his cast less well, it should be removed and the cast changed.

The horse should be kept in a clean, dry box stall, bedded with material that allows some ambulation without hindering forward motion of the cast limb. If straw is all that is available, it should be used sparingly for this reason. The limb should be kept in a cast for approximately 6 weeks. Young animals with ringbone secondary to osteochondrosis will generally show much earlier signs of fusion of the proximal phalanx to the middle phalanx than an adult horse. These cases may require less than 6 weeks in a cast during which time two or three changes of the cast can be anticipated. At each cast change, a radiograph will indicate the degree of fusion.

The last cast should be cut off with the horse standing and lightly tranquilized if necessary. The limb should be maintained in a pressure bandage for 2 to 3 weeks following cast removal to prevent the limb swelling that typically occurs at this time.

Comments

In the authors' experience, the prognosis for complete return to athletic function following arthrodesis of the pastern in the hind limb is 83%. Approximately 60% of horses will be sound if this joint in the forelimb is fused (2).

Since the authors' report (2), another series of 26 animals in which adequate follow-up was available reported a successful outcome in 65%. This included a successful outcome in four of six horses with bilateral arthrodeses. The technique was noted a modification in that the three screws converged. In the six horses in which bilateral arthrodesis was performed, it was successful in the three horses with hind limb arthrodeses (two returned to racing and one to stock work). One horse with bilateral forelimb arthrodesis resumed useful pleasure riding and breeding. Two horses were euthanized because of complications related to infection of the second arthrodesis. Bone grafting was not considered necessary. The glide holes in the first phalanx were drilled retrograde. In assessing the overall difference between forelimbs and hind limbs, this paper's data was combined with the authors' previous publication to give a sample size of 51 limbs and a P value of 0.003. The authors also agreed that prolonged convalescence may be required. Although many horses were considered to have a normal gait 30 days after cast removal, the six horses that resumed racing had a mean lay-off of 10 months. A 1-year convalescent period after arthrodesis is not unexpected.

Complications the authors have seen following this surgical procedure are distal interphalangeal DJD (low ringbone), screw breakage, and excessive formation of callus, all which produced continued lameness. A small number of horses exhibit toe elevation during weightbearing. The authors have also witnessed fracture of the small shelf created on the distal end of the proximal phalanx. The shelf must be made sufficiently high up P1 and be large enough to avoid this (2).

The convalescence after this procedure is long, and it is unusual for the horse to become sound within 1 year of surgery (2). It is also an expensive operation for most owners. It does, however, offer reasonable hope for horses that would otherwise be permanently lame or, at best, require years, if ever, for the joint to ankylose spontaneously (2–9).

The convalescent period of certain middle phalangeal (P2) fractures can be shortened and greater stability can be achieved with the lag screw technique. This technique is limited to the middle phalangeal fracture that is not severely comminuted and has only one or both caudal eminences fractured off, as well as high ringbone. This technique essentially involves an approach similar to that described above. In some instances in which the P2 fracture is severely comminuted, arthrodesis and internal fixation are done using an ASIF T-plate.

Whenever possible, the lag screw technique is preferred for pastern arthrodesis because of less exposure to the coffin joint area.

REFERENCES

1. Schneider JE, Carinine BL, Guffy MM. Arthrodesis of the proximal interphalangeal joint in the horse: a surgical treatment for high ringbone. JAVMA 1978;173:1364.
2. Martin GS, McIlwraith CW, Turner AS, et al. Long term results and complications of arthrodesis of the proximal interphalangeal joint. JAVMA 1984;184:1136.
3. Caron JP, Fretz PB, Bailey JV, et al. Proximal interphalangeal arthrodesis in the horse. A retrospective study and a modified screw technique. Vet Surg 1990;19:196–202.
4. Trotter GW, McIlwraith CW, Norrdin RW, et al. Degenerative joint disease with osteochondrosis of the proximal interphalangeal joint in young horses. JAVMA 1980;180: 1312.
5. Gabel AA, Bukowiecki CF. Fractures of the phalanges. Vet Clin North Am Large Animal Pract 1983;5:233.
6. Genetzky RM, Schneider EJ, Butler HC, et al. Comparison of two surgical procedures for arthrodesis of the proximal interphalangeal joint in horses. JAVMA 1981;179:464.
7. Ellis DR, Greenwood RES. Six cases of degenerative joint disease of the proximal interphalangeal joint of young Thoroughbreds. Equine Vet 1985;17:66.
8. Steenhaut M, Verschooten F, De Moor A. Arthrodesis of the pastern joint in the horse. Equine Vet J 1985;17:35.
9. Turner AS. Large animal orthopaedic surgery. In: Jennings PB, ed. Textbook of Large Animal Surgery. Philadelphia: WB Saunders, 1984:858.

Arthrodesis of the Distal Tarsal Joints

Bone spavin is osteoarthritis (DJD) of the "low-motion joints" of the hock, usually involving the distal intertarsal and tarsometatarsal joints (1). Occasionally the proximal intertarsal joints are involved. Typical radiographic evidence includes subchondral lysis with loss of joint space and periosteal proliferation, most commonly on the medial aspect of the hock. At Colorado State University it is a common cause of hind limb lameness, with usually a progressive course finally rendering the horse unsuitable for its intended use. Currently, nonsurgical treatment has included rest, exercise with or without the use of nonsteroidal anti-inflammatory drugs, intra-articular corticosteriods, and corrective shoeing. Although the authors believe that continued exercise may result in spontaneous ankylosis of the joints and remission of lameness, eventually this is unpredictable, however, and may take a long time (years) (1).

Arthrodesis of these joints is aimed at eliminating pain, presumably by improving joint stability. A technique first reported in 1970 (2) is described here. Numerous surgical techniques have been performed to achieve fusion in these joints, but the easiest and most practical entails destruction of the articular cartilage by means of a drill introduced on the medial side of the joints involved. Earlier reports of this technique revealed a mixed success rate (2, 3). It was recommended that at least 60% of articular cartilage be destroyed (3). Horses frequently suffered pain, weight loss, and continued to be lame. The author of a report subsequent to the initial description encountered such a high incidence of complications that he could not recommend the procedure (4).

The first author reevaluated the technique following the paper by Edwards (5) and a report on a modified technique in the United States (Murray ES, personal communication, 1983). It appears that if one is too radical in removing articular cartilage, then excessive instability occurs and results in the high morbidity observed with the initially described technique. Early postoperative exercise also seems to help the convalescence (Murray ES, personal communication, 1983). The authors now recommend this procedure for the treatment of bone spavin, realizing that an attempt to remove all articular cartilage from these joints is not only contraindicated but is unnecessary for a successful outcome.

Before surgery is attempted, a good clinical examination is indicated to rule out existing lameness. If possible, the authors like to see some response to intra-articular anesthesia of these joints. To place local anesthesia into the tarsometatarsal joint, the needle is placed plantar-laterally between the head of the fourth metatarsal and fourth tarsal bones. By forcing the anesthetic solution under pressure, some may be forced into the distal intertarsal joint because of dissection of the anesthetic material through internal connective tissue spaces, but this does not happen with consistency. Reliable anesthetization of the distal intertarsal joint therefore requires a separate injection done from the medial side of the hock (6). The needle is placed through the gap between the fused first and second tarsal bone and the central tarsal bone. A 1-inch needle is placed as far proximally as possible and advanced almost to the hub so that the tip remains in the joint. Although radiographic osteoarthritis is the typical indication for arthrodesis, the surgery is also appropriate when persistent retracting disease (defined by intra-articular analgesia) of the distal tarsal joints is present.

Both hocks should be radiographed because frequently the condition is bilateral, although worse in one. If both hocks are involved clinically, the authors currently operate on both at the same time. Previously the authors believed that both hocks should be done a week apart because of the possibility that one or both of the operations will produce excessive postoperative pain, but this has not been the case. If there is radiographic evidence of disease in both hocks but the horse is lame in only one, then two options are available: both can be operated on or the lame leg can be operated on and a "wait-and-see" policy adopted for the other limb.

Anesthesia and Surgical Preparation

The surgical procedure is done under general anesthesia with the horse placed in lateral recumbency with the affected limb down or, alternatively, in dorsal recumbency. Before induction of anesthesia, the entire hock region of the horse is clipped if it will tolerate this; otherwise, clipping may be done when the horse is anesthetized. Following positioning of the horse on the appropriate padding (waterbed, inner tubes, air mattress), the upper hind limb is secured in such a way to allow access to the medial side of the affected hock (when the surgery is done in lateral recumbency). The authors use a leg stand and pull the uppermost limb slightly caudad to the one being operated on. Allowance also must be made for positioning of an x-ray cassette caudal to the hock, since one intraoperative radiograph will be necessary to ensure that the joints are located. The authors have found it useful to position the head of the x-ray machine in its approximate location to save time.

When the horse is positioned, the medial side of the hock dorsal to the chestnut is shaved and prepared for surgery in a routine manner. An Esmarch's bandage and a tourniquet are not necessary for this operation.

Additional Instrumentation

Arthrodesis of the distal tarsal joint requires a power drill (e.g., ASIF compressed nitrogen drill, hand drill, or sterilized electric drill, 4.5-mm drill bits, and a drill guide).

Surgical Technique

After draping (sterile plastic adherent drapes are recommended for this procedure), the cunean tendon is identified by deep palpation. A 5-cm vertical skin incision is made slightly caudal to the cranial branch of the medial saphenous vein to expose the cunean tendon (Fig. 5.27*A*). The cunean bursa is entered, and forceps are directed under the tendon. The cunean tendon is severed, and a 1 to 2 cm section of the tendon is removed to provide better access to the joints. The area under the tendon is probed with 20-gauge ½-inch needle to find the distal intertarsal and tarsometatarsal joints (Fig. 5.27*B*). With practice, the surgeon can locate the joints quickly, although if any bony exostosis exists, entry into these joints may be difficult or impossible. Even if the needle has not entered the joint, it can still function satisfactorily as a marker, especially if it is placed securely in soft tissue. A dorsopalmar radiograph is then made.

When the film has been developed, the surgeon may need to either reposition the needles and take another radiograph (if the needles had completely missed the joint) or proceed with the arthrodesis. From the radiographs, not only the *location* of the needles can be checked but also their *direction*; this precaution will enable the drill to be directed *along the plane of the joint* (Fig. 5.27*C*).

Without disturbing the other needle, one needle is removed and the drill positioned and aligned to follow the plane of the joint. An ASIF 4.5-mm drill is used and three drill tracks made through each joint (Fig. 5.27, *D* and *E*). The use of power equipment and a new sharp drill bit is strongly recommended. It is imperative that the drill remain in the joint space. Frequent cleaning of the drill bit is essential to ensure efficient cutting. If the drill hole becomes impacted

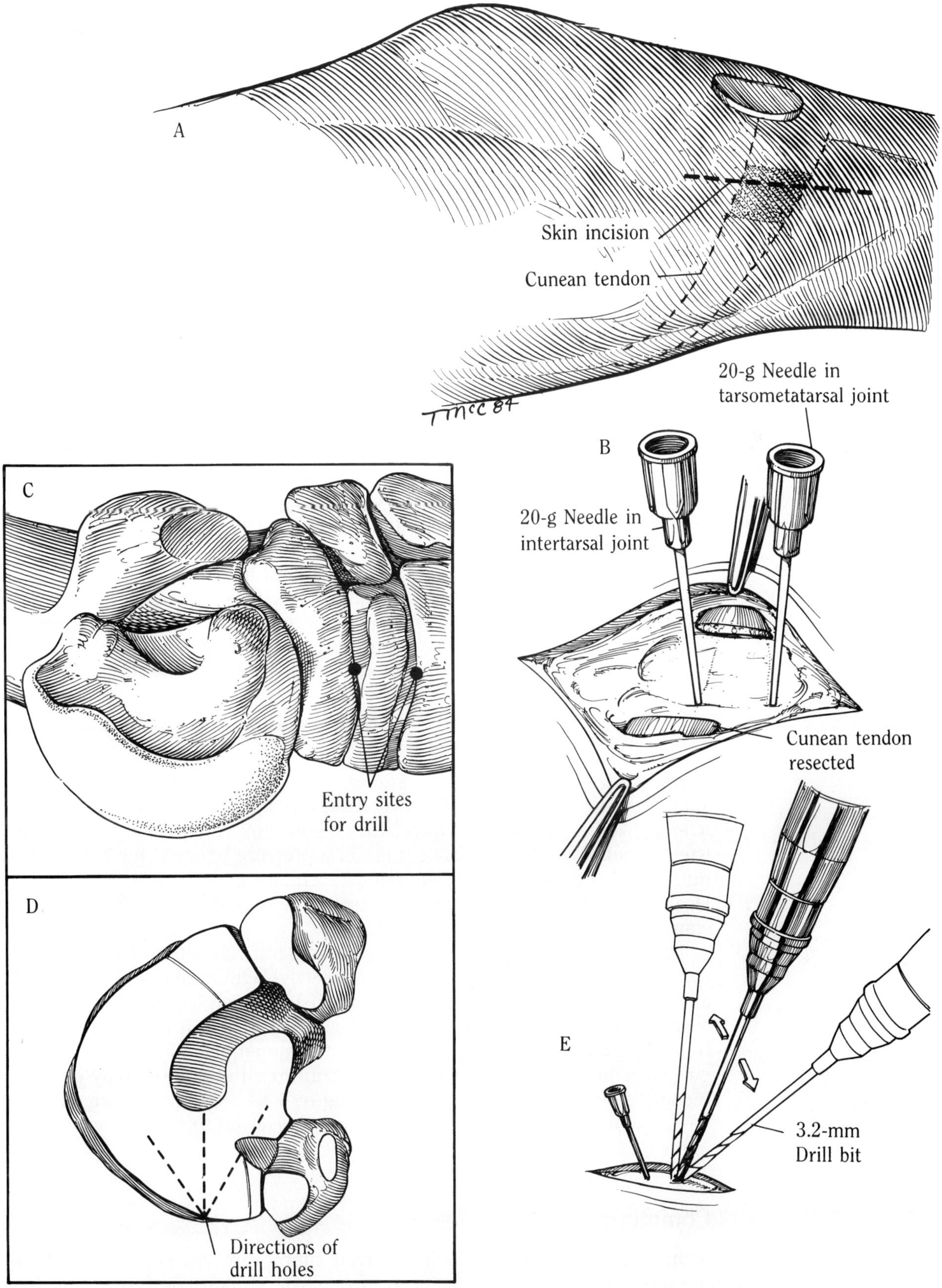

Figure 5.27, A–E. Arthrodesis of the distal intertarsal joint and tarsometatarsal joint.

with bone swarf, binding may occur and the drill bit may break. The risk of this happening is also enhanced when using old drill bits or 3.2-mm drill bits. The first author has broken several 3.2-mm drill bits, but fortunately they all broke close to the skin edge and were easily retrieved with an autoclaved pair of vise grips. If the drill bit broke deep within the joint, its retrieval would be impossible.

The length of each track is somewhat difficult to determine, and the authors believe that 2 to 3 cm depth is adequate. Again, frequent withdrawal of the drill bit and cleaning with mosquito forceps and cotton gauzes is essential. If the drill bit does emerge from outside the articular surface, a periosteal reaction may be stimulated, but no untoward sequelae have been observed (5). The most dorsally located drill track that is directed obliquely across the cranial aspect of the joint is more likely to be overdrilled because it is more difficult to ascertain the exact depth (5).

The procedure is repeated on the other joint. The drill track for each joint enters through one medially located hole under the cunean tendon. Following drilling of both joints, the wound is flushed and bony debris removed. The subcutaneous tissues are closed with simple continuous sutures using a synthetic absorbable suture material of the surgeon's choice. The skin is closed with simple interrupted sutures using a synthetic monofilament nonabsorbable material. A subcuticular suture using an absorbable material can also be used (5), but the authors would recommend this only if there were minimal to no tension on the skin edges at the time of closure. This latter technique obviates the need for suture removal.

A sterile nonadherent dressing is applied and held in position with cotton gauze. The entire hock is bandaged, using an elastic adhesive bandage that will adhere readily to the skin and prevent slippage of the dressing during recovery from anesthesia. The remainder of the limb distal to the hock is wrapped with a firm pressure bandage to reduce limb swelling distal to the surgical site.

Postoperative Management

Postoperative pain is surprisingly minimal. The authors administer phenylbutazone immediately before and for several days after operating if the horse requires it. Most patients require 3 to 4 days of this medication. Antibiotics are not administered routinely. The limb is kept under a pressure bandage for 7 to 10 days, during which time one complete bandage change may be all that is required. Healing is typically uncomplicated despite the difficulty in maintaining constant, firm pressure over the incision.

The horse is discharged 10 to 12 days postoperatively with instructions to the owner to commence hand-walking immediately. Light riding can begin 4 weeks after the arthrodesis. Because no hard and fast rules can be laid down regarding exercise, the authors recommend a judicious approach. It is often possible to return the horse to full work at 12 days if postoperative pain is minimal. If a particular horse has more pain than usual, then the authors may delay the recommendation and begin hand-walking by 1 to 2 weeks. Walking is begun despite a mild lameness because exercise is believed to hasten fusion of the joints (1, 2, 5).

Comments

Arthrodesis of the tarsal joint is relatively simple, and the complications with the technique described have been low. During drilling, profuse hemorrhage has emerged occasionally from one of the drill holes. This is probably caused by trauma to the proximal perforating branch of the cranial tibial artery. Although the bleeding is alarming at first glance, the authors have proceeded with the operation by placing a finger over the drill hole when the drill is removed for cleaning. At the end of the operation the bleeding usually subsides, and in all cases the bleeding has been inconsequential following skin closure.

Theoretically, to hasten fusion, any arthrodesis technique should involve removal of as much articular cartilage as possible to ensure maximum bony contact (7). In the initially described technique, efforts were directed at maximum joint destruction, even to the point of "fanning" the drill bit (2). In the authors' opinion, this is contraindicated because it appears to create severe postoperative pain. Although the authors have no biomechanical evidence of this, they suspect that the more radical techniques produce a greater instability to the joint. It seems that three carefully placed 4.5-mm drill holes through each joint are all that are required.

The authors' results agree with those of Edwards (5), demonstrating that approximately 80% of patients will return to full function after the surgery. The time from surgery to full working soundness varies from a few weeks to a year. Surprisingly, horses have shown improvement soon after surgery even though it has been too early to expect bony union. The authors' recommendation to owners has been to not make a decision on surgical outcome before 12 months.

Several modifications of this surgery do exist. These include packing the holes with cancellous bone, the use of lag screws, ASIF T-plates, and Steinmann pins. These are all designed to either speed fusion or provide quicker stability. From a practical standpoint, the method described is simple and less expensive to the owner. If more radical drilling and removal of tissue is required, the authors agree that some form of fixation (e.g., plate) is appropriate.

Another option for arthrodesis of the distal tarsal joints is chemical fusion with sodium monoiodoacetate. This compares favorably with surgical arthrodesis and medical management for the treatment of bone spavin (8). Some problems include the drug not being currently licensed as a pharmacologic agent for clinical use and the risk of inadvertent transmission of drug into the tibiotarsal joint. In a series of cases of 26 horses, 19 were free of lameness 1 month after treatment (73%) and 4 of 26 had radiographic fusion of the treated distal tarsal joints. Three months after treatment, 19 of 27 horses (70%) were free of lameness, 17 of 27 (63%) had radiographic fusion, and 15 of 27 (56%) were considered successful. Six months after treatment, 21 of 26 horses (81%) were free of lameness, 22 of 26 (85%) had radiographic fusion, and 21 of 26 cases (81%) were considered successful. At 12 months posttreatment, 27 of 29 (93%) were free of lameness, 28 of 29 (97%) had radiographic fusion, and 26 of 29 cases (90%) were considered successful.

REFERENCES

1. Adams OR. Lameness in Horses. 3rd ed. Philadelphia: Lea & Febiger, 1974:326.
2. Adams OR. Surgical arthrodesis for the treatment of bone spavin. JAVMA 1970;157:480.
3. Mackay RCJ, Liddell WA. Arthrodesis in the treatment of bone spavin. Equine Vet J 1982;4:34.
4. Barber SM. Arthrodesis of the distal intertarsal and tarsometatarsal joints in the horse: J Vet Surg 1984;13:227.
5. Edwards GB. Surgical arthrodesis for the treatment of bone spavin in 20 horses. Equine Vet J 1982;14:117.
6. Sack WO, Orsini PG. Distal intertarsal and tarsometatarsal joints in the horse: communication and injection sites. JAVMA 1981;179:355.
7. Turek SL. Orthopaedics, Principles, and Their Application. Philadelphia: JB Lippincott, 1984.
8. Bohanon TC. Chemical fusion of the distal tarsal joints with sodium monoiodoacetate in horses clinically affected with osteoarthrosis. In: Proceedings of the 41st Annual Meeting of the AAEP, Lexington, Kentucky, 1995:148–149.

Arthrodesis of the Fetlock Joint

Arthrodesis of the fetlock joint is indicated for the management of traumatic disruption of the suspensory apparatus either by fracture of the medial and lateral sesamoid bones, disruption of the distal sesamoidean ligaments, rupture of the suspensory ligament, or severe osteoarthritis (DJD) (1–4). (The latter is a less frequent indication because it occurs less frequently and such injuries can often be managed without surgery.)

With disruption of the suspensory apparatus there is an inability to weightbear and abnormal dorsiflexion of the metacarpophalangeal (fetlock) joint in the horse. The diagnosis of the condition is straightforward and obvious, but it is important that a complete set of fetlock radiographs be made to provide complete information with regard to the presence of biaxial sesamoid fractures (as well as the presence of other fractures) or, in the case of distal sesamoidean ligament disruption, proximal displacement of the sesamoid bones (distal displacement of the sesamoid bones in cases of suspensory disruption). Fetlock arthrodesis is also indicated for the treatment of advanced osteoarthritis (DJD) of the fetlock joint. Although osteoarthritis of the fetlock joint usually has a chronic history, the presentation with severe debilitating lameness may be relatively acute. Diagnosis is confirmed with radiographs, and, in cases whereby fetlock arthrodesis is indicated, the most prominent radiographic manifestation is collapse of the joint space. Arthrodesis is indicated for the relief of pain.

Fetlock arthrodesis is also indicated for the treatment of degenerative disruption of the suspensory ligament and in the authors' experience is usually seen in the Peruvian Paso. In all instances of fetlock arthrodesis, the expense involved in surgery as well as postoperative management is considerable. There needs to be clear communication between the surgeon and the owner with regard to the overall costs (particularly in the convalescent period), and potential complications need to be explained.

It is the authors' opinion that with the exception of some instances of suspensory ligament disruption, fetlock arthrodesis is the most predictably effective method of managing the above problems. Casting and splinting have been previously used for traumatic disruption of the suspensory ligament apparatus. External support with casts is associated with a high prevalence of major pressure sores (3). Although a board splint has been described as a method of treatment, complications include laminitis in the opposite forelimb (at a higher incidence than with surgical arthrodesis) and acquired flexural deformities. Marked improvement in the acute management of the patient after suspensory apparatus disruption has decreased the complications of surgery, making arthrodesis an effective treatment.

A number of techniques for fetlock arthrodesis have been described (1–5; Herthel DF, personal communication, 1996), including the use of the dynamic compression plate (DCP) down the dorsal surface together with a figure-8 tension band wire placed on the palmar aspect of the limb (1–4), biaxial bone plates placed on the palmarolateral and palmaromedial aspects of the fetlock (5), and, most recently, the use of a large interlocking nail inserted through the carpus down to the second phalanx (Herthel DF, personal communication, 1996). The technique described here has been used with consistent success by the first author and utilizes a DCP plate without the adjunctive use of wire. As has been previously pointed out by the originator of fetlock arthrodesis, if the suspensory apparatus of the fetlock joint is intact (in such cases as osteoarthritis), transfixing the sesamoid bones and tightening the distal sesamoidean ligaments by extending the joint provides palmar support to aid the plate in resisting extension. The technique described here uses the principle of keeping the dorsal plate straight with adjunctive lag screw fixation across the joint. If there is sufficient sesamoid bone to be used, these are involved in lag screw fixation as well.

The initial acute care after catastrophic injury of the fetlock is critical in the overall success of the procedure. Hyperextension of the fetlock joint results in tension on the palmar nerve vascular structures. If this condition is uncorrected, avascular necrosis of the distal limb may result. Specially designed splints that provide support to the distal limb and prevent fetlock extension (protecting the blood supply of the distal limb) should be routinely available at racetracks. The most commonly used splint is the Legsaver made by Kimsey Welding Works in Woodland, California. Another alternative is the Farley compression boot made by Equine Orthotics Inc, Indian Harbor Beach, Florida. If the above devices are unavailable, a board splint can be used but it is definitely a less desirable choice.

Anti-inflammatory agents such as phenylbutazone (4.4 mg/kg body weight twice daily) is started immediately after surgery and preoperative antibiotics are given. The period of preantibiotic administration is usually longer than normal because of the compromising effect of decreased vascularity. Penicillin and gentamicin are usually used. Surgery is usually performed between 12 to 72 hours after injury (3).

Anesthesia and Surgical Preparation

The surgical procedure is done with the horse under general anesthesia with the affected leg uppermost. The leg is positioned on a leg stand so that intraoperative radiographs can be taken conveniently and without any risk to aseptic technique. The leg is clipped completely from below the carpus distal to the hoof and the dorsal aspect shaved. A tourniquet is not used because of the potential compromising effect on vascularity (nor is it used by the author with elective arthrodesis for osteoarthritis). The area of the surgical incision is prepared for aseptic surgery in a routine manner. Plastic adhesive drapes are also used.

Additional Instrumentation

Instrumentation for DCP plate fixation and lag screw fixation with 4.5-mm cortical bone screws and 5.5 mm-cortical bone screws (see Appendices I–II) are needed. Curets, a chisel (1–2 cm wide), mallet, medium periosteal elevator (Synthes), and equipment for intraoperative radiographs are also required. A 14-hole broad DCP plate is used.

Surgical Technique

A dorsolateral skin incision is made from 4 cm below the carpus, following the center of the common digital extensor tendon, distad to the fetlock joint to immediately proximal to the pastern joint (Fig. 5.28, *A* and *B*). The incision is extended through the subcutaneous tissues and the common digital extensor tendon is split longitudinally (as illustrated in Fig. 5.28*B*). The incision is continued through the periosteum, which is reflected, and the dorsal joint capsule of the fetlock joint is incised longitudinally to immediately proximal to the first phalanx and then horizontally to the lateral collateral ligament. The lateral collateral ligament is incised (Fig. 5.28*C*) so that the fetlock joint can be flexed and luxated to expose the articular surface of the distal metacarpus, proximal first phalanx, and sesamoid bones. The articular cartilage of the distal metacarpus, proximal first phalanx, and (if appropriate) sesamoid bones is removed with a curet (Fig. 5.28*D*). The prominence created by the sagittal ridge of the distal metacarpus is removed with a chisel to facilitate fitting of the plate. The 14-

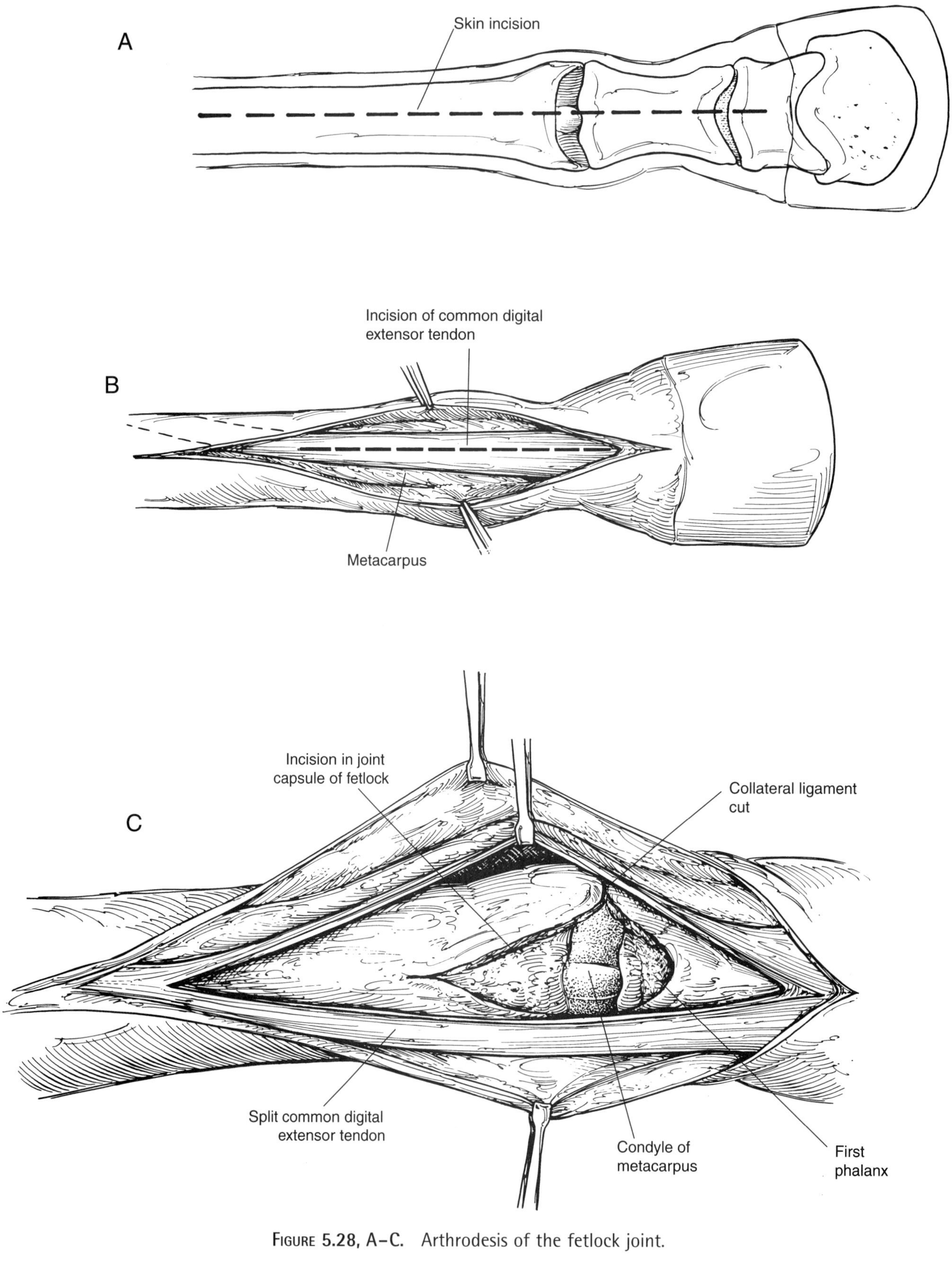

Figure 5.28, A–C. Arthrodesis of the fetlock joint.

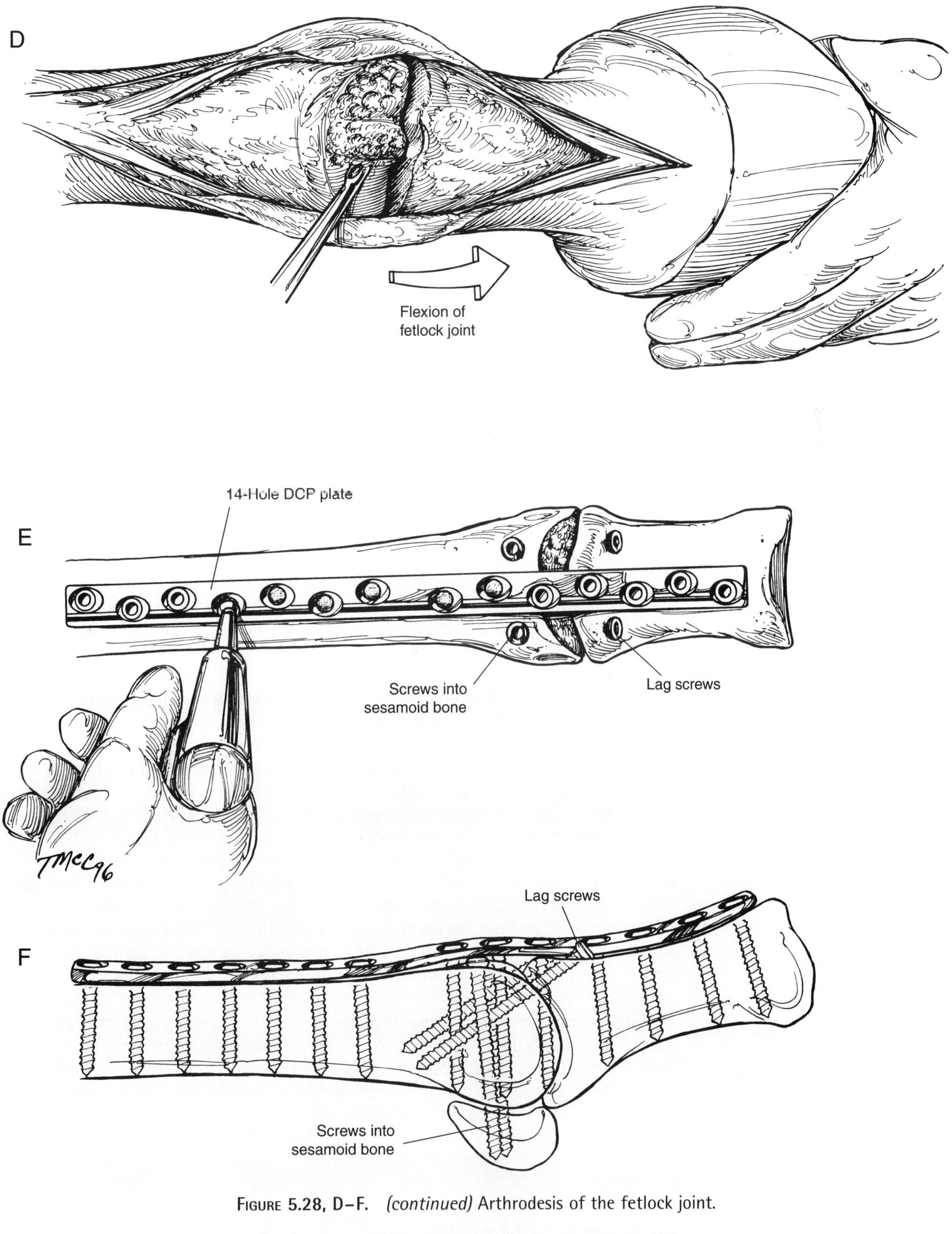

FIGURE 5.28, D–F. *(continued)* Arthrodesis of the fetlock joint.

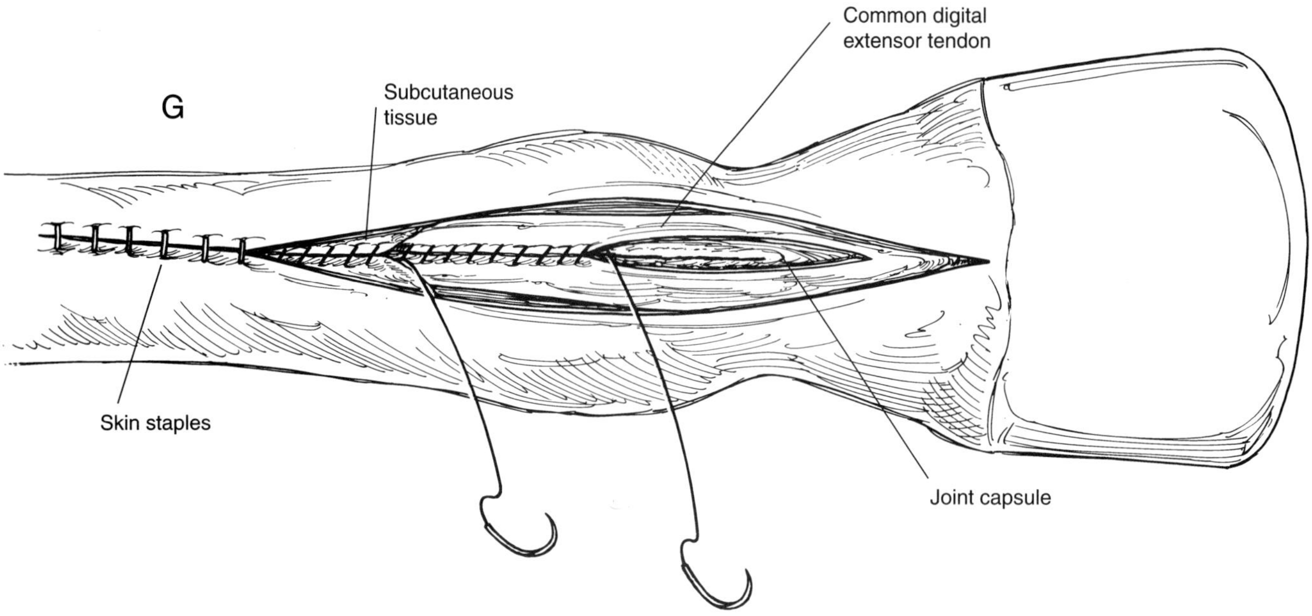

Figure 5.28, G. *(continued)* Arthrodesis of the fetlock joint.

hole DCP bone plate (a 16-hole plate is appropriate in a horse with a long cannon bone) is fitted to the dorsal surface of the bone (Fig. 5.28, *E* and *F*). Although the diagram depicts some contouring, efforts are made to keep the plate relatively straight in an attempt to minimize the compression forces on a hyperextended plate. Attention is paid to ensure the proximal aspect of the plate is below the top of the postoperative cast. The plate is placed so that the foremost distal holes are located over the dorsal surface of the first phalanx for insertion of screws into the first phalanx. In addition to maximum contact of the plate on the dorsal surfaces of the bone, care must be taken to ensure that the fetlock is properly reduced so that there is minimal potential for movement. Cortical bone screws (4.5 mm) are used to fix the plate to both the first phalanx and the distal metacarpus. The first two screws on either side of the plate are placed with 1 mm of lag to provide some compression. After insertion of these screws, two 5.5-mm cortical bone screws are placed in lag screw fashion. These are inserted on either side of the plate through pre-drilled glide holes in the first phalanx, up into the condyles of the metacarpus (Fig. 5.28, *E* and *F*). Two additional 4.5-mm cortical bone screws are placed across into the sesamoid bones (if intact and/or reduced in an appropriate position). After placement of the two 5.5-mm lag screws from P1 to the metacarpus, the sesamoid screws are placed and then the remainder of the screws are placed in the DCP plate (Fig. 5.28, *E* and *F*).

The incision is closed in three layers (Fig. 5.28*G*). The incision in the common digital extensor tendon is closed with a continuous suture of synthetic absorbable suture. The subcutaneous tissue is then closed with a continuous layer of 2/0 synthetic absorbable suture, and the skin is closed with skin staples. Nonadherent dressings are applied and maintained in a position with a cotton gauze such as Kling. A fiberglass cast is then applied to the distal limb for the recovery from anesthesia and to protect the implants from cyclic loading in the postoperative period.

Postoperative Management

The horse is routinely maintained on penicillin and gentamicin for 5 days, but this period of antibiotic administration may be extended depending on the state of damage to the soft tissues (up to several weeks). Phenylbutazone is used postoperatively. The first cast is usually maintained for 2 weeks but if there is any discomfort or concern over the state of the soft tissues, it will be changed earlier. In some instances, one cast has been maintained for 5 weeks and removed standing. In other instances, a second cast is applied.

The horse is maintained in a clean dry box stall for at least 2 months. A larger area can be allowed after that time. Adequate bedding needs to be maintained to encourage the horse to lie down. Return to exercise should be gradual, allowing the horse and its joints to adapt to the new restrictions of a fused fetlock joint.

Comments

In a retrospective study of the results of fetlock arthrodesis, 34 of 52 horses with fusion of the fetlock joint survived and were eventually allowed unrestricted activity (2). The results were better when horses had fetlock arthrodesis as a primary initial treatment, compared with those in which conservative treatment was tried initially and the fetlock arthrodesis was elected as a last resort. The prognosis was also better for horses wherein arthrodesis was used to treat osteoarthritis than for horses with rupture of the suspensory apparatus, which is logical because of the lack of soft tissue compromise with osteoarthritis. In general, the prognosis for cases of osteoarthritis is excellent if the opposing foot has no evidence of laminitis. When there is evidence of laminitis and distal phalanx rotation, the prognosis drops proportionately. With suspensory apparatus breakdown, the prognosis is determined by the severity of the injury and vascular damage. When there is no significant soft tissue injury, the prognosis is similar to that associated with osteoarthritis.

The technique described here does not use a tension band but has yielded good results. It is thought that maintaining the plate and MCIII-P1 angle at 180° causes considerably less cyclic loading on the plate, which is bent 15° from this position when the tension band is used (1). When treating cases of osteoarthritis and distal sesamoidean ligament disruption, adequate adjunctive lag screw fixation can be obtained and presumably contributes markedly to the quality of the repair. When the sesamoids are fractured, no screws are placed across the distal metacarpus into the sesamoid bone, but 5.5-mm diameter screws are used to lag the proximal first phalanx and the distal metacarpus.

Infection around the plate has been observed as a complication and requires removal of the plate. Such infection can cause discomfort and reluctance of the horse to use the limb. Infection of the fixation has been reported as common in cases of traumatic disruption of the suspensory apparatus because in most instances the trauma also damages the skin (1). Implant removal is indicated when infection of the implants causes fistula formation and drainage. The plate is removed when bony fusion of the fetlock has been obtained.

The most significant complication associated with arthrodesis is laminitis of the opposing limb. The development of laminitis is influenced by the severity of the original injury, the immediate postinjury care, the surgery itself, as well as the development of complications at the surgery site. The latter complications could be associated with instability of the fixation, an inadequate repair, or devascularization caused by damage to the blood vessels. Although the vascular injury can be catastrophic, resulting in necrosis of the distal limb and sloughing of the hoof wall, more minor insult causes wound healing delays (1).

REFERENCES

1. Bramlage LR. An initial report on a surgical technique for arthrodesis of the metacarpophalangeal joint in horses. In: Proceedings of the 27th Annual Convention of the American Association of Equine Practitioners. 1981;27:257–261.

2. Bramlage LR. Arthrodesis of the metacarpophalangeal joint. Results in 52 horses. Vet Surg 1984;14:45.
3. Bowman KF, Leith M, Nunamaker DM, et al. Complications during treatment of traumatic disruption of the suspensory apparatus in Thoroughbred horses. JAVMA 1984; 184:706–715.
4. Bramlage LR. Fetlock arthrodesis. In: Nixon A, ed. Equine Fractures. Philadelphia: WB Saunders, 1996:172–178.
5. Nunamaker DM, Bowman KF, Herring ME, et al. A comparative biomechanical study of surgical arthrodesis of the fetlock joint of the horse. Lecture, 18th Ann Mtg.

Decompression of the Suprascapular Nerve

Paralysis of the suprascapular nerve (sweeny) results in atrophy of the supraspinatus and infraspinatus muscles. It is usually caused by direct trauma to the nerve and was frequent in draft horses with poorly fitting collars (1). It has also been seen when there is overstretching of the nerve, as may occur when the shoulder is thrust caudad when an animal slips (1, 2).

In the *acute* stage, the gait of a horse with sweeny is almost unmistakable. During the support phase of the stride there is a rapid outward excursion of the shoulder, observed best when the horse is walked toward the examiner (1, 3, 4). This occurs because the infraspinatus muscle and, to a lesser degree, the supraspinatus muscle contribute to the lateral support of the shoulder. The abnormal gait is frequently seen shortly after injury. Eventually the muscles atrophy and the spine of the scapula becomes obvious. The onset of muscle atrophy is usually evident, within 7 to 14 days following trauma (3).

The outward movement of the scapula during weightbearing is believed to cause intermittent *overstretching* of the suprascapular nerve, resulting in continued trauma. Additionally, scar tissue around the nerve can be responsible for the paralysis because as the collagen in the scar tissue matures, nerve conduction is constricted and impaired (5).

The diagnosis of suprascapular nerve paralysis should be made only after a thorough physical and radiographic examination to rule out fractures and arthritis of the shoulder region and OCD in young horses. When available, electromyography of the infraspinatus and supraspinatus muscles is helpful, particularly in the early case (before muscle atrophy) to identify denervation.

Surgical treatment is aimed at decompression of the suprascapular nerve as it passes over the cranial edge of the scapula and at removal of the surrounding organizing hematoma or scar tissue (neurolysis) (5). Reduction of the tension being exerted on the nerve is achieved by removing a piece of scapula that underlies the nerve. This procedure reduces tension on the nerve created by the abrupt change of its dissection over the cranial edge of the scapula and removes the potential for intermittent tension on the nerve during full weightbearing (1, 4, 6).

Anesthesia and Surgical Preparation

The operation is done with the horse in lateral recumbency with the affected limb uppermost. Before anesthesia, the shoulder region is clipped to reduce anesthetic time. Following induction of anesthesia, the area of surgical incision (Fig. 5.29*A*) is shaved and routine surgical preparation is carried out.

Additional Instrumentation

Decompression of the suprascapular nerve requires a wire bone saw or osteotome, a chisel, and a mallet, curettes, rongeurs, Penrose drain, and tubing (e.g., ¼-inch). An air drill is helpful, if available.

When an osteotome is used, the ventral osteotomy should be made first to reduce the chances of creating a fracture of the supraglenoid tuberosity that could extend into the shoulder joint (6).

Surgical Technique

After draping (the use of sterile plastic adherent drapes is recommended for this procedure), the spine of the scapula is identified. A 15-cm skin incision is made commencing 4 cm proximal to the end of the scapular spine and 1 cm cranial to it and extending distad to the distal end of the cranial spine. The

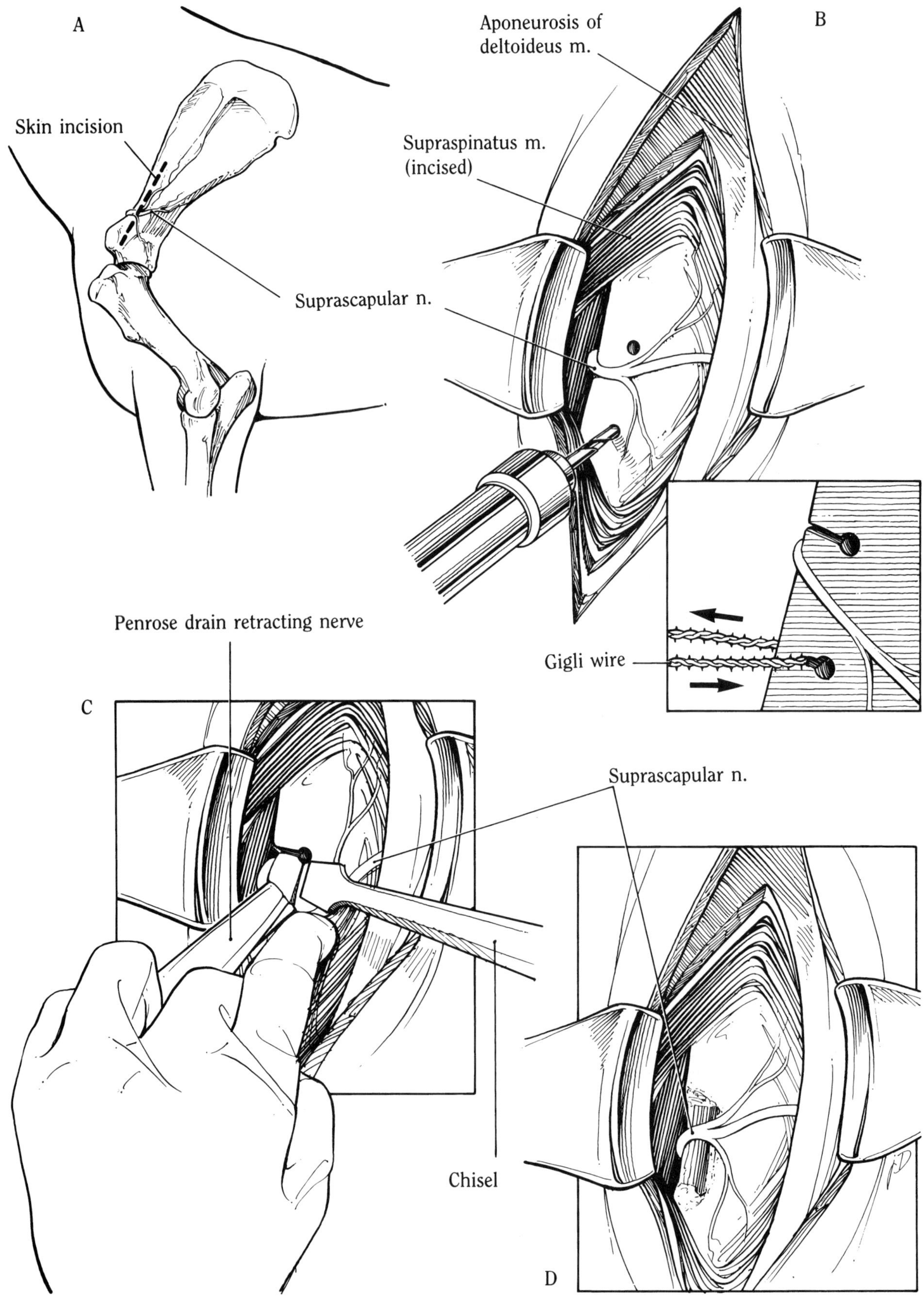

Figure 5.29, A–D. Decompression of the suprascapular nerve for the treatment of sweeny.

dissection plane continues down to the origin of the supraspinatus muscle on the scapular spine (Fig. 5.29*A*). This origin is then incised 1 cm cranial to the scapular spine, and the supraspinatus muscle is reflected craniad to expose the suprascapular nerve.

Organizing hematoma or scar tissue surrounding the nerve is dissected free from the nerve as atraumatically as possible (this procedure is called external neurolysis). Hemostasis should be attended to as hemorrhage arises. All attempts should be made to reduce the inflammatory response and resultant scar tissue that will arise from healing at the surgical site.

When the external neurolysis is complete, the nerve is gently retracted by an encircling Penrose drain, and a piece of bone 1.2 × 2.5 cm lying directly under the nerve is removed using a wire saw, an osteotome, a chisel, or an air drill. If a wire saw is used, holes should be drilled into the neck of the scapula to initiate the path for the saw cuts (Fig. 5.29, *B* and *C*). The vertical component of the saw cuts can be connected by chiseling the fragment of bone away from the parent structure (Fig. 5.29*C*). If an osteotome is used, the vertical osteotomy should be made first to reduce the chances of creating a fracture of the supraglenoid tuberosity that could extend into the shoulder joint (6). The defect created will have sharp edges that must be smoothed or removed with the selected use of bone curettes, rongeurs, or a burr and air drill (Fig. 5.29*D*). When available, an air drill with a medium fluted burr facilitates the removal of a curved piece of bone underlying the suprascapular nerve. The advantages of the burr air drill technique are that it is quicker and, with practice, safer. Because a curved and not rectangular piece of bone is removed, there is less risk of the ventral aspect of the osteotomy site fracturing into the shoulder joint (Stashak TS, personal communication, 1985).

During the closure, a Penrose drain may be inserted under the supraspinatus muscle and anchored by a long horizontal mattress suture that exits near the proximal end of the incision. Subcutaneous tissues and skin are apposed in a routine manner. A stent bandage is sutured over the incision line (1, 6).

Postoperative Management

The Penrose drain is removed in 24 to 48 hours, depending on its rate of decline of exudate productivity. Hand-walking is commenced 1 week following surgery and increased depending on the degree of improvement shown by the horse. The stent bandage is removed 4 to 5 days after the operation. If the surgical procedure has been successful, the horse can be turned out to pasture in 6 weeks.

Comments

It is obvious to any student of wound healing that the surgical manipulation involved in removal of the organizing hematoma or scar tissue from around the nerve, especially dissections of the epineurium, results in reformation of scar tissue. Theoretically, this could result in a secondary re-entrapment of the nerve (3). To avoid this, the nerve should be dissected meticulously, beginning in normal tissue, both proximally and distally if possible, so that all branches of the nerve can be identified and preserved. Dissection then progresses centripetally, exposing the region of nerve damage (5).

It may be argued that decompression of the nerve in chronic cases would be futile. In humans, however, neurogenic muscle atrophy can be reversed in some cases if reinnervation occurs within 20 months (7). Unfortunately, no such time frames are available in horses. The limiting factor for recovery is the ability of the animal to restore the atrophied muscle. It has been recommended that exploratory decompression be performed when soft tissue healing has occurred and a "reasonable period of time" has elapsed for reinnervation of the muscle. Two to four months after the signs have appeared has been the recommended period to wait before attempting surgery (4). One series, however, identified the earliest return to function and best end result in horses operated on *early,* after the acute swelling had decreased and muscle atrophy was first noticed (6). Electromyography can be helpful in identification of early denervation.

Long-term results of decompression of the suprascapular nerve have been encouraging. In another series, 11 of 12 cases of sweeny improved following surgery, and although the muscle mass returned to normal in most horses, it was not uncommon for the dorsal one-half of the supraspinatus muscle to remain atrophied (6).

REFERENCES

1. Stashak TS, ed. Adams' Lameness in Horses. 5th ed. Philadelphia: Lea & Febiger, 1986.
2. Rooney JR. Biomechanics of Lameness in Horses. Baltimore: Williams & Wilkins, 1969: 114.
3. Adams OR, Schneider RK, Bramlage LR, et al. A surgical approach to treatment of suprascapular nerve injury in the horse. JAVMA 1985;187:1016.
4. Stashak TS. The nervous system: specific techniques. In: Jennings PB, ed. Textbook of Large Animal Surgery. Philadelphia: WB Saunders, 1984:1019.
5. Bora FW, Unger A. In: Hunt TK, et al., eds. The Inhibition of Scar After Tendon and Nerve Injury in Soft and Hard Tissue Repair, Vol. 1. Surgical Science Series. New York: Praeger Scientific Publications, 1984:586.
6. Schneider JE, Adams OR, Easley KJ, et al. Scapular notch resection for suprascapular nerve decompression in 12 horses. JAVMA 1985;187:1019.
7. Leffert RD. Surgery of the peripheral nerves and brachial plexus. In: Schmidek HH, Sweet WH, eds. Current Techniques in Operative Neurosurgery. New York: Grune and Stratton, 1977.

"Street Nail" Procedure

Infection of the navicular bursa (bursa podotrochlearis) is caused by penetration by any sharp object (e.g., nail) into the solar surface of the hoof at the middle third of the frog (1). It also has been seen as an iatrogenic infection following injection of corticosteriods or other anti-inflammatory agents into the area of the navicular bursa.

Infection of the navicular bursa produces a severe lameness resembling a fracture of one of the phalanges. The lameness will improve dramatically when the palmar (plantar) nerves are blocked, but the horse will rarely approach complete soundness.

Radiographs are useful to rule out fractures. If a foreign body is present, it should be left in place until radiographs have been taken. They will give the clinician an indication of how close it has come to penetrating the bursa. If the tract made by the penetrating wound is still open, then injection of a suitable contrast agent up the track or insertion of a sterile metal probe also will help determine if the navicular bursa is involved. Infection of the bursa will cause radiographic changes in the navicular bone when the condition is long-standing. A diagnosis of infectious navicular bursitis is usually based on the presence of severe lameness associated with a puncture wound that has not responded to therapy. Horses with puncture wounds of the sole may respond to drainage of the wound within 24 to 48 hours. If improvement is not noticed in this time, and the wound is located in such a region of the sole that puncture of the bursa is possible, septic navicular bursitis osteomyelitis and sepsis of the deep digital flexor tendon can occur (1). Conservative methods of therapy are generally futile because of the location of the septic process, which will extend from the navicular bursa into the deep digital flexor tendon and navicular bone. Surgery for infection of the navicular bursa has historically been called the penetrating "street nail" procedure because of the cause of the infection. It consists of drainage of the bursa through a "window" cut in the frog, digital cushion, and deep flexor tendon (1–4).

Anesthesia and Surgical Preparation

The foot is prepared by trimming the hoof with a pair of good quality nippers and a rasp. The foot is then placed in a medicated bandage and allowed to soak overnight, in preparation for surgery. The entire foot is again prepared for surgery in a routine manner following removal of this bandage. The procedure is best done with the horse under general anesthesia with the affected limb uppermost. A tourniquet placed above the fetlock joint is essential to produce a relatively bloodless field and allow the surgeon to inspect the flexor tendon and navicular bone for damage.

Additional Instrumentation

A Stryker or similar oscillating saw or osteotome set and mallet and hoof-trimming equipment (knife, nippers, and rasp) are required. A shoe with a removable steel plate will be necessary later in the convalescence.

Surgical Technique

A square hole is cut in the center third of the frog (Fig. 5.30, *A* and *B*). In horses with a soft pliable frog, a sharp scalpel will be adequate. Horses in dry parts of the country will have a hard, tough frog and will require a Stryker or similar oscillating saw or osteotomes (Fig. 5.30*C*). The procedure should begin with

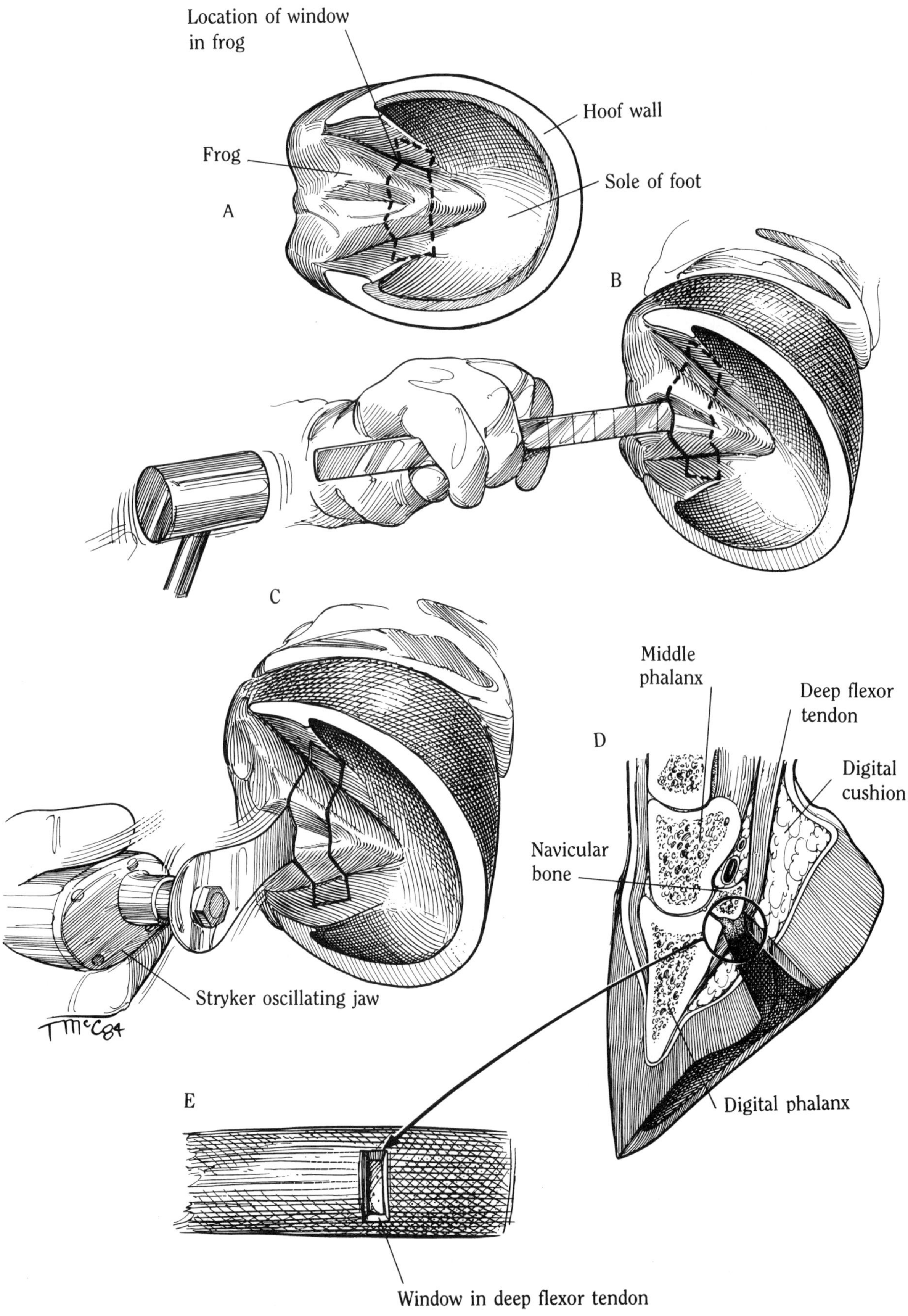

Figure 5.30, A–E. "Street nail" procedure for septic navicular bursitis.

transverse incision through the frog at the junction of the caudal and middle third of the frog; external and perpendicular to the bearing surface of the frog. Another transverse incision is made as shown in Figure 5.30*A* and then connected with the first incision by two lateral incisions. The loosened portion of the frog and digital cushion are dissected free. The aperture should measure 7.5 × 2 cm and taper down to a smaller one, as shown in Figure 5.30*D*. The authors have found that an external aperture smaller than this will result in a smaller internal aperture (in the deep flexor tendon), which will seal over and not provide adequate drainage. When the "core" of the frog and digital cushion have been removed, the condition of the deep flexor tendon will be evident. A small rectangular window is made in the deep flexor tendon, to complete the entry into the navicular bursa, by initially making two transverse incisions (Fig. 5.30*E*). A culture of the infected bursa should be taken at this time. Visibly obvious necrotic tendon should be removed at this point. This can result in a larger defect in the tendon. Care should be taken not to incise dorsal to the navicular bone, thus injuring the distal sesamoid impar ligament, which will result in immediate entry into the distal interphalangeal (coffin) joint.

The flexor (distal) surface of the navicular bone will be visible, and its hyaline cartilage covering should be inspected by flexing and extending the distal interphalangeal joint. The defect in the frog and digital cushion should be vigorously flushed to remove tissue debris. It is then packed with gauze soaked with an antibacterial solution.

Postoperative Management

The convalescent period is long and will require almost daily attention for several weeks. Antibiotics are usually administered for 1 week postoperatively. Penicillin and an aminoglycoside antibiotic have been recommended (1). Nonsteroidal anti-inflammatory drugs will be required for at least 1 week to control pain because it is usually severe, at least initially. Tetanus prophylaxis must be provided.

The medicated gauze that has been placed in the defect is changed daily until a good healthy bed of granulation tissue has appeared. This will take 10 to 14 days. After this time, the dressing can be changed less frequently, depending on the amount of suppuration that is present initially. Nerve blocks may be required if the horse is very sensitive. Equally important during this time is to provide a good waterproof, durable bandage around the hoof to prevent contamination of the surgical site. The horse should be kept in a clean dry stall, free of any moisture if possible.

When the defect has completely filled with granulation tissue and there is no evidence of fistula formation, a shoe with a removable steel plate can be applied. This will drastically reduce the amount of bandage material required to keep the foot clean and enable the horse to be turned out into a less restricted area. It is also useful in horses that do not tolerate the bandage or bandage changes well. Eventually, the regrown frog that has bridged the defect must be toughened sufficiently to allow the horse to be without the special shoe. Drying agents such as tincture of iodine are useful at this stage. Finally, a shoe with a leather pad can be applied and reset much like a normal shoe, depending on the amount of sole growth.

Comments

The prognosis for future soundness for a penetrating wound of the navicular bursa should always be guarded to poor (1). Frequently it is difficult to save the horse even for breeding purposes. Rotational laminitis in the opposite limb often leads to the demise of the horse. The key to success in the operation is *early* surgery as soon as penetration of the bursa is diagnosed or even suspected. The authors are aware of several horses that may have been saved if diagnosis had been made sooner. If the operation has been successful, the horse will gradually begin to put weight on the limb. It is important that nonsteroidal anti-inflammatory drugs not mask the signs of uncontrolled infections, further tissue necrosis, and overall patient deterioration. Although the authors recommend antibiotics, the key to success in this operation is ventral drainage of what is a "closed cavity" infection.

If the horse is still nonweightbearing some days after the operation, then continued necrosis of the deep flexor tendon and/or infectious arthritis of the coffin joint should be suspected. Development of an ascending cellulitis proximad indicates involvement of the tendon sheath, and additional surgery (including drainage) should be considered. Advanced cases of tendon sheath involvement can result in rupture of the deep digital flexor tendon (1).

REFERENCES

1. Richardson GL, O'Brien TR, Pascoe JR, et al. Puncture wounds of the navicular bursa in 38 horses. A retrospective study. Vet Surg 1986;15:156.
2. Frank ER. Veterinary Surgery. 7th ed. Minneapolis: Burgess Publishing Company, 1964:222.
3. Guard WF. Surgical Principles and Technics. Columbus, OH: WF Guard Publisher, 1953:131.
4. Kersjes AW, Nemeth F, Rutgers LJE. Atlas of Large Animal Surgery. Baltimore: Williams & Wilkins, 1985:90.

Surgery For Fibrotic Myopathy (After Bramlage)

Fibrotic myopathy in the horse refers to a gait abnormality that results from fibrosis of the semitendinosus muscle, with occasional involvement of the semimembranosus and biceps femoris muscles (1, 2). Fibrotic myopathy involving the gracilis muscle also has been reported (3), and trauma with subsequent inflammation and fibrosis is considered the initiating factor (1). External trauma can result in fibrotic myopathy, but the condition also may be work-related, particularly in Quarter horses (1, 2). If bone forms in the affected tissues, the condition is termed ossifying myopathy (1). Examination of case histories of 18 horses with fibrotic myopathy at the authors' hospital revealed that 5 had developed the lameness secondary to intramuscular injections (2). In this series, all 5 had involvement of the left hind limb, which may reflect that horses are handled from the left side and left-sided injections may have been given more commonly (2). The condition may also be congenital (4).

Earlier treatments described for these conditions included semitendinosus tenotomy and resection of the affected tissue, with surgical removal of restrictive adhesions (1). This procedure was, in the authors' practice, associated with a high incidence of complications. These complications included acute disruption of the skin incision, dehiscence of the wound during healing, prolonged hemorrhage from the wound, and necrosis under the quill sutures that were used to relieve tension across the skin incision (2).

The authors have subsequently used a modified technique first described by Bramlage et al. (4). This technique entails a tenotomy of the tendinous insertion of the semitendinosus muscle. It is technically an easier procedure than partial myotenotomy and seems to be more effective in treatment of fibrotic myopathy of the semitendinosus muscle (3).

Anesthesia and Surgical Preparation

The surgical procedure is done with the patient under general anesthesia in lateral recumbency with the affected limb down. The area immediately caudodistal to the femorotibial joint is clipped and surgically prepared.

Surgical Technique

The semitendinosus tendon of insertion is palpated over the proximal medial tibia, caudal to the medial saphenous vein, and overlying the gastrocnemius muscle (Fig. 5.31*A*). An 8-cm vertical skin incision is made over the tendon, and the incision is carried through the subcutaneous and crural fascia until the tendon is exposed (Fig. 5.31*B*). A large forceps, such as curved Kelly or Crile forceps, is passed under the tendon to isolate it from the muscle, and the tendon is transected (Fig. 5.31*C*). Fascial layers are closed with interrupted synthetic absorbable sutures, and the skin is closed with interrupted nonabsorbable suture material. Tension sutures or support sutures are also recommended.

Postoperative Management

The use of antibiotics is optional. No special treatment of the skin incision is required or recommended. The incision is too proximal to recommend pressure bandaging. Occasionally, a seroma may form at the surgical site. If the seroma is large, it may require needle aspiration under aseptic conditions. Because of the high mobility of the skin in this area, partial dehiscence of the skin incision

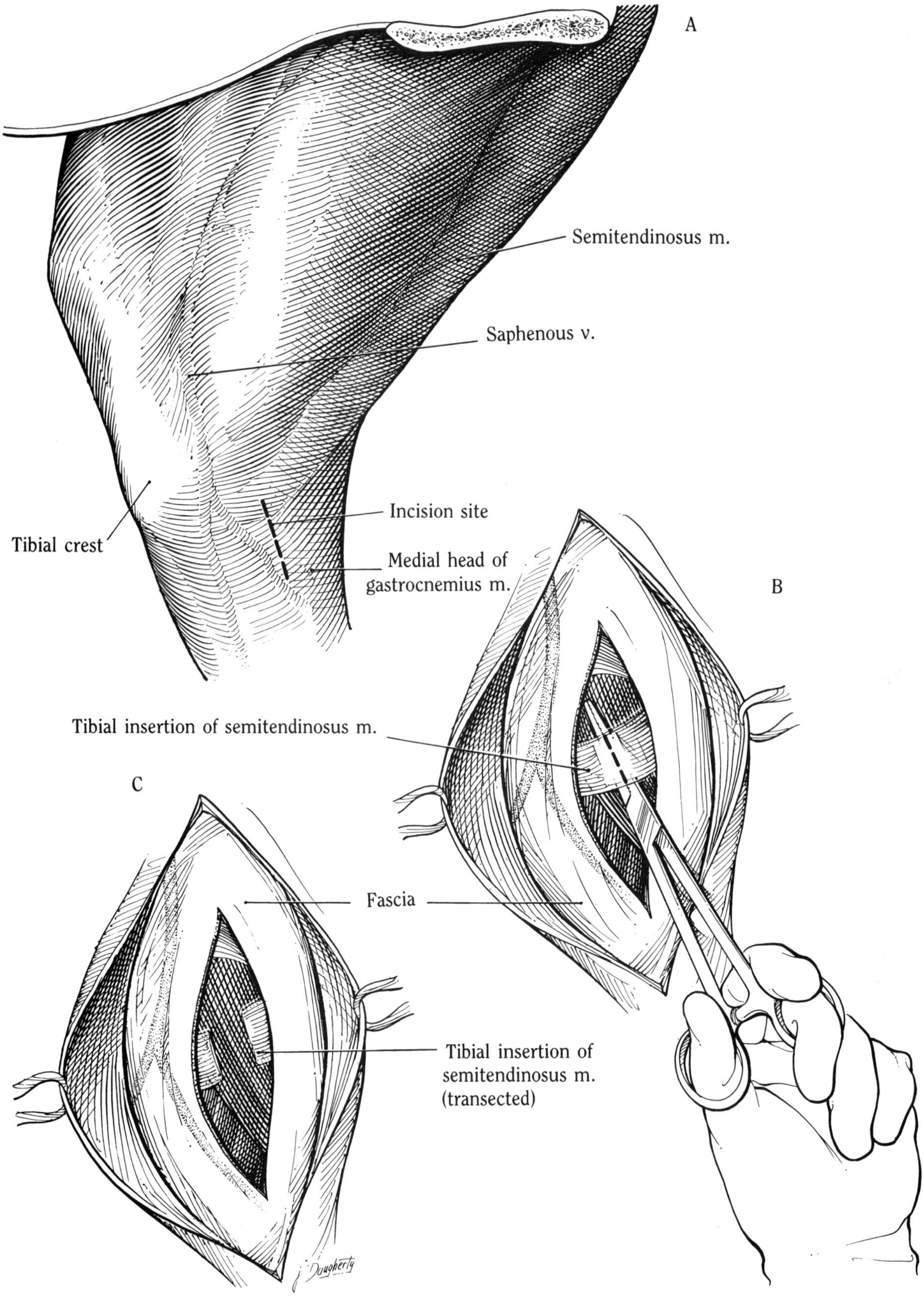

Figure 5.31, A–C. Tenotomy of the tendinous insertion of the semitendinosus muscle for fibrotic myopathy.

may occur, but uneventful healing by second intention usually follows. Phenylbutazone (2 to 3 g) is administered intravenously to reduce postoperative pain, although it would be ill-advised to recommend or encourage too much activity for the horse in the immediate postoperative period. Mild exercise can begin at 2 weeks with unrestricted exercise allowed after 6 weeks (4). Skin sutures are removed 12 to 14 days after the operation.

Comments

The authors' initial experience with this technique was encouraging. Certainly the consequences of skin dehiscence of this smaller incision are not nearly as great as with the myotenotomy procedure previously described (1, 2). The surgical procedure is much less extensive, and there is less predisposition to reformation of a scar that can result in recurrence of the gait abnormality (4). However, more cases must be accumulated to compare the effectiveness of this technique with earlier methods.

REFERENCES

1. Adams OR. Lameness in Horses. 3rd ed. Philadelphia: Lea & Febiger, 1974:320–322.
2. Turner AS, Trotter GW. Fibrotic myopathy in the horse. JAVMA 1984;184:335.
3. Bishop R. Fibrotic myopathy in the gracilis muscle of a horse. Vet Med Small Animal Clin 1972;67:270.
4. Bramlage LR, Reed SM, Embertson RM. Semitendinosus tenotomy for treatment of congenital and acquired fibrotic myopathy in the horse. JAVMA 1985;186:565.

6

SURGERY OF THE UPPER RESPIRATORY TRACT

Prosthetic Laryngoplasty

The use of a prosthetic device for surgical correction of laryngeal hemiplegia was first described in 1970 (1) and is now a time-honored technique, although various modifications are used by individual surgeons (2–8). The principle of the technique is to place a suture or sutures between the caudodorsal aspect of the cricoid cartilage and the muscular process of the arytenoid cartilage to abduct the arytenoid cartilage and simulate the action of the paralyzed cricoarytenoideus dorsalis muscle. To date, the technique is generally considered the best procedure to alleviate exercise intolerance and respiratory noise associated with laryngeal hemiplegia, particularly when endoscopic examination has revealed that the corniculate process of the arytenoid cartilage is displaced axially from the normal resting or intermediate position and there is a significant loss of arytenoid abductor function. The technique of laryngoplasty is usually augmented with a unilateral or bilateral ventriculectomy.

Although the success rates reported for laryngoplasty and ventriculectomy range from 5 to 90%, an experienced surgeon can expect that 50 to 75% of the operated horses will show marked improvement following surgery (9). The outcome is dependent on the skill of the surgeon and on case selection. The majority of horses show marked improvement in respiratory capacity and will not produce noise during exercise (5), but this assessment is controversial (10). Experimentally, laryngoplasty has been shown to alleviate flow limitations and reduce the inspiratory resistance associated with laryngeal hemiplegia (11). Even when the arytenoid cartilage is abducted less than desired, the success rate exceeds that of ventriculectomy alone.

Anesthesia and Surgical Preparation

A prosthetic laryngoplasty is done under general anesthesia. The horse is placed in lateral recumbency with the affected (usually left) side up. The head and neck must be fully extended, and a pad is placed under the laryngeal region to improve the surgical presentation (Fig. 6.1*A*). After completing the laryngoplasty, the horse is moved to dorsal recumbency for the laryngeal ventriculectomy.

Before surgery, phenylbutazone can be administered to minimize postoperative laryngeal edema. Intravenous penicillin and gentamicin sulfate are also given preoperatively, and tetanus toxoid is administered. The neck is clipped before surgery, and the immediate surgical site is shaved either just before or just after induction of anesthesia.

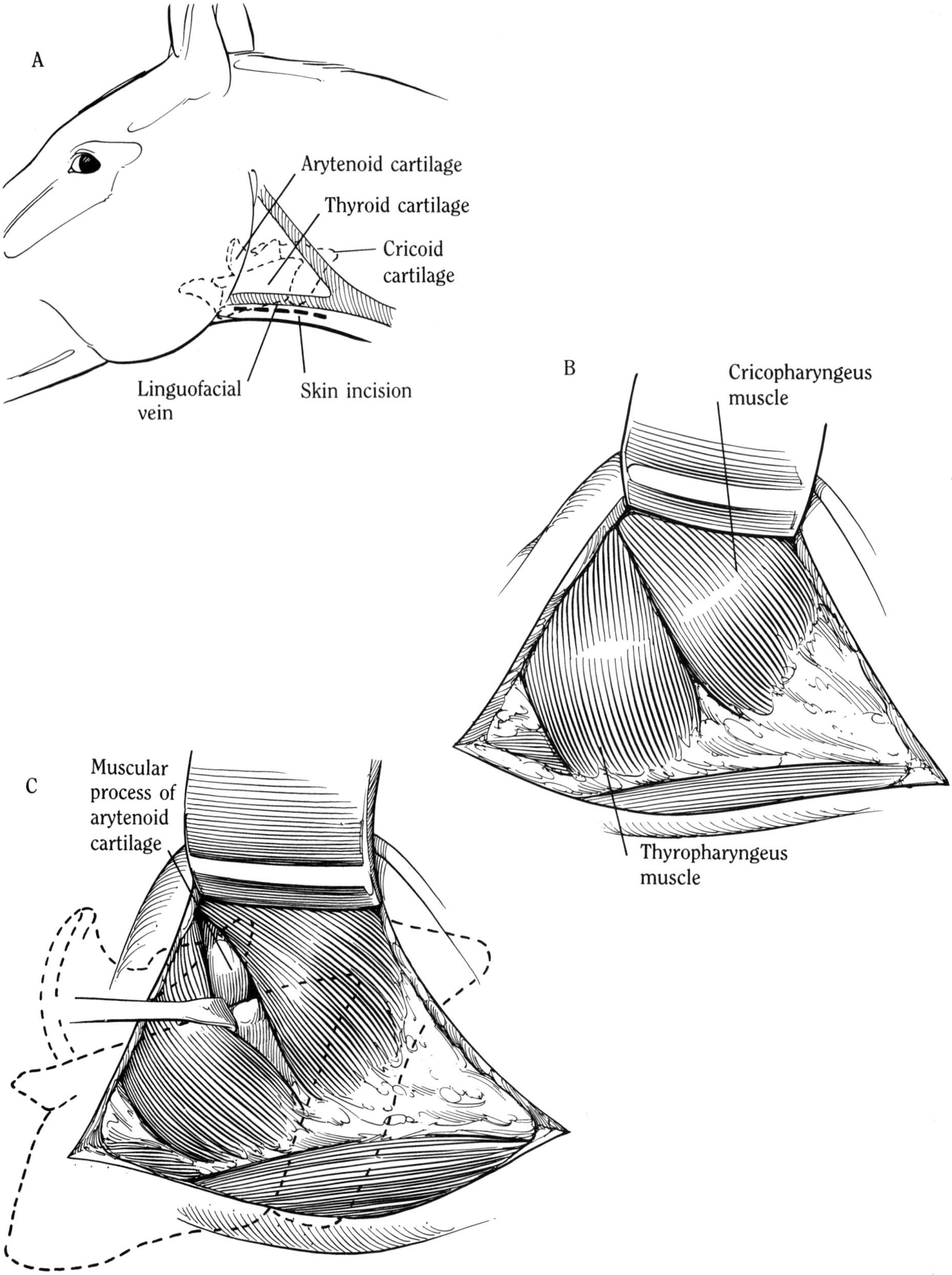

Figure 6.1, A–C. Prosthetic laryngoplasty.

Surgical Technique

A 10- to 12-cm skin incision is made parallel and ventral to the linguofacial vein extending rostrad from the sternomandibularis muscle (Fig. 6.1*A*). Electrocautery or ligation is used to control hemorrhage. The incision is continued through the fascia to establish a plane of dissection below the linguofacial vein and dorsal to the omohyoideus muscle. This plane of dissection can be continued bluntly with the use of scissors and finger dissection to expose the lateral aspect of the larynx with the overlying thyropharyngeus and cricopharyngeus muscles. The cleavage plane between these two muscles can be identified (Fig. 6.1*B*). A malleable retractor is used dorsally to facilitate surgical exposure. Care is taken to avoid the thyrolaryngeal vascular pedicle. The fascial septum between the thyropharyngeus and cricopharyngeus muscles is then divided, first using Metzenbaum scissors and then bluntly with digital dissection, to expose the muscular process of the arytenoid cartilage in the more dorsal part of the incision (Fig. 6.1*C*). Fascia over the dorsal caudal portion of the cricoid cartilage is then bluntly separated digitally to expose the most axial portion of the cricoid cartilage. Necessary portions of the larynx are now exposed and ready for placement of the prosthetic suture.

A number of suture materials have been and can be used for the prosthesis, but the material should be nonabsorbable, and some attention to tissue reactivity is appropriate to minimize the risk of postoperative infection. The elastic material Lycra, which was initially described (1), has been replaced by most surgeons with nonelastic materials such as no. 5 Polydek (Deknatel) or a double strand of no. 2 Mersilene.

Different suture configurations have been used. In many instances a single suture is placed, but some evidence suggests two sutures are more advantageous (10). In some instances the two sutures are passed through a single hole in the muscular process, but in others they are placed through two separate holes. A technique using one suture (a double strand of no. 2 Mersilene) with the material placed through the cricoid cartilage first and the muscular process of the arytenoid cartilage second will be described. Other surgeons place the suture in the muscular process first; these are merely differences in technique.

The landmark for placement of the suture in the cricoid cartilage is a notch immediately adjacent to the dorsal midline of the larynx, which can be palpated with a finger. Placement of the suture (or one of the sutures if a double technique is used) through this area is important to mechanically achieve maximum abduction of the arytenoid cartilage. Research shows that better abduction can be obtained with less tension if the prosthesis is anchored in the cricoid cartilage close to its dorsal midline (10). If the prosthesis is placed too laterally, it begins to produce adduction of the vocal cord as well as inadequate abduction of the corniculate portion of the arytenoid cartilage. This is apparently related to the complex range of movement of the cricoarytenoid joint. A round-bodied, ½ circle, trocar point needle is threaded, and the tip is placed behind the cricoid cartilage in the region of this axial notch and carefully advanced submucosally along the inner surface of the cricoid cartilage to avoid penetration of the laryngeal mucosa (Fig. 6.1*D*). The cricoid cartilage is penetrated approximately 1 to 1.5 cm rostral to the caudal border. The carotid artery and the esophagus are reasonably close to the dorsal aspect of the larynx. They are easily avoided if a large malleable retractor is used by an assistant and the left index finger of the surgeon is placed on the dorsal spine of the cricoid cartilage, pushing the esophagus away from the anticipated point of needle penetration. If the needle penetrates a laryngeal vessel during this process, bleeding initially may be profuse but can be controlled with sponges and pressure.

The needle is then cut off the suture and the leading end of the double strand of suture is drawn cranially under the cricopharyngeus muscle using a large

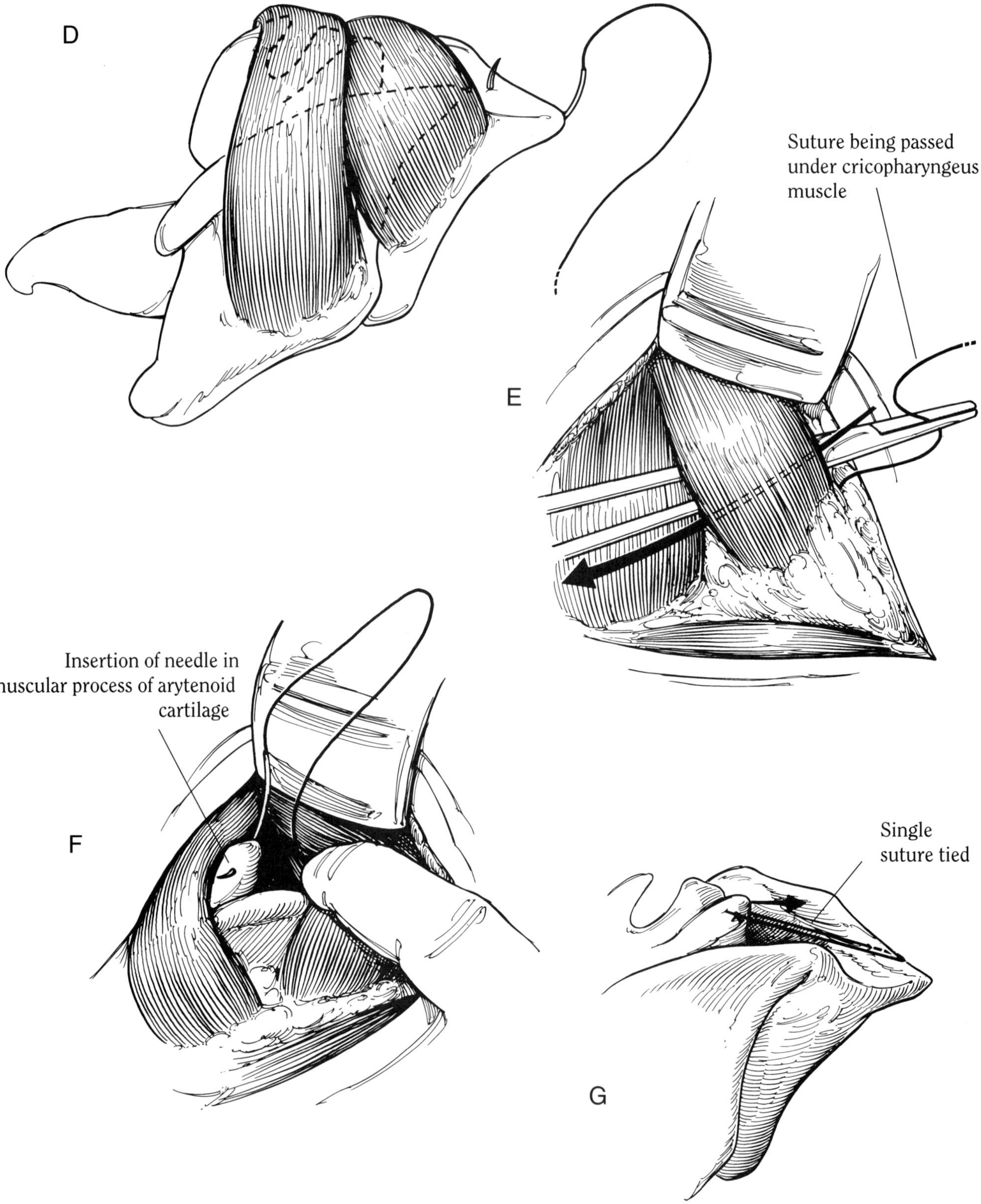

Figure 6.1, D–G. *(continued)* Prosthetic laryngoplasty.

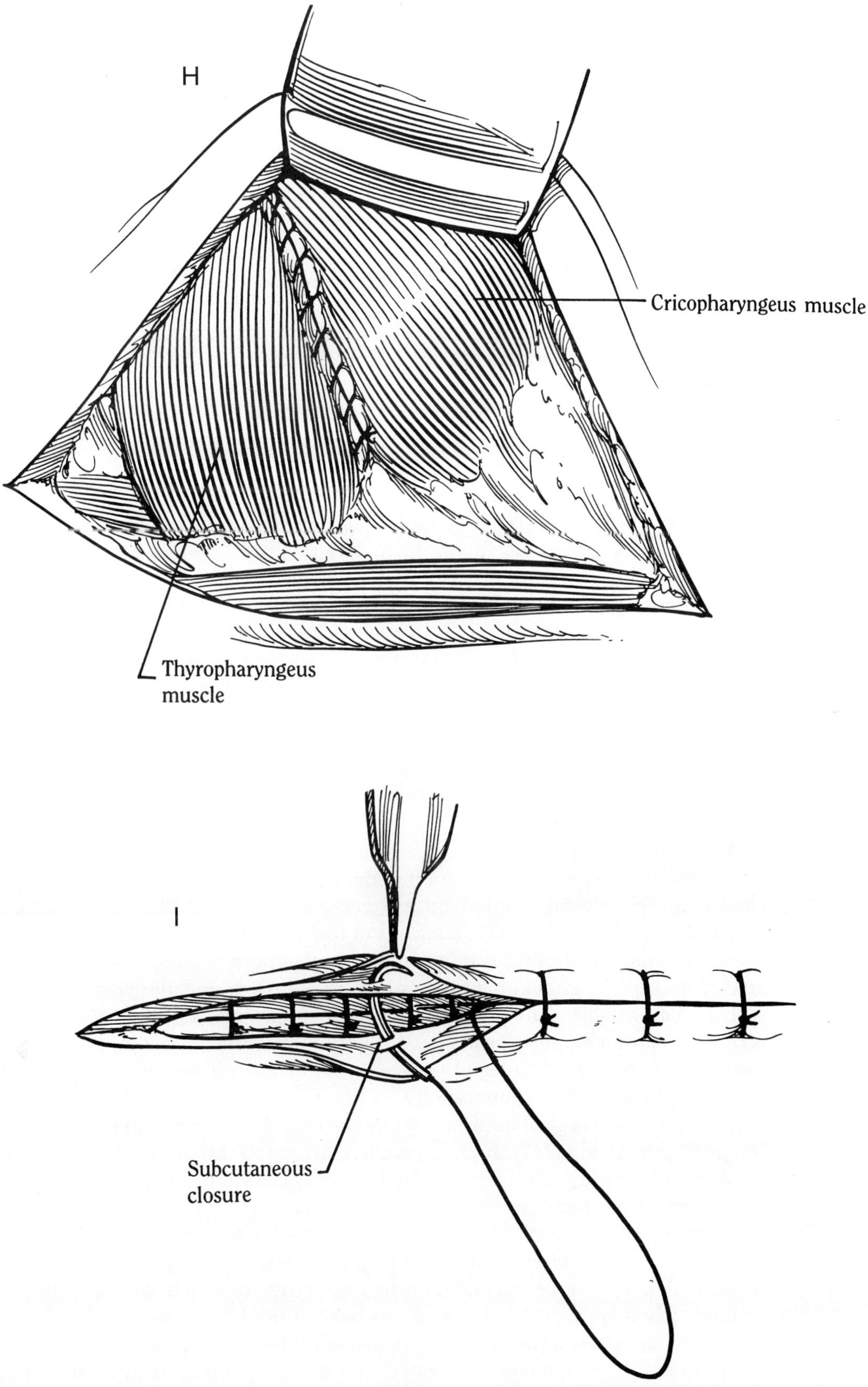

FIGURE 6.1, H–I. *(continued)* Prosthetic laryngoplasty.

hemostat (Fig. 6.1*E*). The suture is then rethreaded on a new trocar point needle. A new needle is used because the trocar point of the first needle is often damaged when it is grasped with needle holders at its point of emergence in the cricoid cartilage. A smaller needle also can be used to pass the suture through the muscular process. The surgeon then positions the point of the needle on the medial side of the muscular process and passes it laterally and in a slightly caudal to rostral direction (Fig. 6.1*F*). The needle should penetrate the lateral aspect of the muscular process above the level of the wing of the thyroid cartilage. The needle should be placed closer to the base of the muscular process than to its apex, ensuring the suture will be firmly embedded in cartilage. The surgeon's left index finger can be used to retract the cricopharyngeus muscle to provide better access to the muscular process. Another way to provide better access to the muscular process is to place a small sharp retractor over the wing of the thyroid cartilage and have an assistant rotate the larynx toward the surgeon. Directly grasping the muscular process with an instrument to facilitate exposure is traumatic and should be discouraged. Once the suture is drawn through the muscular process it is pulled tight to ensure that there is no hidden slack. The trailing end of the suture is then drawn under the cricopharyngeus muscle.

The first throw is placed on the prosthetic suture and is pulled tight. An assistant maintains tension by grasping the throw with a needle holder while the surgeon completes the square knot. Two or three additional square knots are usually added for knot security. The assistant should be cautioned against crushing the suture material with excessive pressure from the jaws of the needle holder. The amount of tension desired varies among surgeons. More tension is generally required to abduct the arytenoid cartilage in older patients. Some surgeons assess the degree of arytenoid abduction intraoperatively with a videoendoscope, which is secured in position before surgery. This can be particularly useful in assessing the degree of abduction achieved in a horse undergoing a second laryngoplasty. In such situations, it is important to know if the arytenoid is pulled into a more abducted position because if it is not, an arytenoidectomy can then be done in dorsal recumbency (9). Figure 6.1*G* illustrates the position of the suture once it is tied.

The incision between the thyropharyngeus and cricopharyngeus muscles is closed with simple interrupted sutures using 2/0 synthetic absorbable suture material (Fig. 6.1*H*). The fascia adjacent to the linguofacial vein and omohyoid muscle is re-apposed using a simple interrupted pattern of 2/0 synthetic absorbable material. The subcutaneous tissue is re-apposed, and the skin is closed with nonabsorbable suture material using a simple interrupted pattern (Fig. 6.1*I*) or with skin staples. Dead space is left between the larynx and the fascia associated with the linguofacial vein and omohyoid muscle, but the use of a drain prophylactically is unnecessary.

An alternative surgical approach to the larynx, dorsal to the maxillary vein, has been described (1, 12). It gives excellent access to the muscular process of the arytenoid cartilage, but it is a more difficult approach to the cricoid cartilage and therefore not recommended.

Following completion of the laryngoplasty, the horse is positioned in dorsal recumbency while a laryngotomy and laryngeal ventriculectomy are performed (described in a previous text, 13). During the laryngotomy, a brief check should be made to ensure that the laryngeal mucosa has not been penetrated with the prosthetic suture. If a previous ventriculectomy has been performed and the ventricle is not completely obliterated, the healed opening of the saccule is incised and as much mucosa removed as possible. At the completion of the ventriculectomy, the laryngotomy incision is not sutured.

Postoperative Management

The laryngotomy incision is cleaned twice daily with a moist gauze sponge until it is healed. The laryngoplasty incision skin sutures are removed in 10 days. The horse is confined to a stall for 30 days but can be hand-walked daily for exercise. Depending on the surgeon's preference, and based on the circumstances surrounding the surgery and on the owner's schedule for the horse, the horse can receive an additional 2 weeks' stall rest or can resume light exercise after 30 days.

The authors prefer to limit the use of antibiotics to the perioperative period unless the horse develops incisional swelling in conjunction with a fever in the recuperative period. Intravenous broad-spectrum antibiotic therapy should then be initiated and continued for at least 72 hours or until the horse's temperature returns to normal. Most horses will develop some degree of seroma formation in the laryngoplasty incision but few will require drainage. Drainage of the laryngoplasty surgical site is indicated if infection is suspected. The indications for drainage are fever, increased swelling at the surgical site with increased sensitivity on digital palpation, and leukocytosis. The skin sutures are removed, the incision area is sterilized, and a small hemostat or teat cannula is introduced through the laryngoplasty incision into the seroma. Fluid is immediately released; some of the fluid should be collected for culture and cytology. The opening is then enlarged using scissors and blunt digital separation of the tissues. Care must be taken not to tear or lacerate the linguofacial vein. Fibrin clots can be gently removed from the operative area using a gloved index finger.

The incisional opening must be kept open to allow drainage. An incisional infection can resolve without having an associated infection of the laryngoplasty suture; however, if the suture does become infected, a chronic draining fistula may develop.

Potential Complications and Comments

Potential complications of laryngoplasty include wound infection, infection of the synthetic implant, development of a chronic cough, and expulsion of water or food material from the nose. The likelihood of wound infection is minimized with good technique and the use of perioperative antibiotics. Infection of the prosthesis would lead typically to the formation of a chronic sinus tract and usually results in a failure of laryngoplasty. A chronic cough is generally attributed to the lateral fixation of the arytenoid cartilage and the inability of the larynx to protect the trachea from the aspiration of ingesta (1, 14–16). Pharyngeal dysfunction associated with surgical trauma could be a factor in some instances (14). Excessive arytenoid abduction is believed to interfere with the flow of ingesta in the lateral food channel and allow spillage of ingesta into the larynx during swallowing. Occasionally a horse will aspirate food material following a laryngoplasty that has positioned the arytenoid cartilage in only moderate abduction. Coughing was noticed in 26 of 68 (38%) horses in one series (17). If nasal return of food or water occurs, it is likely caused by pharyngeal dysfunction (14).

The suture can pull through the laryngeal cartilage, and long-term success is dependent on some degree of permanent adhesion/fibrosis to maintain abduction should the prosthesis fail to provide tension between the arytenoid and cricoid cartilages. Secure placement of the suture in the cricoid and the muscular process of the arytenoid cartilage will minimize the degree of migration through the cartilage. The value of a second suture is debatable. If a second suture is used, it should be placed through the cricoid cartilage just lateral to the first suture and above or below the position of the first suture.

When a laryngeal prosthesis fails, repeating the operation is an alternative that can be successful (9, 16, 18). Alternatively, a partial arytenoidectomy is performed (18). Partial arytenoidectomy or subtotal arytenoidectomy should not be used as a primary treatment for laryngeal hemiplegia (19). In horses that have an unacceptable amount of coughing or aspiration of food into the airway following laryngoplasty, the prosthetic suture can be removed in the hope of alleviating the problem.

There have been reports of a nerve muscle pedicle graft technique being used to successfully treat left laryngeal hemiplegia (20, 21). Clinical validation of the technique will be required before it can be considered a viable alternative to laryngoplasty.

REFERENCES

1. Marks D, MacKay-Smith MP, Cushing LS, et al. Use of a prosthetic device for surgical correction of laryngeal hemiplegia in horses. JAVMA 1970;157:157.
2. Baker GJ. Laryngeal hemiplegia in the horse. Compend Cont Educ 1983;5:S61.
3. Cahill JI, Goulden BE. Diseases of the larynx. In: Equine Medicine and Surgery. Vol 1. 4th ed. Goleta, CA: American Veterinary Publications Inc, 1991:411.
4. Haynes PF. Surgical complications in upper respiratory surgery. In: Proceedings of the AAEP, St. Louis, MO, 1978:223.
5. Haynes PF. Surgery of the equine respiratory tract. In: Jennings PB, ed. The Practice of Large Animal Surgery. Philadelphia: WB Saunders, 1984:388–487.
6. Merriam JP. Laryngoplasty—An evaluation of three abductor muscle prostheses. Proceedings of the 19th Meeting of the American Association of Equine Practitioners, Las Vegas, NV, 1974:123–131.
7. Speirs VC. Laryngeal surgery—150 years on. Equine Vet J 1987;19:377.
8. Speirs VC, Tulleners EP, Ducharme NG, et al. Larynx. In: Auer JA, ed. Equine Surgery. Philadelphia: WB Saunders Co, 1992:460.
9. Robertson JT. Pharynx and Larynx in Equine Respiratory Disorders. Philadelphia: Lea & Febiger, 1991:331.
10. Speirs VC, Bourke JM, Anderson GA. Assessment of the efficacy of an abductor muscle prosthesis for treatment of laryngeal hemiplegia in horses. Aust Vet J 1983;60:294.
11. Shappell KK, Derksen FJ, Stick JA, et al. Effects of ventriculectomy, prosthetic laryngoplasty, and exercise on upper airway function in horses with induced laryngeal hemiplegia. Am J Vet Res 1986;49:1760.
12. Johnson JH. Laryngoplasty for advanced laryngeal hemiplegia. VM/SAC 1970;65:347.
13. Turner AS, McIlwraith CW. Techniques in Large Animal Surgery. 2nd ed. Philadelphia: Lea & Febiger, 1989.
14. Greet TRC, Baker GJ, Lee R. The effect of laryngoplasty on pharyngeal function in the horse. Equine Vet J 1979;11:153.
15. Johnson JH. Complications in equine laryngeal surgery. Arch Am Coll Vet Surg 1975; 4:9.
16. Raker CW. Complications related to the insertion of the suture to retract the arytenoid cartilage to correct laryngeal hemiplegia in the horse. Arch Am Coll Vet Surg 1975; 4:64.
17. Goulden BE, Anderson LG. Equine laryngeal hemiplegia. III. Treatment by laryngoplasty. NZ Vet J 1982;30:1.
18. Tulleners EP. Management of failed laryngoplasty: 25 horses (1988–1993). In: Proceedings of the 29th Annual Scientific Meeting. Washington, DC: ACVS, 1994:24.
19. Williams JW, Pascoe JR, Meagher DM, et al. Effects of left recurrent laryngeal neurectomy, prosthetic laryngoplasty, and subtotal arytenoidectomy on upper airway pressure during maximal exertion. Vet Surg 1990;19:136.
20. Fulton IC, Derksen FJ, Stick JA, et al. Treatment of left laryngeal hemiplegia in Standardbreds using a nerve muscle pedicle graft. Am J Vet Res 1991;52:1431.
21. Fulton IC, Derksen FJ, Stick JA, et al. Histological evaluation of nerve muscle pedicle graft used as a treatment for left laryngeal hemiplegia in Standardbreds. Am J Vet Res 1992;53:593.

Partial Arytenoidectomy

Partial arytenoidectomy is indicated to increase airflow through the larynx in cases of chondritis or chondroma of the arytenoid cartilage(s), in ossification of the laryngeal cartilages, and in some cases of laryngeal neoplasia (1–7). It is also indicated in cases of laryngeal hemiplegia that have not responded to the conventional treatments of laryngoplasty and ventriculectomy (1, 2, 4). It is not indicated as an alternative to laryngoplasty for initial treatment of laryngeal hemiplegia. Currently, the most common indication for arytenoidectomy is chondritis of the arytenoid cartilage.

The object of partial arytenoidectomy is to remove the body and corniculate portions of the diseased cartilage to enlarge and streamline the lumen of the larynx (2, 8). The muscular process of the arytenoid is retained. Partial arytenoidectomy is preferable to subtotal arytenoidectomy, in which the corniculate process is retained for improvement of upper airway airflow in performance horses (4, 9). There is concern that removing the corniculate portion of the arytenoid can lead to aspiration and coughing; however, these undesirable complications can be minimized by carefully dissecting and preserving the mucosa overlying the corniculate process as a cuff of tissue that helps to protect against aspiration (2, 8).

Mild cases of chondritis in which there is some residual abduction of the affected cartilage may respond to focal excision of intraluminal lesions (10). This may provide transient improvement as long as the underlying chondritis remains quiescent. This surgery can be done under general anesthesia via a laryngotomy and is often done in concert with a ventriculectomy on the affected side. Intralaryngeal granulation tissue can also be excised in the standing horse using a Nd:YAG laser (11). Nonsurgical management, which includes rest, systemic antibiotics, and anti-inflammatory medications, can improve swelling associated with some cases of chondritis; however, resumption of training usually will cause further irritation and recrudescence of the problem.

Partial arytenoidectomy is used in an attempt to return a racing or performance horse to athletic performance and also as a salvage procedure in other cases wherein the extent of the condition compromises the patient's ability to breathe, even at rest. The condition is usually discovered and diagnosed much earlier in racehorses because of close observation and the need for maximal airflows to sustain performance. Even seemingly small chondritic lesions can cause respiratory noise and affect exercise tolerance.

Bilateral arytenoidectomy can be done as a single procedure in cases of bilateral chondritis (1). Alternatives include performing a unilateral arytenoidectomy on the most severely affected side and leaving the other side alone; treating the other arytenoid less aggressively with local excision of intralaryngeal masses and delicate curettage of fistulous tracts in the diseased cartilage; or removing the second arytenoid at a later date (staged unilateral arytenoidectomy) (3). As a salvage procedure, a permanent tracheostomy could be considered as an alternative to bilateral arytenoidectomy or unilateral arytenoidectomy in the horse with advanced chondritis and concurrent upper airway abnormalities (3).

Anesthesia and Surgical Preparation

Preoperative treatment includes phenylbutazone, tetanus toxoid, and prophylactic antibiotics such as penicillin and gentamicin. The ventral throat and neck area is clipped prior to induction, and the final preparation of the surgical sites is done after induction of anesthesia.

Partial arytenoidectomy is performed through a laryngotomy incision with the horse positioned in dorsal recumbency. Inhalation anesthesia is administered by an endotracheal tube placed through a midcervical tracheostomy incision. In patients with serious respiratory compromise at rest, preoperative placement of a tracheostomy tube may be necessary. In patients without respiratory compromise at rest, the tracheostomy is performed immediately following induction of anesthesia. If an endotracheal tube has been placed through a tracheostomy incision in the standing horse before anesthesia, and the anesthesiologist wishes to replace it with a larger diameter tube for maintenance of anesthesia, keep in mind that it may be difficult to reinsert because the skin and soft tissue and tracheal openings may not have the same relationship since the horse is now in dorsal recumbency. This may necessitate lengthening of the incision over the trachea. Forceful insertion of a stiff endotracheal tube could produce a tracheal mucosal laceration.

Surgical Technique

Directly following induction of anesthesia, the midcervical region is quickly prepared, a tracheostomy incision is made between the tracheal rings, and a cuffed endotracheal tube is inserted (Fig. 6.2*A*). The laryngotomy site is then aseptically prepared for the operation.

A ventral laryngotomy is performed and self-retaining Weitlaner retractors are placed into the larynx. Although trauma to the cricoid cartilage should be avoided during a routine laryngotomy, the authors routinely incise the cricoid cartilage on ventral midline to increase the surgical exposure to the affected arytenoid cartilage (8). Splitting the thyroid cartilage may also increase exposure, but it is rarely necessary. A submucosal injection of 1:10,000 epinephrine to help control oozing and assist in elevation of the mucous membrane during the operation may be made at this time. However, it has minimal effectiveness when there is extensive chondritis and adhesion of the laryngeal mucosal membrane to the arytenoid cartilage. A vertical mucosal incision is made rostrally over the corniculate cartilage and extended over the ventral and caudal aspect of the arytenoid cartilage, creating a large, three-sided mucosal flap (Fig. 6.2*B*). Other patterns for mucosal incision have been described (Fig. 6.2*C*) (2, 12).

The mucous membrane over the luminal side of the arytenoid cartilage is then elevated away from the cartilage with a nasal or periosteal elevator (Fig. 6.2*D*). The dissection is continued forward over the corniculate portion. All efforts are made to preserve the mucosa, but it is easily disrupted in regions of pathologic change. When the mucosa has been freed from the luminal side of the involved arytenoid cartilage, the lateral (abaxial) surface of the cartilage is dissected free of the soft tissues (vestibularis, vocalis, and cricoarytenoideus lateralis muscles and lateral ventricle) using scissors (Fig. 6.2*E*). Dissection around the corniculate portion is completed using a combination of dissection with sharp scissors and blunt digital separation of the mucosa from the cartilage. The arytenoid cartilage is then grasped with forceps and retracted in a rostral direction to enable separation of the cartilage immediately below the level of the muscular process and articular facet. If possible, the arytenoid cartilage is disarticulated from the cricoid at the articular facet. Alternatively, a portion of the articulation may be left behind when the arytenoid is amputated. This separation usually requires heavy, sharply curved scissors. Retraction is continued in a rostral direction while the remaining soft tissue attachments along the dorsal surface of the arytenoid cartilage are divided with scissors to complete removal of the arytenoid cartilage (Fig. 6.2*F*). The latter maneuvers may involve removal of the arytenoid cartilage in more than one portion. Any remaining cartilage in the dorsal portion of the larynx can be carefully removed with a set of rongeurs or grasped with forceps and dissected free with scissors (Fig. 6.2*G*).

Following removal of the arytenoid cartilage, the lateral ventricle on that side is also removed. The free edge of the corniculate mucosa is retracted slightly

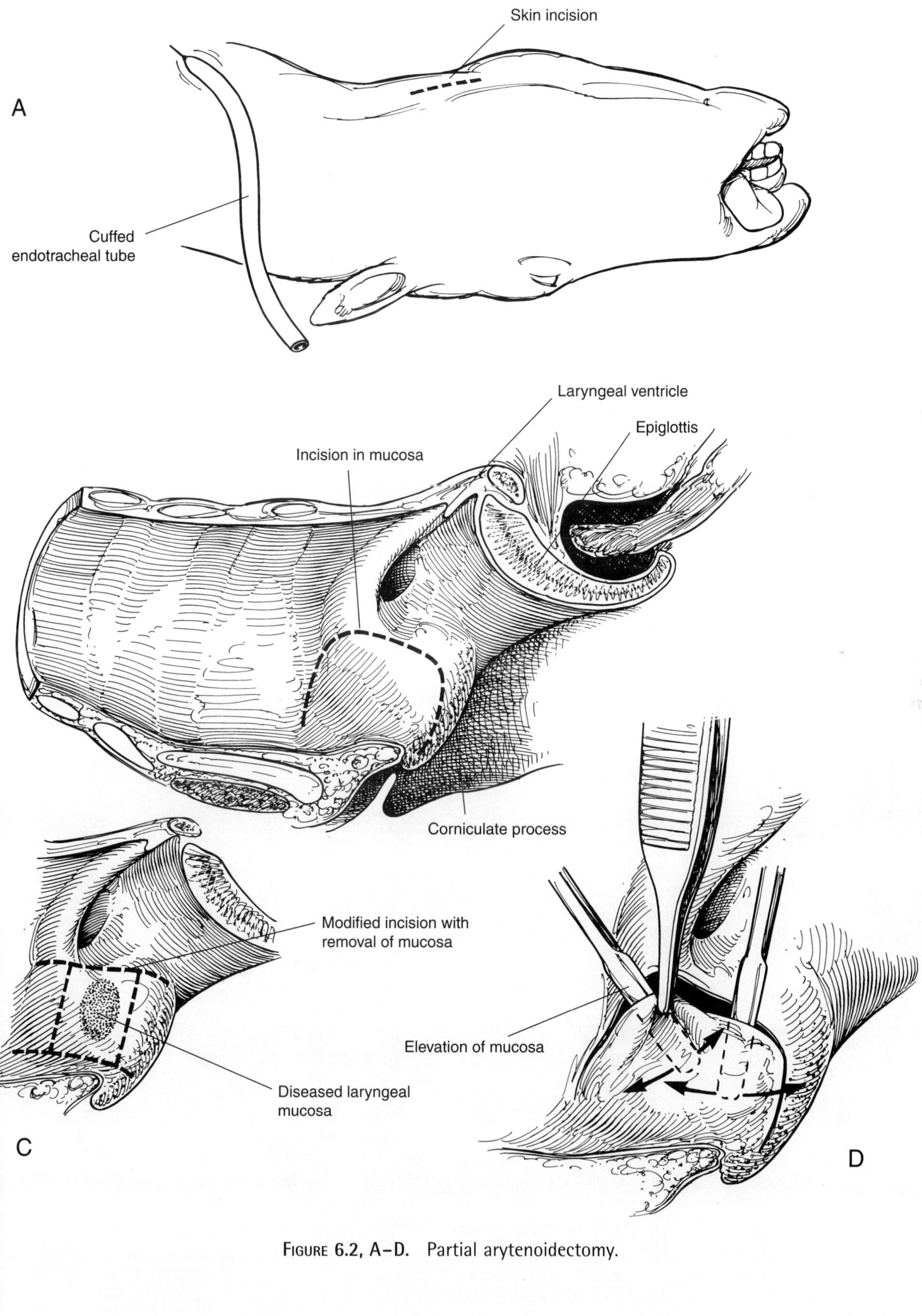

FIGURE 6.2, A–D. Partial arytenoidectomy.

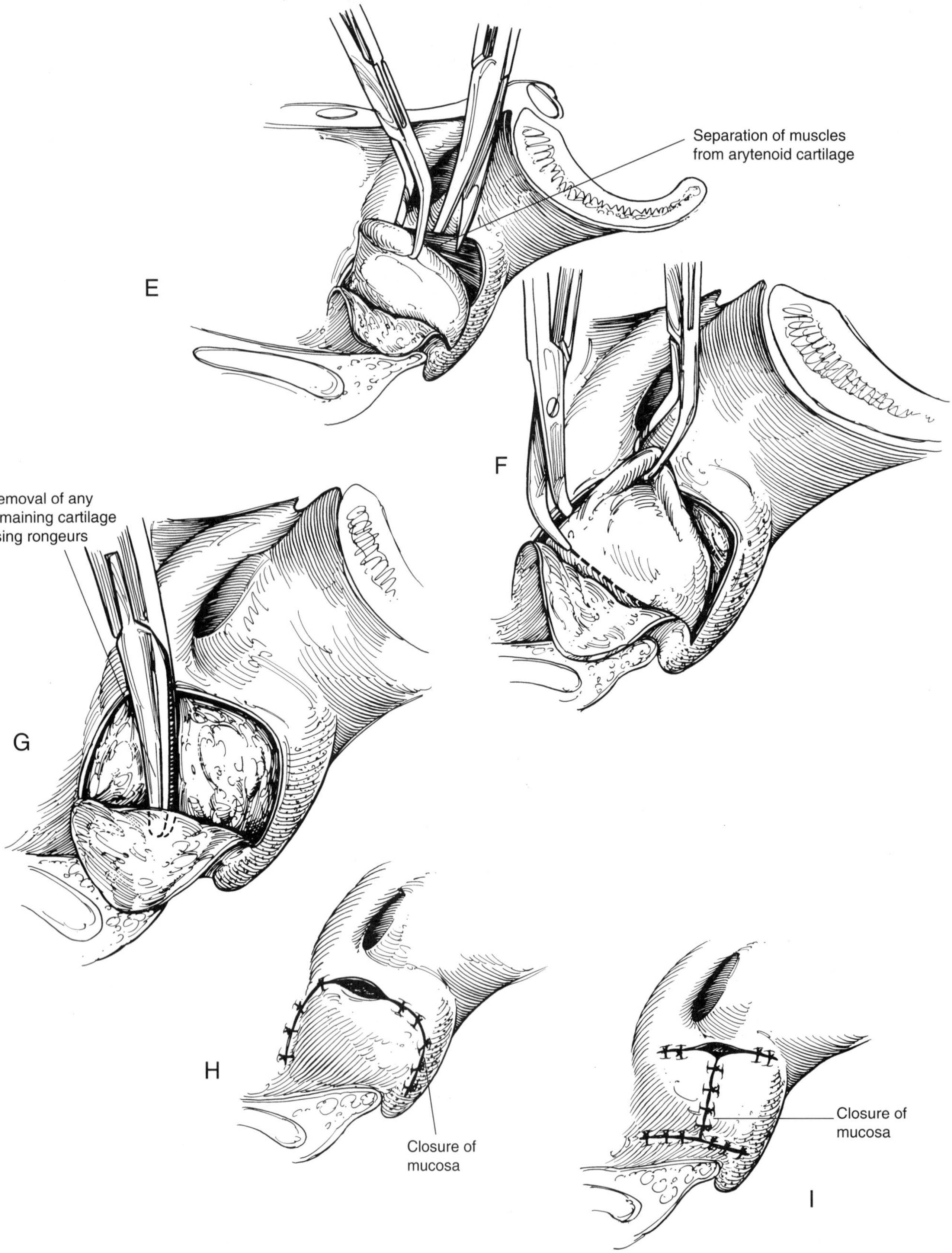

Figure 6.2, E–I. *(continued)* Partial arytenoidectomy.

caudally and sutured laterally to the remaining soft tissue to form a cuff of tissue that is protective to the airway yet does not obstruct airflow (8). In the authors' opinion, excessive caudal retraction of this mucosa to streamline the airway and help cover mucosal defects created during resection is contraindicated and will produce more problems with aspiration postoperatively (2, 8). The mucosal incision is then closed in a simple interrupted pattern using 3/0 polyglactin 910 (Vicryl) swaged on a small taper-point, half-circle needle (Fig. 6.2, *H* and *I*). If possible, suture knots should be buried and not exposed to the lumen. Efforts should be made to tack the mucosal flap, created during the resection, laterally to help limit the dead space in the wound and minimize hematoma formation.

Also, in most cases of advanced chondritis, there will be mucosal defects following cartilage removal that do not allow for complete mucosal closure. These defects are of no concern because they will heal well by second intention (13). Complete mucosal closure should not be attempted because an opening must be maintained ventrally to allow for drainage from beneath the mucosal flap (Fig. 6.2, *H* and *I*). The ventral laryngotomy incision is allowed to heal by second intention. If the cricoid cartilage was incised, the soft tissues immediately adjacent to the cartilage are sutured, providing a tight apposition of the cartilage ends. There is no need to put suture material through the cartilage; in fact, that might induce chondroma formation.

Postoperative Management

A tracheostomy tube is secured in place during recovery. This tube is generally removed within 24 hours of surgery. Swelling of the intraluminal laryngeal surgical site can be anticipated to reach a maximal extent at 48 to 72 hours postsurgery. A nonsteroidal anti-inflammatory agent can be administered as required. Feeding is resumed after full recovery from anesthesia. Sequential endoscopic examinations can be done to assess the airway. Some dehiscence of the suture line may occur within a few days to a week after surgery, particularly when there has been marked compromise of the mucosa. These sites will heal, however, generally without complication. Endoscopically, the arytenoidectomy site should appear healed with minimal inflammation at 45 to 60 days. If inflammation still exists or there are still areas where granulomas have formed around the mucosal sutures, more convalescent time is required.

Comments

To date, no clinical studies compare the results following partial versus subtotal arytenoidectomy for treatment of arytenoid chondropathy or failed laryngoplasty. The available experimental and clinical data, however, suggest that partial arytenoidectomy is preferable for improving upper airway function in the performance horse (1, 4, 9). The risk of aspiration of ingesta can be minimized by using appropriate technique (2, 8). Also note that one should not be overly concerned with the immediate postoperative appearance of the surgical site, as this will improve considerably on subsequent examinations over a 2-month period.

A risk of bilateral arytenoidectomy is dorsal glottic stenosis. If the dorsal laryngeal mucosa is not preserved, granulation tissue will cover the defect and result in a constrictive web formation (14).

REFERENCES

1. Tulleners EP, Harrison IW, Raker CW. Management of arytenoid chondropathy and failed laryngoplasty in horses: 75 cases (1979–1985). JAVMA 1988;192:670–675.

2. Speirs VC. Partial arytenoidectomy in horses. Vet Surg 1986;15:316–320.
3. Dean PW, Cohen ND. Arytenoidectomy for advanced unilateral chondropathy with accompanying lesions. Vet Surg 1990;19:364–370.
4. Lumsden JM, Derksen FJ, Stick JA, et al. Evaluation of partial arytenoidectomy as a treatment for equine laryngeal hemiplegia. Equine Vet J 1994;26:125–129.
5. Haynes PF, Snyder TG, McClure JR, et al. Chronic chondritis of the equine arytenoid cartilage. JAVMA 1980;177:1135–1142.
6. Shapiro J, White NA, Schlafer DH, et al. Hypertrophic ossification of the laryngeal cartilages of a horse. J Equine Med Surg 1979;3:370–374.
7. Trotter GW, Aanes WA, Snyder SP. Laryngeal chondroma in a horse. JAVMA 1981;178:829–830.
8. Robertson JT. Pharynx and larynx. In: Beech J, ed. Equine Respiratory Disorders. Philadelphia: Lea & Febiger, 1991:331–387.
9. Belknap JK, Derksen FJ, Nickels FA, et al. Failure of subtotal arytenoidectomy to improve upper airway flow mechanics in exercising Standardbreds with induced laryngeal hemiplegia. Am J Vet Res 1990;51:1481–1487.
10. Haynes PF. Surgery of the equine respiratory tract. In: Jennings PB, ed. The Practice of Large Animal Surgery. Philadelphia: WB Saunders, 1984:388–487.
11. Hay WP, Tulleners EP. Excision of intralaryngeal granulation tissue in 25 horses using a Nd:YAG laser (1986–1991). Vet Surg 1993;22:129–134.
12. Speirs VC. Laryngeal surgery—150 years on. Equine Vet J 1987;19:377–383.
13. Tulleners EP, Harrison IW, Mann P, et al. Partial arytenoidectomy in the horse with and without mucosal closure. Vet Surg 1988;17:252–257.
14. Harrison IW, Raker CW. Dorsal glottic stenosis after bilateral arytenoidectomy in two horses. JAVMA 1988;192:202–204.

Surgical Relief of Epiglottic Entrapment

Epiglottic entrapment is the envelopment of the apex and lateral margins of the epiglottis by the arytenoepiglottic folds (1). The arytenoepiglottic folds extend from the lateral aspect of the arytenoid cartilage to the ventrolateral aspect of the epiglottis. This fold of respiratory mucosa is continuous with the glossoepiglottic fold in the subepiglottic area, and the latter also contributes to the entrapping tissue (1).

Surgical treatment of an epiglottic entrapment is indicated if the diagnosis coincides with a history of poor performance. Some horses can race successfully with an entrapped epiglottis. In fact, epiglottic entrapment may be found as an incidental endoscopic finding in horses with neither decreased exercise tolerance nor abnormal respiratory noise (2). Horses with hypoplasia of the epiglottis and those with epiglottic abnormalities associated with an entrapment are more likely to develop intermittent dorsal displacement of the soft palate (DDSP) following correction of the entrapment (1–4). Also, if there is preoperative evidence of concurrent intermittent DDSP, DDSP is likely to persist after epiglottic surgery.

It is difficult to estimate the overall size, shape, and consistency of the epiglottis when it is enveloped in the aryepiglottic tissue. Preoperative radiographs of the pharyngeal region with placement of markers of known size allow for measurement of epiglottic length. Short thyroepiglottic lengths have been found in horses with epiglottic entrapment as well as with DDSP (5). Thyroepiglottic length, the measured length from the body of the thyroid cartilage to the tip of the epiglottis, is 8.76 (0.44 cm in healthy Thoroughbreds) (5).

Transoral Axial Division

There are basically two ways to surgically correct an entrapped epiglottis: axial division of the entrapping membrane or resection of the arytenoepiglottic tissue (6). Most owners and trainers prefer some form of axial division of the entrapment because a laryngotomy or pharyngotomy incision is not required and the horse can generally return to training within 2 weeks. With axial division there is less likelihood of developing persistent DDSP postoperatively. However, because the aryepiglottic tissue is not resected, there is a greater likelihood of recurrence of the entrapment.

Currently, one of the most popular methods for axial division of the entrapping membrane can be accomplished transendoscopically in the standing horse using the Nd:YAG laser. This method, in the hands of an experienced operator, is safe and effective and has a very low recurrence rate (5%) (4). A disadvantage is the expensive equipment required. Another technique done in the standing, sedated horse is splitting the entrapping tissue with a long-handled bistoury introduced per nasum and under endoscopic guidance (7). This technique, which is generally successful, can result in catastrophic incisions in the soft palate or in other tissues if the horse rears unexpectedly (7, 8).

The entrapping membrane can be split more safely if the cutting instrument is passed per os in the anesthetized horse (6, 9, 10). Transoral axial division of the entrapping membrane greatly reduces the possibility of accidental laceration of the soft palate. The operation can be done under endoscopic guidance with the endoscope passed into the oropharynx, or blindly with manual positioning of the bistoury. The authors prefer the manual technique for hook placement and division of the entrapping membrane. The major limitation of this technique is a narrow oral cavity and oropharynx, or a large hand. Contrary to the opinion of one group of authors (9), manual positioning of the hook does allow for precise placement of the hook on midline, provided the operator is experienced. It is also important to perform the procedure quickly once the horse is anesthetized, because the longer the procedure, the more likely the horse is to start swallowing. If swallowing is a problem, a short-acting barbiturate can be administered.

A secure dental speculum is necessary for transoral axial division. The epiglottic bistoury can be obtained commercially or custom-fashioned to the surgeon's specifications. The design of the hooked bistoury is important (6, 9, 10). The length of the hook should be slightly longer than the length of the entrapping membrane, as measured from the caudal edge of the membrane to the apex of the epiglottis. This ensures that the hook securely engages the entrapping membrane before the tissue is cut and produces a complete division of the entrapping membrane. If the hook is short, much of the entrapment will role off the tip of the epiglottis before the hook engages, and only the caudal margin will be cut, increasing the likelihood of recurrence. The pointed tip of the hook should be blunt enough so as not to cause trauma to the epiglottis. The cutting edge, situated on the inside curve of the hook, should be sharp enough that even swollen and fibrotic aryepiglottic tissue can be incised rather than torn.

Anesthesia and Surgical Preparation

The authors recommend perioperative antibiotics, such as penicillin and gentamicin. A nonsteroidal anti-inflammatory agent is also given before surgery, particularly if the procedure is done on an outpatient basis. The horse is sedated with xylazine (1.1 mg/kg, IV), and anesthesia is induced with glycerol guaiacolate (15–30 g, IV) and ketamine (2.2 mg/kg, IV) (10). The addition of glycerol guaiacolate relaxes the horse and appears to reduce swallowing. The horse is positioned in lateral recumbency, the speculum is placed, and the tongue is pulled gently out of the mouth to allow passage of the endoscope or the operator's hand (6, 9, 10). With either technique, the soft palate must be displaced prior to hook placement.

Surgical Technique

The bistoury is introduced into the oropharynx and the hook is passed between the caudal border of the entrapment and the dorsal surface of the epiglottis (Fig. 6.3, *A* and *B*) and advanced rostrally until the tip engages the membrane overlying the tip of the epiglottis (Fig. 6.3*C*). The pointed tip should penetrate the entrapping membrane on midline, immediately adjacent to the tip of the epiglottis (Fig. 6.3, *D* and *E*). An asymmetric incision in the entrapping membrane appears to predispose to recurrence. The membrane is engaged and divided as the hook is pulled in a rostral direction (Fig. 6.3*E*). The hook can be guarded with the operator's hand to prevent accidental penetration of the tongue (Fig. 6.3*F*). At this point, if the axial division was done under endoscopic guidance, the surgery is complete. The authors prefer to make two additional but smaller slits in the aryepiglottic tissue after the initial axial division. This can be accomplished by grasping and elevating the aryepiglottic tissue on one side of the epiglottis with the thumb and index finger; rotating the hook through 90° with the other hand; hooking the flap of tissue at a point approximately .5 cm caudal to the apex and immediately adjacent to the lateral margin of the epiglottis; and putting tension on the bistoury to produce an incision. The procedure is repeated on the opposite side.

Postoperative Management

Regardless the method of axial division, most horses benefit from 7 to 10 days of stall rest, with hand-walking following the surgery. Phenylbutazone can be administered daily to reduce inflammation (9). In the authors' experience, transoral axial division using manual placement may produce a good deal of

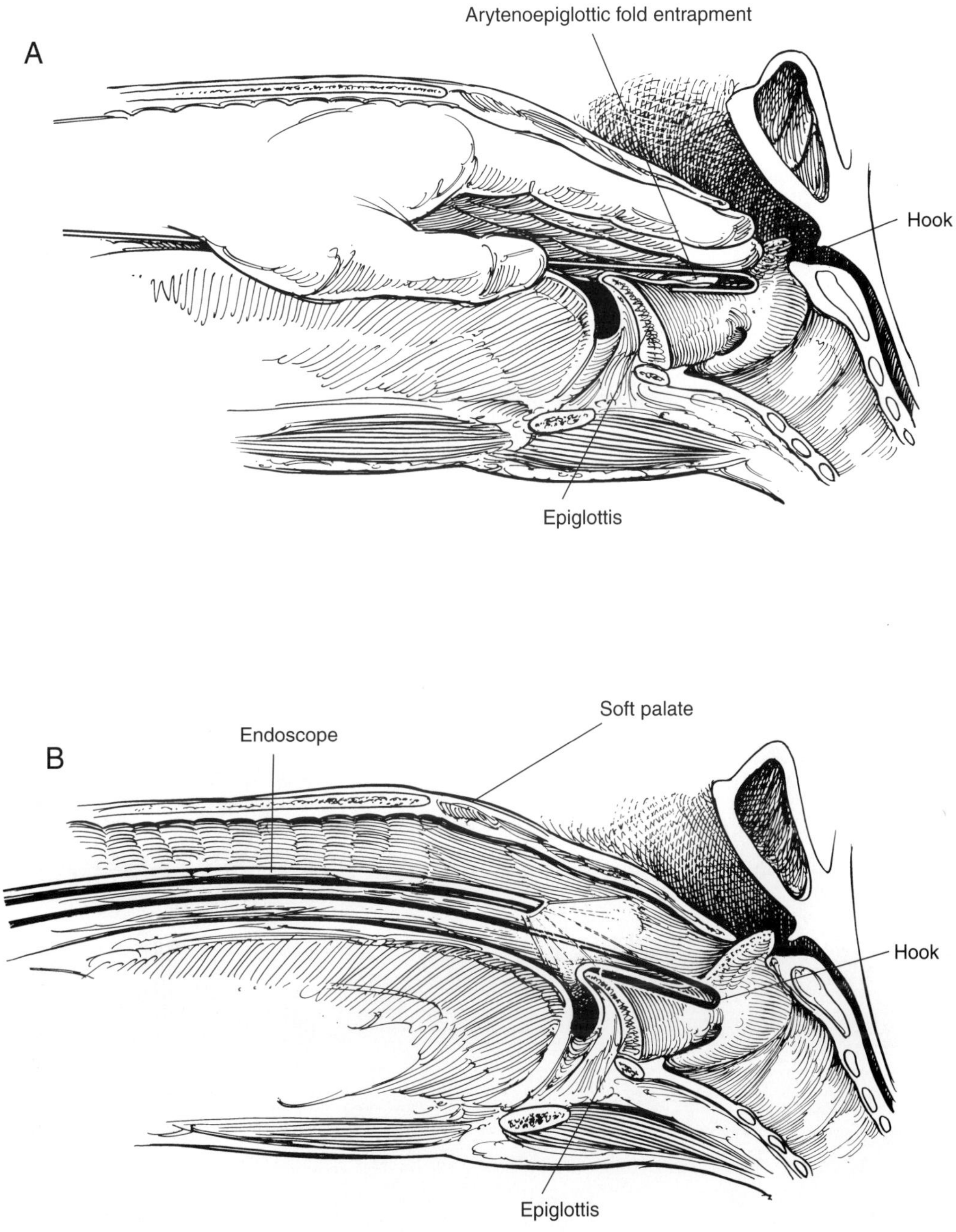

Figure 6.3, A–B. Surgical relief of epiglottic entrapment.

inflammation and resultant subepiglottic granulation tissue that takes 2 to 3 weeks to completely subside. If a horse develops intermittent DDSP when training is resumed and there is residual epiglottic or subepiglottic inflammation, a short rest period and treatment with an anti-inflammatory throat spray or nebulizer solution will usually resolve the problem. If the DDSP problem persists, a sternothyrohyoid myectomy and staphylectomy are indicated. If an epiglottic deformity exists as a result of a prolonged entrapment, excessive inflammation, or an injury associated with the entrapment surgery, the prognosis is poor.

Comments

As previously stated, the recurrence rate is approximately 5 to 10% following axial division of the entrapping tissue. If a surgeon is experiencing a higher rate,

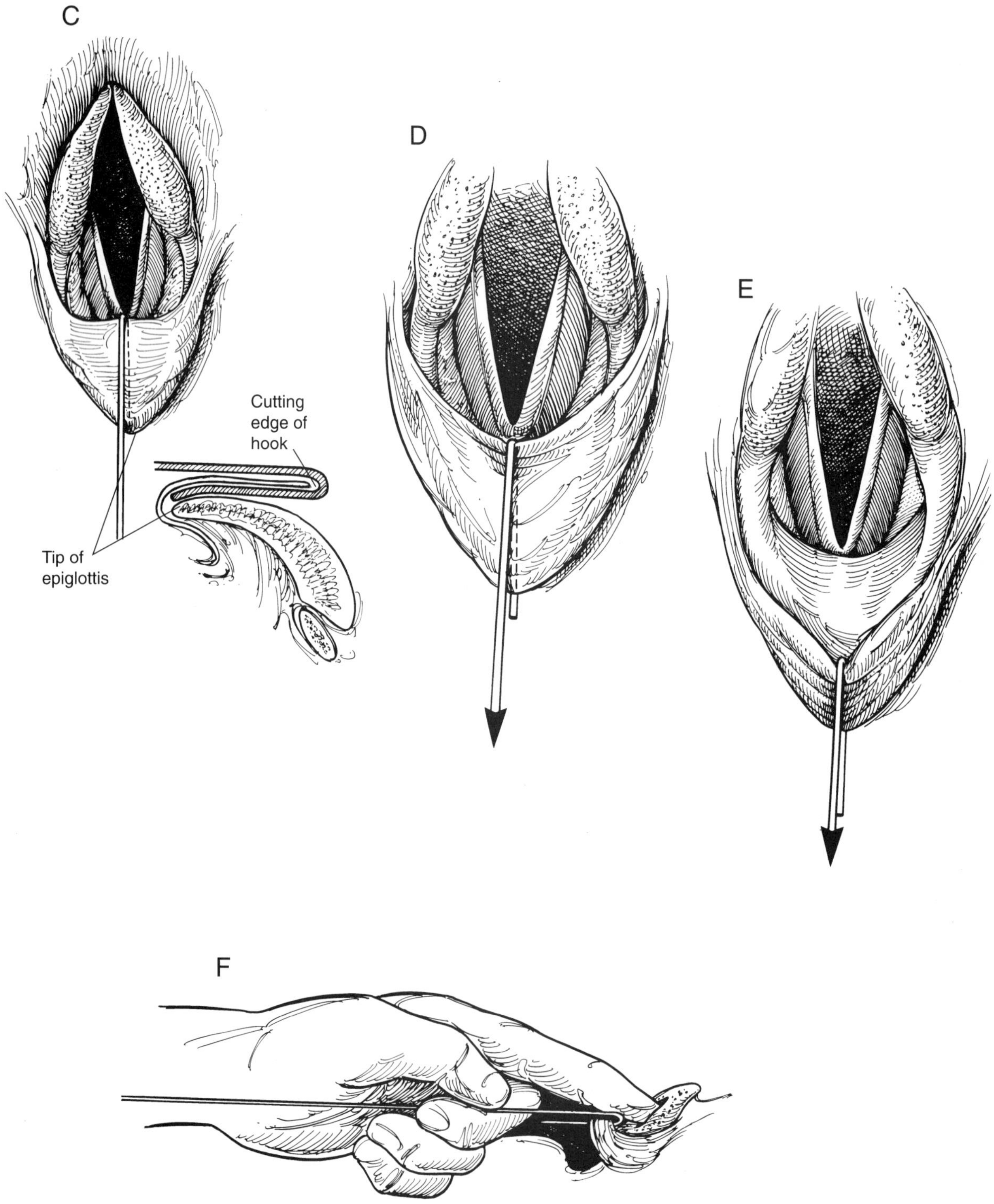

Figure 6.3, C–F. *(continued)* Surgical relief of epiglottic entrapment.

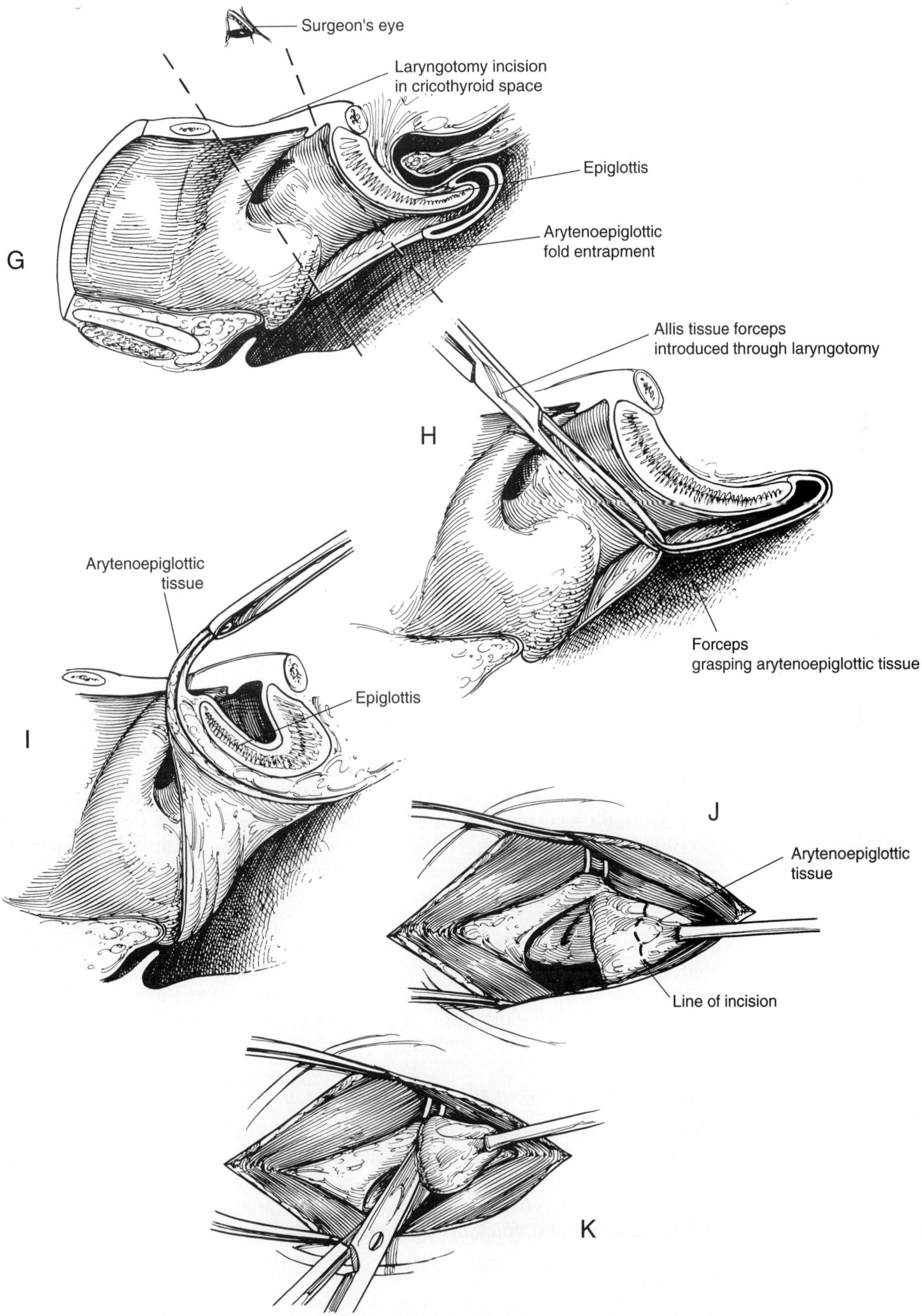

Figure 6.3, G–K. *(continued)* Surgical resection of the arytenoepiglottic tissue.

the technique or design of the bistoury should be reviewed. Also, the degree of inflammation or ulceration of the entrapping membrane does not appear to affect either the recurrence rate or the incidence of postoperative DDSP following intraoral axial division, provided the epiglottic cartilage remains normal.

Surgical Resection of the Arytenoepiglottic Folds

Some surgeons prefer to correct the epiglottic entrapment by resecting the aryepiglottic tissue through a laryngotomy incision. This may be done as a primary treatment, particularly in the case of an intermittent entrapment (which is unusual) or as an alternative approach if the entrapment has recurred following axial division.

Anesthesia and Surgical Preparation

The horse is placed under general anesthesia in dorsal recumbency. The procedure can be done under intravenous anesthesia or with inhalation anesthesia, the tube being withdrawn after the laryngotomy has been completed. Antibiotics (such as intravenous penicillin and gentamicin) and tetanus toxoid are administered perioperatively. Phenylbutazone is optional.

Surgical Technique

A ventral laryngotomy is performed. The epiglottis and entrapping arytenoepiglottic folds lie rostral and deep to the laryngotomy incision but are clearly visible (Fig. 6.3*G*). The entrapping arytenoepiglottic tissue is grasped on midline with Allis tissue forceps (Fig. 6.3*H*), and traction is then used to evert the apex of the epiglottis (it will come with the entrapping fold because of its attachment to the epiglottis) into the laryngotomy opening (Fig. 6.3*I*). If the epiglottis is not entrapped at this time, the epiglottis is retroverted with a finger or curved sponge forceps and the aryepiglottic tissue is grasped with Allis tissue forceps (see "Epiglottic Augmentation"). The arytenoepiglottic folds are then excised with scissors. Only the central portion of the fold is excised, rather than a complete excision from the margins (Fig. 6.3*J*). Figure 6.3*K* illustrates an axial "notching" incision commencing on one side and extending across to the opposite side. Resection of more of the fold can potentiate epiglottic dysfunction and the development of DDSP. Care is also taken that the incision line is at least 5 mm away from the junction of the arytenoepiglottic fold with the epiglottis to ensure that the epiglottic mucosa or the cartilage is not traumatized. Such damage could potentially lead to epiglottic cartilage deformity. As the entrapping folds are removed, the epiglottis will return to its normal position. The laryngotomy is left to heal by second intention.

Postoperative Management

The laryngotomy wound is cleaned once or twice daily until it has healed (approximately 2 weeks). During this time, the horse should be confined to stall rest with hand-walking for exercise. Training can resume when the laryngotomy incision is closed, provided an endoscopic examination shows normal laryngopalatal function and epiglottic inflammation is subsiding.

Comments

The most common postoperative complication associated with surgical removal of an epiglottic entrapment is the development of DDSP postoperatively (1, 3). The relationship of DDSP to epiglottic entrapment and epiglottic shortening has been documented, and it is likely that DDSP will occur with higher frequency in epiglottic entrapment cases when the epiglottis is hypoplastic (3, 5). The occurrence of DDSP postoperatively may be associated simply with reducing the "bulk" of the epiglottis by removing the enveloping aryepiglottic tissue. This in turn leaves an epiglottis (particularly if it is hypoplastic) that allows the soft palate to displace easily. It is also possible that formation of subepiglottic scar tissue associated with resection of the aryepiglottic tissue may interfere with proper epiglottic function and promote intermittent or even persistent DDSP.

Postoperative DDSP may resolve spontaneously in 10 to 14 days (1) or it may persist. If the condition does persist, surgical intervention to correct the DDSP should be considered but may be unrewarding. Because of the frequency of DDSP as a sequel to resection of the entrapping tissue, trimming of the soft palate at the same time the epiglottic entrapment is corrected has been recommended (5). Removal of less tissue at the time of the entrapment operation is likely the key in preventing the problem (assuming the epiglottis is functionally normal) (11). A sternothyrohyoid myectomy can also be done concurrently with the aryepiglottic fold resection and the staphylectomy (this technique is described separately in this text). If DDSP is recognized preoperatively, the surgeon should seriously consider performing an axial division of the entrapping membrane in conjunction with a sternothyrohyoid myectomy. The prognosis in an uncomplicated entrapment (normal epiglottis and no evidence of DDSP) is good. In patients with concurrent DDSP or in those predisposed to DDSP because of a hypoplastic epiglottis, the prognosis is guarded.

Re-entrapment may also occur as a postoperative complication. Although it may be suggested that an adequate amount of tissue had not been resected, the situation has occurred in animals following consistent technique (12). Granuloma formation characterized by tissue proliferation in the area of the epiglottis (probably from excessive tissue resection) has also been seen as a complication. Resection of any such masses generally carries a poor prognosis.

REFERENCES

1. Haynes PF. Surgery of equine respiratory tract. In: Jennings PB, ed. The Practice of Large Animal Surgery. Philadelphia: WB Saunders, 1984.
2. Raphel CF. Endoscopic findings in the upper respiratory tract of 479 horses. JAVMA 1982;181:470.
3. Haynes PF. Dorsal displacement of the soft palate and epiglottic entrapment: diagnosis, management and interrelationship. Comp Cont Educ 1983;5:S379.
4. Tulleners EP. Transendoscopic contact neodymium:yttrium aluminum garnet laser correction of epiglottic entrapment in standing horses. JAVMA 1990;196:1971–1980.
5. Linford RL, O'Brien TR, Wheat JD, et al. Radiographic assessment of epiglottic length and pharyngeal and laryngeal diameters in the Thoroughbred. Am J Vet Res 1983; 44:1660.
6. Robertson JT. Pharynx and larynx. In: Beech J, ed. Equine Respiratory Disorders. Philadelphia: Lea & Febiger, 1991:331–387.
7. Honnas CM, Wheat JD. Epiglottic entrapment: a transnasal surgical approach to divide the aryepiglottic fold axially in the standing horse. Vet Surg 1988;17:246–251.
8. Holcombe SJ, Robertson JT, Richardson L. Surgical repair of iatrogenic soft palate defects in two horses. JAVMA 1994;205:1315–1317.
9. Ross MW, Gentile DG, Evans LE. Transoral axial division, under endoscopic guidance, for correction of epiglottic entrapment in horses. JAVMA 1993;203:416–420.
10. Lumsden JM, Stick JA, Caron JP, et al. Surgical treatment for epiglottic entrapment in horses: 51 cases (1981–1982). JAVMA 1994;205:729–735.
11. Jann HW, Cook WR. Transendoscopic electrosurgery for epiglottal entrapment in the horse. JAVMA 1985;187:484–492.
12. Haynes PF. Surgical failures in upper respiratory surgery. Proceedings of the 24th Annual Convention of the American Association of Equine Practitioners, St. Louis, MO, 1978. 1979:223.

Surgical Treatment For Intermittent DDSP

Midcervical Myectomy of the Sternothyroid and Sternohyoid Muscles

Myectomy of the sternothyroid and sternohyoid muscles is a simple procedure for treatment of intermittent DDSP (1). The rationale behind this procedure is based on the concept of laryngopalatal subluxation in the pathogenesis of the majority of cases of intermittent DDSP. It has been suggested that excessive contraction of the sternothyrohyoid and omohyoid muscles during forced inspiration might lead to an overretraction of the larynx, resulting in laryngopalatal subluxation (2). The hypothesis also correlates with the observed movements of the larynx during forced inspiration induced by nasal occlusion (3). The sternothyroid and sternohyoid muscles originate on the cartilage of the manubrium and extend along the ventral aspect of the neck to insert upon the thyroid cartilage of the larynx and the basihyoid bone. The omohyoid muscle originates from subscapular fascia and inserts on the basihyoid bone. The abnormally vigorous contraction of these muscles may be a reaction in a horse suffering from other respiratory disease, or may be the result of overreaction or spasm of the muscle in a normal horse caused by nervous excitement when a willing horse is suddenly asked to give its best (2).

It was originally suggested that myectomy of the omohyoid and sternothyrohyoid muscles close to their insertion may prevent laryngeal retraction that results in DDSP (3). Today, most surgeons perform only a sternothyrohyoid myectomy in the midcervical region. The omohyoid myectomy creates more dead space, increases the likelihood of hemorrhage, and usually necessitates placement of a Penrose drain. Practically, there appears to be no additional benefit to performing the omohyoid myectomy. The actual value of the myectomy is somewhat controversial, but the authors consider that it offers a relatively benign initial treatment for intermittent DDSP. The horse can continue training and the benefits of the surgery will be realized soon after surgery. The myectomy procedure can be coupled with a staphylectomy if the surgery is done under anesthesia (4). Performing a staphylectomy in conjunction with the myectomy may have an added benefit in some horses, particularly if there is ulceration on the caudal border of the soft palate.

The midcervical myectomy can be done on the standing horse or in dorsal recumbency under anesthesia (1). A standing midcervical sternothyrohyoid myectomy will be described.

Anesthesia and Surgical Preparation

Perioperative broad-spectrum antibiotics and tetanus toxoid are administered. The standing myectomy is done with the horse sedated and with its head elevated and neck extended to place some tension on the ventral cervical muscles and facilitate their identification. The ventral portion of the neck is clipped, and a surgical site is prepared over the juncture of the cranial and middle thirds of the neck. Local anesthesia is administered in the form of a line block. The incision should be placed at a point where the sternothyrohyoideus bundle is easily palpated and caudal to the area where the sternothyrohyoideus diverges from the sternohyoid muscle (between the eighth and twelfth tracheal rings) (1). Performing the surgery more cranially toward the larynx in the standing horse makes it more difficult to locate the sternothyroid muscles. A common mistake made during this myectomy is to resect only a portion of the sternohyoideus and leave the sternothyroid muscles intact.

Surgical Technique

A 12- to 15-cm midline skin incision is made through the skin, subcutaneous tissue, and cutaneous colli muscle to expose each of the paired sternohyoideus muscles (Fig. 6.4*A*). A 6- to 7-cm segment of the sternothyrohyoideus muscle bundle is bluntly dissected free from the surrounding tissues and fascia on the ventral aspect of the trachea (Fig. 6.4*B*). A Péan clamp is placed across the muscle bundle (Fig. 6.4*C*). Using the clamp to apply traction, the muscles are sharply incised at the proximal and distal limits of the incision (Fig. 6.4*D*). The severed ends of the muscles retract, leaving a considerable dead space. Usually there is minimal hemorrhage; however, it may be necessary to ligate bleeding vessels. It is not necessary to place a Penrose drain, provided the operative site has not been contaminated. The subcutaneous fascia and cutaneous colli muscle are closed with a simple interrupted suture of 2/0 polyglactin 910 (Vicryl). The skin is closed with simple interrupted sutures of nonabsorbable material (2/0 nylon) or skin staples (Fig. 6.4*E*). The neck is then bandaged to apply moderate pressure over the surgical site. This minimizes postoperative hemorrhage into the dead space and prevents hematoma and seroma formation.

Postoperative Management

The neck bandage is maintained for 3 days and the horse is stall-rested for 7 to 10 days. Sutures are removed at 10 days postsurgery, and training is resumed. Some swelling may develop at the site when the horse resumes exercise. Usually, no treatment is necessary.

Comments

Some surgeons still prefer to resect an axial portion of each omohyoid muscle in addition to the sternothyrohyoid muscles. The additional resection of the axial portion of the omohyoid muscle is an attempt to nullify any potential retraction action of this muscle on the larynx. Although it is recognized that the more lateral portions of the muscle are necessarily left intact, the muscle fibers run obliquely, and it is thought that some effect of the muscle is negated by transection of the axial portion. These opinions are, however, subjective.

Opinions vary on the success rate of the sternothyrohyoid myectomy for correcting DDSP. This is understandable because the diagnosis of DDSP is frequently subjective, and it should be recognized that DDSP is a multifactorial problem. In addition to the myectomy, many of these horses receive concurrent medical treatment, making it difficult to assess the effect of surgery. In recent reports, the success rate of the sternothyrohyoid myectomy approximates 60% (1, 4).

A study of sternothyrohyoid myectomy on upper airway mechanics in normal, exercising horses showed decreased airway patency and increased resistance—a somewhat paradoxical result (5). The effect of this myectomy on the upper airway function if a horse is suffering from intermittent DDSP remains unknown.

Sternothyroid Tenectomy, Myectomy, and Tenectomy, and Sternohyoid Myectomy

Although many surgeons still perform the midcervical sternothyrohyoid myectomy, others have developed different approaches and procedures. Currently, the most popular procedure in North America is a simple sternothyroid tenectomy at its point of insertion on the thyroid cartilage of the larynx (Fig. 6.4*F*). This is done with the horse under intravenous anesthesia and can be performed quickly by the experienced operator (Llewellyn HR, personal communication, 1992). A variation of this technique that the authors prefer is to remove the tendon and a 3- to 4-cm portion of the sternothyroid muscle (6).

Some surgeons limit the surgery to the sternothyroid muscle, while others

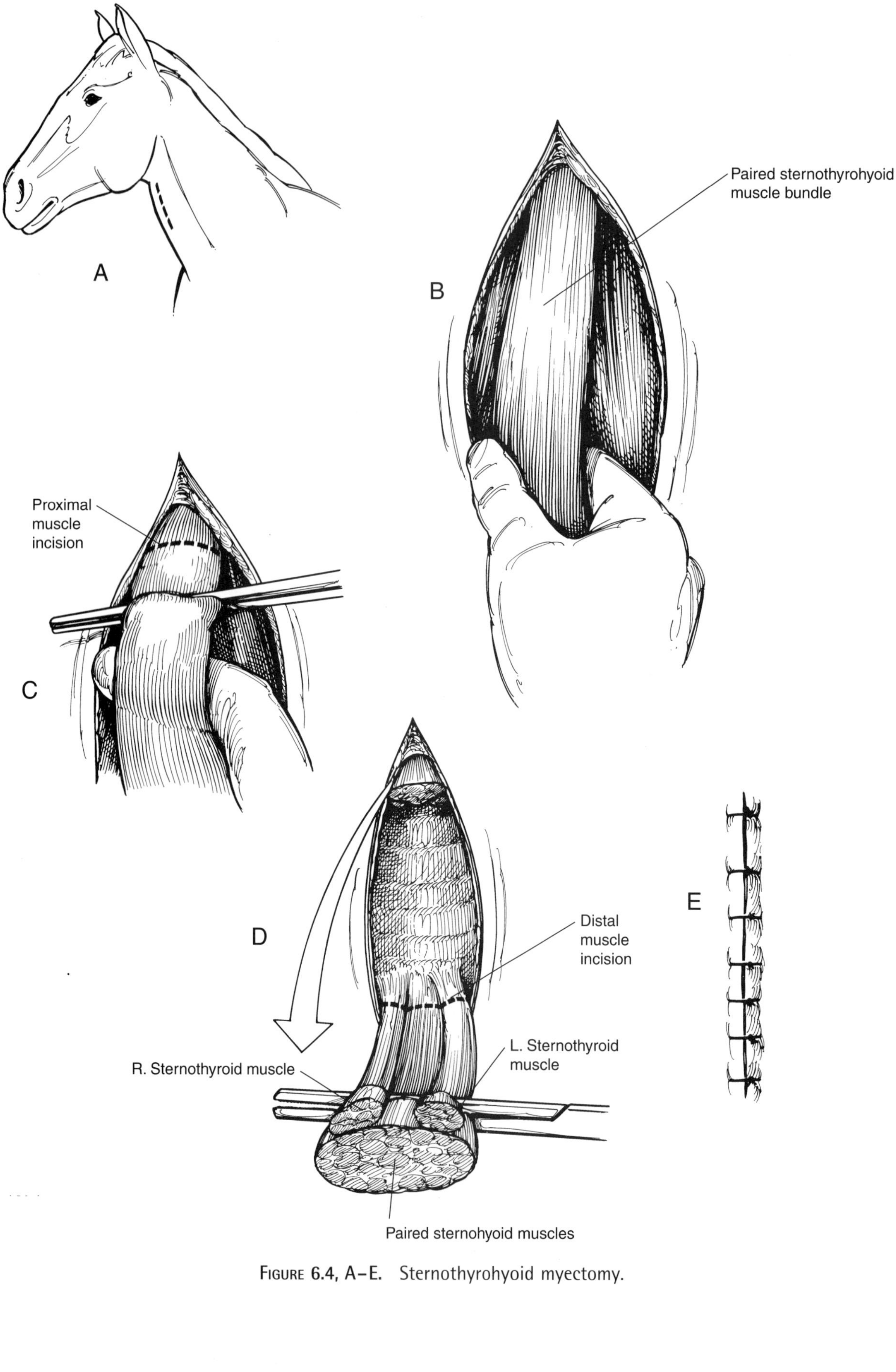

Figure 6.4, A–E. Sternothyrohyoid myectomy.

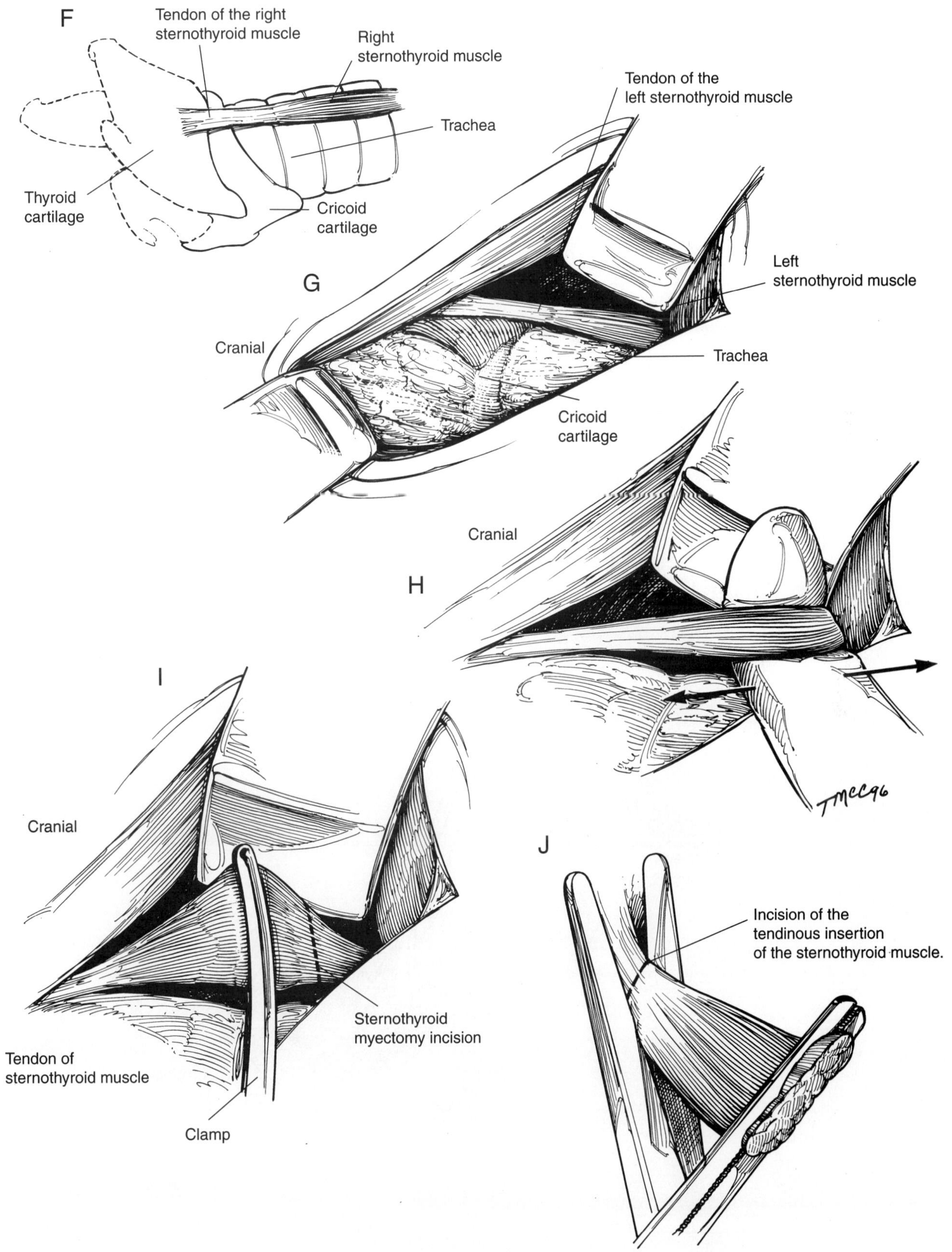

Figure 6.4, F–J. *(continued)* Sternothyroid tenectomy and myectomy.

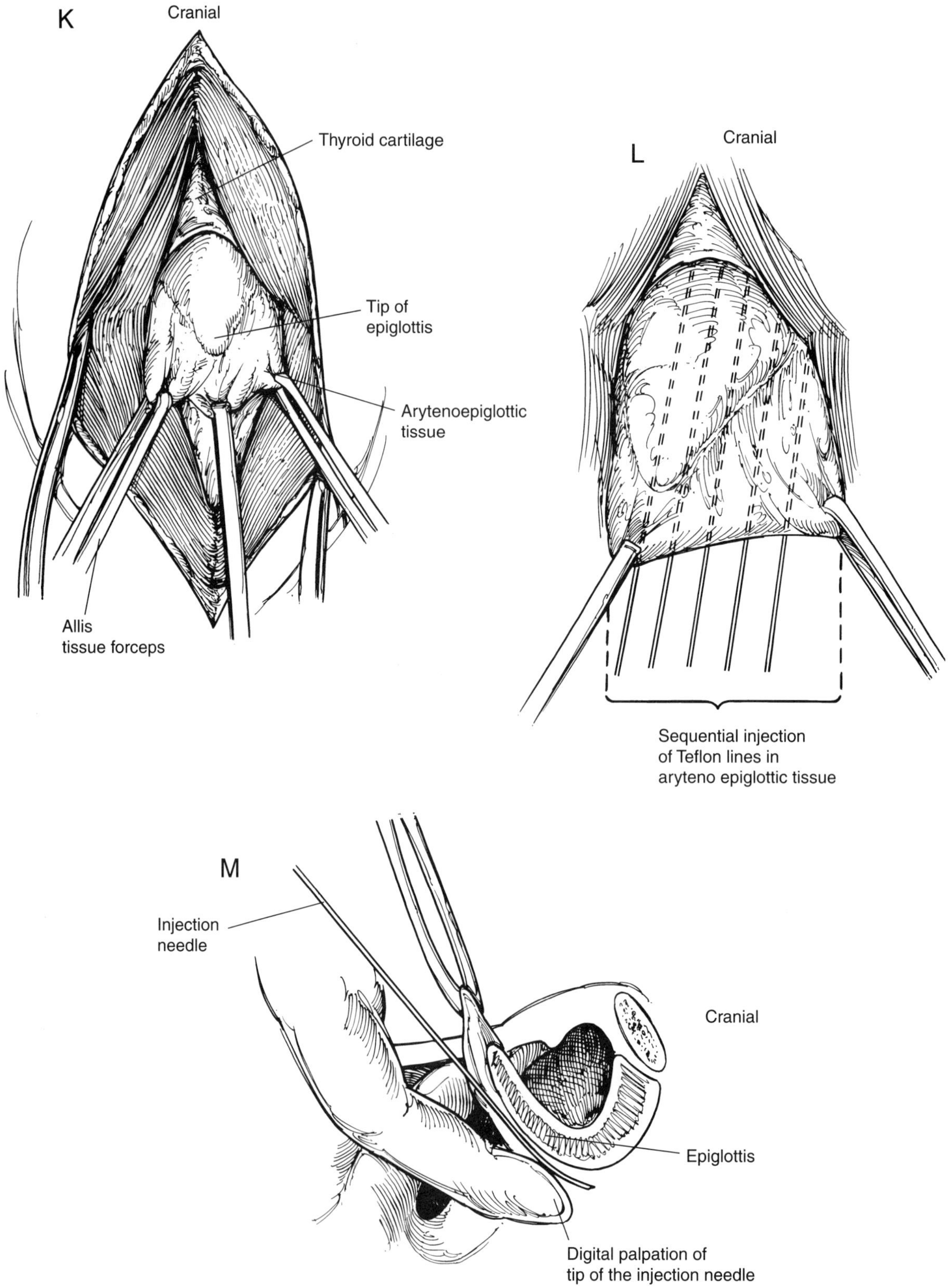

Figure 6.4, K–M. *(continued)* Epiglottic augmentation.

remove a segment of the sternohyoid as well. This seems to be purely surgeon preference, as there is no published work showing the efficacy of either the sternothyroid tenectomy or the sternothyroid tenectomy and myectomy in combination with a sternohyoid myectomy.

Anesthesia and Surgical Preparation

The horse is given intravenous anesthetics and placed in dorsal recumbency. The area over the larynx is surgically prepared. Preoperative broad-spectrum antibiotics are advised and tetanus toxoid is given.

Surgical Technique

An 8- to 10-cm midline skin incision is made over the larynx and extended caudally to the level of the first tracheal ring. The sternohyoideus muscles are bluntly separated on midline with scissors, exposing the ventral aspect of the larynx and the cricotracheal space (Fig. 6.4*G*). The musculotendinous portions of the sternothyroid muscles are located with blunt digital dissection and bluntly separated from their fascial attachments (6) (Fig. 6.4*H*). All dissection should be carefully limited to the area immediately adjacent to the sternothyroid muscles and their attachments to avoid inadvertent damage to other structures. The sternothyroid tendon can be simply incised, or the tendon and a segment of muscle can be removed by incising the muscle distally (Fig. 6.4*I*) and the tendinous insertion on the thyroid cartilage proximally (Fig. 6.4*J*). The authors believe that the benefit of removing a portion of the sternothyroid muscle, as well as performing a tenectomy at its point of insertion on the thyroid cartilage, is that it reduces the likelihood of reattachment of the muscle through the scar, thereby reducing the possibility of having to repeat the procedure.

At the level of the larynx, the paired sternohyoid muscles are closely associated with the omohyoideus muscles laterally. The junction of the sternohyoid and the omohyoid muscles can be palpated with the thumb and index finger. A 5-cm segment of each of the paired sternohyoid muscles can be excised on each side of the incision to complete the myectomy. The incision is left open to heal by second intention.

Postoperative Management

The incisional area is cleaned daily and heals within 2 weeks. Most horses can resume exercise or training within a few days of having this type of myectomy, and many have raced 7 to 10 days after surgery.

Comments

There are some advantages to performing the myectomy/tenectomy procedures at the level of the larynx. A bandage is not necessary and training can be resumed within a few days of surgery. Wound care is simple and when healed, there is no blemish.

Partial Resection of the Soft Palate (Staphylectomy)

A staphylectomy may be done if a myectomy procedure fails to produce improvement, or it may be done in conjunction with a sternothyroid tenectomy or a sternothyroid tenectomy/myectomy and sternohyoid myectomy. The staphylectomy may offer additional benefits in horses that have ulceration of the soft palate. Provided only a thin strip of palate mucosa is resected, there is little likelihood of producing permanent dysphagia.

Anesthesia and Surgical Preparation

Preoperative broad-spectrum antibiotics and tetanus toxoid are administered. The surgery is done under intravenous or general anesthesia, depending on what other procedures are done in conjunction with the staphylectomy. The area over the larynx is surgically prepared. A gauze sponge, folded in fourths, is grasped with sponge forceps and soaked with approximately 20 mL of 2% lidocaine. This is used to swab the lumen of the larynx, the palate, and the nasopharynx once the laryngotomy is completed.

Surgical Technique

A laryngotomy is performed and self-retaining retractors are placed into the larynx. If an endotracheal tube is in place, it must be withdrawn to gain access to the caudal margin of the soft palate. If the procedure is done under intravenous anesthesia, it may be necessary to displace the palate with a finger or curved sponge forceps. Swabbing the lumen of the larynx and the palate and nasopharynx with a local anesthetic reduces the propensity for swallowing. A surgery light or head lamp is positioned over the laryngotomy incision so that the palate is visible. Long-handled Allis tissue forceps are used to grasp the mucosa of the soft palate on midline on the caudal free border. A crescent-shaped segment of mucosa, widest at midline and tapering laterally, is excised using long-curved Metzenbaum scissors. The excised strip of mucosa need not be any wider than .5 to 1 cm at midline to be beneficial. The laryngotomy incision is left to heal by second intention.

Postoperative Management

The laryngotomy incision is cleaned once a day with saline or water-moistened gauze sponges. Usually, horses can successfully resume exercise once the laryngotomy incision is closed. Occasionally, following a staphylectomy, a horse will develop a temporary but persistent DDSP. If exercise is resumed before this is allowed to resolve, the recuperative period may be prolonged for as long as 6 to 8 weeks. Although it is not recommended, some trainers resume exercising these horses within days of the staphylectomy.

Epiglottic Augmentation

Intermittent DDSP may be associated with a hypoplastic epiglottis (7–9). The diagnosis of a hypoplastic epiglottis is based on both objective (measurement of length) and subjective (endoscopic) assessment of the epiglottis. The normal thyroepiglottic length was found to be 8.76 (0.44 cm in 24 healthy Thoroughbreds) (9). Horses with significantly shorter thyroepiglottic lengths of 6.43 (0.4 cm) had associated DDSP. An epiglottis that is flaccid and appears to lack the rigidity required to hold the soft palate in a subepiglottic position might be considered hypoplastic, regardless of its length. Endoscopic assessment of the epiglottis can be made at rest during nasal occlusion, immediately upon cessation of training, or during an exercise test on a treadmill.

If the epiglottis is marginally hypoplastic, a sternothyroid tenectomy, or sternothyroid tenectomy and myectomy, and a sternohyoid myectomy and staphylectomy may improve the horse. If these simple procedures fail or if the epiglottis is obviously hypoplastic and DDSP has become a consistently repeatable event, epiglottic augmentation may be necessary. Most horses with a hypoplastic epiglottis will experience DDSP during training or racing in their 2-year-old year.

As young horses develop, the epiglottis will mature. However, beyond 2 years of age, significant change or improvement in a hypoplastic epiglottis is unlikely. Injection of polytetrafluoroethylene paste into the subepiglottic and aryepiglottic tissues increases epiglottic thickness and creates an inflammatory response that produces fibrosis and increased rigidity (7, 8).

Anesthesia and Surgical Preparation

Preoperatively, the horse should receive tetanus prophylaxis, intravenous broad-spectrum antibiotics, and a nonsteroidal anti-inflammatory agent. The horse is anesthetized with an inhalation anesthetic. Once the laryngotomy incision is made, the endotracheal tube is usually withdrawn to allow the augmentation procedure to proceed. The anesthetist should be prepared to deliver intravenous anesthesia for the duration of the procedure. If necessary, the procedure could be halted temporarily while the endotracheal tube is replaced to allow further delivery of inhalation anesthesia. A tracheostomy is not necessary for placement of an endotracheal tube to deliver the anesthetic, provided the surgery is completed in an efficient manner.

Additional Instrumentation

An intracordal injection set (such as Arnold-Bruening intracordal injection set, Storz Instrument Co., St. Louis, MO) is required. The injection set is comprised of a pressure syringe, a loading adapter, and two injection needles that have an 18- or 19-gauge tip. One tube (7 mL) of polytetrafluoroethylene paste (Teflon, Polytef paste, Mentor O & O Inc., Norwell, MA) is also required.

Surgical Technique

The horse is placed in dorsal recumbency. If a myectomy is being done in conjunction with the augmentation, the authors prefer to do the sternothyroid tenectomy and myectomy before making the laryngotomy incision. Self-retaining retractors are placed in the larynx and the endotracheal tube is withdrawn into the oral cavity. The larynx and nasopharynx can then be swabbed with local anesthetic to reduce the likelihood of swallowing. Curved sponge forceps are hooked around the lateral edge of the epiglottis near its base to retrovert the epiglottis toward the incision. Using long Allis tissue forceps, the aryepiglottic tissue close to the tip of the epiglottis is grasped and the tip of the epiglottis is everted into the larynx. Through manipulation of the aryepiglottic tissue with the Allis tissue forceps, the aryepiglottic tissue is symmetrically extended from the apex of the epiglottis. One forcep is used to grasp the tissue on midline, while two others are placed approximately 1.5 cm to each side (Fig. 6.4*K*). In effect, most of the epiglottis is suspended in the larynx by a "sling" of aryepiglottic tissue. The epiglottis is positioned in much the same fashion as it would be for surgical resection of an aryepiglottic fold entrapment.

With an assistant holding the aryepiglottic tissue on one side of the epiglottis taut between two Allis tissue forceps, the surgeon inserts the injection needle between the two mucosal layers on the leading edge of the aryepiglottic tissue, and then advances the needle within the tissue toward the base of the epiglottis. The authors prefer to begin injections at the lateral aspect of the aryepiglottic tissue and work toward midline (Fig. 6.4*L*). The surgeon can palpate the tip of the needle as it is advanced to ensure that it does not penetrate the mucosa (Fig. 6.4*M*). The paste is injected as the needle is slowly withdrawn. Laterally, much of the paste is deposited into the aryepiglottic tissue, while axially it is deposited primarily between the epiglottic cartilage and the subepiglottic mucosa. However, when the epiglottis is released at the completion of the surgery, the aryepiglottic tissue will retract to occupy a subepiglottic position. When one side is completed, the aryepiglottic tissue on the opposite side is tensed and the procedure is repeated.

The objective is to deposit a total of 5 to 7 mL of paste, uniformly, in approximately 10 lines that run parallel to the long axis of the epiglottis. The key to success is even distribution of the paste.

On completion of the augmentation, a small triangular piece of arytenoepiglottic tissue is excised at the apex of the epiglottis to prevent postoperative development of an epiglottic entrapment (7). A staphylectomy can also be done at this time, as well as a sternohyoid myectomy.

Postoperative Management

The laryngotomy (and myectomy) wound is cleaned daily. Many horses that have epiglottic augmentation are febrile for 2 to 3 days after surgery, and most show some degree of dysphagia in the immediate postoperative period. Systemic antibiotics and nonsteroidal anti-inflammatory drugs can be used at the surgeon's discretion. Endoscopic examination in the immediate postoperative period may reveal a persistent DDSP or an epiglottis that appears extremely inflamed. A persistent DDSP may be present for as long as 6 to 8 weeks; however, function will return once the inflammation in the region subsides. A minimum of 6 weeks stall rest is recommended following this surgery.

Comments

When healing is complete, there may be some endoscopic evidence of the augmentation such as focal thickening of the arytenoepiglottic tissue. In some horses, the gross appearance of the epiglottis is much as it was before surgery; however, functionally it is improved. Approximately 60–65% of the horses that have epiglottic augmentation, often in conjunction with other soft palate-related techniques, can be expected to improve (7, 10). It is the authors' opinion that horses responding best to this procedure are those that were able to train to a point close to racing speed or were able to start some races as 2-year-olds, and in which the epiglottis appears to be flaccid but has a length that is close to the normal range.

Scarring of the aryepiglottic tissues greatly reduces the prognosis for epiglottic augmentation. As a result of fibrosis, the tissue is relatively immobile and it is not possible to distribute the paste in a uniform fashion. Also, an epiglottis that is deformed as a result of a previous surgery cannot be improved with any type of augmentation.

REFERENCES

1. Harrison IW. Sternothyrohyoideus myectomy in horses. JAVMA 1988;193:1299–1302.
2. Cook WR. Some observations on form and function of the equine upper airway in health and disease: the pharynx. In: Proceedings of the 27th Annual Convention of the American Association of Equine Practitioners in 1981, New Orleans, LA, 1982:5.
3. Heffron CJ, Baker GJ. Observations on the mechanism of functional obstruction of the nasopharyngeal airway in the horse. Equine Vet J 1979;11:142.
4. Tulleners EP. Surgical management of dorsal displacement of the soft palate. In: Proceedings of the 23rd Annual Surgical Forum, Chicago: 1995:141–145.
5. Holcombe SJ, Beard WL, Hinchcliff KW, et al. Effect of sternothyrohyoid myectomy on upper airway mechanics in normal horses. J Appl Physiol 1994;77:2812–2816.
6. Carter BG, Robertson JT, Beard WL, et al. Sternothyrohyoideus myectomy, tenectomy and staphylectomy for the treatment of dorsal displacement of the soft palate in horses. In: Proceedings of the 28th Annual ACVS Scientific Meeting, 1993:5.
7. Koch C. Augmentation of the equine epiglottis in the Teflon paste. In: Proceedings of the 36th Annual Conference of the AAEP, Lexington, KY, 1990:541–545.
8. Tulleners E, Hamir A. Evaluation of epiglottic augmentation by use of polytetrafluoroethylene paste in the horse. Am J Vet Res 1991;20:1908–1916.
9. Linford RL, O'Brien TR, Wheat JD, et al. Radiographic assessment of the epiglottic length and pharyngeal and laryngeal diameters in the Thoroughbred. Am J Vet Res 1983;44:1660.
10. Tulleners E, Stick JA, Leitch M, et al. Epiglottic augmentation for treatment of dorsal displacement of the soft palate in racehorses: 59 cases (1985–1994). JAVMA 1997; 211:1022–1028.

Surgical Treatment of a Subepiglottic Cyst

Subepiglottic cysts are generally thought to be congenital cysts that originate from embryologic remnants of the thyroglossal duct (1). It has also been suggested that in some foals the cyst may have an inflammatory etiology (2). The cyst enlarges as the horse grows, although the rate of cystic development is variable. A large cyst in a foal, in addition to producing airway obstruction, will produce dysphagia that can cause aspiration pneumonia (2). In horses older than 1 year, the common complaint is an abnormal respiratory noise associated with exercise. The cyst may produce some dysphagia in the older horse but not aspiration pneumonia. A subepiglottic cyst may be found in conjunction with an entrapped epiglottis.

The diagnosis of subepiglottic cyst is based on endoscopic observation of the cyst. The size of the cyst can vary greatly from approximately 1 to 5 cm in diameter, and at times the cyst may not be visible if it is positioned ventral to the caudal border of the soft palate. Usually, if the horse is made to swallow, the cyst will come into view. A subepiglottic cyst will also be hidden from view if there is a DDSP. A lateral radiograph of the pharynx and larynx will usually demonstrate the subepiglottic cyst, although in most cases it provides only additional ancillary information.

Surgical resection of a subepiglottic cyst can be done through a ventral midline laryngotomy or a ventral pharyngotomy approach (3). An advantage of surgical resection through one of these approaches is that the mucosa surrounding the cyst can be preserved. This may reduce the likelihood of scarring in the subepiglottic area, which could interfere with epiglottic function and lead to intermittent or persistent DDSP (4). If the cyst is punctured during the resection, it can be difficult to resect the remaining adherent portion of the cyst. It is important that all secretory tissue be removed to prevent recurrence.

Another method for removing a subepiglottic cyst is to use a wire snare passed through the mouth, and simply excise the cyst (5, 6). The snare can be placed manually over the cyst, or with endoscopic guidance and the use of long forceps. Contact Nd:YAG laser-assisted excision of subepiglottic cysts has been described (5). The method of removal of a subepiglottic cyst is based on operator preference. The authors prefer snare excision per os.

Anesthesia and Surgical Preparation

Laryngotomy or ventral pharyngotomy is done under general anesthesia with the patient in dorsal recumbency. The ventral aspect of the pharynx, caudal mandibular, and laryngeal area is clipped and prepared.

For snare excision of the cyst per os, the horse needs only intravenous anesthesia and is placed in lateral recumbency. A snare can be fashioned using obstetric wire passed through two artificial insemination pipettes that are taped together. Two pairs of pliers are necessary to grasp the obstetric wire. If the horse's mouth is too small to allow a hand, an endoscope (preferably a videoendoscope) will be required to visualize the cyst for snare placement. A long set of grasping forceps is useful (5).

Phenylbutazone, intravenous broad-spectrum antibiotics, and tetanus toxoid are administered preoperatively.

Surgical Techniques

Resection of Subepiglottic Cyst Via Laryngotomy

A routine laryngotomy is performed and the endotracheal tube is temporarily withdrawn into the oropharynx to allow manipulation of the epiglottis. Using curved sponge forceps, which are introduced through the laryngotomy and curled under the base of the epiglottis, the epiglottis is everted into the larynx and the cyst is brought into the field by applying traction with Allis tissue forceps on the aryepiglottic and subepiglottic tissues. Great care should be taken not to traumatize the epiglottic cartilage. Once the cyst has been exposed, it can be digitally elevated and the endotracheal tube reinserted into the trachea. Using a scalpel, the mucosa overlying the cyst is incised and the cyst is dissected free from its surrounding connective tissue with Metzenbaum scissors. Inadvertent perforation of the cyst during this dissection can make completion of the resection difficult. Once the cyst is removed, the mucosa can be apposed with a few simple interrupted sutures of 3/0 synthetic absorbable suture material, burying the knots. If an entrapped epiglottis is associated with the cyst, resection of a portion of the aryepiglottic tissue is indicated. The laryngotomy is left open to heal by second intention.

Resection of a Subepiglottic Cyst Via Ventral Pharyngotomy

Ventral pharyngotomy has been suggested as a possible alternative approach to a subepiglottic cyst, but in the authors' opinion, it offers no significant advantage over a laryngotomy approach (3). The pharyngotomy incision is deep with limited visibility. However, because this approach does offer direct access to the subepiglottic surface, there may be surgical situations in which this approach could be useful (3, 7, 8). Therefore, the authors have included it in this text.

A ventral midline incision is made rostral to the body of the thyroid cartilage (immediately rostral to the site for ventral laryngotomy) (Fig. 6.5*A*). The incision is continued between the sternohyoid muscles to expose the deeper omohyoid muscles. These are also separated axially, and the incision is continued through the thyrohyoid ligament (Fig. 6.5*B*). The hyoepiglottic muscle is divided on the midline deep within the incision. This division reveals the glossoepiglottic fold, and an incision through this fold enables entry into the oropharynx (Fig. 6.5*C*). Figure 6.5*D* illustrates the surgical entry in cross section. The rostral extent of the incision is limited by the basihyoid bone, and division of this to obtain additional exposure for cleft palate repair has been reported by one author (7). Weitlaner retractors facilitate exposure during the surgical approach.

If a subepiglottic cyst is the indication for the pharyngotomy, the surface mucosa is grasped with a pair of Allis tissue forceps and the mucosa divided. Submucosal dissection is then performed to enucleate the cyst. Rupture of the cyst is avoided if at all possible. Following removal of the cyst, excessive mucosa may be trimmed, and the wound can be left to heal by granulation. Because of poor surgical exposure, the subepiglottic surface is not closed. The pharyngotomy incision is left to heal by second intention.

Snare Excision of a Subepiglottic Cyst Via Peroral Approach

When the horse is anesthetized, a large mouth speculum is placed securely on the horse's head. If a hand can be comfortably passed into the oropharynx, the snare is introduced into the oropharynx and the loop is placed over the cyst. Assistants apply tension to the two wires and the snare is tightened around the cyst while the operator maintains digital contact with the cyst and also stabilizes or directs an assistant to stabilize the snare conduit. As the snare is tightened, the end of the snare conduit is kept in a position immediately adjacent and ventral to the cyst. The operator must ensure two things when placing and tightening the snare: that the snare is completely around the base of the cyst and that the epiglottic cartilage is not incorporated into the snare. When the

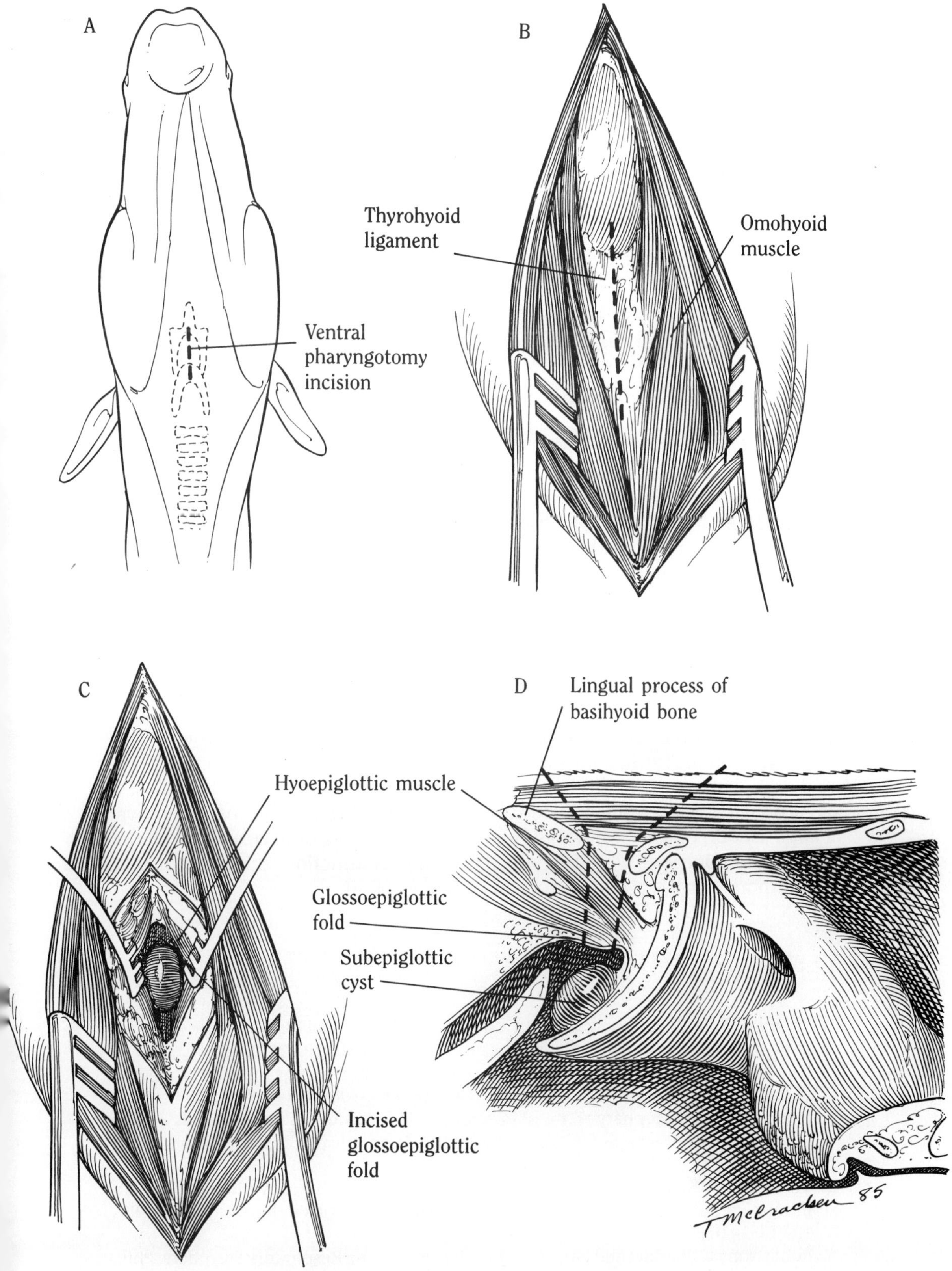

FIGURE 6.5, A–D. Ventral pharyngotomy and excision of subepiglottic cyst.

cyst is tightly ensnared, the obstetric wires are pulled alternately until the cyst is amputated.

If an entrapment of the epiglottis is associated with the cyst, the authors prefer to first slit the entrapping membrane per os and then follow with cyst excision. If the cyst is not associated with an entrapment, the authors will still perform an axial division of the aryepiglottic tissue that remains because after a simple snare excision of a subepiglottic cyst, frequently an entrapment of the epiglottis will develop.

If the small size of a horse's head does not allow passage of a hand into the oropharynx, or the patient is a foal or weaning, the snare excision must be done under endoscopic guidance, using long grasping forceps to manipulate the snare over the cyst (5).

Postoperative Management

A ventral laryngotomy or a pharyngotomy incision should be cleaned daily with a clean moist gauze sponge until it is healed, within approximately 10 to 14 days. Obviously, with a peroral snare excision no wound care is required. Regardless the method used for cyst removal, training or turn-out exercise should not resume until the inflammation surrounding the epiglottis subsides. This usually takes 10 to 14 days. Nonsteroidal anti-inflammatory medication can be administered if swelling at the site of the cyst removal becomes excessive and there is clinical evidence of airway obstruction.

Comments

The authors have encountered many complications following subepiglottic cyst removal in foals, regardless the technique used. Some foals will have epiglottic deformity that predisposes to DDSP, and this becomes evident in the postoperative period. In the immediate postoperative period, foals seem to be more prone to developing upper airway obstructive problems and must be observed closely.

Although it was originally stated that the snare technique, because it removed a large section of mucosa, would predispose to subepiglottic cicatrix formation that would contribute to eliminate soft palate dysfunction, this has not been the authors' experience in performance horses (4, 6).

REFERENCES

1. Koch EB, Tate LP. Pharyngeal cysts in horses. JAVMA 1978;173:858.
2. Stick JA, Boles C. Subepiglottic cyst in three foals. JAVMA 1977;177:62.
3. Haynes PFL. Surgery of the equine respiratory tract. In: Jennings PB, ed. The Practice of Large Animal Surgery. Philadelphia: WB Saunders, 1984:388–487.
4. Raker CW. The nasopharynx. In: Mansmann RA, McAllister ES, Pratt PW, eds. Equine Medicine and Surgery. 3rd ed. Santa Barbara, CA: American Veterinary Publications, 1982:747.
5. Tulleners EP. Evaluation of peroral transendoscopic contact neodymium:yttrium aluminum garnet laser and snare excision of subepiglottic cysts in horses. JAVMA 1991; 198:1631–1635.
6. Robertson JT. Pharynx and larynx. In: Beech J, ed. Equine Respiratory Disorders. Philadelphia: Lea & Febiger, 1991:331.
7. Cook WR. Some observations on diseases of the ear, nose, and throat in the horse, and endoscopy using a flexible fiberoptic endoscope. Vet Rec 1974;94:533.
8. Speirs VC. Entrapment of the epiglottis in horses. J Equine Med Surg 1977;1:267.

Extradiverticular Ligation and Balloon Catheter Occlusion: Techniques For Treatment of Guttural Pouch Mycosis

Guttural pouch mycosis can produce spontaneous and severe epistaxis (1). Usually, there is a premonitory episode of bleeding before fatal exsanguination. The most common fungus involved is *Aspergillus* spp., but the underlying cause behind initiation of the fungal growth is unclear (2). These mycotic lesions tend to be located over the major arteries of the guttural pouch. An underlying defect of the artery, such as an aneurysm, may create favorable conditions for initiation of growth of fungi that normally reside in the pouch, but this has not been substantiated (3). The internal carotid artery is most commonly involved; however, the external carotid artery and its branches may also be affected in approximately one third of cases (4, 5).

Other clinical signs seen in association with guttural pouch mycosis can be attributed to involvement of various nerves that run adjacent to the pouches. These signs include pharyngeal paralysis, dysphagia, laryngeal hemiplegia, DDSP, Horner's syndrome, and facial paralysis (1). Guttural pouch mycosis may also manifest as nasal catarrh, abnormal head posture, mild colic, and subparotid abscessation (1). The signs of the infection are variable and will depend on which nerve or blood vessel is affected. Endoscopic examination of the interior of the guttural pouch will usually demonstrate the lesion on the roof of the diverticulum. The lesion may vary in extent, color, and texture. Some have a black or white furry appearance; others consist of a flat brown diphtheritic plaque, slightly elevated above the mucosa of the guttural pouch.

In horses that have recently bled or are actively bleeding, endoscopic assessment of the lesion may be virtually impossible. Nevertheless, attempts should be made to examine the interior of the pouch to localize the lesion and determine, if possible, which artery (or arteries) is affected. It cannot be simply assumed that the bleeding is originating from the internal carotid artery.

Occasionally, a horse with a unilateral mycotic lesion will exhibit bilateral epistaxis and endoscopically will have blood coming from both guttural pouch openings as a result of erosion of the median septum. Because bilateral mycotic infections can occur, both guttural pouches should be inspected in all cases.

If the horse has a history of an acute profuse epistaxis, conservative therapy (flushes, antifungal agents [topical and systemic]) is usually unsatisfactory. To delay surgical treatment only increases the likelihood of a fatal hemorrhagic episode. The authors therefore recommend operating as soon as practical. However, successive bouts of hemorrhage will make the horse anemic and a high-risk candidate for anesthesia and surgery.

Surgical treatment for guttural pouch mycosis by arterial ligation has been reported (6–8). It was originally proposed that ligation of the internal carotid artery on both sides of the lesion was necessary, because ligation on the cardiac side of the area of fungal growth did not take into account the retrograde blood flow from the cerebral arterial circle and the intercarotid artery (9). Continued hemorrhage could lead to exsanguination and death. Because of the anatomic difficulty and the risks associated with ligating the internal carotid artery on both sides of the lesion, an extradiverticular (without opening the pouch) approach to ligation of the internal carotid artery at its origin was adopted (7, 8). Ligation of the internal carotid artery on the cardiac side of the lesion is believed to help avert further hemorrhage by promoting thrombus formation that extends to the cranial side of the lesion, thereby preventing retrograde bleeding. However, experimental work has shown that these beneficial effects of this proximal ligature are not immediate, and for at least 3 days following the ligation there is no decrease in blood pressure distal to the ligature (9). Fatal hemorrhage will still occur in some horses (7, 8).

Another technique of managing hemorrhage from the internal carotid artery is to use a balloon-tipped catheter (10, 11). The catheter is introduced distal to a ligature on the internal carotid artery close to its origin. The tip is advanced beyond the site of infection, then the balloon is inflated so that the affected segment of artery is isolated from the cerebral vascular system. This technique is probably the ideal method of treatment because it greatly reduces the risk of fatal hemorrhage.

Methods have also been devised to occlude the external carotid and maxillary arteries with balloon catheters on both sides of the eroded segment (12). The technique now favored for managing hemorrhage from the external carotid artery or its branches involves passing balloon-tipped catheters in retrograde fashion through the major palatine and the transverse facial arteries.

The horse that is actively bleeding from a guttural pouch and appears in danger of bleeding to death poses quite a challenge to the surgeon. Endoscopic identification of the source of bleeding may be impossible because of the active hemorrhage. If support staff or equipment are not immediately available, a standing ligation of the common carotid artery can be performed in an attempt to save the horse's life. Preferably the horse is anesthetized, and in the absence of a definitive localization of the lesion to a specific artery, one must be prepared to occlude the internal carotid artery as well as the external carotid artery. This is best achieved using the occlusion techniques described by Freeman (10–12). An alternative to the occlusion technique to reduce flow in the external carotid artery is ligation of the external carotid artery at its origin, to stop normograde flow and ligation of the major palatine artery just rostral to the second maxillary premolar to prevent retrograde flow. The major risk of these ligations when performed in conjunction with internal carotid artery occlusion is blindness on the affected side (13, 14). It does, however, offer the surgeon who is less experienced with the external carotid and maxillary artery occlusion techniques a simple alternative in an emergency situation if fatal exsanguination is imminent. The authors recommend that the reader consult appropriate reference material before performing the occlusion techniques (10, 12). The relevant anatomy is illustrated in Figure 6.6*A*.

Ideally, to ascertain the exact location of the arterial lesion(s) and to identify any aberrant blood vessels, a carotid arteriogram can be done first (3, 15). Practically, this is usually not done for a number of reasons. First, the technique is technically demanding and significantly prolongs anesthesia time. Second, if the lesion can be localized endoscopically to the internal carotid artery, the source of hemorrhage is obvious. Third, if a large mycotic plaque covers the internal carotid and extends over the area of the external carotid or maxillary arteries, the safest approach to prevent fatal exsanguination is to occlude the internal and external carotid arteries with balloon catheters.

Anesthesia and Surgical Preparation

The horse with guttural pouch mycosis can lose large volumes of blood in a very short time. Patients that develop shock should receive intravenous fluids rapidly, as well as hypertonic saline. A suitable blood donor should be located through cross matching and blood collection. A horse in shock will benefit from a transfusion. If the horse has bled several days previously, and the PCV is above 20, an immediate transfusion may not be necessary. Blood collection and storage is still advised in preparation for surgery should hemorrhage occur during the procedure. Both simple ligation of the internal carotid artery and carotid occlusion techniques are done under general anesthesia with the patient

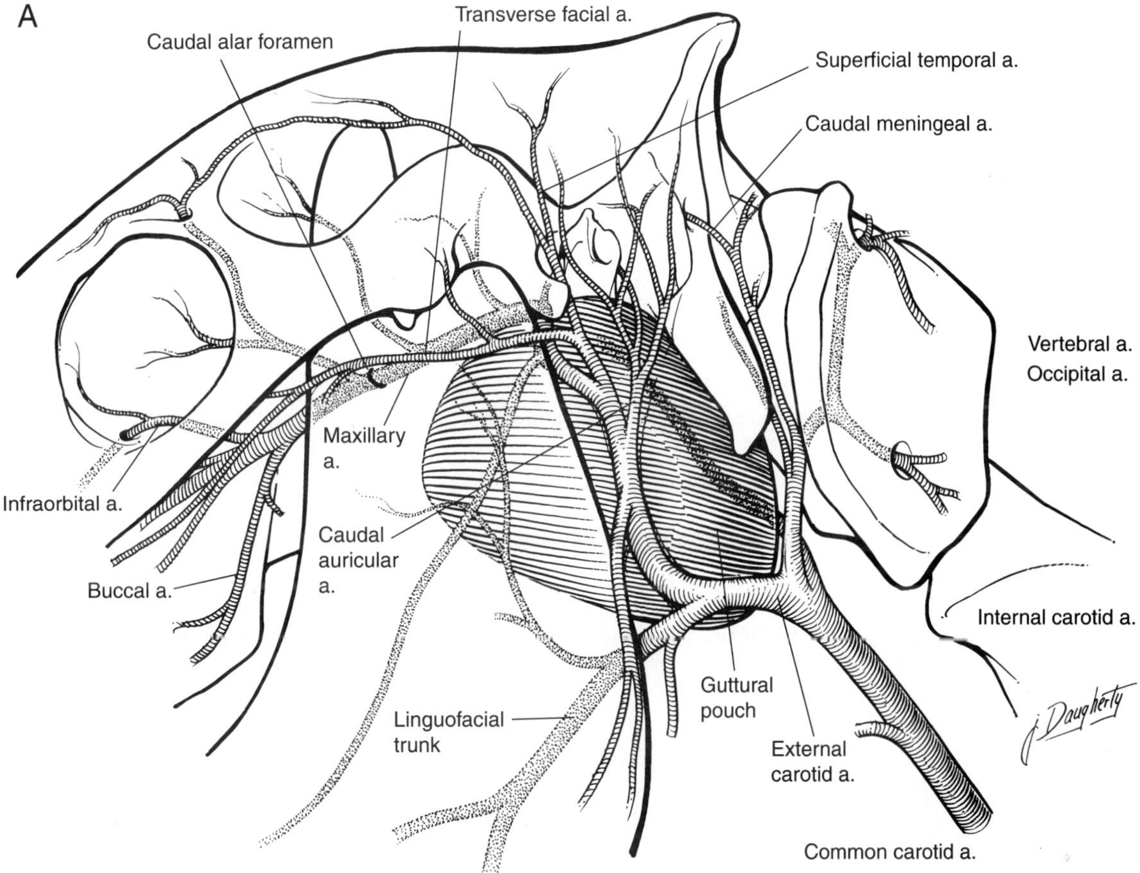

Figure 6.6, A. Distribution of branches of the common carotid artery in relation to the guttural pouch.

in lateral recumbency and the affected side uppermost. Perioperative broad-spectrum antibiotics are administered before surgery, as are phenylbutazone and tetanus toxoid.

Additional Instrumentation

Additional instruments used include self-retaining or malleable retractors, 5F, 6F, and 7F venous embolectomy catheters, and injection caps for the catheters.

Surgical Technique

Arterial Ligation

The surgical approach to the internal carotid artery at its origin from the carotid is similar to the hyovertebrotomy approach to the guttural pouch, except that the incision is slightly more ventral and caudal (6). An 8- to 10-cm incision is made parallel and just cranial to the wing of the atlas (Fig. 6.6*B*). The skin incision exposes the parotid salivary gland and the overlying parotidoauricular muscle. The ventral part of the parotidoauricular muscle is incised, and a dissection plane for the parotid gland is established by incising the fascia on its caudal border. The parotid gland is reflected cranially. The caudal auricular nerve crosses obliquely in the dorsal aspect of the surgical field and is reflected caudally, if necessary. Reflection of the parotid gland reveals the occipitohyoid and

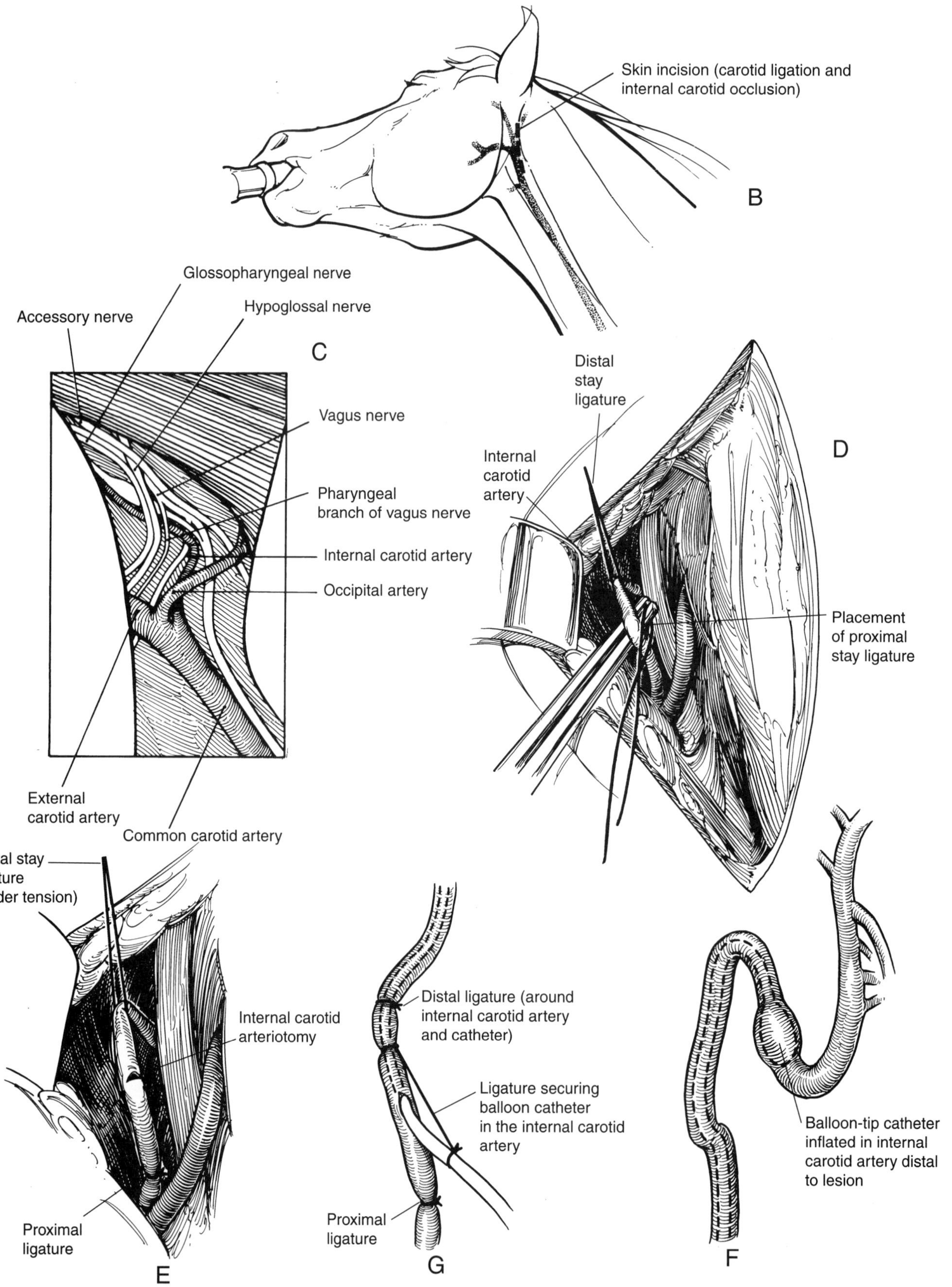

Figure 6.6, B–G. *(continued)* Extradiverticular ligation and balloon catheter occlusion of the internal carotid artery.

digastric muscles craniodorsally, and the rectus capitis cranialis muscle caudodorsally. The mandibular salivary gland is identified ventrally. Blunt dissection through areolar tissue exposes the dorsolateral wall of the guttural pouch and the pharyngeal branch of the vagus nerve. In most cases, the ventral dissection will reveal the origin of both the internal carotid and the occipital arteries (Fig. 6.6*C*).

The origin of the internal carotid artery from the common carotid artery is proximal to the occipital artery, but anatomic variability may make it difficult to distinguish the internal carotid from the occipital artery. The occipital artery is usually more superficially located in the surgical site and tends to be larger. Occasionally, these two arteries will be found originating from a common trunk. If the internal carotid artery cannot be identified with certainty, both the occipital and internal carotid arteries should be ligated to ensure against inadvertent ligation of the wrong one. Identification of the arteries as one dissects through the areolar tissue can be facilitated by palpation of pulsation in the vessel with the index finger. The artery(ies) is individually identified and freed from the surrounding fascia and nerves. Each vessel is double-ligated at a convenient location above its origin from the common carotid artery. Absorbable suture materials may be used; however, the authors prefer to use no. 0 silk for vessel ligation.

Because the ligation procedure does not enter the lumen of the guttural pouch, the wound can be regarded as a sterile one, and primary intention healing can be anticipated. Closure of the hyovertebrotomy incision utilizes a synthetic absorbable suture in the fascia associated with the parotid gland, and the skin is closed with a monofilament nonabsorbable suture material or stainless steel staples.

Balloon Catheter Occlusion of the Internal Carotid Artery

The surgical approach to the internal carotid artery for balloon catheter occlusion is the same as described for simple ligation. The artery is bluntly dissected free from its surrounding fascia and as much as possible is exposed to identify any aberrant branches (15). Once the artery is isolated, it is ligated at its origin from the common carotid artery with no. 0 silk. Two loops of no. 0 silk are placed around the artery and used to isolate and retract a 1.5-cm segment of the artery distal to the ligation in preparation for an arteriotomy (Fig. 6.6*D*). The segment of artery isolated between the two loops of suture is elevated slightly, and a small transverse arteriotomy is made using a hooked scalpel blade (Fig. 6.6*E*). There will be some retrograde bleeding, but a 6F or a 7F catheter can be quickly introduced into the arteriotomy and advanced approximately 13 cm (in adults) until it impacts between the two flexures of the sigmoid portion of the artery. The balloon is then inflated with saline, which is injected through an injection cap on the end of the catheter. If an endoscope is in place in the affected guttural pouch, the catheter may be seen advancing in the artery. Preferably, a video-endoscope can be used so the surgeon can observe the artery and passing of the catheter. Inflating the balloon slightly at some point on the cardiac side of the lesion may allow visual confirmation of its position in the artery, but it may also be a dangerous maneuver if the balloon is in the vicinity of the mycotic plaque. Once the catheter is positioned and the balloon inflated (Fig. 6.6*F*), the distal loop of silk suture is tied over the artery (Fig. 6.6*G*), securing the catheter in position to prevent the catheter from backing out or to prevent retrograde hemorrhage at the arteriorotomy site if the balloon deflates. The excess length of catheter is coiled into the dead space of the incision, and the incision is closed primarily as previously described. Cutting or kinking the catheter should be avoided because it may result in leakage of saline from the balloon.

If there is uncertainty regarding whether the catheter has been placed in the internal carotid artery or in the occipital artery, an intraoperative radiograph can be taken to determine its location because the catheter is radiopaque. A problem the authors have encountered is sudden severe hemorrhage as a result of having passed the catheter tip through the wall of the artery at the site of the lesion. In this case, the surgeon's index finger was introduced into the guttural pouch through a hastily prepared hyovertebrotomy incision, the catheter tip was withdrawn proximal to the lesion, and then advanced beyond the lesion while maintaining digital pressure over the lesion. When the balloon was inflated, the hemorrhage stopped. Alternatively, the balloon can be inflated and the catheter withdrawn until the balloon occludes the hole. A second catheter can then be passed alongside the first and the inflated balloon will prevent the second catheter from passing through the hole in the artery (Freeman DE, personal communication, 1997).

Aberrant branches of the internal carotid artery can exist, and passage of the balloon-tipped catheter into such a branch can result in a failure to prevent hemorrhage because retrograde flow is not arrested (15). In a review of 39 cases of guttural pouch mycosis in which the internal carotid artery was surgically occluded, one horse died as a result of inadvertent occlusion of an aberrant branch (5). During the dissection, as much of the internal carotid artery as possible should be exposed without entering the guttural pouch, to identify branching or bifurcation of the artery (15). The aberrant branch should be ligated and the continuation of the internal carotid artery should then be occluded (15).

Balloon Catheter Occlusion of the External Carotid and Maxillary Arteries

Occlusion of the external carotid and maxillary arteries using balloon-tipped catheters can be accomplished by one of three different methods. These methods for occlusion of the external carotid and maxillary arteries are described and illustrated in detail by Freeman et al. (12). The method currently recommended involves insertion of catheters into the major palatine and the transverse facial arteries (Freeman DE, personal communication, 1997). A major advantage of the technique is that these vessels are relatively superficial and can be approached without a difficult or deep dissection (12). The catheter inserted into the major palatine artery is advanced in a retrograde fashion until the balloon tip is in the maxillary artery just caudal to the caudal alar foramen. The transverse facial artery catheter is directed in a retrograde fashion into the external carotid artery.

A thorough knowledge of the regional vascular anatomy is required to successfully complete the surgery. The authors recommend that our readers refer to the detailed original descriptions of these occlusion techniques if they need to perform occlusion of the external carotid and maxillary arteries.

Postoperative Management

Postoperative antibiotics could be justified with the catheter occlusion techniques because the catheters are in close proximity to or in contact with the arterial lesion. An occlusion catheter in the internal carotid artery may not need to be removed provided signs of incisional infection do not develop. If the horse develops a fever and painful incisional swelling, the catheter should be removed. A secure, occlusive thrombus likely will have formed distal to the catheter tip 7 to 14 days after catheter placement. General anesthesia is recommended for internal carotid artery catheter removal. Catheters placed into the transverse facial and palatine arteries are always removed, and anesthesia is not required (12).

The fungal lesion within the guttural pouch usually resolves after appropriate arterial ligation or occlusion. Concurrent medical treatment may not be necessary but usually consists of local lavage and application of antifungal preparations, as well as the oral administration of thiabendazole (16). Fiberoptic examination of the lesions on the roof of the pouch as early as 1 week postsurgery frequently reveals greatly diminished fungal growth. Once healing is complete, there is usually some evidence of mucosal scarring.

The horse should be confined to a box stall until the fungal lesion is resolved. Stress should be minimized, particularly if a ligation technique alone was employed. Horses that are dysphagic as a result of cranial nerve injury can show improvement, but it may take up to 1 year. It is unlikely that a horse with laryngeal hemiplegia as a result of the mycosis will show significant improvement in laryngeal function.

Comments

The question arises about the potential interference to circulation of the brain when a case of bilateral guttural pouch mycosis is presented for surgical treatment. Both internal carotid arteries can be ligated without neurologic sequelae if the lesion is bilateral (7). Certainly, unilateral ligation or occlusion of the internal carotid artery has no apparent neurologic effects, nor do unilateral internal carotid artery, external carotid, and maxillary artery occlusion using balloon catheters (12). The effects of bilateral occlusion techniques are unknown. As previously mentioned, ligation of the external carotid and palatine arteries has the potential to produce blindness (13). Long-term ligation of both common carotid arteries can produce severe neurologic signs (5).

Surgical debridement of the fungal lesion following ligation or occlusion is not necessary and, in fact, increases the risk for fatal hemorrhage and cranial nerve damage (16).

REFERENCES

1. Cook WR. Observations on the etiology of epistaxis and cranial nerve paralysis in the horse. Vet Rec 1996;78:396.
2. Cook WR, Campbell RSF, Dawson C. Pathology and etiology of guttural pouch mycosis. Vet Rec 1968;83:422–428.
3. Colles CM, Cook WR. Carotid and cerebral angiography in the horse. Vet Rec 1983; 113:483–489.
4. Freeman DE, Ross MW, Donawick WJ, et al. Occlusion of the external carotid and maxillary arteries in the horse to prevent hemorrhage from guttural pouch mycosis. Vet Surg 1989;18:39–47.
5. Feeman DE, Robertson JT, et al. Management of hemorrhage caused by diseases of the guttural pouch. In: Proceedings of the 40th Annual AAEP, Vancouver, British Columbia, 1994:85–86.
6. Owen R ap R. Epistaxis prevented by ligation of the internal carotid artery in the guttural pouch. Equine Vet J 1974;61:143–149.
7. Church S, Wyn-Jones G, Parks AH, et al. Treatment of guttural pouch mycosis. Equine Vet J 1986;18:362–365.
8. Greet TRC. Outcome of treatment in 35 cases of guttural pouch mycosis. Equine Vet J 1987;19:483–487.
9. Freeman DE, Donawick WJ, Klein LV. Effect of ligation on internal carotid artery blood pressure in horses. Vet Surg 1994;23:250–256.
10. Freeman DE, Donawick WJ. Occlusion of internal carotid artery in the horse by

means of a balloon tipped catheter: evaluation of a method designed to prevent epistaxis caused by guttural pouch mycosis. JAVMA 1980;176:232–235.

11. Freeman DE, Donawick WJ. Occlusion of internal carotid artery in the horse by means of a balloon tipped catheter: clinical use of a method to prevent epistaxis caused by guttural pouch mycosis. JAVMA 1980;176:236–240.
12. Freeman DE, Ross MW, Donawick WJ, et al. Occlusion of the external carotid and maxillary arteries in the horse to prevent hemorrhage from guttural pouch mycosis. Vet Surg 1989;18:39–47.
13. Hardy J, Robertson JT, Wilkie DA. Ischemic neuropathy and blindness after arterial occlusion for treatment of guttural pouch mycosis in two horses. JAVMA 1990;196: 1631–1634.
14. Freeman DE, Ross MW, Donawick WJ. "Steal phenomenon" proposed as the cause of blindness after arterial occlusion for treatment of guttural pouch mycosis in horses. JAVMA 1990;197:811–812.
15. Freeman DE, Staller GS, Maxson AD, et al. Unusual internal carotid artery branching that prevented arterial occlusion with a balloon-tipped catheter in a horse. Vet Surg 1993;22:531–534.
16. Freeman DE. Guttural pouches. In: Beech J, ed. Equine Respiratory Disorders. Philadelphia: Lea & Febiger, 1991:305–330.

Surgical Management of Guttural Pouch Tympany (Tympanitis)

Tympany (tympanitis) of the guttural pouch usually results from a failure of the pharyngeal orifice of the eustachian tube to allow escape of air; the defective orifice acts much like a one-way valve, with air entering the pouch but unable to leave it (1–6). The condition is seen in foals and young horses and is considered to be a congenital defect of the pharyngeal opening. The exact cause has been attributed to excessive mucous membrane attached to the medial lamina of the auditory tube cartilage or an abnormally large and redundant plica salpingopharyngea (2). The condition has a higher incidence in fillies (1, 7). It is usually unilateral, but bilateral cases have been observed (5). The animal usually has a nonpainful tympanic swelling of the parotid region. It may be difficult to determine which is the affected guttural pouch because distension will appear on both sides, especially if severe, and may lead the surgeon into thinking the problem is bilateral (1). Percussion of the tympanic swelling will enable one to determine that the swelling is gas and not fluid.

The foal is usually bright and alert with a normal temperature, pulse, and respiration. On exertion there may be signs of upper airway obstruction if the distension is great. Nursing foals may have dysphagia in severe cases, resulting in an accompanying aspiration pneumonia (with fever and moist rales). Milk may appear from the nostrils and a guttural pouch fluid line may be evident on lateral radiographs (1). A dorsoventral radiograph may help determine which side is involved.

Examination of the pharynx with a fiberoptic endoscope will reveal a bulging of the pharyngeal walls. Catheterization of the affected pouch during endoscopic examination will result in immediate reduction in the size of the parotid swelling. The pouch will gradually reinflate when the catheter is removed. If swelling in the parotid area is still evident following deflation of one side, a bilateral condition should be considered (5).

The surgical treatment most commonly employed involves creation of a fistula between the right and left pouches by excising a portion of the medial septum (4, 7). This technique allows the pharyngeal orifice on the healthy side to provide atmospheric pressure to both guttural pouches. In addition, the pharyngeal orifice on the affected side can be enlarged by digitally stretching the opening or by excising mucosa at the opening (4, 7, 8). Bilateral cases are managed with a combination of septal fenestration and excision of mucosa at the pharyngeal orifice (7, 8).

Transendoscopic Nd:YAG laser fenestration of the medial septum has been described and has the advantage of requiring no surgical approach to the guttural pouch (9, 10). There is, therefore, less risk of inadvertent cranial nerve damage. The Nd:YAG laser can also be used to create a salpingopharyngeal fistula caudal and dorsal to the pharyngeal opening of the guttural pouch (10). A combination of medial septum fenestration and salpingopharyngeal fistula formation has been used to treat bilateral tympanitis.

Anesthesia and Surgical Preparation

The conventional fenestration technique is done under general anesthesia. The animal is positioned in dorsal recumbency if a modified Whitehouse approach is made, or in lateral recumbency with the affected side up if the approach is through Viborg's triangle (1, 4, 8). The authors prefer the modified Whitehouse approach because it allows greater access to the guttural pouch.

Preoperative antibiotics should be administered, particularly if aspiration pneumonia is suspected. The surgical area (as illustrated in Figure 6.7, *A* and

B) is clipped and prepared for surgery in a routine manner. Tetanus toxoid is given.

Additional Instrumentation

The procedure requires a flexible fiberoptic endoscope or rigid catheter with an angled tip that can enter the normal guttural pouch. The endoscope or catheter is passed through the nostril of the "normal" side and directed into the "normal" guttural pouch. Malleable retractors will facilitate visualization of the interior of the guttural pouch once the pouch is entered surgically.

Surgical Technique

The guttural pouch classically has been approached through Viborg's triangle, which is the area defined by the tendon of the sternomandibular muscle, the linguofacial (external maxillary) vein, and the caudal border of the vertical ramus of the mandible. A 4- to 6-cm skin incision is made (the size of the skin incision will depend on the size of the patient) just dorsal to and parallel with the linguofacial vein from the border of the mandible caudad (Fig. 6.7, *A* and *B*). The subcutaneous tissue is separated, and the base of the parotid gland is reflected dorsad. Care should be taken to avoid trauma to the parotid gland, linguofacial vein, and the branches of the vagus nerve ventral to the floor of the guttural pouch. In the distended tympanic state, identification of the wall of the guttural pouch is greatly facilitated. Entry into a normal uninflated pouch is difficult. The guttural pouch membrane is grasped and incised with scissors (Fig. 6.7, *C* and *D*).

A modified Whitehouse approach (Fig. 6.7*E*) is made with the foal in dorsal recumbency and the head and neck extended straight out from the body. A 6.8-cm skin incision is made over the distended pouch medial and parallel to the linguofacial vein. The linguofacial vein is separated from thc omohyoideus muscle medially using blunt scissors. The wall of the distended pouch is identified and incised with scissors.

When the affected guttural pouch is entered, the pouch will collapse immediately. At this time, if the opposite pouch appears to remain tympanitic, a bilateral condition should be suspected. With the illumination of the endoscope, its tip will be identified shining through the thin medial septum between the pouches. Alternatively, the angled tip of the mare's catheter is rotated medially and is located by palpation of the catheter through the medial septum. The medial septum is grasped with a pair of Allis tissue forceps, and a generously sized fistula (2 cm $\times$ 2 cm) is created by resecting a portion of the septum with Metzenbaum scissors (Fig. 6.7*D*).

If the condition is bilateral, a long (9-inch) pair of Allis tissue forceps or sponge forceps is passed rostrad through the auditory tube to its pharyngeal orifice. The cartilaginous flap is palpated with the index finger and then grasped with the forceps. A piece of tissue (2.5 cm $\times$ 1.5 cm) is resected. Failure to remove enough tissue and subsequent inflammation and swelling of the new orifice will result in a recurrence of the condition and possibly empyema. This surgical procedure is done in addition to fenestration of the septum. Primary closure of the guttural pouch can be considered; however, the authors prefer to leave the incision open for drainage and allow the wound to heal by second intention.

Postoperative Management

The incision site should be cleaned daily. Irritating solutions should never be flushed into the guttural pouch because of the risk of damage to the major

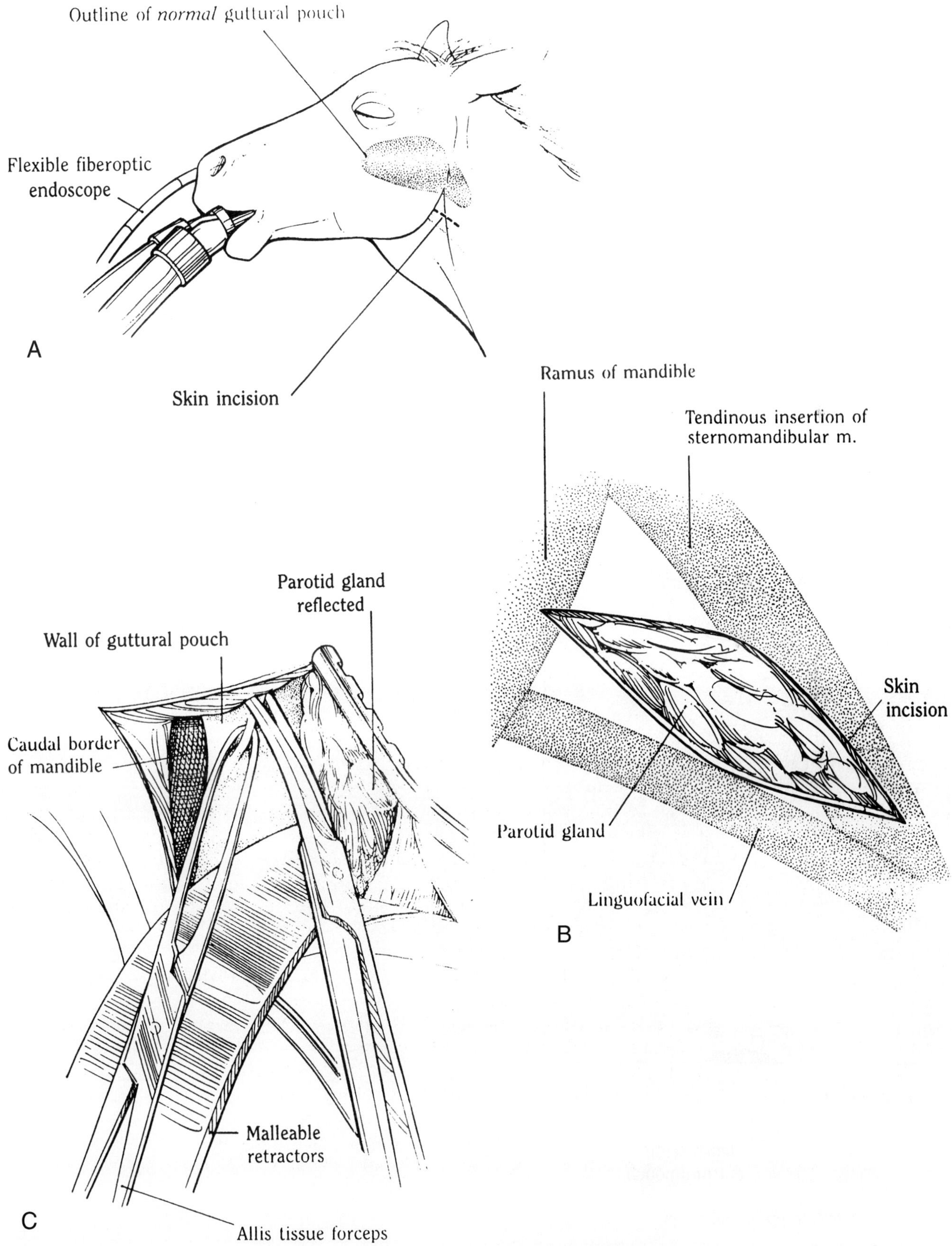

FIGURE 6.7, A–C. Surgical correction of guttural pouch tympany. Approach through Viborg's triangle.

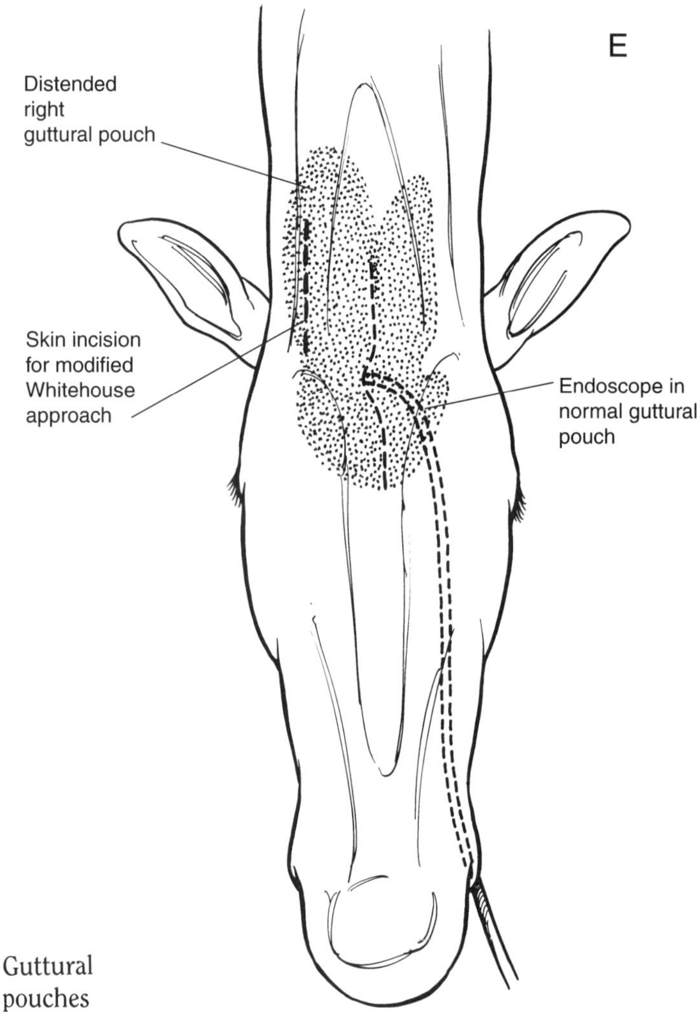

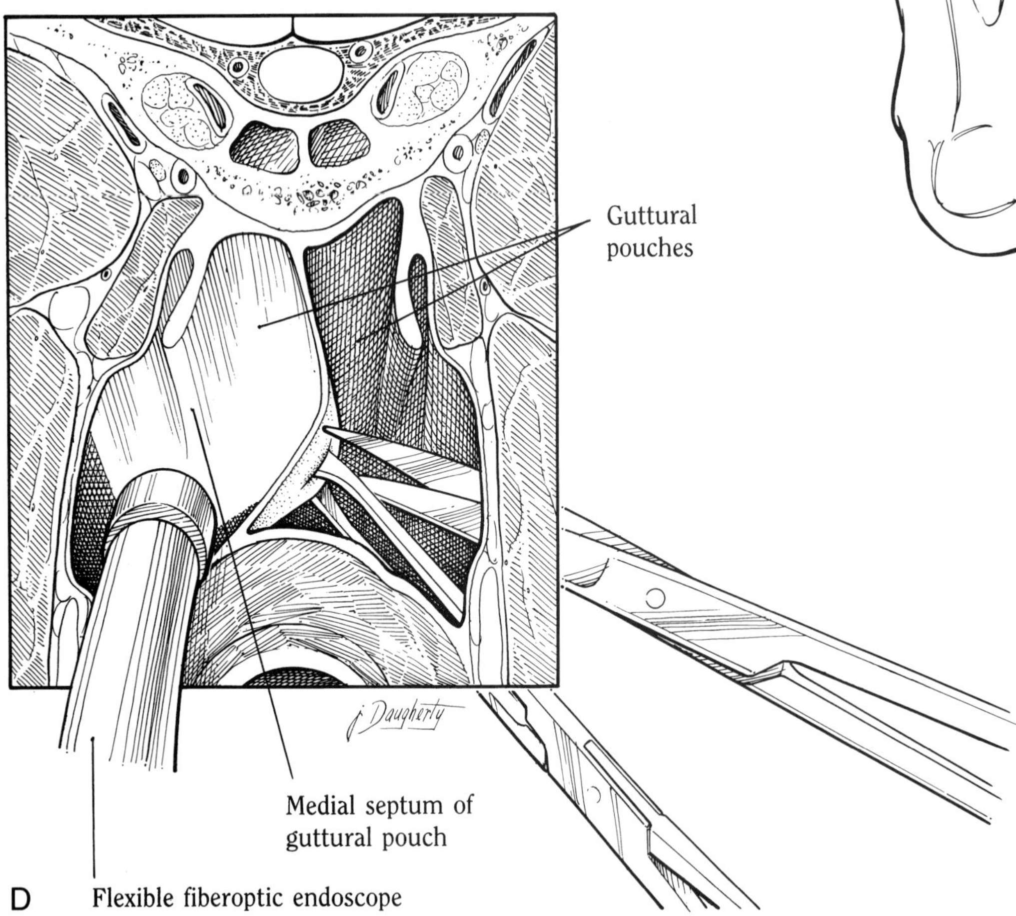

Figure 6.7. *(continued)* **D.** Surgical correction of guttural pouch tympany. **E.** Modified Whitehouse approach to guttural pouch.

nerves and blood vessels that are in close proximity to the guttural pouch. In a case uncomplicated by aspiration pneumonia or guttural pouch empyema, postoperative antibiotics are optional. Postoperative broad-spectrum antibiotics would be required if these conditions did exist.

Comments

In the absence of pneumonia or guttural pouch empyema, the prognosis for successful resolve of a unilateral tympanitis is excellent. The surgical procedure is relatively quick and easy to perform, and an immediate improvement will be noticed if sufficient fenestration between the pouches has been created. If immediate improvement in the foal's condition is not evident, then bilateral involvement should be suspected (1). If initial improvement is observed but the condition recurs, closure of the medial septum should be suspected. This can occur if a small septal window is created and the defect closes as the tissue heals. This could be confirmed by endoscopy of the guttural pouches.

The surgery, regardless the surgical approach or technique used to create the medial septum fenestration, has the potential to produce cranial nerve damage that can produce dysphagia or dyspnea, particularly if the larynx is affected. These neurologic effects may be temporary and improve as inflammation subsides, or they can be permanent. Clients must be informed of the risks of this surgery and warned of the possibility of neurologic damage as a result of surgery.

REFERENCES

1. Freeman DF. Diagnosis and treatment of diseases of the guttural pouch. I. Compend Con Educ Pract Vet 1980;2:503.
2. Haynes PF. Surgery of the equine respiratory tract. In: Jennings PB, ed. Textbook of Large Animal Surgery. I. Philadelphia: WB Saunders, 1984:462.
3. Mason TA. Tympany of the eustachian tube diverticulosis (guttural pouch) in a foal. Equine Vet J 1972;4:153.
4. Milne DW, Fessler JF. Tympanitis of the guttural pouch in a foal. JAVMA 1972;161: 61.
5. Raker CW. Diseases of the guttural pouch. Mod Vet Pract 1976;57:549.
6. Wheat JD. Tympanitis of the guttural pouch of the horse. JAVMA 1962;140:453.
7. McCue PM, Freeman DE, Donawick WJ. Guttural pouch tympany: 15 cases (1977–1986). JAVMA 1989;194:1761–1763.
8. Freeman DE. Guttural pouch tympany. In: White NA, Moore JN, eds. Current Practice of Equine Surgery. Philadelphia: JB Lippincott, 1990:249–251.
9. Tetens J, Tulleners EP, Ross MW, et al. Transendoscopic contact neodymium:yttrium aluminum garnet laser treatment of tympany of the auditory tube diverticulum in two foals. JAVMA 1994;204:1927–1929.
10. Tate LP, Blikslager AT, Little EDE. Transendoscopic laser treatment of guttural pouch tympanitis in eight foals. Vet Surg 1995;24:367–372.

Nasal Septum Resection

Resection of the nasal septum is indicated if septal thickening or deviation is causing upper airway obstruction. The causes of thickening of the nasal septum in the horse are chronic inflammation secondary to trauma, infection, congenital cystic degeneration, or, rarely, neoplasia (1). In athletic horses during strenuous exercise, high airflow through the nasal passages is essential. Narrowing of the nasal passages will produce abnormal noise and exercise intolerance. Fiberoptic examination and radiographic evaluation of the septum are important adjuncts to the physical examination when such a case is encountered. This should enable the surgeon to evaluate the extent and site of the septal deformity (1–3).

Anesthesia and Surgical Preparation

Because the surgical procedure is accompanied by considerable hemorrhage, preoperative physical evaluation should include a complete blood count and a hemogram. A cross match for blood transfusion is indicated *in every case.* For marginally anemic horses, blood should be taken from the appropriate donor and be readily available in the surgery (1, 3). Blood may also be obtained from the patient and stored for autotransfusion (1). Anemic horses should receive a blood transfusion or, alternatively, the cause of the anemia should be diagnosed, treated, and corrected before surgery is performed. The procedure is an elective one, and practice on a cadaver head is recommended. This will enable the surgeon to proceed as rapidly as possible to minimize blood loss. There is no other surgery that exemplifies the adage "time is of the essence" more than nasal septum removal in the horse. In addition, all horses, regardless the anesthetic risk, should receive judicious fluid replacement in the form of balanced polyionic solutions throughout the operation to minimize hypotension. Preoperative antibiotics and phenylbutazone should be administered. Tetanus toxoid is also given preoperatively.

Nasal septum resection is done under general anesthesia with the patient in left or right lateral recumbency. The area between the medial canthi of the eyes and rostral ends of the facial crests is clipped in preparation for the trephination of the nasal cavity and surgically prepared. The midcervical area should be clipped in preparation for a tracheostomy.

Additional Instrumentation

This procedure requires a guarded chisel. These chisels may not be readily available from commercial instrument manufacturers but are readily made by any metal worker/blacksmith (Fig. 6.8*A*). Also needed are a 1-inch trephine, Ochsner or Doyen forceps, sterile cotton gauze, a tracheostomy tube, and vulsellum forceps. Obstetrical wire, long instruments, flexible artificial insemination pipettes, and an endoscope equipped with biopsy forceps are required for an alternative technique that will also be discussed.

Surgical Technique

An 8- to 10-cm skin incision is made exactly on the midline of the face commencing immediately rostral to the frontal sinuses (where the nasal bones begin to diverge slightly caudal to the level of the rostral aspect of the facial crest) (1, 3) (Fig. 6.8*B*). The skin edges are retracted with towel clamps, and the periosteum is quartered and reflected. A 25-mm (1-inch) circular trephine hole is made directly on the midline of the face, and the bone is removed and discarded. The nasal septum will now be visible. Ochsner or Doyen forceps are then inserted through the trephine hole, perforating mucous membrane with each blade on either side of the septum, until the floor of the nasal passage is felt. The forceps

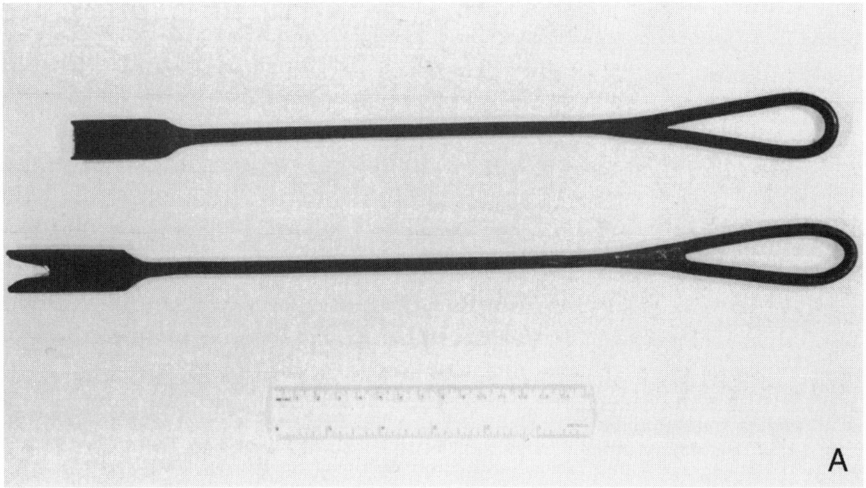

FIGURE 6.8, A. Two different types of guarded chisels that are suitable for nasal septum removal.

should be directed perpendicularly and then closed on the nasal septum (Fig. 6.8*C*).

Moving to the external nares, the surgeon palpates the nasal septum through the uppermost nostril to determine how much of the rostral portion of the septum is unthickened and can be preserved. Incising the lateral ala of the uppermost nostril can be performed to gain better access to the rostral portion of the septum. The surgeon then incises through the rostral aspect of the septum from dorsal to ventral, just caudal to the alar cartilages. This incision should be convex, with the convex surface facing rostrally. This will maintain the support to the alar cartilages (Fig. 6.8, *D* and *E*). If the surgeon wishes to have more exposure of the cranial portion of the nasal septum to facilitate making the rostral septal incision and placement of the guarded chisel, the lateral ala of the external nares can be incised (4).

At this point, surgery must proceed rapidly, as hemorrhage will be profuse. With the guarded chisel, the dorsal and ventral attachments of the septum are severed by forcing the chisel along the nasal septum until it meets the forceps. This may take a few attempts because the chisel may slip off the septum or the septum may be sufficiently thickened that several firm thrusts of the instrument are required to completely sever all dorsal and ventral attachments (Fig. 6.8*F*).

The caudal attachment is severed rostral to the Ochsner or Doyen forceps with a chisel or osteotome. The septum is then grasped firmly with vulsellum forceps and extracted from the nasal cavity. If the septum is still firmly anchored in the nasal cavity, further attempts should be made to sever it dorsally and ventrally with the guarded chisel. Attachments at the caudal end of the septum can be severed with scissors or with an osteotome introduced into the trephine hole.

An alternative technique for incising the nasal septum has been used by the authors, particularly if it is necessary to remove as much of the septum as possible. The principles of the surgery are the same as with the technique just described; however, the dorsal, ventral, and caudal incisions are made using obstetric wires placed after the trephine opening is made. A more oblique cut is made in the caudal septum, just rostral to the ethmoid and sphenopalatine sinus (Fig. 6.8*G*). Three wires are preplaced using long instruments, flexible AI pipettes, and an endoscope equipped with biopsy forceps. The first wire is passed up one nasal passage into the nasopharynx, then grasped and drawn out through the nasal passage and nostril of the opposite side. This wire will be used to sever the ventral attachment of the septum. This wire should be

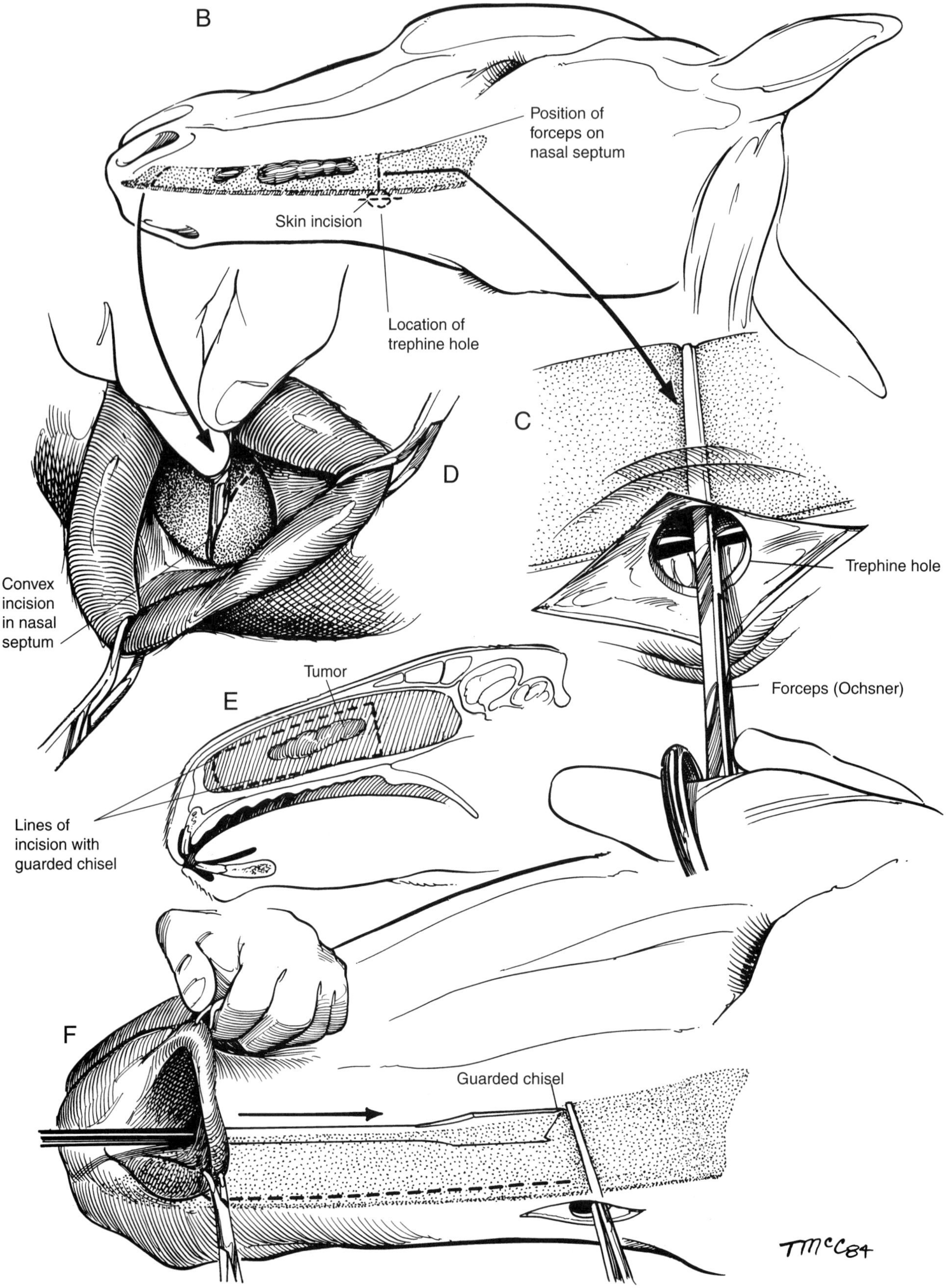

Figure 6.8, B–F. *(continued)* Nasal septum removal.

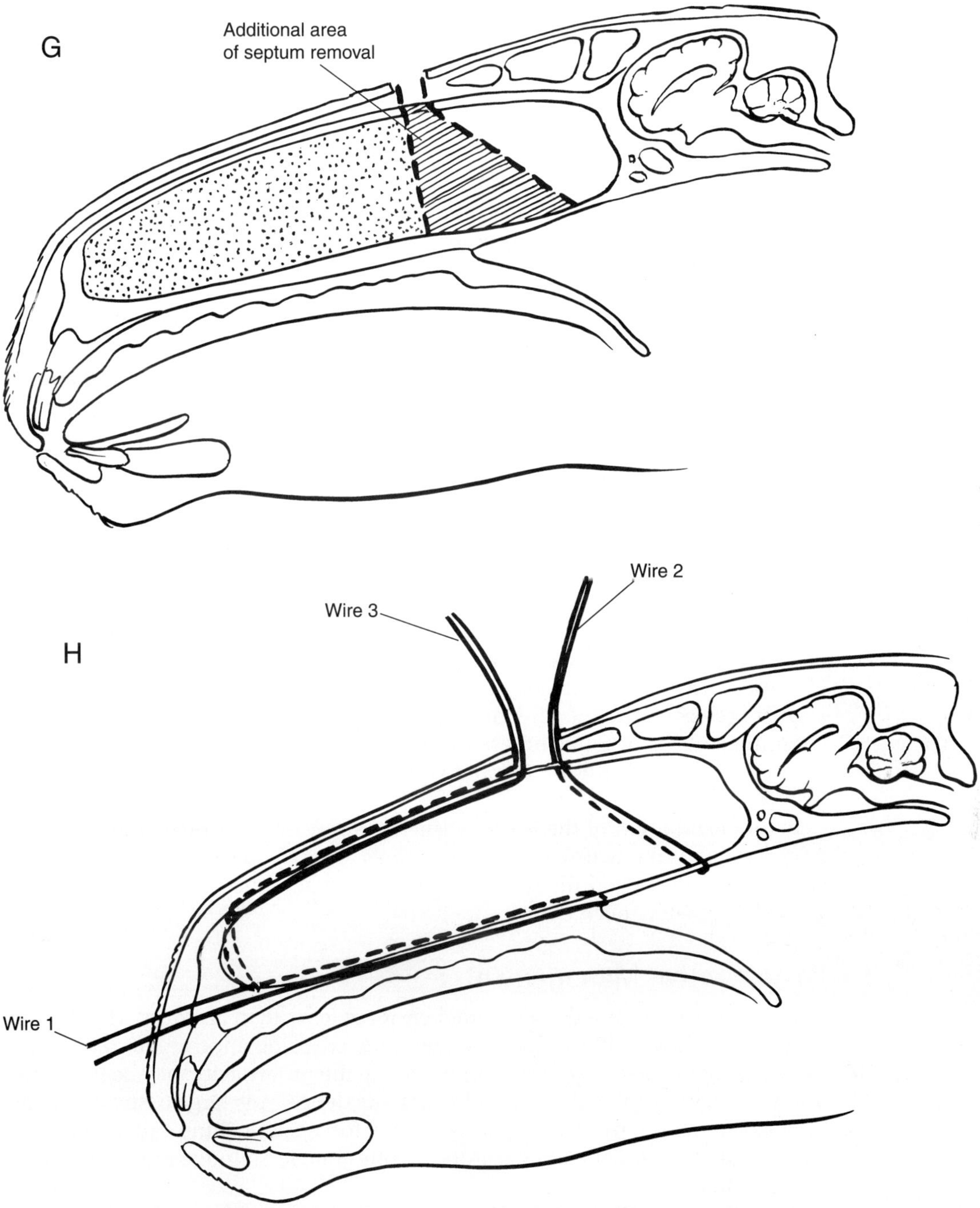

FIGURE 6.8, G–H. *(continued)* Nasal septum removal.

passed before the trephination is made. A second wire is passed through the trephine hole in a caudal and ventral direction, adjacent to the nasal septum, passed under the nasal septum, then grasped and drawn out through the trephine hole on the opposite side of the septum. One end of a third wire is passed forward through the trephine opening into the nasal cavity on the down side and brought out that nostril. The incision on the rostral aspect of the septum is then made with a scalpel, and the end of the third wire is drawn through the most dorsal aspect of this incision and passed up the nasal passage of the up side, then grasped and drawn out through the trephine opening (Fig. 6.8*H*).

This wire will sever the dorsal attachments of the septum. Flexible AI pipettes can be used as conduits to pass wires 2 and 3. The end of the ventral wire that is exiting from the nostril of the down side is passed through the most ventral aspect of the rostral septal incision in preparation for cutting. In turn, each of these wires is pulled in a sawing motion using handles, and the amputation of the septum is completed.

Gauze is then packed into the nasal cavity from the trephine hole and through the external nares. The packing should be inserted as tightly as possible to achieve a tamponade effect to reduce the hemorrhage. The gauze can be anchored at the nostrils by horizontal mattress sutures using no. 2 nylon, but it should not require anchoring at the trephine hole.

If the more caudal portion of the nasal septum is resected, it is more difficult to pack gauze against the caudal stump to reduce the hemorrhage. There is a risk of the packing falling into the nasopharynx and the possibility of the horse swallowing some of the gauze. This problem can be avoided if a closed-ended stockinette is pushed through the trephine opening and the packing then pushed with sponge forceps into the open end of the stockinette. The stockinette will expand as more gauze is pushed into the opening, and eventually enough gauze is introduced to put pressure on the caudal stump. Gauze packing can also be introduced into the nasal passages through the nose.

The alar folds can be resected in conjunction with the nasal septal resection in a further attempt to streamline airflow. A few interrupted sutures of 2/0 synthetic suture material can be used to appose the skin and mucous membrane over the alar cartilage. Each nostril can be packed with gauze to prevent hemorrhage. If the nostril on the upper side of the horse was incised as part of the procedure, it must be reconstructed. The inner layer of the nostril is sutured with a simple continuous layer of 2/0 synthetic absorbable suture material. The remaining layers are apposed with interrupted vertical mattress sutures of size 0 polypropylene.

Before extubation of the horse, a tracheostomy is performed, and a suitable tracheostomy tube is inserted and *anchored securely* in place. If the tracheostomy tube is dislodged the horse may be asphyxiated because the nasal cavity will be completely occluded.

Postoperative Management

Antibiotics are continued postoperatively for at least 48 to 72 hours. The packing should be removed 48 to 72 hours after surgery, using appropriate restraint of the horse. Some bleeding will occur. Flushing the nasal cavity may be indicated. This will aid removal of dried blood and tissue debris. Any large tissue fragments or clots can be removed gently with sponge forceps. Flushing can be achieved using water at ambient temperature or physiologic saline solution in a bulb syringe (3).

The trephine hole is cleaned once or twice daily with gauze sponges and allowed to heal by second intention. The tracheostomy site is managed similarly. Horses that have been scheduled for athletic endeavors should be examined with a fiberoptic endoscope to monitor the healing process. The horse will require approximately 2 months' rest before returning to work (3).

Comments

Complications following nasal septum resection are common. In the largest series of cases published to date, complications included persistence of noise and respiratory difficulty, excessive granulation tissue and adhesions at the caudal incised edge, and inability to remove the entire resected septum (3). In an attempt to minimize these complications, it has been recommended that the caudal edge of the septum be amputated by making a *more oblique cut*, ensuring removal of more septum (Fig. 6.8, *G* and *H*). The oblique cut edge is just rostral to the ethmoid and sphenopalatine sinus and dorsal to the soft palate. Excessive granulation tissue in this region is less likely to cause narrowing or adhesions to the conchae, which would result in airflow turbulence, because the nasal passage is much wider at this point (3). If the original cause of thickening of the nasal septum was a neoplastic process, recurrence of the tumor is always a possibility.

The complication arising from the removal of too much cartilage rostrally is a flattening of the bridge of the nose near the nasal diverticula. Nasal deformity is likely to occur if nasal septal surgery is performed in foals under 6 months of age, regardless how much cartilage is left rostrally. Occasionally it is necessary to remove portions of the nasal septum in foals with a congenital nasal septal cyst or during correction of a severe wry nose.

REFERENCES

1. Haynes PF. The respiratory system. In: Jennings PB, ed. The Practice of Large Animal Surgery. Philadelphia: WB Saunders, 1984:400.
2. Stilson AE, Herring DS, Robertson JT. Contribution of the nasal septum to the radiographic anatomy of the equine nasal cavity. JAVMA 1985;186:590.
3. Tulleners EP, Raker CW. Nasal septum resection in the horse. Vet Surg 1983;12:41.
4. Nickels FA, Tulleners EP. Nasal passages. In: Auer JA, ed. Equine Surgery. Philadelphia: WB Saunders, 1992:433.

Paranasal Sinus Exploration

The paranasal sinuses can be examined endoscopically with a 4.0-mm arthroscope introduced through portals in the frontal, caudal maxillary, or rostral maxillary sinuses (1, 2). Endoscopic examination of the sinuses can provide useful diagnostic information and can even be combined with therapeutic debridement, lavage, and aspiration if the lesion is amenable to such an approach. The procedure can be done in the standing sedated horse using local anesthesia.

Surgical treatment of extensive sinus diseases is best accomplished with the use of a bone flap or flaps (3, 4). Compared to the traditional trephine technique, creating a bone flap allows for greater exposure of the paranasal sinus region. The end result is more satisfactory cosmetically than multiple trephine holes in which the circular pieces of bone and skin are discarded. The bone flap technique is preferred for gaining surgical access in cases of chronic primary sinusitis complicated by accumulation of inspissated exudate, particularly within the ventral conchal sinus; in horses with secondary sinusitis in which exposure of the tooth roots is required for tooth repulsion; and in horses with ethmoid hematomas, sinus cysts, and other sinus masses, including cryptococcal granulomas and neoplasms (3–6).

Bone Flap Technique: Anesthesia and Surgical Preparation

The surgery is performed with the horse under general anesthesia with the affected side uppermost. The surgical site(s) over the affected sinus(es) is clipped and prepared for surgery in a routine manner. It is imperative that the cuff on the endotracheal tube be inflated adequately to prevent the drainage of blood and exudate down the trachea. If a great deal of bleeding is expected, blood can be collected from a suitable cross-matched donor for intraoperative transfusion. Broad-spectrum preoperative antibiotics are indicated, regardless the type of sinus surgery. Tetanus prophylaxis is also provided.

Additional Instrumentation

The bone flap technique requires an osteotome or chisel, a small mallet, stainless steel wire, a hand drill, and a small drill bit. Sterile gauze packing should be available in abundance. A mare's catheter should also be available. An oscillatory bone saw can be used to create the bone flap as an alternative to creating it with the osteotome or chisel. Other instruments such as dental punches, rongeurs, and curettes may be required depending on the disease.

Surgical Technique

Maxillary Sinus Flap

A curved skin incision is made to create a three-sided flap as shown in Figure 6.9*A*. The incision is made over the rostral, ventral, and caudal borders of the maxillary sinus. The skin and subcutaneous tissues are left attached. Frequently, branches of the facial vessels that cross the proposed cranial incision line must be ligated and divided. Usually the levator labii superioris and levator nasolabialis muscles are reflected dorsad rather than incised. The subcutaneous tissues and the periosteum are incised on the same three sides as the skin incision. There is no need to do any periosteal elevation or reflection. The bone is then cut along the same margins.

A variety of instruments have been recommended to cut the bone. An oscillat-

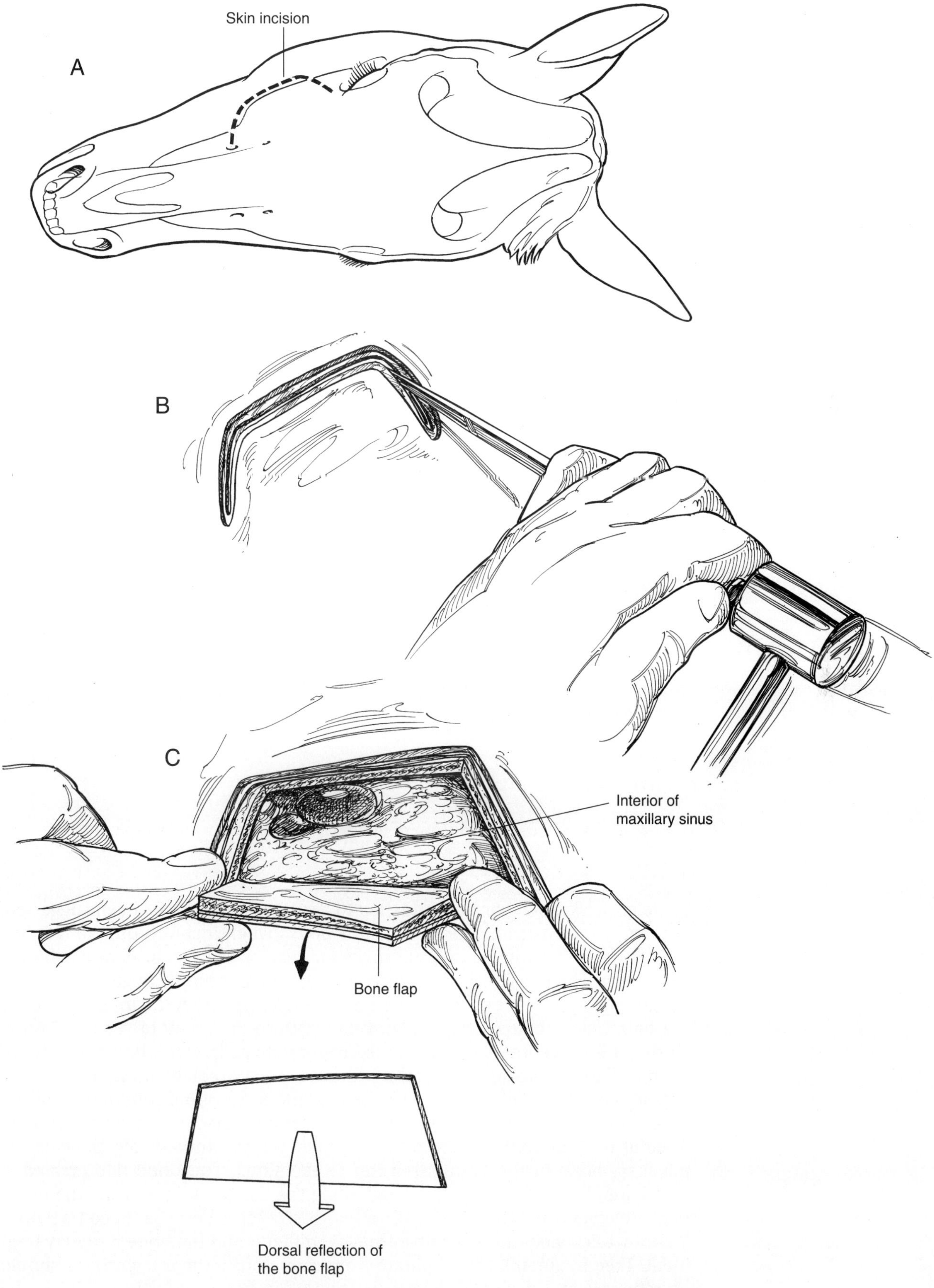

FIGURE 6.9, A–C. Bone flap technique for sinus exploration.

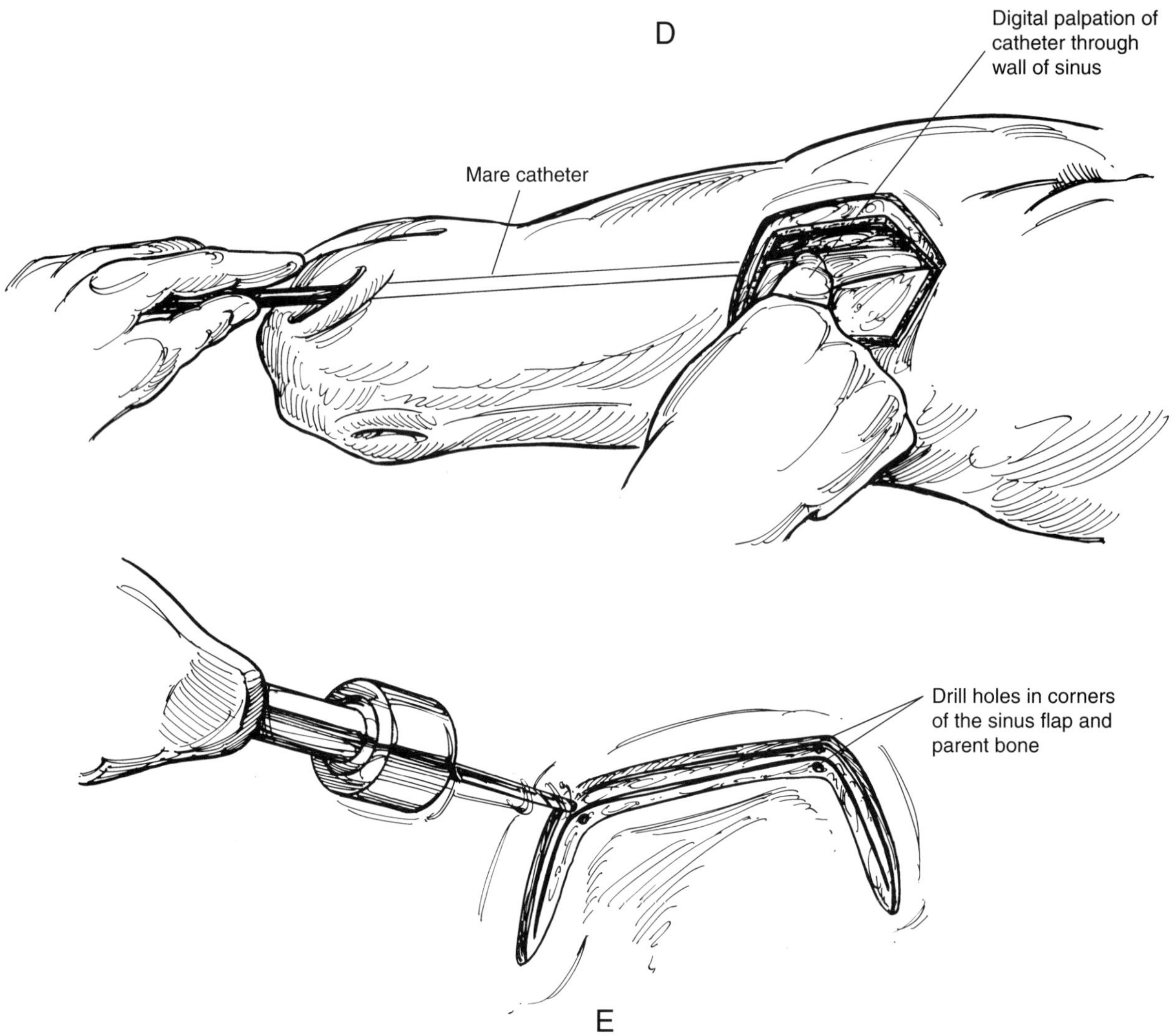

Figure 6.9, D–E. *(continued)* Bone flap technique for sinus exploration.

ing (e.g., Stryker) saw or burr attached to a surgical air drill has been suggested, but both these instruments leave a bony defect when it comes time to reattach the bone flap. A simpler way is to make an incision with a chisel or osteotome (Fig. 6.9*B*). The incision by the chisel is made on an oblique angle to the bone surface such that the external surface is slightly larger than the inner surface of the flap. This produces a better dovetail pattern and a more secure closure. During this procedure care should be taken not to go beyond the boundaries of the maxillary sinus and damage the osseous nasolacrimal duct, which is located dorsally in the maxillary sinus, or damage the intraorbital foramen or nerve. Care should also be taken, particularly in a young horse, not to incise into the alveolus over the root of a cheek tooth, which may lay immediately beneath the maxillary bone in the cranial portion of the sinus. The bone flap created is then carefully elevated and fractured along the dorsal margin, using the intact periosteum and soft tissues as a hinge (Fig. 6.9*C*). If the bone has become pathologically thickened, this maneuver may be difficult and the bone flap may fragment. Free fragments that separate from their soft tissue attachments should be removed and discarded. Once the bone flap has been reflected back, the sinus can be examined and surgery within the sinus can be carried out. Proce-

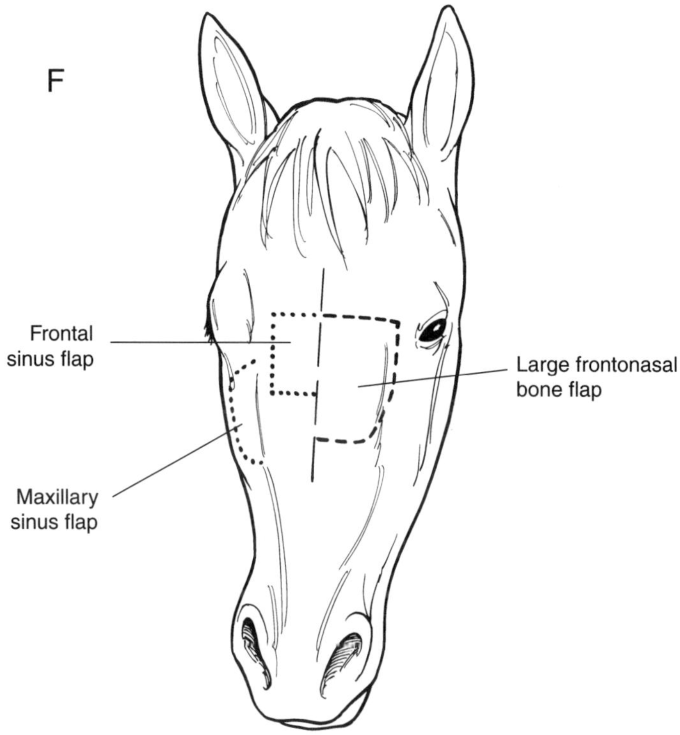

FIGURE 6.9, F. *(continued)* Bone flap technique for sinus exploration.

dures such as tooth repulsion, ablation of a sinus cyst, removal of hypertrophic sinus mucosa, and culture and biopsy can be done. This approach does allow access to the ventral conchal sinus through a narrow space over the infraorbital canal, but evacuation of inspissated material is difficult, especially in younger horses with reduced space. A window can be created in the bony plate beneath the intraorbital canal to allow access to the ventral conchal sinus. In a young horse, where the reserve crowns extend high into the bony plate beneath the infraorbital canal, such a window is only possible after tooth repulsion (3, 4).

It is critical for success of a sinus procedure to ensure adequate postoperative and long-term drainage. In long-standing cases of sinusitis, it is usually necessary to create an opening between the maxillary sinus and the nasal passage. This can be achieved by placing a finger through the conchomaxillary opening (over the infraorbital canal) into the ventral conchal sinus and palpating the medial conchal wall. A mare's catheter is passed up the nasal cavity on the same side and manipulated so that the curved tip is palpable through the wall (Fig. 6.9*D*). The catheter tip is then forced through the conchal wall. This usually creates a great deal of hemorrhage. The opening can be enlarged by spreading scissors or by attaching a length of gauze (seton) to the end of the catheter and then drawing the gauze through a new (or reopened) orifice exiting out the external nares. Drawing the gauze back and forth a number of times will enlarge a new opening and ensure long-term patency. The sinus can then be packed with gauze, which can be connected to the nasal seton and ultimately removed through the nose, or, alternatively, the sinus packing can be exited through a small opening rongeured on one corner of the bone flap. The nasal packing should be secured with a suture to the nostril.

Small gauge wires are passed through holes drilled in the corners of the flap (Fig. 6.9*E*), and the parent bone and the ends are twisted. The wires should not be tightened so vigorously that they cut through the bone, and the ends of the wire sutures should be bent down toward the bone using a needle holder. The periosteum and subcutaneous tissues are apposed with 2/0 absorbable suture material, simple interrupted pattern, and the skin is closed using a suture material and pattern of the surgeon's choice or skin staples.

Frontonasal Bone Flap

A large frontonasal bone flap (6 cm wide × 10 cm long) can be created to allow access to the frontal and conchofrontal sinus as well as to the caudal maxillary sinus, the ventral conchal sinus, and the sphenopalatine sinus (4). The frontonasal bone flap is more versatile than either the maxillary or frontal bone flaps and is useful for exposure and treatment of extensive conditions such as sinus cyst, ethmoidal hematoma, fungal lesions, neoplasia, and empyema, particularly sinusitis complicated by inspissated exudate in the ventral conchal sinus. This flap does not provide access to the rostral compartment of the maxillary sinus. Therefore, the fourth premolar and first molar must be accessed through a maxillary sinus flap.

The base of the frontonasal flap is on the dorsal midline and its margins are as follows: caudally, a line at right angles to dorsal midline and situated midway between the supraorbital foramen and the medial canthus of the eye; laterally, 2 to 2.5 cm medial to the medial canthus of the eye and angling medially as it approaches the nasolacrimal duct rostrally (the course of the nasolacrimal duct can be approximated by drawing a line between the medial canthus of the eye and the nasoincisive notch); rostrally, the margin is a line at right angles to dorsal midline, approximately 10 cm from the caudal margin (Fig. 6.9*F*). The flap is elevated and fractured along its base.

Following the corrective surgery, gauze packing is usually required to control hemorrhage. If a large sinus or ethmoidal mass has been removed, there is frequently a direct communication between the sinus and the nasopharynx. Care should be taken not to push the packing into the nasopharynx. The packing can exit through the nose or through an opening created in the bone flap. Flap closure is similar to that described for a maxillary flap.

Frontal Sinus Flap

A smaller flap can be created over the frontal sinus to gain access to a lesion that is confined solely to the frontal sinus, or it can be used in conjunction with a maxillary sinus flap for access to a lesion that involves both sinuses (Fig. 6.9*F*).

Postoperative Management

The gauze packing should be left in place for a minimum of 48 hours and then removed completely. Hemorrhage may follow gauze removal; however, if the horse is left alone, the bleeding will soon stop. If the horse hemorrhages a great deal during surgery, it is advisable to check the PCV and total protein level before pulling the packing. Leaving the packing in place for 72 hours may reduce some of the bleeding. If flushing of the sinus is required, a small lavage tube can be passed through a hole at the corner of the flap and anchored to the face with nonabsorbable retention sutures.

Sinuses can be irrigated twice daily until the discharge becomes noticeably less purulent. Very dilute povidone-iodine (Betadine) solution is satisfactory, although the mechanical rinsing and draining is probably more important than the content of the flush.

Phenylbutazone may be indicated in certain patients following surgery. Antibiotics may be continued postoperatively in cases of sinus infection.

Comments

The location and size of a bone flap(s) is determined preoperatively based on the clinical and radiographic findings and on the anticipated location and extent of the lesion. Occasionally during surgery it will be determined that access through one flap is not satisfactory and a second flap is required. In such a case, the surgeon should be considerate of the blood supply to the areas of both flaps and not compromise the vascular integrity of either area. Practically, it is always better to create a flap that may be larger than required than to be compromised by a flap that is too small. Healing of the bone flap and the associated skin is usually excellent regardless the size of the flap. It is important, however, that the flap is secured firmly to the parent bone and remains stable and that the soft tissue attachments to the flap are left intact to avoid sequestration. If the bone flap is not secure or the bone sequestrates and sloughs, an unsightly depression can occur at the site.

REFERENCES

1. Ruggles AJ, Ross MW, Freeman DE. Endoscopic examination of normal paranasal sinuses in horses. Vet Surg 1991;20(6):418–423.
2. Ruggles AJ, Ross MW, Freeman DE. Endoscopic examination and treatment of paranasal sinus disease in 16 horses. Vet Surg 1993;22(6):508–514.
3. Freeman DE. Paranasal sinuses. In: Beech J, ed. Equine Respiratory Disorders. Philadelphia: Lea & Febiger, 1991:275–303.
4. Freeman DE, Orsini PG, Ross MW, et al. A large frontonasal bone flap for sinus surgery in the horse. Vet Surg 1990;19:122–130.
5. Schumaker J, Honnas C, Smith B. Paranasal sinusitis complicated by inspissated exudate in the ventral conchal sinus. Vet Surg 1987;16:373–377.
6. Lane JG, Longstaffe JA, Gibbs C. Equine paranasal sinus cysts: a report of 15 cases. Equine Vet J 1987;19:537.

Surgical Repair of Depression Fractures of the Skull

Fractures of the facial bones and cranial vault are seen occasionally in horses. Fractures of the cranial vault are usually fatal because of the associated neurologic problems (1, 2). Fractures of the facial bones in horses are amenable to various reconstructive techniques (2–11).

Nasofacial fractures that remain closed with minimal displacement can be managed conservatively without surgery. Open fractures of the facial bones with considerable displacement should be repaired because facial deformity, bone sequestration, and sinusitis may occur. Cosmetic results are important in show animals. Reconstruction should be preferably an elective procedure when the animal has been physiologically stabilized (7). The exception would be orbital or periorbital fractures causing pressure on the globe, or excessive tension on the optic nerve because the eye is being proptosed. Bone fragments can project into the orbit causing damage to the globe. In such circumstances, emergency reconstruction of the orbital rim and return of the eye to its socket are required to minimize the chance of permanent blindness and to prevent further damage to the eye (2, 9, 10). The other indication for immediate surgery is a fracture of the cranium with a deterioration in vital signs, progressive pupillary dilation, and depressed consciousness, or an open fracture extending into the cranial vault (1, 2).

Anesthesia and Surgical Preparation

Epistaxis frequently occurs when the nasal mucosa has been torn; hence, blood loss may make the animal an anesthetic risk. In such cases, the horse should be stabilized before surgery. Correction of any fluid or electrolyte imbalance before anesthesia is important. Blood transfusions are generally not necessary in most skull fractures, but those with extensive trauma should at least be cross matched with a suitable available donor, and a thorough neurologic evaluation should be performed.

Anesthesiologists should be aware that there may be an undetectable brain injury that could affect the horse in the perioperative or postoperative period. Certain anesthetic measures can be taken to minimize the possibility of increased intracranial pressure during the perioperative period. Some horses with intracranial hemorrhage associated with the original injury appear stable and nonneurologic preoperatively, but deteriorate neurologically in the postoperative period as a result of increased intracranial pressure (12).

Most depression fractures of the facial bones are open because the mucous membrane of the sinus or nasal cavity is frequently lacerated. It is advisable to begin antibiotic therapy, especially if surgery is to be delayed while the horse is being stabilized. Because of the rich blood supply to the head, it is the authors' opinion that surgical management (debridement, fracture reduction, irrigation, and wound closure) is the key to success in such fractures. Broad-spectrum perioperative antibiotics are advised.

If there has been severe impairment of nasal cavity function as a result of displacement of bone and soft tissues, tracheostomy may be indicated. The tracheostomy site should be clipped and prepared for surgery in a routine manner. Following induction of anesthesia, the horse can then be intubated through the tracheostomy. Alternatively, intubation can be done in the normal manner through the mouth and a suitable tracheostomy tube inserted through a tracheostomy when the horse is standing following the recovery from anesthesia.

The procedure is always done with the horse under general anesthesia and in lateral recumbency. The location of the depression fracture will dictate whether the horse will be positioned in right or left lateral recumbency (Fig. 6.10*A*).

Additional Instrumentation

This procedure requires periosteal elevators, a bone hook or elevator, 18- or 20-gauge stainless steel wire, wire twisters, a hand drill, and small drill bits.

Surgical Technique

Because of the variability in the configuration of depression fractures, it is impossible to describe a standard technique. Instead, we discuss general principles.

Large curvilinear skin incisions or generous S-shaped incisions extending well beyond the margins of the involved bones should be used to expose the fracture site (7) (Fig. 6.10*A*). Reduction of the fracture with the aid of a periosteal elevator should be done patiently, being careful not to detach bone fragments from their blood supply (Fig. 6.10*B*). The authors have found that during reduction of the fracture it is advantageous to elevate using as many points of contact under the fragment as possible to minimize the chances of the fragment splitting into smaller pieces. Once reduction is achieved, if the fragments are unstable they can be maintained in position with 18- to 20-gauge stainless steel wire (Fig. 6.10, *C* and *D*). Holes should be drilled in the loose fragments with the appropriately sized drill bit, approximately 0.5 cm from the fracture edge. The fragment(s) should be supported during the drilling process. Corresponding holes in the surrounding stable bone also should be drilled. Pieces of wire should now be inserted and preplaced. Reduction of the fracture can now be commenced. When reduction of the fracture is satisfactory, the wire sutures are secured by twisting. The wire twists should be bent over and be smooth to the touch, thereby avoiding pressure necrosis on the overlying skin flap. Care must be taken not to twist the wire too tightly or it will cut through the fragile bone. Small pieces of bone devoid of periosteum that cannot be rigidly stabilized should be discarded because of potential formation of sequestra. Defects may exist when the repair is completed, but the final appearance is usually satisfactory if the surrounding bones are flush with the normal contours of the face.

If a large defect exists because bone fragments have become loose and devoid of periosteum or are missing, the surgeon may consider filling the defect with synthetic mesh. This technique has also been used for filling a defect remaining after removal of an everted sinus in a horse (8). To secure the mesh, holes are drilled around the edge of the defect, and the mesh is sutured in place using interrupted horizontal mattress sutures of a suitable braided synthetic suture material, such as Mersilene. The sutures are placed through the mesh and the holes. The edges of the mesh can be sutured to the subcutaneous tissue with a synthetic absorbable suture material (8).

Following reduction of the fracture or implantation of the mesh, the skin is sutured. The use of a synthetic intradermal suture improves the cosmetic appearance. However, this pattern can be used only when tension of the incision has been relieved by a strong subcutaneous suture layer and the wound edges are almost in apposition before beginning this suture (7).

Fractures of the orbital rim also can be reconstructed by the principles described above. It is important to be sure that no retrobulbar fracture fragments remain after reduction of the fracture. This can be determined by digital palpation of the conjunctival fornix during surgery.

A noninvasive technique for reduction of simple closed zygomatic process fractures has been described. With the horse under general anesthesia and the

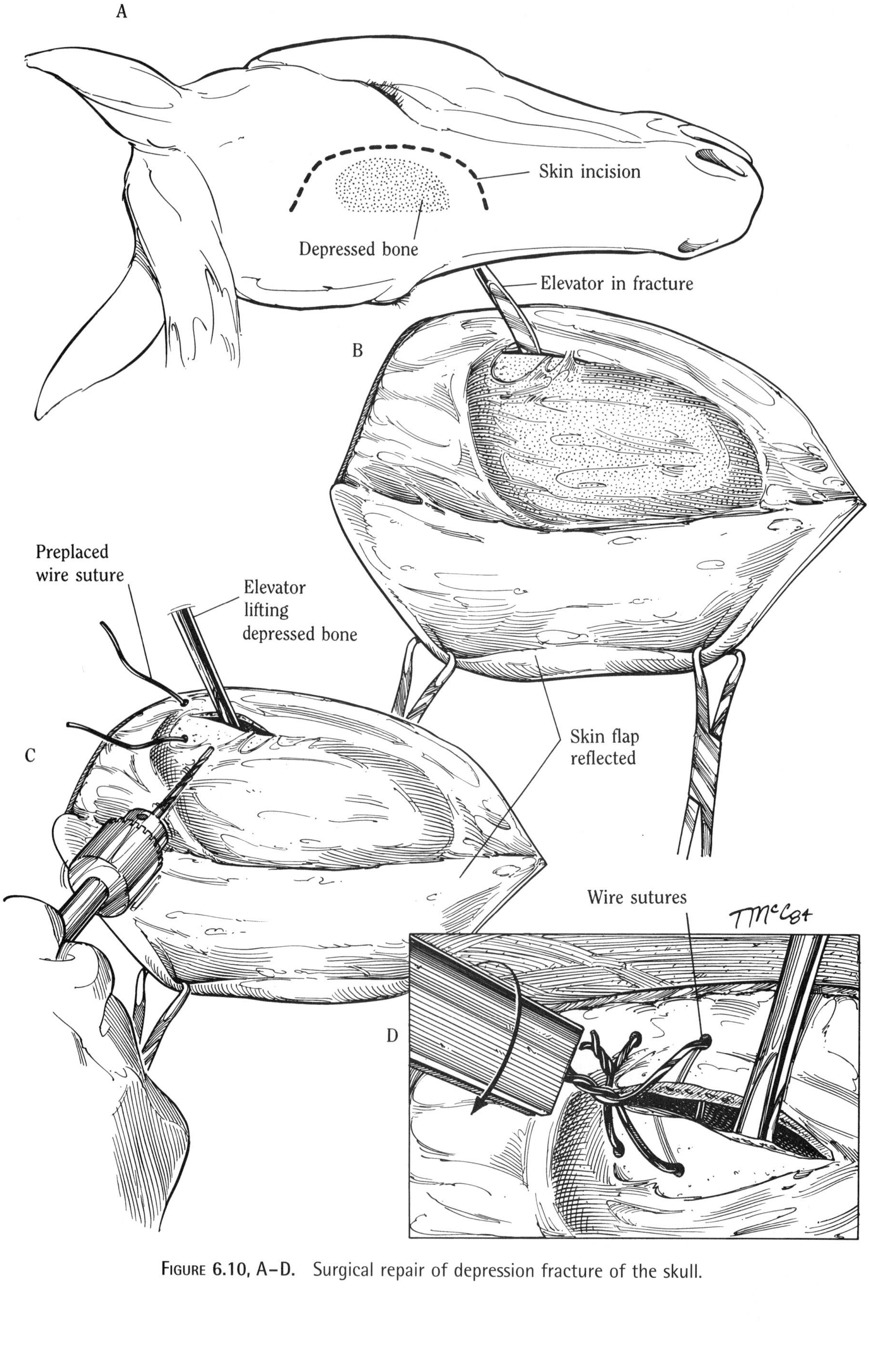

Figure 6.10, A–D. Surgical repair of depression fracture of the skull.

area surgically prepared, a surgical bone hook is carefully guided into the fornix and placed under the fractured zygomatic bone. With the hook firmly seated under the fractured segment of the zygomatic process, firm traction is exerted in a dorsolateral direction to elevate the fracture fragment and thereby reduce the fracture. No further stabilization is necessary. This technique was successful in 12 of 13 cases (9).

It is possible with some fractures of the frontomaxillary region to elevate the fracture fragments and reduce the fracture without having to surgically expose the fracture site. An elevator is introduced into the sinus through a small opening created in the fractured area or immediately adjacent to it, and the elevator is used to elevate the fractured bone (2). If the bone fragments appear stable after the fracture is reduced, further fixation is generally not required. This minimally invasive type of repair will succeed only if there is a minimum of comminution, little damage to the skin over the fracture site, and if the fracture site appears stable after fracture reduction.

Postoperative Management

During the early postoperative period, in those cases where open fracture reduction and stabilization has been performed, head bandages are recommended. A nonadherent dressing is applied and held in position with a cotton gauze bandage that is applied to the head in a figure-eight pattern. This is then covered with elastic adhesive bandage. The bandage should allow normal mastication, maintain firm even pressure along the surgical site, and keep dust and feed material from entering the wound. The bandage will also help to minimize chances of subcutaneous emphysema that is caused by air escaping from the nasal cavity. The bandage should be monitored carefully to ensure that it does not slip and cause mechanical irritation to the eyes. The bandage should be removed in 4 to 5 days.

Antibiotics should be continued until the bandage is removed and the surgeon has had an opportunity to assess the healing of the incision(s). If sinusitis and nasal discharge develop, antibiotic therapy may be indicated for longer periods. If a nasal discharge persists for longer than 2 to 3 weeks, radiographs may be indicated to rule out the possibility of formation of sequestra or the presence of a foreign body.

REFERENCES

1. Stashak TS. The nervous system: specific techniques. In: Jennings PB, ed. Textbook of Large Animal Surgery. Philadelphia: WB Saunders, 1984:1005.
2. Blackford JT, Blackford LAW. Surgical treatment of selected musculoskeletal disorders of the head. In: Auer JA, ed. Equine Surgery. Philadelphia: WB Saunders, 1992: 1075–1092.
3. Turner AS. Surgical management of depression fractures of the equine skull. Vet Surg 1979;8(29):1979.
4. Levine SB. Depression fractures of the nasal and frontal bones of the horse. J Equine Med Surg 1979;3:186.
5. Koch DB, Leitch M, Beech J. Orbital surgery in two horses. Vet Surg 1980;9:61.
6. Little CB, Hilbert BJ, McGill CA. A retrospective study of head fractures in 21 horses. Aust Vet J 1985;62:89.
7. Turner AS. Large animal orthopedic surgery. In: Jennings PB, ed. Textbook of Large Animal Surgery. Philadelphia: WB Saunders, 1984:897.
8. Martin GS, McIlwraith CW. Repair of a frontal sinus eversion in a horse. Vet Surg 1981;10:149.

9. Blackford JT, Hanselka DV, Heitmann JM, et al. Noninvasive technique for reduction of zygomatic process fractures in the horse. Vet Surg 1985;14:21–26.
10. Caron JP, Barber SM, Bailey JV, et al. Periorbital skull fractures in five horses. JAVMA 1986;188:280–284.
11. Burba DJ, Collier MA. T-plate repair of fracture of the nasal bones in a horse. JAVMA 1991;199:909–912.
12. LeBlanc PH, Brunson DB. Anesthetic management of equine head trauma: a case report. Vet Surg 1986;15:279–282.

Modified Forssell's Operation For Cribbing

Crib biting in the horse is a vice characterized by the placement of the upper incisors on a solid object, arching of the neck, depressing the tongue, elevating the larynx, and pulling backward. If the horse swallows air, the vice is called wind sucking. There is usually an audible grunt. The sequelae to these habits are poor performance, weight loss, erosion of incisor teeth, and flatulent colic. Above all, it is a vice that is objectionable and irritating to most owners. Why horses commence cribbing or wind sucking is unknown. It is a vice that is learned or acquired, and the most common cause cited is boredom or frustration. In our experience, one of the most common reasons for presentation of a horse that crib bites is owner annoyance rather than weight loss, colic, and property destruction (the more traditional side effects of the vice) (1).

Surgical methods of treatment have included the Forssell's procedure, which involves removal of portions of the sternomandibular, omohyoid, sternohyoid, and sternothyroid muscles. This technique has since been modified and is described here. Creation of a therapeutic buccal fistula (buccostomy) has also been described. The disadvantages of this procedure include spontaneous closure of the buccostomy or daily care of the tube used to prevent such closure. The surgical technique involving sectioning of the ventral branch of the accessory nerve (cranial nerve XI) has been used (2). This nerve innervates the sternomandibular muscle, the largest and most powerful muscle involved in cribbing. The nerve is transected bilaterally. The disappointing results with this method obtained by various surgeons in the United States and overseas (3) prompted the authors to adopt the modification of Forssell's procedure, whereby excision of a portion of the sternothyrohyoid and omohyoid muscles is combined with bilateral removal of a 10- to 12-cm section of the accessory nerves (1).

Anesthesia and Surgical Preparation

The modified Forssell's technique is done with the horse under general anesthesia and in dorsal recumbency with the head positioned at approximately a 30° angle to the horizontal. The ventral neck and throat region is clipped, shaved, and scrubbed for aseptic surgery in a routine manner. Perioperative broad-spectrum antibiotics are administered as well as tetanus toxoid.

Additional Instrumentation

This procedure requires malleable retractors (1-inch width), a 1-inch Penrose drain, and a hand towel (the latter will be used as a stent bandage to minimize incisional swelling).

Surgical Technique

A skin incision approximately 30 cm long is made on the ventral aspect of the neck, and the skin edges are reflected laterad (Fig. 6.11*A*). This exposes the ventral surfaces of the paired bellies of the omohyoid and sternothyrohyoid muscles (Fig. 6.11*B*), as well as the cranial ends of the sternomandibular muscles. Hemostasis is controlled by electrocoagulation or torsion and ligation.

A plane of dissection is established on the medial side of the sternomandibular muscle, approximately 5 cm caudal to the musculotendinous junction (Fig. 6.11, *B* and *C*). The ventral branch of the accessory nerve is located on the dorsomedial aspect of this muscle by carefully rolling the muscle belly laterad. To aid in locating the nerve, one can dissect down to the aponeurosis of the sternomandibular muscle and identify a constant muscular branch from the

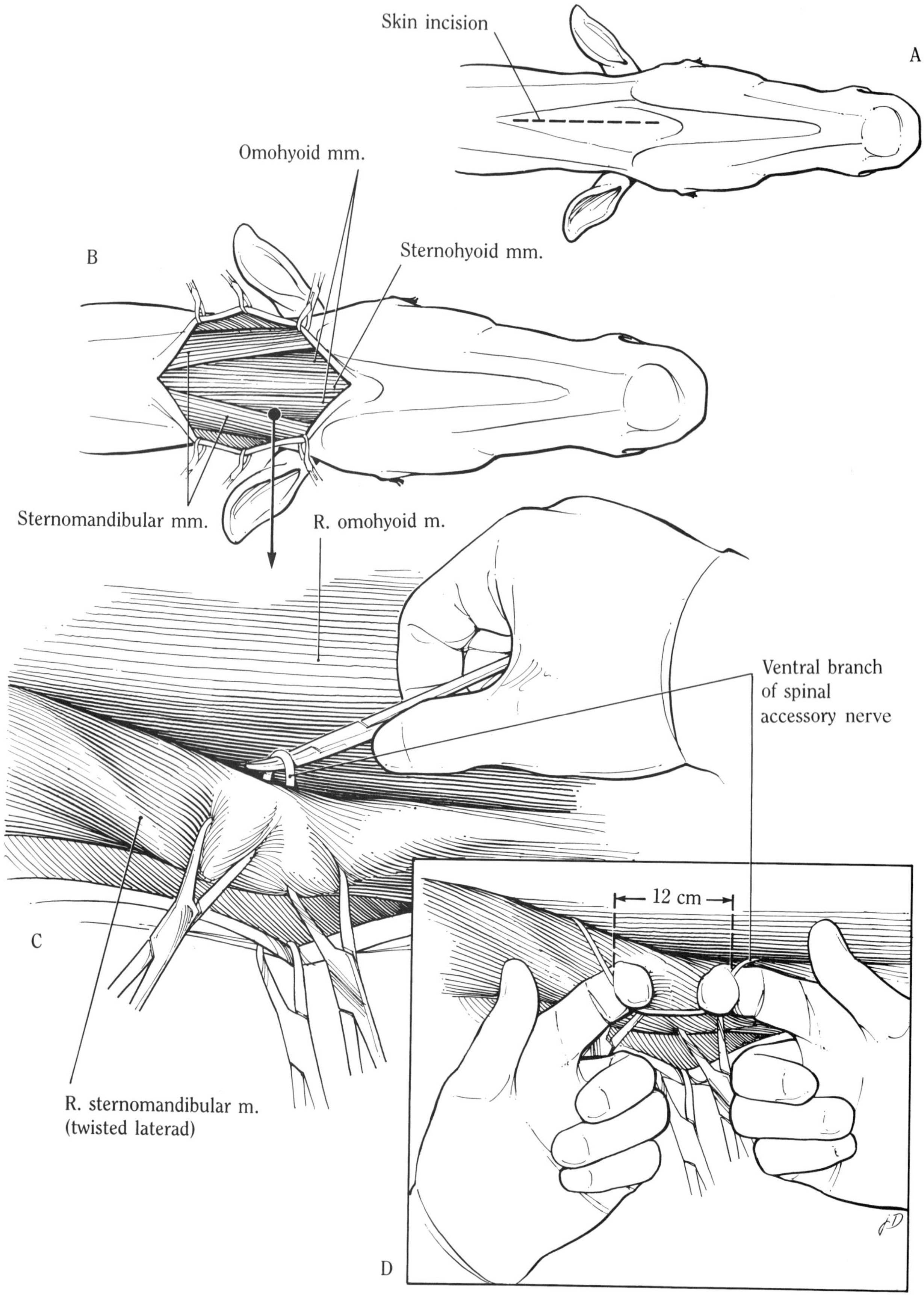

Figure 6.11, A–D. Modified Forssell's operation for cribbing.

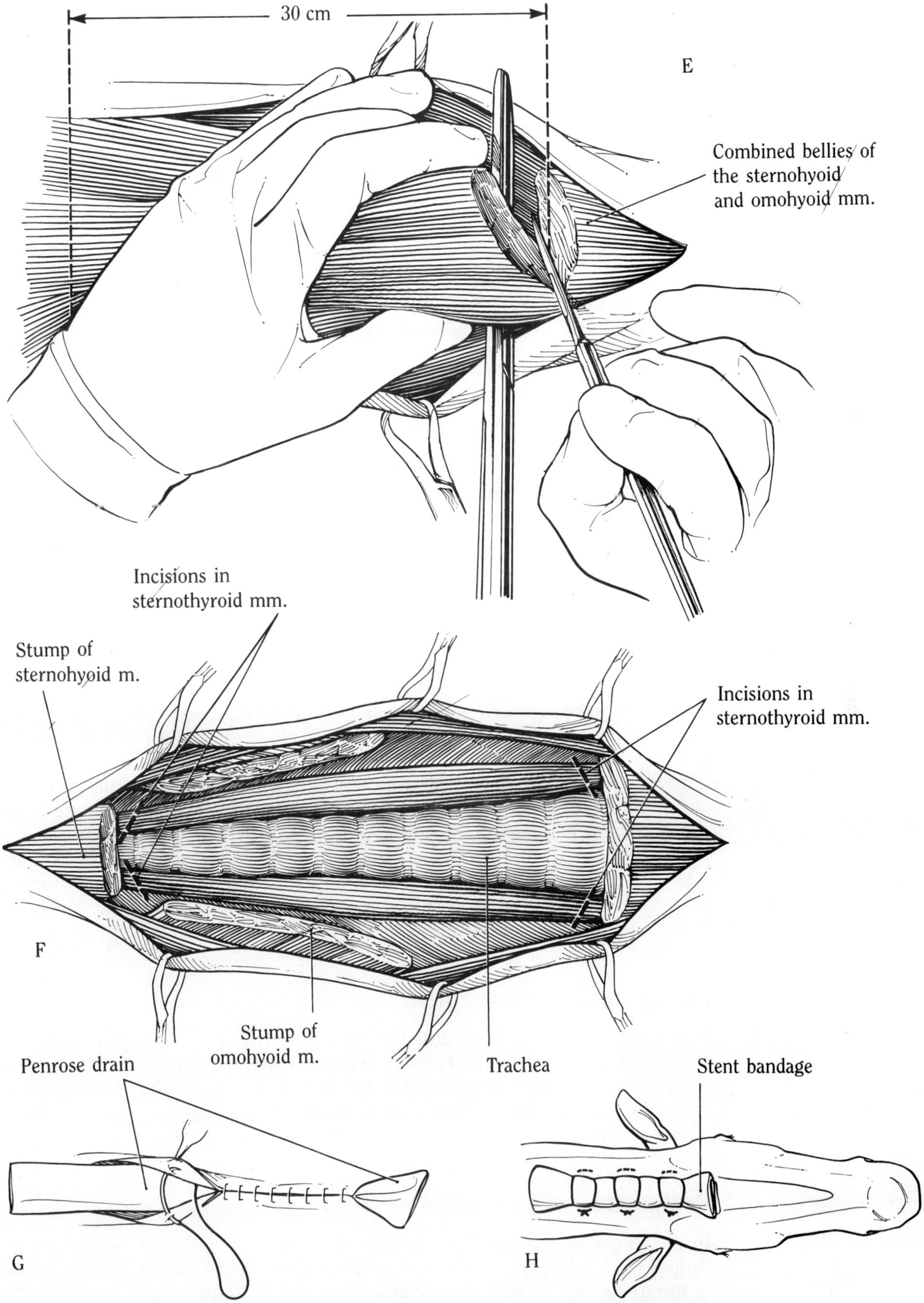

Figure 6.11, E–H. *(continued)* Modified Forssell's operation for cribbing.

common carotid artery, which crosses between the sternomandibular and omohyoid muscles. Just beneath this vessel, the ventral branch of the accessory nerve emerges from within the neck and extends laterad (1). Sudden contracture of the sternomandibular muscle can be initiated by gently pinching the nerve with a hemostat. This indicates that the nerve has been located.

Curved hemostats are placed under the nerve (Fig. 6.11*C*). The nerve is then elevated until both fingers can be inserted under the nerve. By forcefully elevating and separating the fingers, a sizable portion of the nerve can be exteriorized and removed (at least 12 cm) (Fig. 6.11*D*). This maneuver is then done on the opposite side. Maintaining hemostasis up to this point minimizes staining of the areolar tissue and fascial planes, thus simplifying location and identification of the nerve.

Following bilateral neurectomy, the myectomy is performed. A 30-cm section of the combined bellies of the omohyoid and sternothyrohyoid muscles is removed. These muscle bellies are isolated in the cranial end of the incision, immediately ventral to the larynx. The muscles are freed from the larynx and fascial attachments to the linguofacial vein and thyroid gland. A pair of straight scissors, Ochsner, or similar forceps is passed under the muscle bellies before transection to ensure inclusion of all parts of the muscle bellies (Fig. 6.11*E*). The muscle bellies are then grasped and "peeled" caudad, and areolar connective tissue attaching them to the trachea is sharply dissected away. The bellies of the sternothyroid muscles and the ventral aspect of the trachea are then visible. The omohyoid muscles are now sectioned obliquely and the sternohyoid muscles are sectioned at the caudal extremity of the incision (Fig. 6.11*F*). The sternothyroid muscles on the ventral surface of the trachea (Fig. 6.11*F*) are then removed, using scissors or a scalpel.

Closure consists of a simple continuous suture in the subcutaneous tissue with synthetic absorbable material, along with insertion of a 1-inch diameter Penrose drain. The Penrose drain can emerge from the incision itself (Fig. 6.11*G*), but a better surgical principle is to place the ends through generous stab incisions at either end of the incision. Skin closure is performed with nonabsorbable suture material in an interrupted pattern of the surgeon's choice. The authors routinely use skin staples to reduce the operative time associated with closure of this long incision, and find them satisfactory. To help eliminate dead space, a stent bandage (hand towel) can be sutured over the incision, using nonabsorbable suture material in a horizontal or vertical mattress pattern (Fig. 6.11*H*) (1). An alternative to the stent bandage is to apply a neck bandage immediately after anesthetic recovery. This bandage can be changed as needed and maintained for 3 to 5 days.

Postoperative Management

After surgery, the horse is confined to a box stall. The stent bandage is removed 3 to 4 days after surgery. The Penrose drain is maintained for 3 to 7 days. Antibiotics are continued for 24 hours after the drain is removed. The drain sites are cleaned daily, and skin sutures or staples are removed approximately 2 weeks after surgery.

Comments

In a retrospective study of 35 horses, 20 (57%) were not cribbing 1 year following surgery (1). Marked improvement was noted in another 11 (noticeable reduction in the frequency of crib biting). Some horses in this latter group would apply the incisor teeth to an object but did not arch the neck and go through the motions of cribbing. Four of thirty-five horses returned to cribbing in the same manner as before surgery. One of these would arch the neck but not make the characteristic "grunt." This horse gained considerable weight after surgery. Several cribbing brood mares had lost considerable weight and had failed to ovulate. After surgery they either stopped cribbing or continued to crib at a much reduced frequency and gained weight. They began to have regular estrous cycles and some were bred successfully. In 34 cases, the final cosmetic result was regarded as excellent by the owners. One owner reported that the "scar" from surgery was still visible (1).

The modified myectomy and neurectomy technique appears to be superior to neurectomy alone. The poor results achieved with neurectomy alone are believed attributable to the variable innervation of the sternomandibular muscle, which receives additional ventral cervical branches beyond the site of section of the ventral branch of the accessory nerve (3).

This method differs slightly from a modification of this technique wherein myectomy is performed before neurectomy (4). The authors believe the ventral branch of the spinal accessory nerve is identified more readily before the surgical field has become obscured by blood from the transected stumps of the muscle bellies. Similarly, the authors believe meticulous control of hemorrhage is important until the nerves are located. The outstanding advantage with this method is that good cosmetic results and quicker wound healing can be achieved when compared with the original, more radical Forssell's technique. Virtually all owners questioned were pleased with the cosmetic appearance of the surgical site (1). The Forssell procedure produces a thin neck and a steplike defect where the sternomandibular muscle bellies are transected distally.

It is interesting to note, however, in a report from Sweden comparing the results of the Forssell's procedure with the combined myectomy-neurectomy technique that the Forssell's procedure had better long-term results (5). In that study, the best prognosis with either technique was in young animals with a short history of cribbing. Although with careful dissection the recurrent laryngeal nerves are avoided, the client should probably be warned of the possibility of surgical trauma producing laryngeal hemiplegia. An endoscopic examination of the horse before surgery is recommended.

REFERENCES

1. Turner AS, White NA, Ismay J. Modified Forssell's operation for cribbing in the horse. JAVMA 1984;184:309.
2. Firth EC. Bilateral ventral accessory neurectomy in windsucking horses. Vet Rec 1980; 106:30.
3. Huskamp B, Henschel E, Arenhoevel H. Technik and Ergebnisse einer modernen Kopperoperation. Prak Tierarz 1983;64:110.
4. Greet TRC. Windsucking treated by myectomy and neurectomy. Equine Vet J 1982; 14:299.
5. Hakansson A, Franzen P, Pettersson H. Comparison of two surgical methods for treatment of crib-biting in horses. Equine Vet J 1992;24:494.

Permanent Tracheostomy

Horses with permanent and inoperable stenosis of the upper airway causing respiratory distress are candidates for permanent tracheostomy (1, 2). Conditions that may necessitate permanent tracheostomy include neoplasia, arytenoid chondritis, nasopharyngeal cicatrization, and cranial nerve damage that results in dysphagia and bilateral arytenoid paralysis (1–3; Hardy J, personal communication, 1996). Permanent indwelling tracheal cannulae can be surgically placed but may need to be removed and cleaned daily to prevent obstruction from accumulation of tracheal secretions. Permanent tracheostomy is an alternative to having to maintain a tracheal cannula. The technique has few complications and is best done under general anesthesia. The procedure can also be done in the standing horse if there are financial constraints or if general anesthesia poses too great a risk (1, 2).

Anesthesia and Surgical Preparation

Perioperative broad-spectrum antibiotics are administered. Tetanus toxoid is given. The horse is placed under general anesthesia in dorsal recumbency. If the upper airway obstruction is so severe that the horse cannot be intubated, it may be necessary to perform a temporary tracheostomy at a site separate and distant from the proposed permanent tracheostomy site, in order to place the endotracheal tube. If a temporary tracheostomy is placed before surgery, the permanent tracheostomy site should be selected at a site distant (proximal or distal depending on the location of the temporary tracheostomy), where the tissues are not inflamed. It is preferable to situate the permanent tracheostomy in the proximal third of the cervical trachea. The ventral cervical area is clipped and shaved and surgically prepared.

If the procedure is done in the standing horse, the horse is sedated and restrained in stocks with its head and neck extended in cross ties (2). The surgical area is infiltrated in an inverted U pattern dorsal and lateral to the surgical site (second through the fifth tracheal ring) with local anesthetic.

Surgical Technique

In the anesthetized patient, a 10-cm skin incision is made on ventral midline over the proximal one third of the cervical trachea. The incision should be placed immediately over the level of the proposed tracheostomy. The first tracheal ring should be left intact and the tracheostomy constructed at a site distal to that ring. The incision is extended through the subcutaneous tissue and the cutaneous colli muscle. The paired sternothyrohyoid muscles are dissected free of their surrounding fascia and can be incised at the proximal and distal limits of the incision, thereby exposing the underlying trachea. Bleeders should be found and ligated. Four tracheal rings are identified and a ventral midline and two paramedian incisions are made through each of these four rings on their ventral surface (Fig. 6.12*A*). These incisions do not extend through the tracheal mucosa. Each of these rectangles of tracheal cartilage are then dissected free of the underlying tracheal mucosa and discarded (Fig. 6.12*B*). When planning where to make the tracheal cartilage incisions, it is important that the resultant defect not exceed $\frac{1}{4}$ to $\frac{1}{3}$ of total circumference of the tracheal ring. A larger defect could result in tracheal collapse.

The tracheal mucosa is then incised in a double-Y pattern, creating flaps of mucosa with a triangular flap at each end of the tracheostomy (Fig. 6.12*C*). The mucosa and submucosa at the edges of these mucosal flaps are then sutured to the skin with simple interrupted sutures of 2/0 polypropylene (Fig. 6.12*D*).

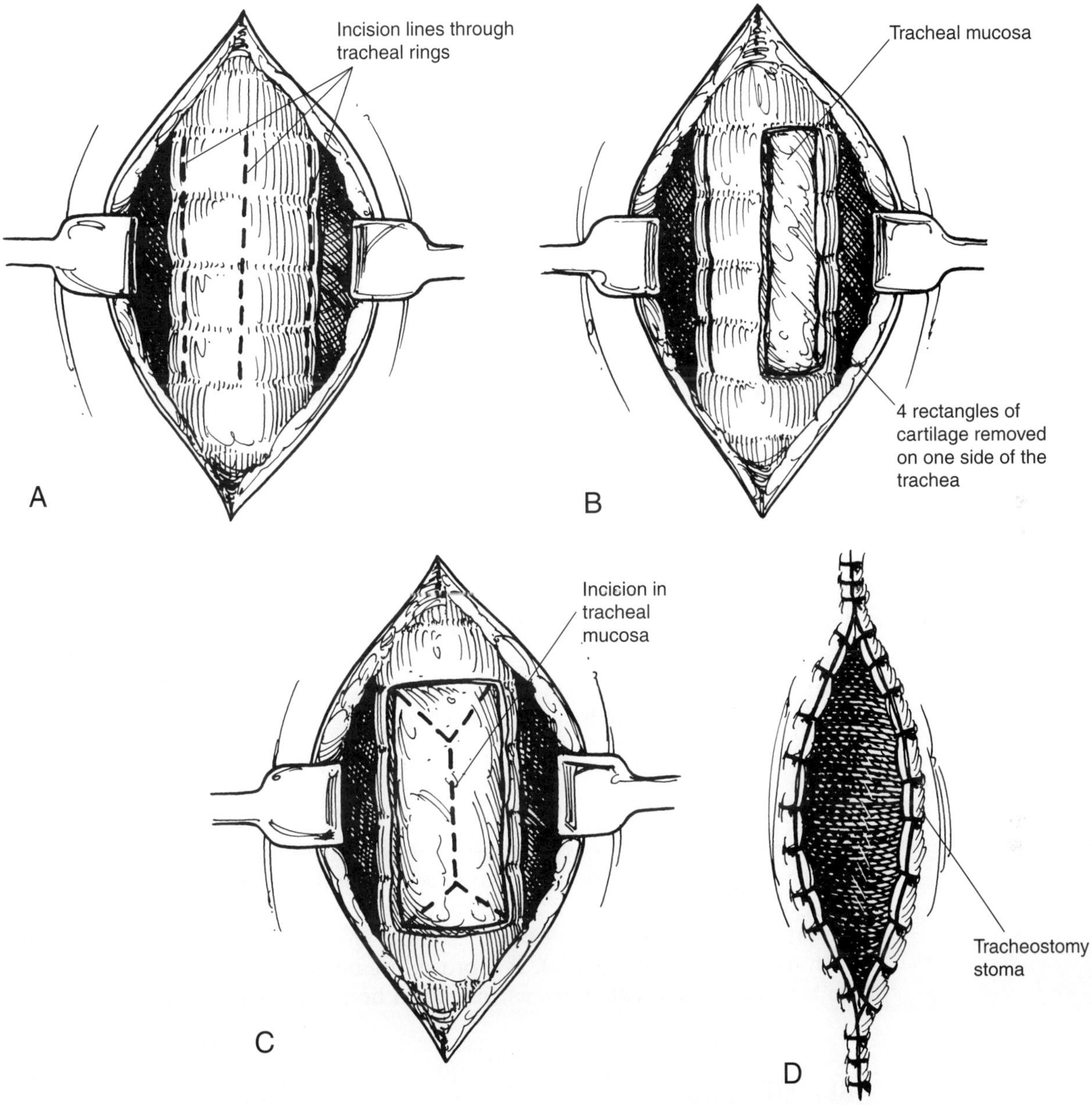

FIGURE 6.12, A–D. Permanent tracheostomy. (Adapted from Shappell KK, Stick JA, Derksen FJ, et al. Permanent tracheostomy in equidae: 47 cases (1981–1986). JAVMA 1988;192: 939–942.)

If the skin incision has extended beyond either end of the tracheostomy stoma, the subcutaneous tissue is closed with simple interrupted sutures of 2/0 synthetic absorbable suture material and the skin with simple interrupted sutures of 2/0 polypropylene (Fig. 6.12*D*).

The technique described for permanent tracheostomy in the standing horse differs slightly from that in the anesthetized horse (2). A 3 cm × 6 cm segment of skin and subcutaneous tissue is removed from ventral midline of the neck over the proposed tracheostomy site. The sternothyrohyoid muscles are isolated, clamped, and incised, proximally and distally. Removing the portion of the skin allows better exposure of the trachea without the need for retraction, and may prevent the collapse of soft tissues over the tracheal stoma in the postoperative period, particularly in a thick-necked horse. Before making the tracheal ring incisions, the tracheal mucosa is desensitized by inserting a needle into the lumen of the trachea proximal to the tracheostomy site and irrigating the tracheal mucosa with 30 mL of 2% lidocaine. This reduces the likelihood of coughing and of the horse becoming restless during the procedure. The rest of the tracheostomy construction is similar to that already described. Dead space can be reduced before mucocutaneous closure by suturing the subcutaneous tissue to the tracheal fascia adjacent to the tracheostomy with size 0 synthetic absorbable suture material in a single interrupted pattern.

Postoperative Management

The tracheal stoma is cleaned daily, for 2 to 3 weeks, with gauze sponges moistened with saline. Careful removal of crusted secretions and exudate is necessary so as not to disrupt the mucocutaneous suture line. Some dehiscence of the mucocutaneous suture line may occur, but generally no repair is required. Swelling of the site will occur, and if abscesses develop in the dead space adjacent to the stoma, drainage is required. This can usually be accomplished by removing one or two of the ventral mucocutaneous sutures.

The amount of exudate that accumulates daily around the stoma will vary between horses. Horses with preexisting pulmonary disease will have more tracheal exudate. Every effort should be made to keep a horse with a permanent tracheostomy in a relatively dust-free environment. Also, these horses should not be allowed near a body of deep water where the tracheal stoma could become submerged. Permanent tracheostomy has been performed in brood mares that have subsequently foaled uneventfully (2).

Comments

Based on the results of two reports, stomal stricture following permanent tracheostomy appear to pose no problem in ponies and horses. This technique provides a long-term, functional airway that is cosmetically acceptable. The complication rate associated with the procedure is low even if the procedure is done with the horse standing (1, 2). The procedure has been performed successfully on brood mares and stallions as well as on horses used for riding.

REFERENCES

1. Shappell KK, Stick JA, Derksen FJ, et al. Permanent tracheostomy in Equidae: 47 cases (1981–1986). JAVMA 1988;192:939–942.
2. McClure SR, Taylor TS, Honnas CM, et al. Permanent tracheostomy in standing horses: techniques and results. Vet Surg 1995;24:231–234.
3. Dean PW, Cohen ND. Arytenoidectomy for advanced unilateral chondropathy with accompanying lesions. Vet Surg 1990;19:364–370.

7

SURGERY OF THE GASTROINTESTINAL TRACT

Caudal Molar Extraction

Removal of teeth is indicated in cases of infundibular necrosis, fractures, abscesses, periodontal disease, and chronic ossifying periostitis. Infection of the teeth may occur secondary to fractures of the skull (mandible and maxilla) that involve the roots of the teeth. When the disease involves the mandibular teeth, swelling and chronic drainage from the ventral border of the mandible is usually present. Involvement of the caudal molar (sixth cheek tooth) of the mandible is unusual because of the extreme caudal location of this tooth. Removal is performed in a slightly different manner than that for the more rostral teeth. Because of the unique problems associated with repulsion of the caudal molar, the authors have included this surgery in this chapter.

Anesthesia and Surgical Preparation

Repulsion of the caudal molar of the mandible should be done with the horse under general anesthesia and with the affected tooth uppermost. A mouth speculum is placed securely in the horse's mouth and opened sufficiently to allow admission of the surgeon's hand. The hair is clipped over the entire masseter muscle on the affected side, and a routine surgical preparation is performed (1). Perioperative antibiotics and phenylbutazone are administered, as well as tetanus toxoid.

Additional Instrumentation

Caudal molar extraction requires a mouth speculum, mallet or hammer, chisels or osteotomes, curved dental punches, umbilical tape, and gauze or dental wax.

Surgical Technique

The location of the sixth lower cheek tooth necessitates trephination over the lateral surface of the mandible. A line is drawn from the center of the table surface of the tooth to the point of greatest curvature of the ramus of the mandible (Fig. 7.1*A*). An incision is made on this line through the skin and masseter muscle in the direction of its fibers. The incision should be liberal enough to allow the muscle to be separated from the bone. The skin and muscle incision is terminated at least 4 cm from the border of the mandible to avoid severing the branches of the facial nerve and maxillary artery that spread out over the surface of the masseter muscle from above, ventrad and rostrad. This dissection can be difficult if there is a masseteric abscess present or if there is a fistula with a great deal of associated soft tissue inflammation. The root of the sixth cheek tooth can be identified by its bulging appearance. To gain access to the tooth root, an opening is made with a chisel. The opening is further elongated to give better direction for the punch and lessen the chances of fracturing the medial bony plate of the mandible (Fig. 7.1*B*). With careful guidance of the chisel, it is possible and preferable to provide access to the root of this tooth without ever using a trephine. When sufficient lateral bony plate of the mandible has been removed, the surgeon introduces one hand into the mouth, locates the diseased tooth, and determines the tooth's path in the jaw. The punch is then placed onto the root of the tooth, and an assistant begins to tap the punch with a mallet. The first few blows with the mallet should be sufficient to seat the punch into the root of the tooth (Fig. 7.1*C*). To allow the punch access to the diseased tooth, the opening may have to be enlarged by removing a little more of the lateral cortex of the mandible with the chisel or a curette.

Once the punch is seated, the assistant delivers steady blows to the punch. The mallet blows will produce a characteristic ringing sound when the punch is seated properly, and the surgeon will feel the vibrations of these blows transmitted through the tooth to his or her hand. If the punch slips off the tooth, it must be repositioned. After some time, the surgeon will feel the gradual loosening of the tooth with the hand that is in the horse's mouth. Subsequent blows with the mallet should be less forceful because the tooth is being driven from the alveolus. Removal of the crown of the tooth with molar cutters may be required in young horses before it can be removed from the mouth.

Following tooth repulsion, any fragments should be removed from the alveolus with forceps or a curette. The alveolus may require curettage if diseased bone surrounds the tooth. To prevent the socket from being packed with food substances, it should be filled with a suitable material such as dental wax, dental acrylic, gutta-percha, or gauze rolls until the socket is almost filled with granulation tissue. If gauze rolls are used, a roll that will fit snugly into the hole is made and tied around the center with umbilical tape, leaving two long ends. The ends are passed through the socket and trephine hole, the gauze is wedged firmly into the cavity, and the umbilical tape is brought to the exterior. The umbilical tape is then secured to the skin by tying it to another gauze roll. The ends should be kept long so that the gauze roll in the alveolus can be replaced without having to thread the new piece of umbilical tape back through the trephine hole.

Vinyl polysiloxane impression material (Reprosil, Dentsply International, Inc., Milford, DE), commonly known as dental wax, is preferred by the authors for packing the alveolus. It is prepared by mixing a putty base and catalyst together, and is then packed into the top half of the socket from the oral side and flared over the gingival margins medially and laterally for approximately .5 cm while it has a dough-like consistency. It hardens within minutes.

After the socket has been attended to, the dorsal two thirds of the masseter muscle is opposed with synthetic absorbable sutures. The dorsal two thirds of the skin incision is closed with synthetic monofilament nonabsorbable sutures, leaving the ventral aspect open to ensure drainage. To completely close the incision in the masseter muscle would be inviting problems because the potential contamination from the oral cavity could result in abscessation and/or cellulitis if the incision were not free to drain.

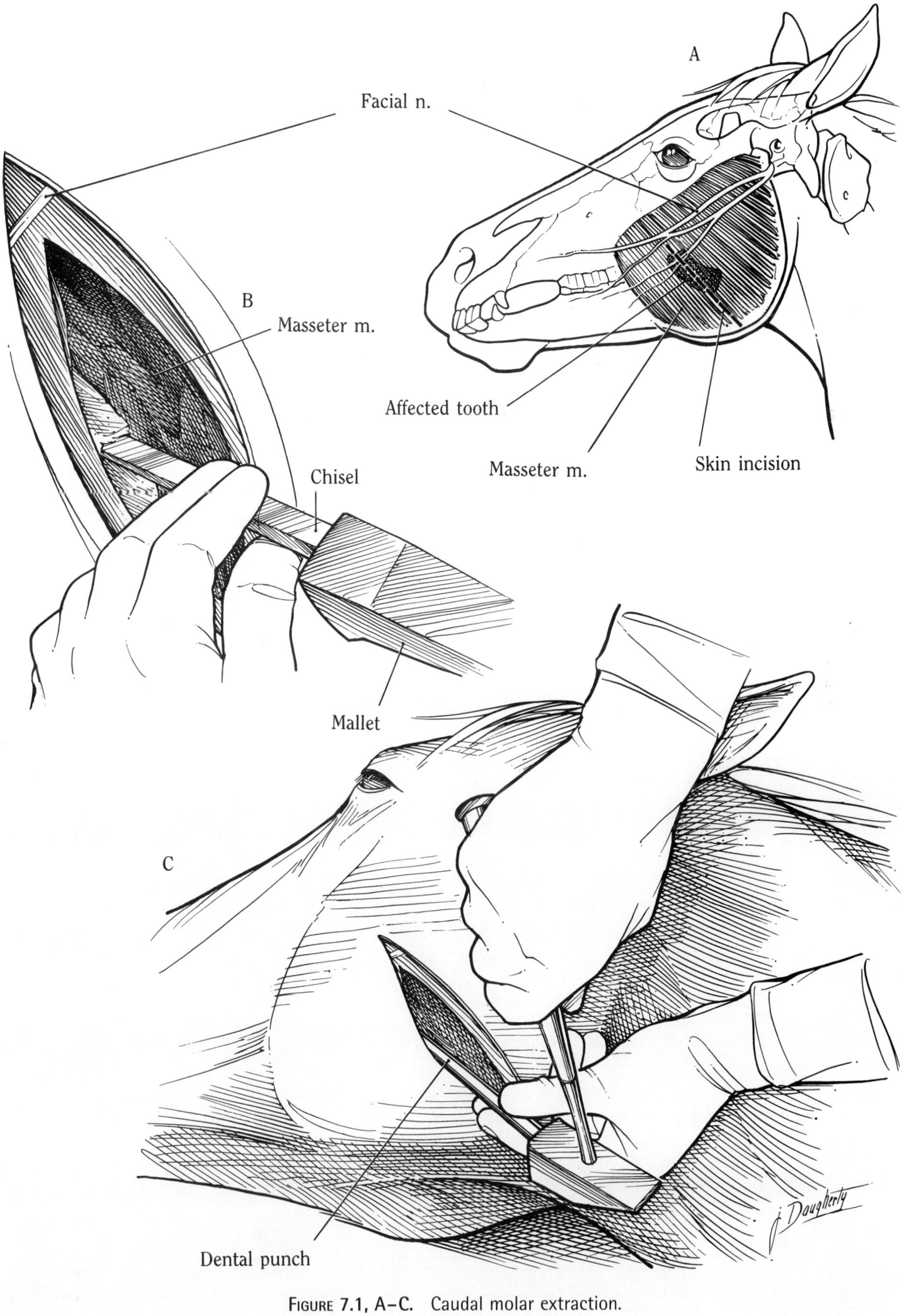

FIGURE 7.1, A–C. Caudal molar extraction.

Postoperative Management

The decision to use postoperative antibiotics is based on the surgeon's assessment of the condition of the surgical site following tooth repulsion. If a gauze pack has been placed in the alveolar socket, it should be changed every other day for 2 weeks. Following removal of the gauze, the socket should be flushed with warm antiseptic solution. The new gauze should be tied to the umbilical tape, wedged back into the socket, and secured to the skin by tying it to another gauze roll. This maneuver is best done with a secure mouth speculum in place and sedation with a drug such as xylazine, xylazine and butorphanol combination, or detomidine. The maneuver necessitates placing the hand into the mouth to grasp the old gauze roll and reposition the new gauze roll. This does present a management problem, and the procedure is not without risk to the surgeon if the horse resents manipulation in this area. For these reasons, packing the socket with dental wax or acrylic at the time of surgery is preferred as a more practical solution. The socket eventually fills with granulation tissue extruding the plug. If the alveolar plug loosens and falls out prematurely, the horse must be reanesthetized, the socket flushed and all feed material removed, and a new plug reinserted.

REFERENCES

1. Turner AS, McIlwraith CW. In: Techniques in Large Animal Surgery. 2nd ed. Philadelphia: Lea & Febiger, 1989.

Esophagotomy For Removal of an Esophageal Foreign Body

Treatment of esophageal obstruction can involve medical, manipulative, and surgical methods; a fixed protocol is not appropriate. Many cases of obstruction with feed materials will resolve themselves spontaneously or with simple medical support. Gentle manipulation with a stomach tube combined with lavage can be useful in clearing feed obstructions. However, the long-term presence of an impaction can cause pressure necrosis of the esophageal mucosa and subsequent stricture formation; overzealous manipulations with a stomach tube can have similar effects and even cause perforation of the esophagus. Foreign bodies should be definitively identified by radiographic and/or endoscopic examination (1). Inert, firm, rough-surfaced, or sharp foreign bodies may need to be removed surgically to avoid extensive esophageal damage.

Longitudinal esophagotomy with primary closure of the incision results in minimal complications when performed in a region of normal esophagus (2, 3). The surgeon should always remember that a well-performed esophagotomy is less traumatic than prolonged pressure and bruising to the esophageal wall. The reader is reminded that the esophagus has properties quite distinct from the remainder of the GI tract and these are important surgically. The esophagus is not covered by serosa (this tissue layer promotes a rapid seal as a result of exudation of fibrin following intestinal surgery). The musculature of the esophagus is weak and holds sutures poorly, but the mucosa is relatively strong (in the remainder of the GI tract, the mucosa is weak and the submucosa is the strongest layer). Nonabsorbable suture material is used to close the mucosa, and some surgeons now use polypropylene for all layers (3). Blood vessels to the esophagus are short and easily damaged, requiring care and imposing limitations in mobilizing the esophagus.

Anesthesia and Surgical Preparation

The esophagotomy is done under general anesthesia with the horse placed in dorsal recumbency. Before induction of anesthesia, the horse's neck is clipped for a ventral midline approach. The horse should be carefully evaluated for any evidence of aspiration pneumonia secondary to choke. Perioperative antibiotics are administered, as well as tetanus toxoid.

A nasogastric tube is also placed as far as the foreign body to facilitate identification of the esophagus during the surgical approach. When the horse is anesthetized, the midline of the neck is shaved, and a routine surgical preparation is performed.

Surgical Technique

An 8- to 10-cm skin incision is made on the ventral midline over the area of the obstruction. This will provide sufficient exposure to make a 5-cm incision in the esophagus. The paired sternohyoid muscles are divided on the midline to expose the trachea. The fascia on the left side of the trachea is then bluntly dissected to locate the esophagus (Fig. 7.2*A*). The ventral wall of the esophagus is exposed with careful dissection of adventitial tissue, and the left carotid sheath containing the carotid artery and vagus nerve is identified and gently retracted laterad (Fig. 7.2*A*). The surrounding tissues are packed off with moist towels and a longitudinal incision is made through the esophagus with a scalpel (Fig. 7.2*B*). The surgeon attempts to incise a normal esophageal wall, but this will depend on the site, mobility, and extent of the obstruction.

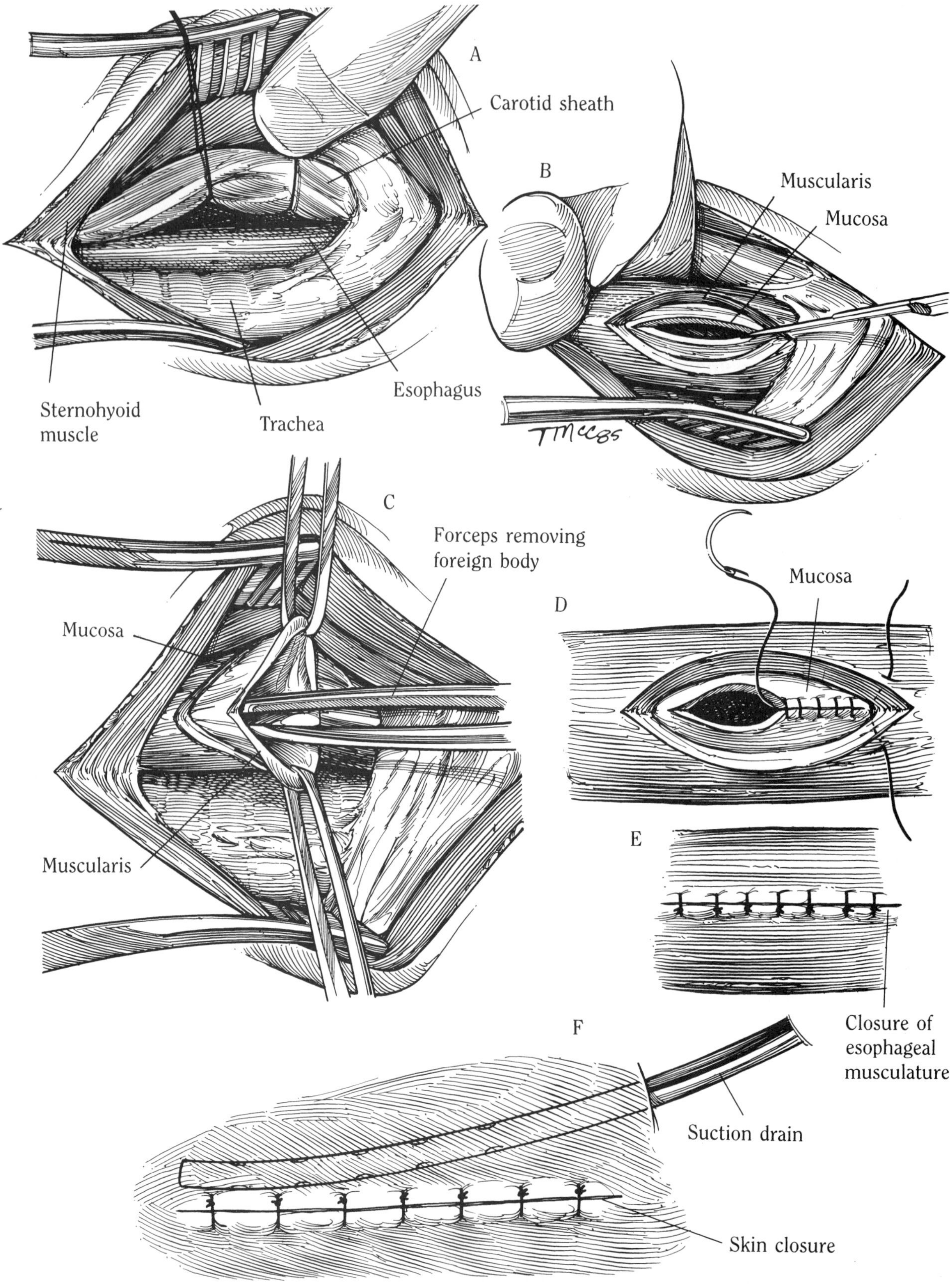

Figure 7.2, A–F. Esophagotomy.

Following removal of the foreign body (Fig. 7.2*C*), the mucosa of the esophagus is examined. If it appears normal, it is closed with 3/0 polypropylene or nylon suture material in a simple continuous pattern, with the knots tied within the lumen (Fig. 7.2*D*). The esophageal musculature is closed with 2/0 nonabsorbable monofilament material or synthetic absorbable material in a simple interrupted pattern (Fig. 7.2*E*). A ¼-inch fenestrated suction drain (Snyder Hemovac middle-perforated tubing, ¼-inch, 19 Fr. OD, Zimmer, Dover, OH) is placed beside the esophagus and exited through the skin caudal to the skin incision (Fig. 7.2*F*). It is maintained for 48 hours to remove serum and blood from the surgical site. Retention of the drain beyond this period is contraindicated unless salivary leakage is present. The muscle and fascia of the neck incision are closed with synthetic absorbable material in a simple interrupted pattern. The skin is closed with simple interrupted sutures of nonabsorbable material (Fig. 7.2*F*).

If removal of the foreign body is necessary through an obviously diseased segment of the esophagus, the esophagotomy incision is not closed and the muscle and tissue of the neck are only partially closed, leaving an opening for ventral drainage. An esophagotomy tube may be placed directly through the esophagotomy incision.

Postoperative Management

Broad-spectrum antibiotics are administered for 3–5 days following surgery. When an esophagotomy with a primary closure has been performed through healthy mucosa, extraoral alimentation is not used postoperatively. Food is withheld for 48 hours, and then small quantities of pelleted feed in a slurry are given. The progression of healing is directly dependent on the form of feed given in the postoperative period (3). First-intention healing can occur if pelleted mash feed is given for 8 to 10 days following surgery. After this time, normal feeding can be resumed. As discussed previously, the drain is removed in 48 hours unless saliva is leaking from the drain. Detection of salivary leakage heralds the occurrence of dehiscence. If this does occur, the incision is opened to avoid spread of infection down into the thorax (a major potential complication). In the early convalescent period, parenteral electrolyte solutions may be used to maintain hydration if necessary.

If the esophagotomy is done through a compromised esophagus, extraoral alimentation is given through either an esophagostomy tube placed through a separate aboral incision or an esophagostomy tube placed directly into the initial esophagotomy incision. Cervical esophagostomy has been documented as a safe and convenient means of tube feeding in the horse (4, 5). A complete pelleted diet (7 g/kg in 5 L water, t.i.d.) is satisfactory for extraoral alimentation (5). Ten days of extraoral alimentation is sufficient in most esophageal surgery cases. The tube is removed, and the stoma is left to heal by second intention.

Comments

The use of a primarily sutured esophagotomy through healthy mucosa has definite advantages. It heals significantly faster than a nonsutured esophagotomy, and the latter also tends to develop a traction diverticulum (2, 3). Even with careful attention to tissue handling in this area, laryngeal hemiplegia can be a sequelae to esophageal surgery.

REFERENCES

1. Stick JA. Surgery of the esophagus. Vet Clin North Am Large Animal Pract 1982;4:33.
2. Stick JA, Krehbiel JD, Kunze DJ, et al. Esophageal healing in the pony: comparison of sutured vs. non-sutured esophagotomy. Am J Vet Res 1981;42:1506.

3. Stick JA, Slocombe RF, Derksen FJ, et al. Esophagotomy in the pony: comparison of surgical techniques and form of feed. Am J Vet Res 1983;44:2123–2132.
4. Freeman DE, Naylor JM. Cervical esophagostomy to permit extraoral feeding of the horse. JAVMA 1978;172:314.
5. Stick JA, Derksen FJ, Scott EA. Equine cervical esophagostomy: complications associated with duration and location of feeding tubes. Am J Vet Res 1981;42:727.

Surgical Correction of Displacements and Abnormalities of the Small Intestine

In keeping with the concept of this text as a surgical atlas, the presentations of this and the next section will be limited to a brief description of specific abnormalities and the manipulations to correct them. The inexperienced surgeon needs to augment this material with more detailed discussions of the pathogenesis, pathophysiology, diagnosis, and medical management of these conditions available elsewhere in textbooks (1–3) and in journal publications.

When a specific procedure such as enterotomy or jejunocecal anastomosis is given as a treatment method (or part of the treatment), the reader is referred to the sections where these techniques are specifically presented. When the surgical diagnosis and manipulative treatments for a condition are straightforward and diagrams are considered unnecessary, only a brief summary of the presentation and treatment will be given.

Simple Obstruction of the Small Intestine

Impaction of the Small Intestine

Primary impactions of the small intestine are of two types: impaction of the ileum with feed material (1, 4, 5) and generalized impaction of the small intestine with *Parascaris equorum* (2, 6).

Cases of ileal impaction with feed material present with clinical signs of simple obstruction of the small intestine. At laparotomy, ingesta are found impacted from the ileocecal orifice orad for 30 to 90 cm (4). The small intestine cranial to the impaction will be distended with gas and fluid. Treatment in most cases involves massage of the feed material into the cecum with or without prior injection of saline solution into the mass to soften the ingesta. In occasional severe cases, enterotomy may be necessary to remove the impacted feed material. In severe cases, ileocecal bypass (side-to-side anastomosis) or resection and jejunocecal anastomosis (if bowel compromise is present) may be necessary. Conservative management in early cases may be feasible (1, 5). Some degree of postoperative ileus can be anticipated following surgical correction.

Ascarid impaction usually occurs shortly after antihelminthic treatment. The small intestine may be partially or completely obstructed with these worms, and rupture of the intestine can occur in severe cases. Surgical relief of the obstruction through enterotomy is indicated for complete obstruction or for any obstruction that has not responded to administration of mineral oil. In some cases laparotomy reveals that the intestine has already ruptured. In addition to the normal physiologic changes associated with small intestinal obstruction and fluid sequestration, it has been suggested that dead ascarids cause a toxic or allergic effect that may exacerbate any systemic deterioration. The prognosis for survival in foals and horses treated surgically is poor (6).

Pedunculated Lipoma

Pedunculated lipomas of the small intestinal mesentery may cause simple obstruction when the long pedicle of the lipoma encircles the small intestine; however, they more commonly cause a strangulating obstruction. They are a problem of older horses. Laparotomy is needed to confirm the diagnosis of obstruction caused by a pedunculated lipoma, and whether it is simple or strangulated (7).

Adhesions

Adhesions may cause simple obstruction of the small intestine. They are most commonly seen following peritonitis or abdominal surgery. Simple obstructions associated with adhesions are commonly partial, and there may be a history of recurrent colic. Treatment of the adhesions usually involves either separation or cutting of the adhesions to reestablish a patent lumen and normal bowel configuration. In other instances, intestinal resection and anastomosis (in some cases, a side-to-side anastomosis leaving the strictured bowel in situ is the most appropriate method) are performed. The severed or separated surfaces must be oversewn to minimize further adhesion formation. The prognosis is always guarded because of the potential for adhesion reformation.

Abdominal Abscesses

Abdominal abscesses may produce compression or stricture of a portion of the small intestine. The majority of abdominal abscesses involve the mesentery, and systemic spread from respiratory infection is considered the most common cause of the abscessation (8). *Streptococcus equi, Streptococcus zooepidemicus,* and *Corynebacterium pseudotuberculosis* are the most common isolates. The condition is commonly a medical one, and long-term administration of penicillin has been used successfully in the treatment of internal abdominal abscesses (8). Surgical treatment is indicated in some instances if a surgical colic is deemed to be present and if abscesses can be drained intraoperatively or marsupialized without peritoneal contamination. Intestinal resection and anastomosis with abscess removal may be appropriate in selected cases of localized obstruction associated with abscessation (9).

Muscular Hypertrophy of the Ileum

Muscular hypertrophy of the distal ileum (at the ileocecal valve) may cause intestinal obstruction. The condition has been associated with stenosis of the ileum secondary to a mucosal lesion, strongyle larvae migration, neurogenic stenosis with prolonged closure of the ileocecal valve, and ileocecal intussusception (10). The condition is classified as primary idiopathic hypertrophy when predisposing lesions are not found at necropsy (11). The clinical signs will vary depending on whether the obstruction is incomplete or complete. Diagnosis is confirmed at laparotomy. Ileal myotomy has been used as a treatment (10), but jejunocecal anastomosis is used more frequently.

Neoplasia

With the exception of pedunculated lipomas, neoplasms of the intestines are rare. Lymphosarcoma can involve the small intestine and small intestinal mesentery, and squamous cell carcinoma may metastasize throughout the abdomen, involving the small intestine and small intestinal mesentery. These situations are not considered surgical cases, but surgery may be the means by which diagnosis is achieved. Solitary nonmetastatic tumors of the small intestine may be amenable to resection.

Duodenitis-Proximal Jejunitis Syndrome (Anterior Enteritis)

The duodenitis-proximal jejunitis syndrome is well recognized in Europe and the United States (12–15). There are clinical signs of a simple cranial obstruction of the small intestine with gastric reflux of fluid. There is a functional ileus of the proximal small intestine with a secondary overloading of the stomach (13). The irony of this condition is that although the clinical signs suggest a lesion requiring surgical intervention, the stresses of general anesthesia and surgical manipulation may produce a higher morbidity or mortality rate than when conservative therapy is used (12, 15). The condition can be suggested on rectal examination by palpating a distended transverse duodenum. It may be difficult to differentiate the condition from other causes of small intestinal obstruction, and diagnosis can be achieved only at surgery in some cases (15). Conservative management is generally considered the treatment of choice and includes systemic antibiotics, flunixin meglumine (Banamine) for relief of pain and to combat the effects of endotoxin, endoserum, and supportive fluid therapy. Some horses required up to 10 days of critical care before gastric reflux ceased and normal eating was allowed (12). Clostridiosis or salmonellosis have been suggested etiologic factors, but as yet no definitive cause is known.

A technique of duodenocecostomy has been described to facilitate drainage of accumulating fluid into the cecum in several cases and has been reported as a successful procedure (13). If performed, it involves a right flank approach between the 17th and 18th ribs with removal of the 18th rib. A side-to-side anastomosis of the duodenum to the base of the cecum is performed, using two layers of sutures in the serosa and muscularis and a cutting suture in the mucosa. The originator of the technique suggests that early closure of the stoma is facilitated by not involving mucosa in the suture line (13). Gastro-jejunostomy has also been described for successful management of acute proximal enteritis in an adult horse (16).

Gastroduodenal Obstruction

Gastroduodenal obstruction is an uncommon condition that has been reported in foals 4 months of age and younger (17, 18). The condition also occurs in the adult horse, but rarely (19, 20). Although congenital stricture of the pylorus or duodenum is possible, most obstructions are acquired as a result of chronic gastroduodenal ulcer disease (17, 18).

The clinical signs include mild to moderate colic with gastric reflux, salivation, bruxism, depression, anorexia, and unthriftiness. The diagnosis is generally confirmed with positive-contrast radiography, which will demonstrate retention of contrast in the stomach for at least 1 hour (17). Foals with associated cholangitis and pancreatitis have a grave prognosis (17).

Various surgical procedures have been discussed for relief of pyloric or duodenal obstructions. Simple pyloromyotomy may be effective for congenital stricture of the pylorus (21). Bypass procedures that have been reported for obstructions related to ulcer disease include gastroduodenostomy to bypass pyloric stenosis; gastroduodenostomy after partial resection of the stomach, pylorus, and a small segment of duodenum; duodeno-jejunostomy followed by jejuno-jejunostomy to bypass duodenal stricture beyond the hepaticopancreatic ampulla; and gastro-jejunostomy followed by jejuno-jejunostomy to bypass extensive stricture of the duodenum (17). Hepatico-jejunostomy, duodeno-jejunostomy, and jejuno-jejunostomy are the procedures of choice for stricture of the duodenum proximal and distal to the ampulla and for obstruction of the common hepatic duct (22).

The procedure selected to manage gastric outflow obstruction is based on the nature of the lesion (congenital versus inflammatory), the location of the obstruction, its severity, and the accessibility of the affected area. Surgical access to the stomach and proximal duodenum is easier in a foal than in an adult. In a case report of surgical management of duodenal obstruction in an adult horse, a novel J-shaped abdominal incision was made to allow access to the proximal duodenum (19). The cranial aspect of the laparotomy incision was curved and was extended to the right costal arch, creating an abdominal wall "flap." This allowed greater access for the surgeon and assistants for retraction of viscera. A hand-sutured duodeno-jejunostomy was then performed between the duodenal sigmoidal flexure and the jejunum.

Surgical stapling instruments can be used to create the anastomotic stomas, or they can be hand-sutured. A three-layer or three-"tier" construction is preferred for the hand-sutured anastomosis (21). This consists of two layers of seromuscular closure and one layer of mucosal closure. (These techniques are similar in principle to that described for a side-to-side jejunocecal anastomosis on page 340). Contamination is unavoidable but can be minimized by using continuous suction, packing off adjacent viscera with large saline-soaked laparotomy sponges, and draining the stomach before doing the anastomosis.

There is a possibility for development of an internal hernia with incarceration and strangulation of intestine if a potential hernial ring is created during the bypass procedure. This is probably more likely to occur if a gastro-jejunostomy has been done. Blind loop syndrome is also a possible sequela to gastro-jejunostomy or duodeno-jejunostomy. The rationale for performing an adjunctive jejuno-jejunostomy is to provide secretions from the pancreas, liver, and the duodenum an alternative route into the distal jejunum, instead of having to reenter the proximal duodenum or stomach (19).

Strangulating Obstruction of the Small Intestine

Intussusception

An intussusception is the invagination of a segment of intestine (intussusceptum) and its mesentery into the adjacent distal segment of bowel (intussuscipiens) (Fig. 7.3*A*). The small intestine is the most common site of occurrence for this condition, and it can involve the jejunum, ileum, or terminal ileum (ileocecal intussusception). The condition occurs more frequently in young horses (23, 24), but not exclusively so. The initial clinical signs are usually characterized by signs of colic associated with obstruction of the small intestine. The superimposed signs of bowel strangulation develop at later stages. Preoperatively, ultrasonographic examination of the ventral abdomen in foals may demonstrate small intestinal intussusception (25). The condition is easily recognized at laparotomy with systematic exploration of the small intestine starting at the ileocecal valve. Reduction of the intussusception may be possible but can be precluded by excessive swelling of the intussuscipiens or serosal adhesions. While intussusceptions have been treated by reduction alone, the authors recommend that resection of all intussusceptions should be a general consideration even when the intussuscipiens is apparently viable. Progressive mucosal degeneration can still develop (26). The surgeon must remember that the ileal artery, which runs along the mesenteric border of the ileum, is the sole source of blood supply for the ileum if the intussusception involves this area. Peritonitis (from necrosis of the bowel segment), stenosis, or adhesions are all potential developments if the intussuscepted portion is not resected.

For jejunal intussusceptions, resection and end-to-end anastomosis are usually appropriate. If the ileum is involved in the intussusception, a jejunocecal anastomosis is performed.

Ileal intussusception can be successfully managed with reduction and a side-to-side ileocecal bypass performed proximal to the site of the intussusception (24). An ileal resection and jejunocecostomy would obviously be indicated if the viability of the ileum was in question.

The surgical technique selected for correction of an ileocecal intussusception is dependent on whether the condition is acute or chronic, the length of bowel involved and its viability, and whether the intussusception can be reduced (27).

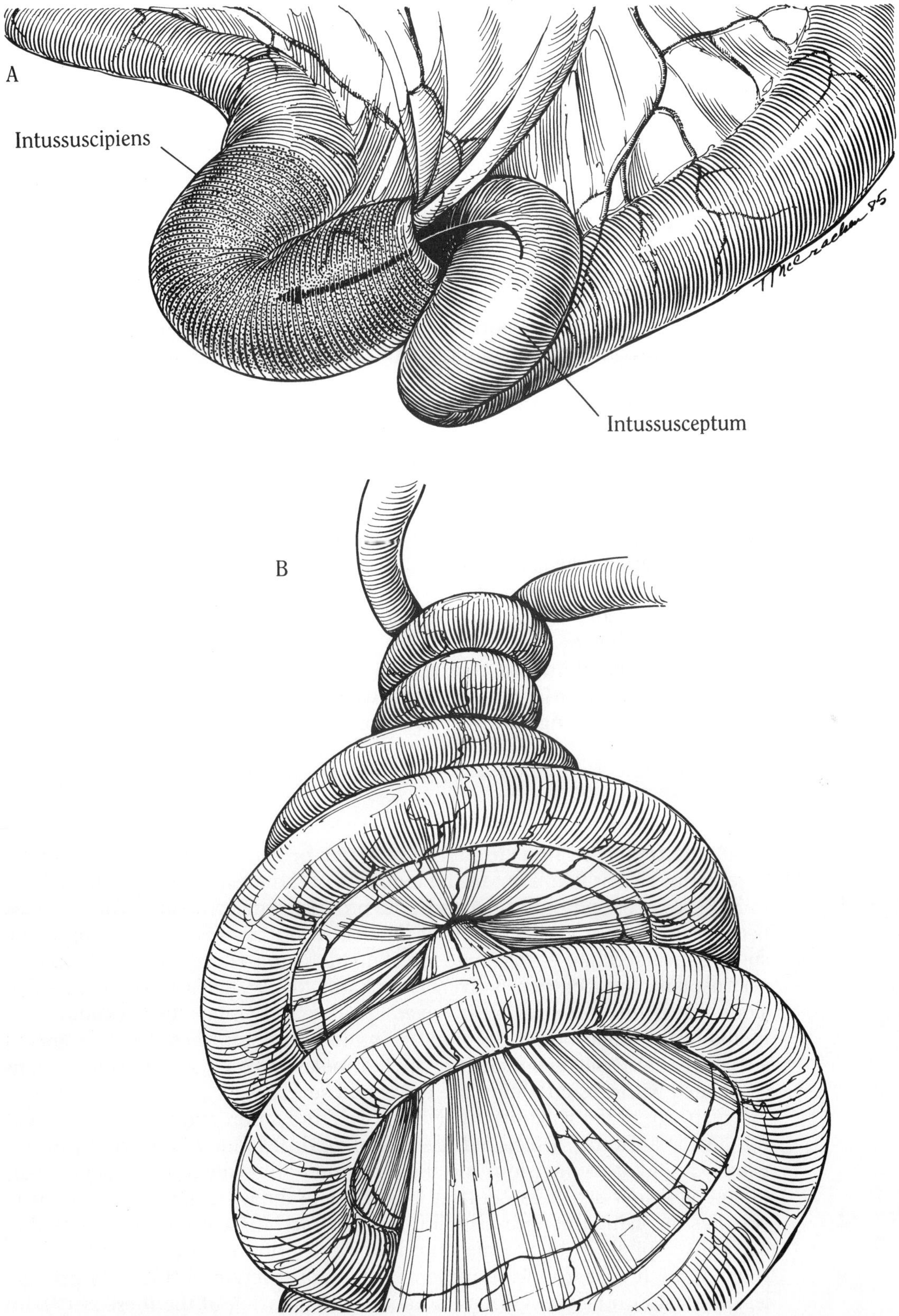

Figure 7.3. Strangulating obstruction of the small intestine. **A.** Intussusception of small intestine. **B.** Volvulus of small intestine.

Most ileocecal intussusceptions produce acute and complete obstruction; however, there are cases of chronic intussusception that produce partial obstruction and recurrent colic. Generally, the chronic ileocecal intussusception involves a shorter length of distal ileum (27).

With an acute ileocecal intussusception, there are a number of options for correction. If the intussusception can be reduced, the ileum and a portion of distal jejunum are resected, the distal ileum is blind-stumped, and a jejunocecostomy is performed. If the intussusception cannot be reduced, there are other possibilities for correction. The ileum or distal jejunum can be amputated as close to the cecum as possible, leaving a blind stump of distal bowel, and a jejunocecal anastomosis performed. The intussusception remains in situ, and if the distal stump becomes necrotic, fatal peritonitis may develop. Regardless, horses treated in this fashion generally have a protracted postoperative ileus and a poor prognosis. Another alternative is to simply leave the intussusception in situ and perform a side-to-side jejunocecal bypass (28). Leaving a large intussusception in the cecum may result in obstruction of the cecocolic orifice (29).

There are reports of resection of the intussusception through a typhlotomy (27, 30). The most recent describes a method for complete resection with closure of the ileocecal orifice from within the cecum (30). A jejunocecostomy was then performed. Distal ileal inversion techniques with and without ileocecal orifice closure have also been described (31). In some horses it may be possible, with the use of stapling devices, to resect the entire distal ileum and place inverting sutures across the ileocecal orifice. This technique should be attempted only if the surgeon is convinced that the distal ileum is nonviable and the horse is small enough to allow this type of access.

Chronic ileocecal intussusception can be successfully treated with a side-to-side ileocecostomy or jejunocecostomy without resection (32).

As with all the strangulating obstructions described in this section, ancillary therapy to combat the effects of ischemia and endotoxemia is important.

Volvulus

Small intestinal volvulus is produced by a 180° or greater rotation of a segment of jejunum and/or ileum about the long axis of the mesentery. Rotations of up to 180° may occur physiologically without producing disturbances. Volvulus may occur as a primary displacement or may be secondary to a preexisting lesion, such as incarceration of the small intestine in the mesentery, epiploic foramen, gastrosplenic ligament, mesodiverticular band, Meckel's diverticulum, or adhesions. The ileum is commonly involved. Incarceration involving the caudal segments of the small bowel (terminal jejunum and ileum) has been assigned a specific name, "volvulus nodosus," by European workers (1). The clinical signs associated with this condition are acute and severe.

Treatment of the volvulus involves surgical reduction and intestinal evacuation. At laparotomy, discolored, thickened, and distended loops of bowel are usually found at the incision, and the direction of the volvulus is usually ascertained by palpating the mesentery at the base of the twist (Fig. 7.3*B*). In severe volvulus involving the entire small intestinal tract, the mesentery is twisted in a cordlike spiral up to the mesenteric root. The more times the intestine is rotated, the higher up in the mesentery the constriction occurs. Any primary lesion must also be recognized and addressed. Tearing of the mesentery with incarceration may also occur secondarily to the volvulus. Which malposition to correct first depends on the individual case. Correction of the volvulus is performed by rotating all affected loops in the appropriate direction. Sectioning of intestine with temporary closure may be necessary to correct the displacement. Following reduction, nonviable bowel is resected and an end-to-end anastomosis or jejunocecal anastomosis performed as appropriate. If resection of greater than 50% of the small intestine is indicated, euthanasia should be considered (33).

The prognosis in cases of volvulus is commonly poor because of the rapid deterioration of the patient and excessive intestinal involvement in many instances.

Internal Hernias

An internal hernia is a displacement of organs through a normal or pathologic opening within the abdominal cavity (34). Internal herniation of the small intestine usually results in incarceration. Herniation may occur through a normal opening (epiploic foramen) or a pathologic opening (acquired or congenital mesenteric defects, tears in the greater or lesser omentum or gastrosplenic ligament, or defects in the broad ligament or foramina formed by fibrous bands or adhesions). Herniation through a tear in the ligament of the ductus deferens also has been described (1). The clinical signs are generally typical of strangulating obstruction of the small intestine. In some instances, however, strangulation has not yet occurred at the time of laparotomy, and the intestine is still viable.

Epiploic Foramen Incarceration

The epiploic foramen that separates the omental bursa from the major peritoneal cavity is bounded dorsally by the caudal lobe of the liver and the caudal vena cava and ventrally by the right lobe of the pancreas, gastropancreatic fold, and portal vein. The foramen is limited cranially by the hepatoduodenal ligament and caudally by the junction of the pancreas and mesoduodenum (35). Herniation of small intestine through the epiploic foramen can occur in a right-to-left direction from the peritoneal cavity through the foramen into the omental bursa (also called herniation from the lateral side) (1), or in a left-to-right direction when the omental bursa is involved in the herniation and the omentum is torn (also called herniation from the medial side). Herniation from right to left is the most commonly recognized form in the United States (12 of 15 cases in one report) (36), but in a European report, incarceration from medial to lateral was reported as more common (1). These hernias are illustrated in Figure 7.3, *C* and *D*. The incarcerated portion of bowel is distended. A special, rare form of epiploic foramen incarceration whereby a portion of the small intestinal wall protrudes through the epiploic foramen from the lateral side has been described in Europe, and has been called a Littré's hernia (1). Incarceration of the large colon through the epiploic foramen can also occur (37).

Surgical treatment of incarceration of small intestine in the epiploic foramen is made difficult because the condition is not always associated with signs typical of intestinal incarceration (38, 39). The degree of pain may be highly variable, but analysis of peritoneal fluid can be useful. Abdominal ultrasonography can also be helpful for revealing small intestinal distension that may not be evident on rectal examination (39). Failure to diagnose the condition early and intervene surgically causes a low success rate (36). Success rates have improved with earlier referral and diagnosis and prompt surgical treatment (39).

The condition is confirmed at laparotomy during systematic exploration of the small intestine. Although the condition may be recognized by palpating the region of the epiploic foramen, the condition is more consistently characterized by locating the ileocecal fold and following the ileum craniad until the incarceration is encountered. The incarceration may involve midjejunum or distal jejunum and/or ileum. A large portion of the small intestine may be incarcerated. If the incarceration is from right to left, reduction is made from the right side of the abdominal cavity and the intestine is pulled out of the omental bursa through the epiploic foramen. Reduction in this fashion is usually possible, but the strangulated intestine can become edematous to the point that reduction

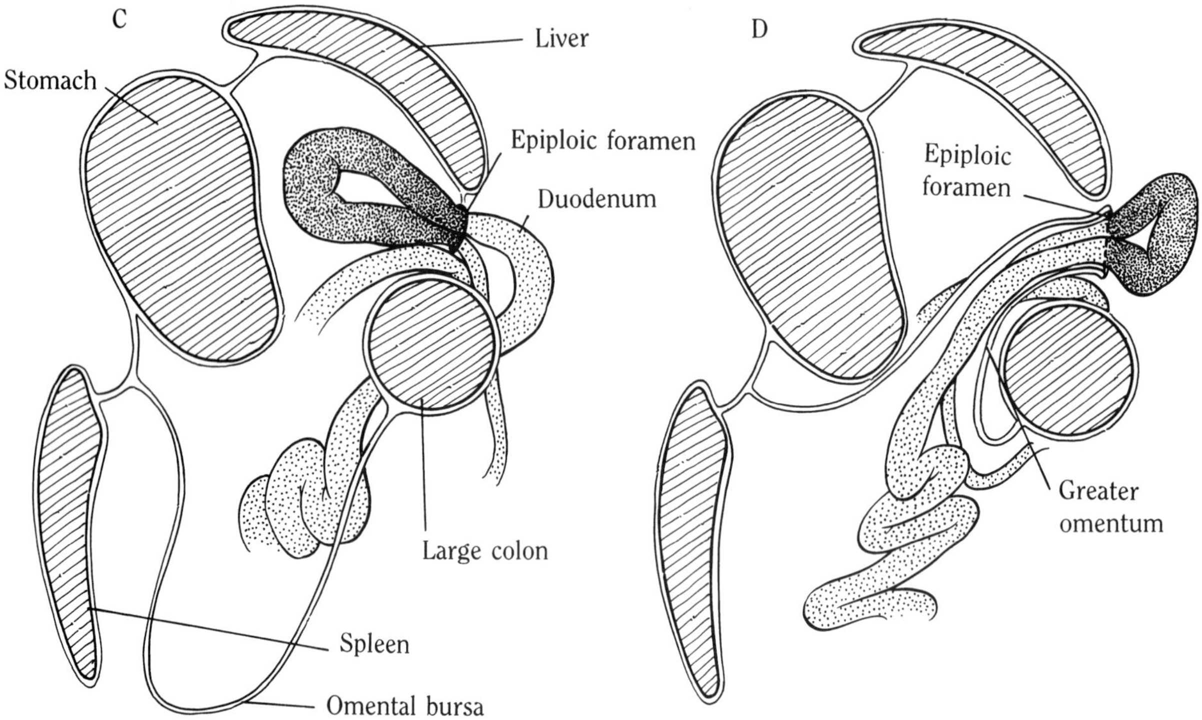

Figure 7.3. *(continued)* **C.** Right-to-left hernia of small intestine through epiploic foramen. **D.** Left-to-right hernia through epiploic foramen.

may not be feasible. Cautious manipulation and traction should be performed because of the risk of rupturing vascular structures associated with the epiploic foramen (40). Prior decompression or even sectioning of the intestine and evacuation may be required in an exceptional case (37). A left-to-right incarceration must be retracted back into the omental bursa side. Resection and anastomosis of devitalized bowel is usually required, and end-to-end anastomosis of jejunum or jejunocecal anastomosis is performed as appropriate. Closure of the epiploic foramen is not practical. The prognosis depends on the promptness of surgical intervention and on the amount of compromised bowel.

Mesenteric Incarceration

Incarceration through an acquired rent in the mesentery usually occurs through the ileal mesentery. It is assumed that these tears occur at the same time as the incarceration. However, spontaneous tears of the mesentery associated with physiologic invaginations of the small intestine as a result of hyperperistalsis may occur. In these cases, the mesentery of the intussusceptum becomes stretched and possibly torn (1). Mesenteric rents may also have been created during a previous colic surgery. The herniated piece of intestine can become incarcerated and strangulated by the hernial ring (Fig. 7.3*E*). Volvulus may occur secondary to this condition (Fig. 7.3*F*). The clinical signs are typical of strangulation obstruction of the small intestine. They will generally be more severe if there is an associated volvulus.

The condition is recognized at laparotomy. If volvulus of the herniated segment of bowel is found, it should be corrected first. Reduction of the mesenteric hernia may require prior evacuation of the herniated portion of the intestine as well as enlargement of the hernial ring. The strangulated jejunum or ileum is resected, and an end-to-end jejunal or jejunocecal anastomosis is performed

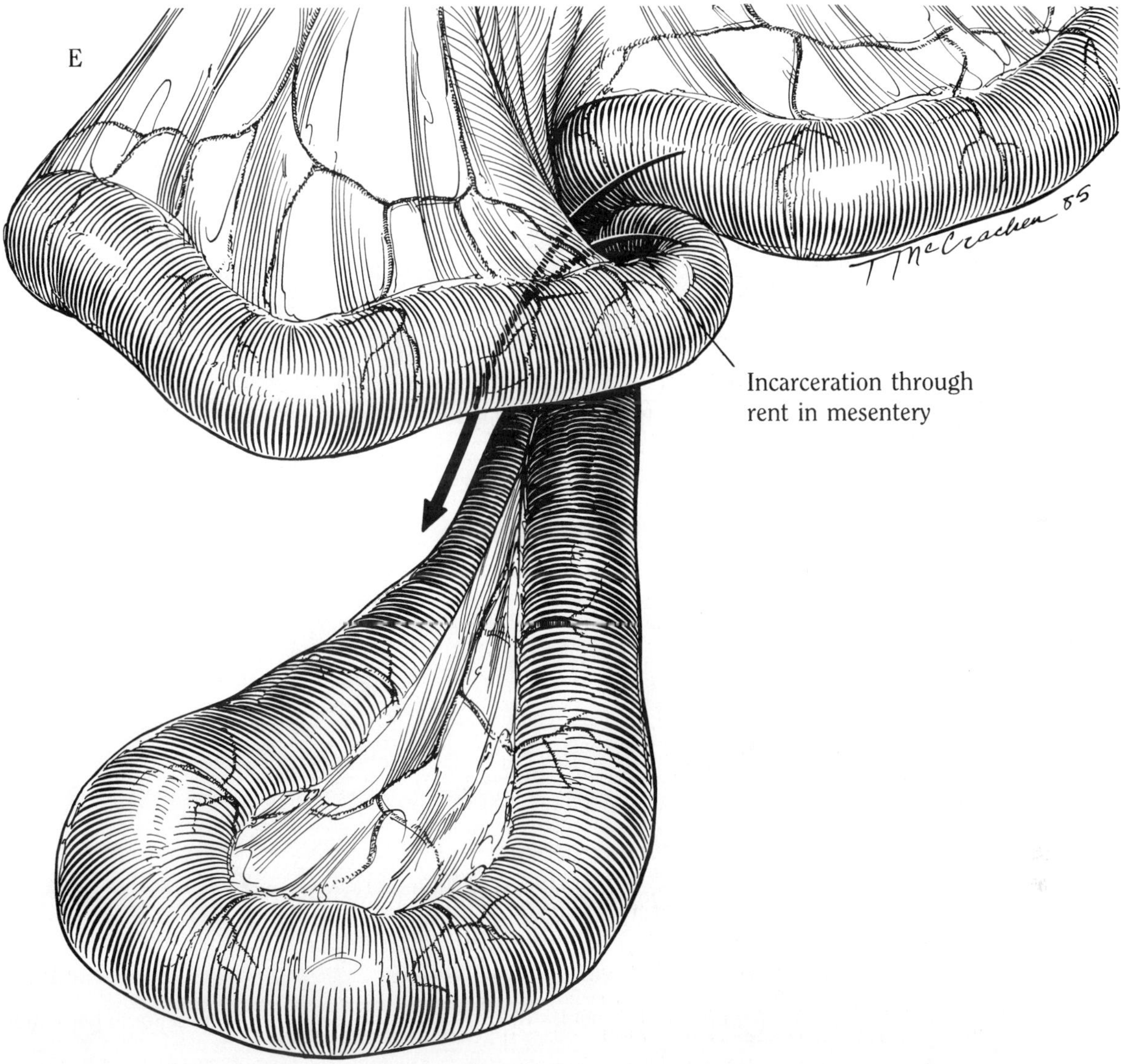

FIGURE 7.3. *(continued)* E. Herniation of small intestine through a mesenteric rent.

as appropriate. Effective closure of the mesenteric rent can be difficult, particularly in foals in which the mesentery is very friable or if the tear extends into the more proximal mesentery. Care must be taken to avoid damaging any mesenteric vessels during mesenteric repair.

Mesenteric Incarceration in Association with an Anomalous Mesodiverticular Band

A mesodiverticular band is formed by persistence of a distal segment of a vitelline artery and its associated embryonic mesentery (Fig. 7.3*G*). The band extends from one side of the small intestinal mesentery to the antimesenteric surface of the intestine (usually jejunum), and a triangular hiatus is thus formed among the mesodiverticular band, jejunal mesentery, and jejunum (Fig. 7.3*G*). Entrapment of intestine in this hiatus can result in herniation of the intestine through the jejunal mesentery (41). Secondary volvulus of the incarcerated portion may also occur. Treatment of this condition consists of reduction of the incarceration and volvulus, and intestinal resection and anastomosis.

F

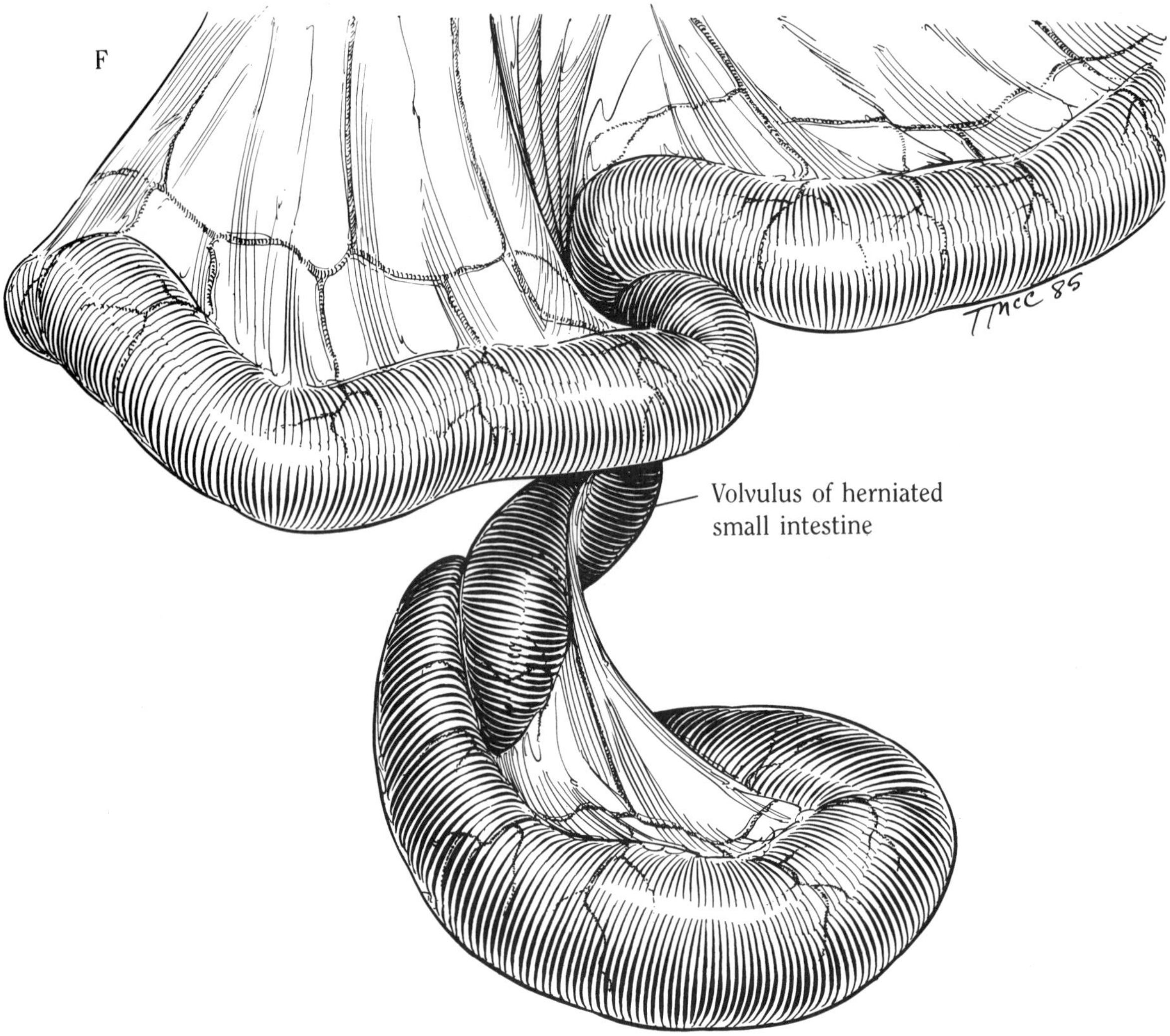

Figure 7.3. *(continued)* F. Volvulus of small intestine secondary to mesenteric herniation.

Herniation Through Omental Defects

The small intestine may herniate through a rent in the greater omentum or a window formed by an omental adhesion (42). It may also herniate through the gastrosplenic ligament (43) or through tears in the lesser omentum (hepatogastric and hepatoduodenal ligament) (1). Clinical signs and surgical management are similar to those for other internal hernias. Defects in the greater omentum are best handled by removal of the offending portion of the omentum. Obliteration of a defect in the lesser omentum is not feasible.

Herniation Through the Broad Ligament

Herniation of small intestine through the broad ligament has been reported, but is uncommon (44). Reduction and resection (and anastomosis, if necessary) are performed. The defect in the mesometrium cannot be closed.

Strangulating Hernia Associated with a Pedunculated Lipoma

Simple obstruction associated with a pedunculated lipoma has been mentioned previously. Strangulating obstruction of the small intestine can occur when the pedicle of a pedunculated lipoma encircles a section of small intestine (Fig.

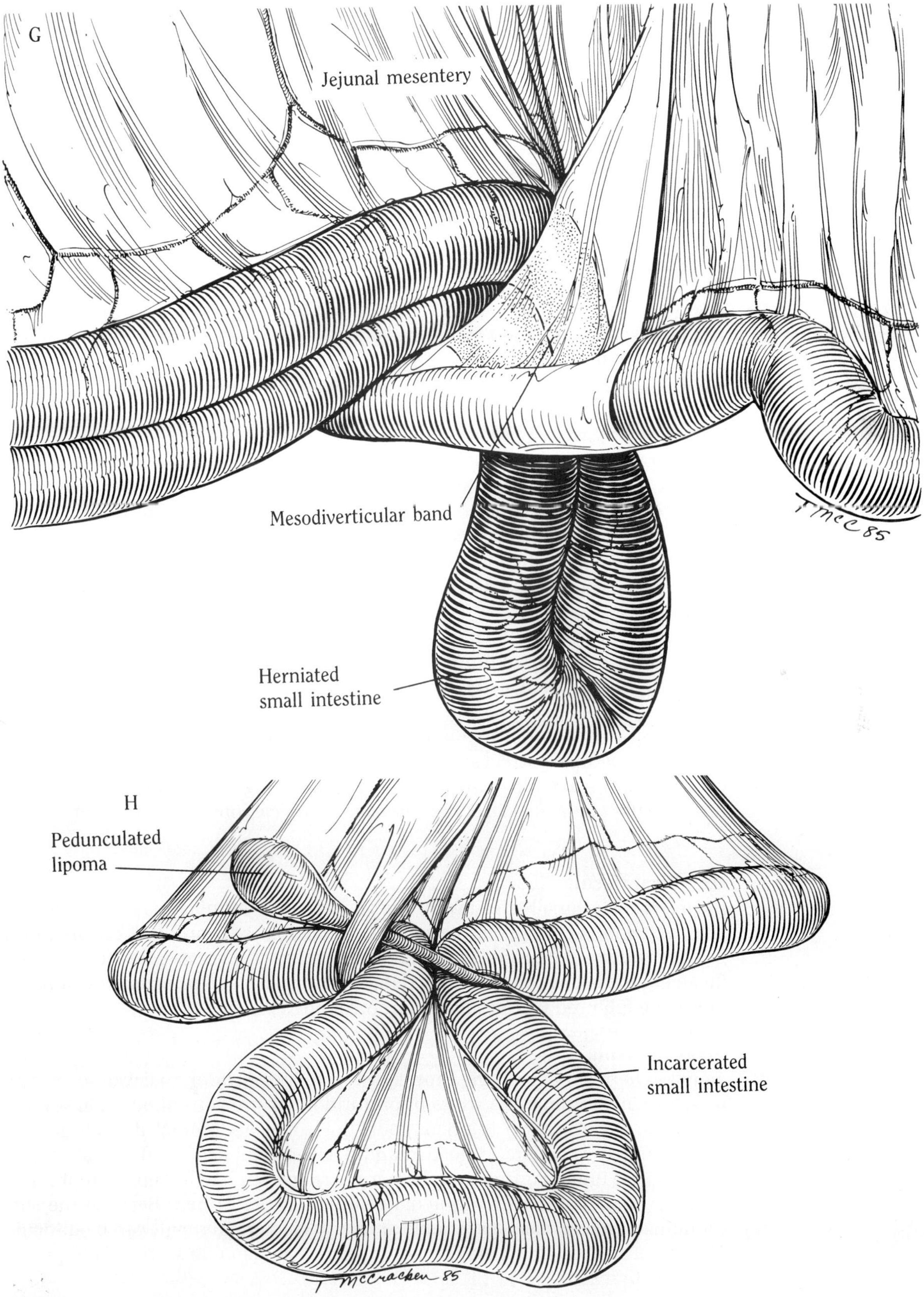

Figure 7.3. *(continued)* **G.** Mesenteric herniation in association with an anomalous mesodiverticular band. **H.** Strangulated obstruction of small intestine caused by a pedunculated lipoma.

7.3*H*). Incarceration of intestine through a ring created by a pedicle of the lipoma can be considered a form of internal hernia. Treatment involves severance of the pedicle, removal of the lipoma, and resection and anastomosis of the intestine.

External Hernias

An external hernia is a displacement of abdominal contents beyond the abdominal cavity. Examples include inguinal hernias, umbilical hernias, ventral abdominal hernias, and diaphragmatic hernias.

Inguinal or Scrotal Hernia

The term *inguinal hernia* is usually used if hernial contents descend into the inguinal canal; if the contents descend into the scrotum, the term *scrotal hernia* is appropriate (34). However, the term *inguinal hernia* is often used to mean either condition. Acquired inguinal hernia is a problem of stallions (45). The condition is usually unilateral and almost always produces an acute strangulating obstruction of the jejunum or ileum. The vaginal ring forms the hernial orifice, and the tunica vaginalis forms the hernial sac (classified as *indirect* hernia). *Direct* herniation as it occurs in man, without involvement of the internal ring, has been reported rarely in the horse (46). Clinical diagnosis of an inguinal hernia is confirmed with a combination of external palpation and rectal palpation of the inguinal rings. Ultrasonographic examination of the swollen scrotum may provide ancillary confirmation of a scrotal hernia. The surgical correction of an inguinal hernia is described in detail in the "Inguinal Herniorrhaphy" section.

Owners should be informed that an inguinal hernia may be an inheritable condition. A higher than normal incidence of scrotal hernia has been reported in certain breeds, such as the Standardbred. Bilateral castration should be considered.

Surgical correction of inguinal hernias in foals is usually not necessary because most of them correct spontaneously as the foal grows. Occasionally, incarceration can result (the intestine can break through the common tunic and migrate subcutaneously in some cases) and surgical intervention becomes necessary.

Umbilical Hernia

Incarceration of small intestine through an umbilical hernia is rare but occasionally occurs. Most umbilical hernias are reducible and produce no problems in their routine repair, as discussed in the authors' previous textbook (47). If incarceration occurs, the hernia is reduced surgically, and resection and anastomosis are followed by umbilical herniorrhaphy (48).

Ventral Hernia

Acquired hernias occur in the ventral or ventrolateral abdominal wall secondary to abdominal trauma, the stress of parturition, or previous abdominal surgery (3). Acute incarceration is uncommon but some abdominal discomfort can occur. Surgery is generally elective and delayed until acute inflammation and infection are under control and the hernial ring is sufficiently fibrosed. If intestinal incarceration occurs, immediate surgery is performed. Because the surrounding tissue is often very friable at this stage, hernial repair can be difficult. The use of surgical mesh may be appropriate (see separate section for repair of hernia with mesh).

Diaphragmatic Hernia

Diaphragmatic hernias are rare. Most cases are acquired (49–51), but congenital hernias do occur (52). The majority of the lesions occur in the tendinous portion of the diaphragm, most commonly where the centrum tendineum blends into the pars costalis. Congenital defects are infrequent, resulting from incomplete fusion of the pleuroperitoneal folds (52).

The clinical signs associated with diaphragmatic hernia are variable and depend on the size of the hernial orifice and on the amount of herniated viscera. Most cases of diaphragmatic hernia have been definitively diagnosed at laparotomy or necropsy. A definitive clinical diagnosis is possible by thoracic radiography and ultrasonographic examination of the thoracic cavity. Successful surgical correction of nonstrangulating diaphragmatic hernia has been reported (52, 53). A ventral midline laparotomy approach is used, and a mesh implant can be incorporated into the repair of the diaphragmatic defect (53). Generally, surgical repair in the adult horse is difficult because of an inaccessibility of the dorsal diaphragmatic rent, inability to retract the viscera, and the friability of the damaged diaphragmatic tissue. A case of peritoneopericardial hernia has been reported in a 3-year-old Standardbred stallion (54). The hernial defect was not closed, and the horse was normal 1 year later (54). An unusual case of a diaphragmatic diverticulum, in which there was no communication between the peritoneal and the pleural or pericardial cavities, was repaired with polypropylene mesh (55).

REFERENCES

1. Huskamp, B, Daniels, H, Kopf, N. Diseases of the stomach and intestine. In: Dietz O, Wiesner E, eds. Diseases of the Horse. Basel: S Karger, 1984:164.
2. White NA, Sullins KE, Robertson JT. Surgery for acute abdominal disease. In: The Equine Acute Abdomen. Philadelphia: Lea & Febiger, 1990:210–307.
3. Steckel RR. Diagnosis and management of acute abdominal pain (colic). In: Auer JA, ed. Equine Surgery. Philadelphia: WB Saunders, 1992:348–360.
4. Embertson RM, Colahan PT, Brown MP, et al. Ileal impaction in the horse. JAVMA 1985;186:570.
5. Hanson RR, Schumaker J, Humbug J, et al. Medical treatment of horses with ileal impactions: 10 cases (1990–1994). JAVMA 1996;208:898.
6. Southwood LL, Ragle CA, Snyder JR, et al. Surgical treatment of ascarid impactions in horses and foals. 42nd Annual Conference Procedures of the AAEP, Denver, CO, 1996:258.
7. Blikslager AT, Bowman KF, Haven ML, et al. Pedunculated lipomas as a cause of intestinal obstruction in horses: 17 cases (1983–1990). JAVMA 1992;201:1249.
8. Rumbaugh GE, Smith BP, Carlson GP. Internal abdominal abscesses in the horse: a study of 25 cases. JAVMA 1978;172:304.
9. Valdez H, McLaughlin SA, Taylor TS. A case of colic due to an abscess of the jejunum and its mesentery. J Equine Med Surg 1979;3:36.
10. Horney FD, Funk KA. Ileal myotomy in the horse. Mod Vet Pract 1971;52:49.
11. Lindsay WA, Confer AW, Ochoa R. Ileal smooth muscle hypertrophy and rupture in a horse. Equine Vet J 1981;13:66.
12. White NA, Tyler DE, Blackwell RB, et al. Hemorrhagic fibrinonecrotic duodenitis-proximal jejunitis in horses: 20 cases (1977–1984). JAVMA 1987;190:311.
13. Huskamp B. Diagnosis of gastroduodenojejunitis and its surgical treatment by a temporary duodenocaecostomy. Equine Vet J 1985;17:314.
14. Johnston JK, Morris DD. Comparison of duodenitis/proximal jejunitis and small intestinal obstruction in horses: 68 cases (1977–1985). JAVMA 1987;191:849.
15. Leeth B, Robertson JT. A retrospective comparison of surgical to medical management of proximal enteritis in the horse. In: The Proceedings of the 34th Annual Conference of the AAEP, San Diego, CA, 1988:69.
16. Gillis JP, Taylor TS, Puckett MJ. Gastrojejunostomy for management of acute proximal enteritis in a horse. JAVMA 1994;204:633.
17. Orsini JA, Donawick WJ. Surgical treatment of gastroduodenal obstruction in foals. Vet Surg 1986;15:205–213.
18. Campbell-Thompson ML, Brown MP, Slone DE, et al. Gastroenterostomy for treatment of gastroduodenal ulcer disease in 14 foals. JAVMA 1986;188:840–844.

19. Ross MW, Bernard WV, Orsini PG. Surgical management of duodenal obstruction in an adult horse. JAVMA 1989;194:1312–1314.
20. Hanson PD, Bartz TA, Stone WC, et al. Use of a modified Roux-en-Y procedure for treatment of pyloroduodenal obstruction in a horse. JAVMA 1993;202:1119–1122.
21. Orsini JA, Doran R, Allen D. In: Auer JA, ed. Small Intestine in Equine Surgery. Philadelphia: WB Saunders Co, 1992:360–378.
22. Orsini JA, Donawick WJ. Hepaticojejunostomy for treatment of common hepatic duct obstruction associated with duodenal stenosis in two foals. Vet Surg 1989;18: 34–38.
23. Rooney JR. Volvulus, strangulation and intussusception in the horse. Cornell Vet 1965;55:644.
24. Greet TRC. Ileal intussusception in 16 young Thoroughbreds. Equine Vet J 1992;24: 81.
25. Bernard WV, Reef VB, Reimer JM, et al. Ultrasonographic diagnosis of small intestinal intussusception in three foals. JAVMA 1989;194:395–397.
26. Owen R ap R, Physick-Sheard PW, Hilbert BJ, et al. Jejuno- or ileocecal anastomosis performed in seven horses exhibiting colic. Can Vet J 1975;165:164.
27. Ford TS, Freeman DF, Ross MW, et al. Ileocecal intussusception in horses: 26 cases (1981–1988). JAVMA 1990;196:121.
28. Maclean AA, Church S, Dyke TM, et al. An alternative approach for treatment of irreducible ileocecal intussusception in six horses. Equine Vet Educ 1991;3:10–12.
29. Schumaker J, Hanrahan L. Ileocecal intussusception as a sequel to jejunocecostomy in a mare. JAVMA 1987;190:303.
30. Beard WL, Byrne BA, Henninger RW. Ileocecal intussusception corrected by resection within the cecum in two horses. JAVMA 1992;200:1978.
31. Vasey JR, Julian RJ. Elective inversion of the distal ileal stump into the cecum of the horse. Equine Vet J 1987;19:223.
32. Scott EA, Todhunter R. Chronic intestinal intussusception in two horses. JAVMA 1985;186:383.
33. Tate LP, Ralston SL, Koch CM, et al. Effects of extensive resection of the small intestine in the pony. Am J Vet Res 1983;44:1187.
34. Nieberle K, Cohrs P. Textbook of Special Pathological Anatomy of Domestic Animals. Oxford: Pergamon Press, 1967.
35. Rooney JR, Sack WO, Habel RE. Guide to the Dissection of the Horse. Ann Arbor, MI: Edwards Brothers, 1967.
36. Turner TA, Adams SB, White NA. Small intestine incarceration through the epiploic foramen of the horse. JAVMA 1984;184:731.
37. Foerner JJ, Ringle MJ, Junkins DS, et al. Transection of the pelvic flexure to reduce incarceration of the large colon through the epiploic foramen in a horse. JAVMA 1993;203:1312–1313.
38. Engelbert TA, Tate LP, Bowman KF, et al. Incarceration of small intestine in the epiploic foramen: report of 19 cases (1983–1992). Vet Surg 1993;22:57.
39. Vachon AM, Fischer AT. Small intestinal herniation through the epiploic foramen: 53 cases (1987–1993). Equine Vet J 1995;27:373–380.
40. Livesy MA, Little CB, Boyd C. Fatal hemorrhage associated with incarceration of small intestine by the epiploic foramen in three horses. Can Vet J 1991;32:434–436.
41. Freeman DE, Koch DB, Boles CL. Mesodiverticular bands as a cause of small intestinal strangulation and volvulus in the horse. JAVMA 1979;175:1089.
42. Norrie RD, Heistand DL. Chronic colic due to an omental adhesion in a mare. JAVMA 1975;167:54.
43. Tennant B. Intestinal obstruction in the horse: some aspects of differential diagnosis in equine colic. Proceedings of the AAEP, Dallas, TX, 1976:426.
44. Becht JL, McIlwraith CW. Jejunal displacement through the mesometrium in a pregnant mare. JAVMA 1980;177:435.
45. Schneider RK, Milne DW, Kohn CW. Acquired inguinal hernia in the horse: a review of 27 cases. JAVMA 1982;180:317.
46. Vasey JR. Simultaneous presence of a direct and an indirect inguinal hernia in a stallion. Aust Vet J 1981;57:418.
47. Turner AS, McIlwraith CW. In: Techniques in Large Animal Surgery. 2nd ed. Philadelphia: Lea & Febiger, 1989.

48. Markel MD, Pascoe JR, Sams AE. Strangulated umbilical hernias in horses: 13 cases (1974–1985). JAVMA 1987;190:692–694.
49. Crowhurst RC, Simpson DJ, McEnery RJ, et al. Intestinal surgery in the horse. J S Afr Vet Assoc 1975;46:59.
50. Pearson H, Pinsent PJN, Polley LR, et al. Rupture of the diaphragm in the horse. Equine Vet J 1977;9:32.
51. Wimberley HC, Andrews EJ, Haschek WM. Diaphragmatic hernias in the horse: a review of the literature and analysis of six additional cases. JAVMA 1977;170:1404.
52. Spiers VC, Reynolds WT. Surgical repair of a diaphragmatic hernia in a foal. Equine Vet J 1976;8:170.
53. Scott EA, Fishback WA. Surgical repair of diaphragmatic hernia in a horse. JAVMA 1976;168:45.
54. Orsini JA, Koch C, Stewart B. Peritoneopericardial hernia in a horse. JAVMA 1981; 179:907.
55. Proudman CJ, Edwards GB. Diaphragmatic (hernia) in a horse. Equine Vet J 1992; 24:244–246.

Surgical Corrections of Displacements and Abnormalities of the Large Intestine

Simple Obstruction of the Large Intestine

Impaction with Ingesta

Impaction of the large intestine is a common cause of intestinal obstruction. It is commonly treated conservatively, but surgical intervention is appropriate when conservative methods fail to solve the problem. Impaction may involve the cecum, the large colon, or the small colon.

Impaction of the Cecum

Impaction of the cecum is normally insidious in onset and the cause is unknown (1–3). It has been postulated that primary cecal outflow dysfunction may precede the development of cecal impaction, and such factors as hospitalization, systemic illness, and previous treatment may be contributory (2, 3). Cecal impaction may also be secondary to a pathologic problem of the cecocolic orifice (4). The course of the condition can be one of intermittent colic for 1 week or longer. Because the cecum is a blind sac, fluid and some ingesta can bypass the obstruction. There are three forms of surgical therapy if the impaction proves unresponsive to medical treatment. Failure to provide surgical treatment can lead to rupture of the cecum in some horses (3).

Surgical intervention may be limited to a laparotomy with exposure of the cecum and injection of saline solution and the surfactant dioctyl sodium sulfosuccinate (DSS) directly into the impacted mass. Manual massage is performed to break up the impacted mass and distribute the injected fluids. In one report, the results of such treatment were poor (1).

Better results have been achieved with typhlotomy at the cecal apex and evacuation of the impacted contents (evacuation is facilitated by the use of a hose). Early surgical intervention and evacuation of the cecum would seem appropriate based on findings in 12 cases of cecal impaction. The duration of clinical signs before rupture ranged from 4 to 96 hours (1). Failure of normal motility to return after cecal evacuation may also be a problem, and reimpaction can occur.

A third surgical procedure, and the most effective procedure for treatment of horses with more severe, prolonged, or recurrent cecal impaction, is an ileal- or jejunocolostomy that completely bypasses the cecum and prevents recurrence of impaction (2). This procedure is done in conjunction with cecal evacuation via a typhlotomy.

Impaction of the Large Colon

Impaction is a frequent cause of simple obstruction of the large colon. An impaction by ingesta usually occurs at the pelvic flexure or the right dorsal colon-transverse colon region, where the large colon becomes narrow. The pelvic flexure has been identified as a region of resistance to aboral flow and is a probable pacemaker site (5). Selective retention of large particles also occurs in the right dorsal colon, and the transverse colon provides more resistance to flow than does the pelvic flexure (6). Factors that may precipitate impaction include poor quality feed, decreased water intake and dehydration, and parasitic damage. Sand impactions are a special problem that occur in the right dorsal or ventral colon. These are associated with the availability of sand or gravel in the feeding of horses off the ground.

Most impactions with ingesta respond to conservative medical management, which includes the administration of mineral oil and/or DSS together with oral and intravenous fluids, if necessary. Medication is used for pain control. If the problem persists, or if there is systemic deterioration or the development of refractory pain and nasogastric reflux, surgical intervention is indicated. If surgery is delayed, devitalization of the large colon may occur, and the large colon will be more friable and prone to rupture when an expiratory laparotomy is finally done.

The surgical manipulations for impactions of the large colon consist of evacuation accompanied by flushing of the large colon. Generally this is done by exteriorizing the pelvic flexure onto a colon tray, creating an enterotomy, and flushing warm water into the colon using a hose as illustrated in the section on enterotomy (4). This technique is preferable to manually milking out dry ingesta, particularly for right dorsal-transverse colon impactions.

Sand impactions are more difficult to treat. Medical management may include the use of the natural fiber laxative psyllium hydrophilic mucilloid (Metamucil). Surgical intervention is indicated if there is no response to medical treatment and is the same as previously described for an ingesta impaction.

Impaction of the Small Colon

Ingesta impactions can also occur in the small colon, and a predisposition in ponies and American Miniature horses has been reported (7, 8). Methods for treating impactions of the small colon include injection into the bowel and massage, retrograde flushing and massage with a hose inserted per rectum (9), or evacuation through an enterotomy. Horses with small colon impaction may be fecal-culture positive for salmonella, especially after surgery (10).

As a final comment, it should be remembered always that impaction can result secondarily whenever bowel stasis develops. Whenever an impaction is identified at surgery, a complete exploration should be performed to ensure other problems do not exist and that the impaction is indeed primary.

Foreign Body Impaction

A special form of impaction may occur in association with the ingestion of nondigestible foreign materials, such as baling twine, braided materials, rubber or nylon products, and even plastic bags. This situation is typically observed in foals and young horses (11, 12), and a particular problem has been experienced in association with ingestion of rubberized fencing material or nylon cording from nylon-based products (11). The impacting material consists of a firm concretion of ingesta surrounding the core of foreign fibrous strands. Long periods between exposure to the material and development of the clinical problem can occur, indicating that strands of cording may be present in the bowel lumen for a long time before amalgamating to cause an obstruction.

The clinical signs are similar to those of impaction. However, because of the nondegradable nature of the impacting mass, medical treatment is of no value or only palliative until the next attack. Surgical removal of the offending material is necessary, and enterotomy and removal are performed at an appropriate location in the bowel. The obstruction typically occurs in the small colon and/or transverse colon, but the material may extend into the right dorsal colon. Surgical exteriorization of the right dorsal colon-transverse colon or immediately adjacent to the small colon is not possible. Therefore, an enterotomy is made in a portion of the right dorsal colon that can be exteriorized or through the small colon distal to the obstruction. In some instances removal may not be possible, and bowel wall devitalization can also lead to rupture during surgical manipulation. The prognosis is fair if the bowel is healthy and if removal can be performed effectively without extensive contamination of the abdominal cavity. Formation of adhesions in the area is a potential complication.

Enteroliths

Enteroliths occur in the large intestine and can remain there for long periods unassociated with clinical signs until they become impacted in the narrow part of the digestive tract. They may cause obstruction in the right dorsal colon, the transverse colon, or the proximal small colon (the latter site is the most common) (13). Large enteroliths are characteristic of the right dorsal colon (14). The enteroliths are generally spherical or tetrahedral in shape. When multiple stones are present, they are usually tetrahedral. Clinical symptoms vary, but horses typically present with a recurrent mild colic. If the enterolith causes an incomplete blockage, the colic is similar to an impaction. Gas, fluid, and mineral oil can still be passed, but there is no solid fecal material. A complete obstruction will cause a colic that increases in intensity as tympany of the colon occurs.

Treatment is surgical removal. At surgery there will be distension of the colon cranial to the enterolith, and the small colon is empty caudal to the obstruction. If the enterolith is present in a portion of the bowel that can be exteriorized, an enterotomy is performed and the concretion removed. More often, the enterolith is in a segment of bowel that cannot be exteriorized (cranial small colon or caudal right dorsal colon). In this instance, the enterolith is moved retrograde until it is positioned in a portion of the dorsal colon that can be exteriorized for enterotomy. Alternatively, if it cannot be moved by external manipulation, an enterotomy is performed in a region of the right dorsal colon that can be exteriorized and packed off with towels, and an arm is inserted within the lumen of the bowel to grasp the enterolith (Fig. 7.4*A*). This can cause considerable contamination if care is not taken. Retrograde flushing with water using a hose inserted up the small colon is a useful adjunctive technique (9), but exercise caution because of weakened ischemic bowel wall where the enterolith is lodged.

The prognosis is fair (47% success rate in one report of 30 cases) (13). Successful surgery depends on removal of the enterolith before bowel devitalization, as bowel rupture associated with removal of the enterolith is not uncommon. In addition, contamination of the abdominal cavity during removal can compromise the results. The prognosis can be improved if the presence of enteroliths is recognized and the surgery can be done on an elective basis, with the horse being fasted prior to the surgery.

Displacement or Nonstrangulating Torsion of the Large Colon

This category includes various conditions that have been generally classified as torsions but are characterized by an abnormal position of the large colon *without* strangulation of the blood supply (15). The normal flow of ingesta is arrested, but viability of the colon is not generally affected. These torsions are surgical conditions but, because of the lack of bowel strangulation, the patient experiences slow systemic deterioration and the success rate with timely surgical intervention is good. The clinical presentation is often acute because of tympany in the cecum and colon. On rectal examination, distension of the large colon will be palpated. Some patients will manifest a degree of colonic impaction. Paracentesis may yield fluid with an elevated protein level.

A number of malpositions can occur (15). The most common displacement involves part or all of the large colon being displaced to the right and caudad, then winding back mediad and craniad around the fixed point formed by the cecum (Fig. 7.4*B*). The pelvic flexure is often displaced into the cranial aspect of the abdomen. This type of malposition may be complicated by torsion as well.

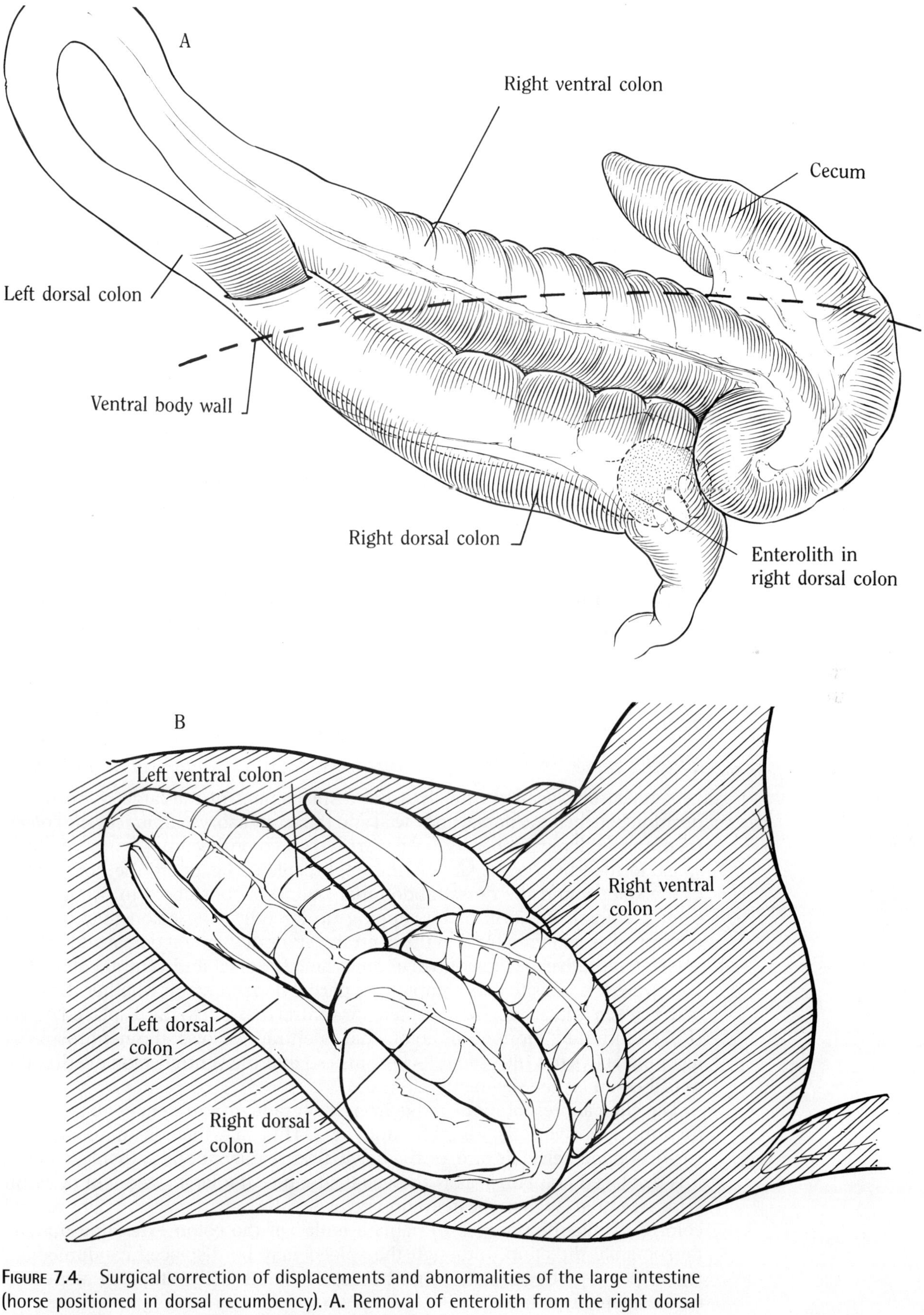

Figure 7.4. Surgical correction of displacements and abnormalities of the large intestine (horse positioned in dorsal recumbency). **A.** Removal of enterolith from the right dorsal colon. **B.** Right dorsal displacement of the large colon.

European equine surgeons have classified such displacement as right dorsal displacement of the large colon (16). In the surgical treatment, the surgeon first attempts to exteriorize the pelvic flexure, and gas and ingesta are then removed as necessary before correction. Ingesta is evacuated through an enterotomy at the pelvic flexure. Reduction is then effected by reversing the pathway in which the pelvic flexure has moved (moving pelvic flexure back around the right side of the base of the cecum and colon) and replacing the sternal and diaphragmatic segments of the colon in their normal cranial position with the pelvic flexure in its caudal position. Effective reduction is ascertained by being able to exteriorize the cecum and large colon normally and visualize the entire cecocolic fold. Such manipulations can be difficult and strenuous because they have to be performed in the depth of the abdomen. Tympany in the colon usually results in an early presentation of these cases, and with timely surgical intervention the prognosis is good.

In the other common form of nonstrangulating obstruction, the pelvic flexure may be in a normal position but the left dorsal and left ventral colon rotate 180° around the sternal and diaphragmatic flexure (Fig. 7.4*C*). Although this is correctly considered as a torsion, it is generally nonstrangulating. Rotations of 90° or less are not clinical problems and are only incidental findings at surgery. The essential feature of the 180° torsion is blockage to the passage of ingesta without compromise of vascularity. With progression of time or with more severe rotations, the condition can become a strangulating one. These patients present with moderately painful colic because of large colon distension, and the distended large colon can be palpated on rectal examination. At surgery the malposition is identified. Edema of the mesentery implies an early vascular obstruction. If indicated, the colon is decompressed before correction of the torsion. The prognosis is generally good in these patients because surgical intervention usually precedes any permanent changes in the intestinal wall or severe systemic deterioration.

Left Dorsal Displacement or Nephrosplenic Entrapment of the Large Colon

Left dorsal displacement involves the displacement of the large colon into a position between the dorsal body wall and the suspensory ligament of the spleen (nephrosplenic ligament) (17) (Fig. 7.4*D*). The colon becomes entrapped in a space formed by the left kidney, the nephrosplenic ligament, the dorsal edge of the spleen, and the dorsal abdominal wall. It is considered to occur either from a cranial direction or by slipping up laterally. The colon may become entrapped as far cranially as in the central regions of the right dorsal and ventral colon. Alternatively, it may involve only the left dorsal and ventral colon. The entrapment is classified as complete or partial depending on whether the edge of the spleen is laterodorsal (complete) or ventral (partial) to the displaced bowel (16). Commonly, the loop of colon that is entrapped over the nephrosplenic ligament is twisted 180° about its long axis so that the ventral colon overlies the dorsal colon on the ligament.

The clinical presentations range from low-grade intermittent colic to refractory unresponsive colic. Rectal findings vary. They may include an impacted or gas-distended pelvic flexure, or the pelvic flexure may not be palpable because it is displaced craniad. This is the usual situation if a larger segment of colon is incarcerated (such as incarceration involving the right dorsal and right ventral colons). It may be possible to palpate teniae of the colon extending up in a dorsocranial direction. Although the spleen may be displaced caudomediad, this is not a pathognomonic sign because dilation of the stomach alone will cause splenic rotation.

Left dorsal displacement of the colon can be treated medically by "rolling"

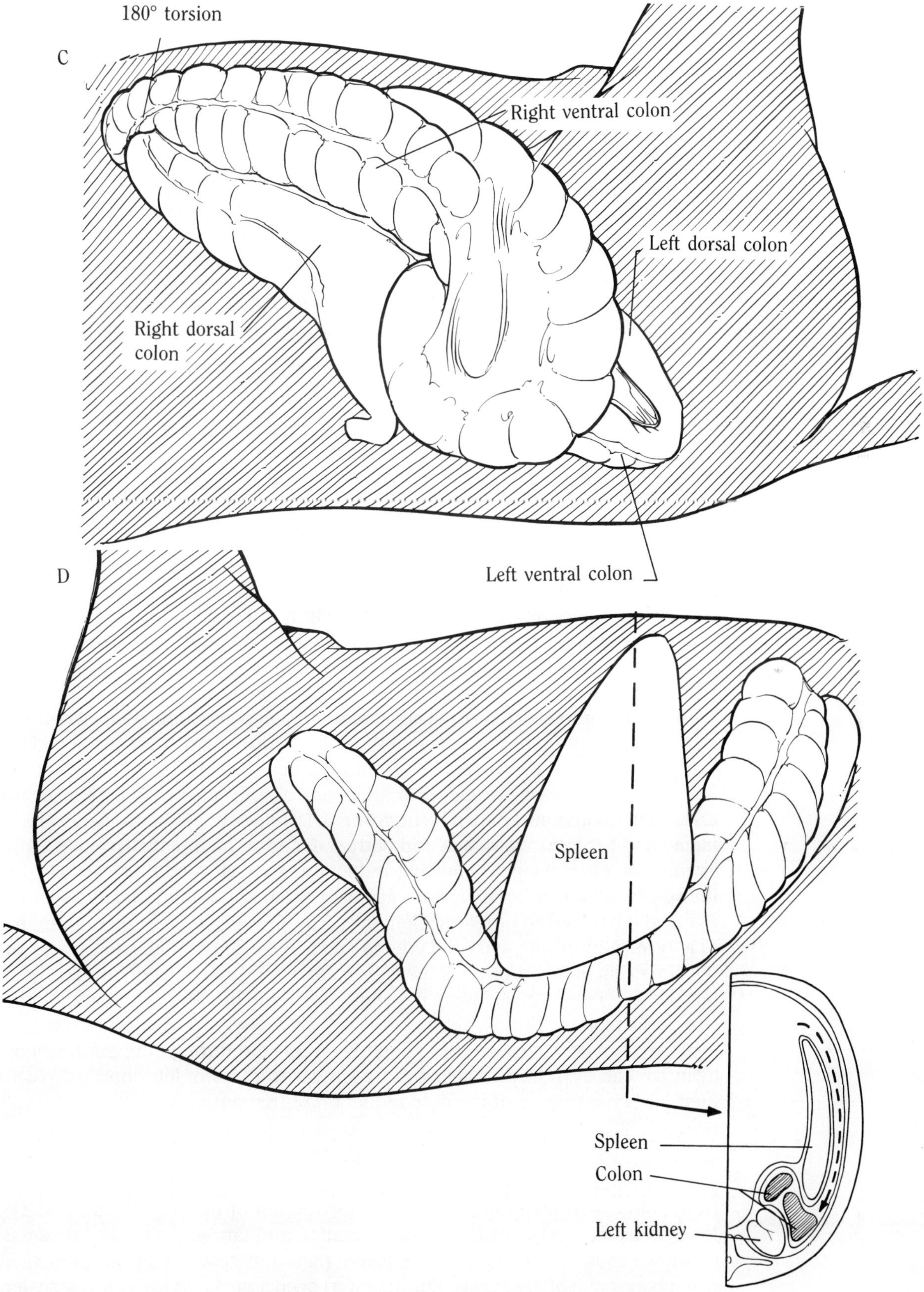

FIGURE 7.4. *(continued)* **C.** 180° torsion of large colon at the sternal and diaphragmatic flexure. **D.** Nephrosplenic incarceration (left dorsal displacement) of large colon.

the horse. This treatment was developed in Europe and is now in common use at some referral centers in North America (18–20). This treatment necessitates a definitive clinical diagnosis per rectum (19). Percutaneous ultrasound examination can be used to substantiate the diagnosis, particularly in horses in which rectal palpation of the nephrosplenic area is difficult (20). It is also useful to monitor its nonsurgical correction. The horse is given intravenous anesthetics and positioned on its right side after anesthetic induction. The hind limbs are hobbled and attached to a hoist and the horse is rolled into dorsal recumbency with its hind quarters elevated. The abdomen is shaken vigorously while the horse is suspended. The horse is then lowered into left lateral recumbency and rolled up into sternal recumbency (18, 19). The horse is examined per rectum to see if the procedure was successful. The procedure can be repeated if necessary. If it is successful, the horse is left in right lateral recumbency to recover. A treatment of intravenous phenylephrine at a rate of 3 ug/kg/min for 15 minutes will induce peak splenic contraction and markedly reduce splenic size (21). Administering phenylephrine before rolling could help facilitate correction of the entrapment.

Another method of nonsurgical treatment recently reported consisted of infusing intravenous phenylephrine at a dose of 2 to 8 mg given over a 10-minute period and followed with 30 minutes of exercise on a long line. This method was successful in four of six horses (22).

Certainly, attempts at nonsurgical correction are not always successful. It is most likely successful in those horses with an uncomplicated left dorsal displacement. It may fail if the horse has moderate to severe colonic distension or if there are preexisting adhesions (18, 19, 23). If evidence of intestinal compromise is present, based on an abdominocentesis, nonsurgical correction is contraindicated. If nonsurgical methods fail to correct the entrapment or another lesion is encountered, surgical treatment should be quickly initiated (19, 24).

In those horses treated surgically, the approach is by midline laparotomy. If excessive distension or impaction of the colon is present, the left dorsal and left ventral colons are evacuated before any reduction. Following closure of the enterotomy and replacement of the left dorsal and left ventral colon in the abdomen, reduction can then be performed. Displacement is corrected by passing a hand between the spleen and body wall and retracting the spleen mediad as the colon is elevated. Following reduction, a check is made to ensure that the spleen is in its normal position against the left abdominal wall and that the reduced colon is free of twists. Generally, compromise to the colon is limited to a localized bruising and mild edema and is inconsequential. However, complications, including rupture of the large colon while reducing the displacement, recurrence of the displacement, degeneration of the bowel wall, and adhesions, can occur (25).

Herniation of the left dorsal and left ventral colon through the gastrosplenic ligament can also occur. The signs are similar to those of left dorsal displacement, and the treatment involves reduction of the hernia.

Intramural Hematoma of the Small Colon

Hematoma is an uncommon cause of obstruction of the small colon (26, 27). It has been associated with chronic ulceration and iatrogenic rectal damage of unknown causes. The horse shows severe pain in excess of that normally seen with obstruction of the small colon. This has been associated with the distension of the intestinal wall associated with the hematoma. Treatment involves resection of the affected portion and an end-to-end anastomosis of the small colon.

Strangulating Obstruction of the Large Intestine

Intussusception of the Cecum

Intussusception of the cecum may occur as either a cecocecal or a cecocolic intussusception (26, 28–32). Afflicted horses typically have subacute colic of several days' duration, but there is considerable variation. Cecocecal intussusception does not completely block the flow of ingesta from the small intestine, but cecocolic intussusception does. On surgical exploration, absence of the cecum is noted and the intussusception can be found by tracing the right ventral colon retrograde until the mass is found. At surgery, it may be possible to manually reduce the cecocolic intussusception by sliding a hand to the cecal apex, grasping the apex, and everting it until the intussusception is reduced (32). If the viability of the cecum is questionable, the apex can be amputated. This can be done by resection and closure of the cecum with a double row of inverting sutures or with the TA-90 stapling equipment. It may be necessary to open the right ventral colon and amputate the cecal apex to be able to reduce the intussusception. It is not possible to use stapling equipment for this amputation because the cecal tissue is very edematous and thick. If the cecolic intussusception is irreducible, an ileocolostomy could be performed to completely bypass the cecum (33).

Torsion of the Cecum

Torsion of the cecum alone is rare (this condition is most commonly associated with torsion of the colon). Incidental displacement of the cecum routinely encountered during surgery is commonly classified as torsion (usually 90°) but is not considered to be a pathologic problem. If true cecal torsion occurs, it presents as an acute colic with a distended cecum but a normal large colon. A discolored, distended cecal apex will be found on surgical exploration and the torsion located. Following decompression of the cecum, the torsion is reduced. Resection will be indicated depending on the vascular compromise. The site of resection will depend on the degree of involvement of the cecum. Complete typhlectomy with ileocolic anastomosis has been described (34), and this condition requires a flank laparotomy.

Torsion (Volvulus) of the Large Colon

The term *torsion* of the large colon implies compromise of the vascular supply, and this typically occurs with a 360° torsion of the entire large colon. This condition constitutes the most severe and rapidly fatal acute abdominal crisis in the horse. Most strangulating torsions are 360° and occur either at the origin of the large colon and involve the cecum or just distal to the cecum in the right colon so that the cecum is not involved (35, 36) (Fig. 7.4*E*). Because these torsions occur near the origin of the large colon, strangulation of the blood supply results in a condition similar to strangulation of the mesenteric root in small intestinal volvulus; hence, this condition is commonly also referred to as volvulus of the large colon. In one report of 124 cases, the twist involved the entire cecal base and the transverse colon in 26 horses (35). Patients with strangulating torsions present with severe unrelenting abdominal pain, severe systemic signs, and marked abdominal distension.

Rapid surgical intervention is of paramount importance if these horses are to be saved. In general, the prognosis for torsions surgically corrected within 2 hours of occurring is good (37). With the typical 360° torsion seen at laparotomy, the colon is grossly distended but the pelvic flexure may appear in a normal

E

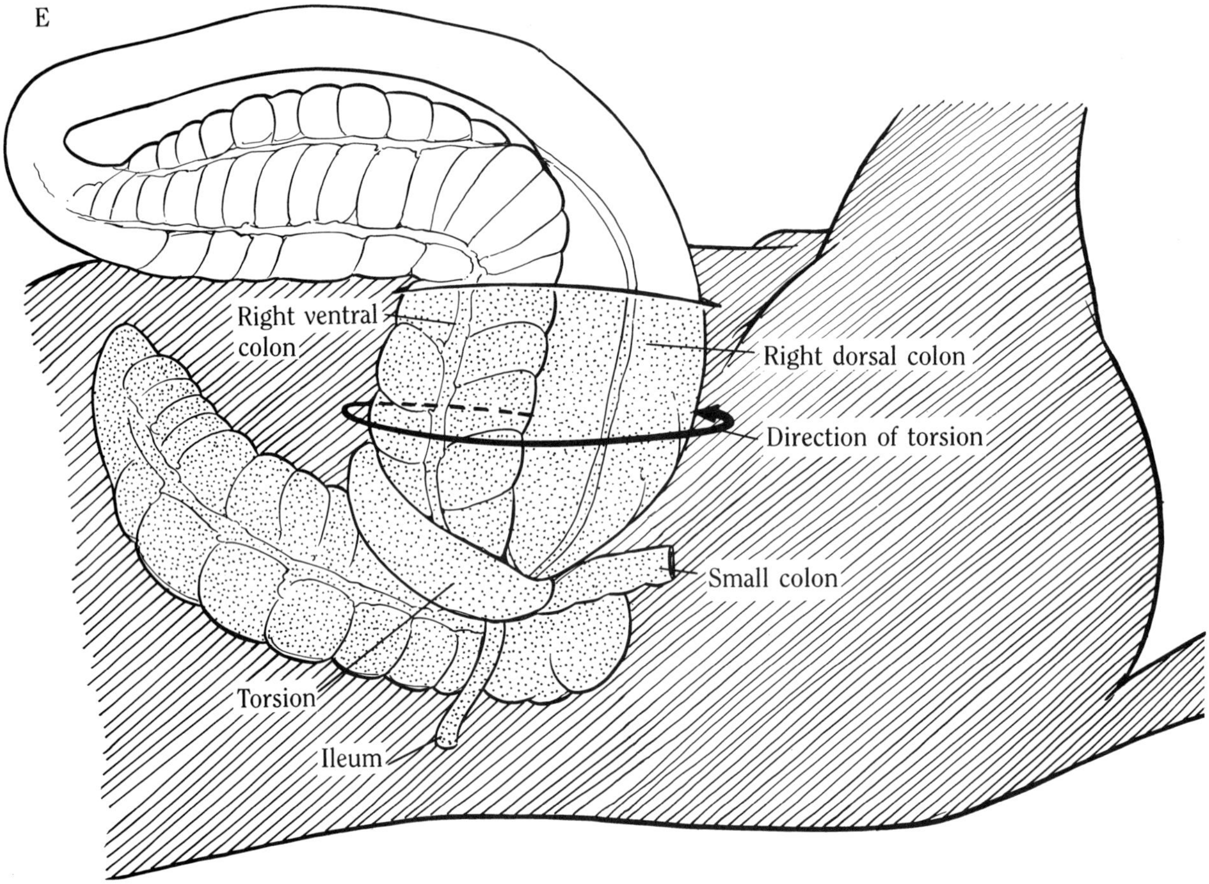

Figure 7.4. *(continued)* E. 360° torsion (volvulus) of the large colon. The torsion is immediately distal to the cecocolic junction.

position because of the complete 360° twist. The color of the serosa varies from white to blue to black, and the wall will be edematous. The large colon can be evacuated before detorsion by an enterotomy at the pelvic flexure and flushing with warm water. This maneuver removes endotoxin that can be potentially absorbed following detorsion, and it also decreases distension before further manipulation of the bowel. At the time of enterotomy, the stage of ischemic necrosis of the colon can be assessed based on the appearance of the mucosa. Dark bloody fluid contents at evacuation constitute another feature of necrosis of the mucosa. The direction of the torsion is then evaluated by palpation at the base of the colon. When the horse is viewed in the ventral surgical position, most torsions at the base of the colon are counterclockwise (Fig. 7.4*E*). With the twisted portion of the colon exteriorized, it is rotated in a clockwise direction to correct the torsion. Exteriorization and visualization of the cecocolic ligament running from the lateral band of the cecum to the right ventral colon is important to ensure that the torsion has been corrected.

The color of the serosal surface typically improves following detorsion, but mucosal evaluation is the more important criterion for assessing potential viability. Surface oximetry has been used to access the viability of the colon following correction of the colonic volvulus and aids in predicting survival (38). The survival rate in these cases, historically, has been low because of the rapid development of bowel ischemia before surgical intervention and the likelihood of development of reperfusion injury following correction of the torsion (39). The surgeon must correct a colon torsion within a few hours of its occurrence to minimize postoperative complications. When the colon is nonviable, resection is an option except when the entire large colon is involved. Techniques have been developed for colon resection, and it is feasible to resect up to 90% of the large colon (see section on large colon resection). However, the surgeon must be able to surgically expose viable colon to perform the resection-anastomosis.

Colopexy

Following successful surgical correction of a large colon volvulus, there is a possibility of recurrence. The recurrence rate may approach 15% (40). Colopexy is a procedure that has been developed to prevent recurrence, and a number of techniques have been described (40–42). The procedure is performed most commonly on brood mares undergoing correction of a large colon volvulus or a right dorsal displacement of the large colon for the second time. Colopexy is not indicated in horses in which the large colon is severely edematous and compromised; nor is it recommended for use in the athletic horse.

Evacuation of the contents of the large colon are recommended for easier correction of the volvulus and to reduce tension on the colopexy suture line during anesthetic recovery. Once the volvulus is corrected, the viscera and large colon are positioned correctly in the abdominal cavity. The subcutaneous space is exposed by blunt dissection for approximately 8 cm to the left of midline over the proposed colopexy site. Using towel clamps to elevate the left edge of the incised abdominal wall, a 25-cm long incision is made in the parietal peritoneum running approximately 8 cm lateral and parallel to the abdominal incision. The retroperitoneal fat is bluntly removed, exposing the internal rectus fascia.

Using interrupted sutures of no. 2 polypropylene in a cruciate pattern, the lateral band of the left ventral colon is sutured to the body wall. Each suture is started in the subcutaneous space and ends in the subcutaneous space, thereby incorporating the tenial band as well as the internal and external rectus fascia. Care is taken not to penetrate the lumen of the colon. The length of the colopexy is approximately 25 centimeters. Once the colopexy is completed, the ventral midline incision is closed in a routine fashion.

Although colopexy of the right ventral colon has been described in conjunction with left colopexy, there appears to be little additional benefit (40).

Postoperative complications associated with the colopexy procedure include colon rupture, abdominal pain that is responsive to treatment, left colopexy dehiscence that may necessitate relaparotomy, severe abdominal adhesions, and subcutaneous fistulous tracts. In one study, the fatality rate attributed to complications associated with the colopexy was 6.8% (40). Some of the complications may be minimized by performing only a left colopexy that penetrates both rectus fascial layers and by not penetrating the lumen of the colon with the pexy sutures.

Intussusception of the Colon

Intussusception of the large colon is rare but has been reported (43–44). In two cases in which the left dorsal colon was involved, the intussusception was resected. An end-to-end anastomosis was performed in one case (44) and a side-to-side anastomosis in the other (43).

Incarceration and Volvulus of the Small Colon

Although the small colon has a long mesentery, both incarceration and volvulus are rare (4, 45). Incarceration can occur through a mesenteric rent or an association with a pedunculated lipoma. Treatment is the same as for a small intestinal incarceration.

REFERENCES

1. Campbell DL, Colahan PC, Brown MP, et al. Cecal impaction in the horse. JAVMA 1984;184:950.
2. Gerard MP, Bowman KF, Blikslager AT, et al. Jejunocolostomy or ileocolostomy for treatment of cecal impaction in horses: nine cases (1985–1995). JAVMA 1996;209: 1287–1299.
3. Ross MW, Martin BB, Donawick WJ. Cecal perforation in the horse. JAVMA 1985; 187:249–253.
4. Foerner JJ. Differential diagnosis and surgical management of diseases of the large intestine. Vet Clin North Am Large Animal Pract 1982;4:129.
5. Sellers AF, Lowe JE, Brondum J. Motor events in equine large colon. Am J Physiol 1979;237:E457.
6. Argenzio RA. Comparative physiology of the gastrointestinal system. In: Anderson NY, ed. Veterinary Gastroenterology. Philadelphia: Lea & Febiger, 1980:172–198.
7. Tennant B. Intestinal obstruction in the horse: some aspects of differential diagnosis in equine colic. Proceedings of the AAEP, Dallas, TX, 1976:426.
8. Dart AJ, Snyder JR, Pascoe JR, et al. Abnormal conditions of the equine descending (small) colon: 102 cases (1979–1989). JAVMA 1992;200:971–978.
9. Taylor TS, Valdez H, Norwood GW, et al. Retrograde flushing for relief of obstruction in the transverse colon in the horse. Equine Pract 1979;1:22.
10. Ruggles AJ, Ross MW. Medical and surgical management of small colon impaction in horses: 28 cases (1984–1989). JAVMA 1991;199:1762–1766.
11. Boles CL, Kohn CW. Fibrous foreign body impaction colic in young horses. JAVMA 1981;179:193.
12. Gay CC, Spiers VC, Christie BA. Foreign body obstruction of the small colon in six horses. Equine Vet J 1979;11:60.
13. Blue MG. Enteroliths in horses—a retrospective study of 30 cases. Equine Vet J 1979; 111:76.
14. Ferraro GL, Evans DR, Trunk DA, et al. Medical and surgical management of enteroliths in Equidae. JAVMA 1973;162:208.
15. Hackett RP. Nonstrangulated colonic displacement in horses. JAVMA 1983;182:235.
16. Huskamp B, Daniels H, Kopf N. Diseases of the stomach and intestine. In: Dietz O, Wiesner E, eds. Diseases of the Horse. Basel: S Karger, 1984:164.
17. Milne DW, Tarr MJ, Lochner FK. Left dorsal displacement of the colon in a horse. J Equine Med Surg 1977;1:47.
18. Sivula NJ. Renosplenic entrapment of the large colon in horses: 33 cases (1984–1989) JAVMA 1991;199:244.
19. Baird AN, Cohen ND, Taylor TS, et al. Renosplenic entrapment of the large colon in horses: 57 cases (1983–1988). JAVMA 1991;198:1423.
20. Santschi EM, Slone DE, Frank WM. Use of ultrasound in horses for diagnosis of left dorsal displacement of the large colon and monitoring its nonsurgical correction. Vet Surg 1993;22:281.
21. Hardy J, Bednarski RM, Biller DS. Effect of phenylephrine on hemodynamics and splenic dimensions in horses. Am J Vet Res 1994;55:1570.
22. Johnston JK. The use of phenylephrine in the treatment of large colon displacement in the horse. Abstract in Proceedings, 31st Annual Scientific Meeting. ACVS, 1996; 13.
23. Moll HD, Schumaker J, Dabareiner RM, et al. Left dorsal displacement of the colon with splenic adhesions in three horses. JAVMA 1993;203:425.
24. Sivula NJ, Trent AM, Kobluk CN. Displacement of the large colon associated with nonsurgical correction of large colon entrapment in the renosplenic space in a mare. JAVMA 1990;197:1190.
25. Markel MD, Orisini JA, Gentile DG, et al. Complications associated with left dorsal displacement of the large colon in the horse. JAVMA 1985;187:1379.
26. Pearson H, Messervy A, Pinsent PJN. Surgical treatment of abdominal disorders in the horse. JAVMA 1971;159:1344.
27. Spiers VC, Van Veenendaal JC, Christie BA, et al. Obstruction of the small colon by intramural haematoma in three horses. Aust Vet J 1981;57:88.

28. Allison CJ. Invagination of the caecum into the colon in a Welsh pony. Equine Vet J 1977;9:84.
29. Cowles RR Jr, Bunch SE, Flynn DV. Cecal inversion in a horse. VM/SAC 1977;72:1346.
30. Robertson JT, Johnson FM. Surgical correction of cecocolic intussusception in a horse. JAVMA 1980;176:223.
31. Sembrad SD, Moore JN. Invagination of the cecal apex in a foal. Equine Vet J 1983; 15:62.
32. Gaughan EM, Hackett RP. Cecocolic intussusception in horses: 11 cases (1979–1989). JAVMA 1990;197:1373.
33. Ward JL, Fubini SL. Partial typhlectomy and ileocolostomy for treatment of nonreducible cecocolic intussusception in a horse. JAVMA 1994;205:325–328.
34. Huskamp B. Some problems associated with intestinal surgery in the horse. Equine Vet J 1977;9:111.
35. Harrison IW. Equine large intestinal volvulus. Vet Surg 1988;17:77.
36. Snyder JR, Pascoe JR, Olander HJ, et al. Strangulating volvulus of the ascending colon in horses. JAVMA 1989;195:757.
37. Embertson RM, Hance SR, Bramlage LR, et al. Large colon volvulus: surgical treatment of 204 horses (1986–1995). Proceedings of the AAEP, Denver, CO, 1996:254.
38. Snyder JR, Pascoe JR, Meaher DM, et al. Surface oximetry for intraoperative assessment of colonic viability in horses. JAVMA 1994;204:1786–1789.
39. Moore RM, Bertone AL, Muir WW, et al. Histopathologic evidence of reperfusion injury in the large colon of horses after low-flow ischemia. Am J Vet Res 1994;55: 1434–1463.
40. Hance SR, Embertson RM. Colopexy in brood mares: 44 cases (1986–1990). JAVMA 1992;201:782–787.
41. Markel MD, Dreyfuss DM, Meagher DM. Colopexy of the equine large colon: comparison of two techniques. JAVMA 1988;192:354–357.
42. Markel MD, Meagher DM, Richardson DW. Colopexy of the large colon in four horses. JAVMA 1988;192:258–359.
43. Robertson JT, Tate LP Jr. Resection of intussuscepted large colon in a horse. JAVMA 1982;181:927.
44. Wilson DG, Wilson WD. Intussusception of the left dorsal colon in a horse. JAVMA 1983;183:464.
45. Adams SB, McIlwraith CW. Abdominal crisis in the horse: a comparison of presurgical evaluation with surgical findings and results. Vet Surg 1978;87:63.

Enterotomy Techniques

Enterotomy is a basic procedure that plays an important role in equine intestinal surgery. The selection of an enterotomy site in different parts of the intestinal tract is dependent on the surgeon's ability to exteriorize the viscus, the distribution of blood supply, the location of the lesion, and the anatomic site involved (1).

Before doing an enterotomy, the viscus is isolated from the peritoneal cavity and other viscera by exteriorization and appropriate draping. Small enterotomies on the small intestine are performed on the long axis along the antimesenteric surface (Fig. 7.5*A*). For the colon, a longitudinal incision on the antimesenteric surface is selected. Enterotomies of the large colon are usually done on the antimesenteric surface in the area of the pelvic flexure (Fig. 7.5*B*). These areas lack teniae, are easily exteriorized, and provide relatively good access for evacuation. The pelvic flexure is the most commonly used area for evacuation of impactions, of both the pelvic flexure and the transverse colon, and the decompression of these cases is facilitated by use of a colon tray and flushing with a hose (2–4). Hard masses in the lumen of the transverse colon, such as an enterolith, can be removed through an enterotomy in the right dorsal colon. This is a compromise because the enterotomy site is still some distance from the lesion, but it is a segment that can be exteriorized and "packed off" to maintain asepsis.

In the small colon, enterotomy is also made parallel to the long axis and on the antimesenteric border (Fig. 7.5*C*). The advantages of performing the enterotomy through the antimesenteric tenia and not off the tenia are that it is easier to perform, there is less hemorrhage, and a larger luminal diameter is maintained long term (5). In the past, there was some debate regarding whether the enterotomy should be made through the antimesenteric tenia or adjacent to it. There is no foundation to the old belief that the tenia is relatively avascular (6).

The authors prefer using an assistant's hands to stabilize the bowel for enterotomy rather than stay sutures or forceps. The enterotomy is made with a scalpel (Fig. 7.5*A*). In the case of the small intestine, excess intraluminal fluid can be aspirated with suction or induced to flow by extraluminal pressure applied with a gloved hand. Evacuation of small intestine through an enterotomy incision is difficult. Evacuation through a piece of intestine later to be discarded (if appropriate) is preferable in controlling contamination. Most evacuations of the large colon (those performed through the pelvic flexure) involve placing the pelvic flexure in a colon tray and evacuating fluid directly out through the enterotomy site. A hose is usually used to facilitate evacuation of the large colon (2, 3) (Fig. 7.5*B*). An assistant inserts the hose through the enterotomy into the lumen of the dorsal or ventral colon. Water is flushed into the lumen, and the water is mixed with ingesta and then allowed to run out. By moving the hose further into the bowel and milking the mixture out, the large bowel can be almost completely emptied. The procedure can then be repeated on the opposite colon. This technique is particularly useful for the evacuation of ingesta or sand impactions in which manual manipulation of rough, dry ingesta imposes considerable trauma to the wall of the colon. A second hose can be used to continuously lavage the serosal surface of the colon (3).

When bowel evacuation is complete, the bowel is prepared for closure by rinsing the enterotomy site with sterile polyionic fluid. Small intestinal enterotomies can be closed with a single continuous inverting layer (Cushing or Lembert pattern) using 2/0 absorbable suture, a two-layer inverting pattern, or one single interrupted layer using a Cushing or Gambee suture pattern of 2/0 absorbable suture material. Two-layer closures cause more inversion of tissue but are recommended for closure of the large colon and small colon enterotomies (4, 5, 7). A synthetic absorbable suture material such as polyglactin 910 is recommended.

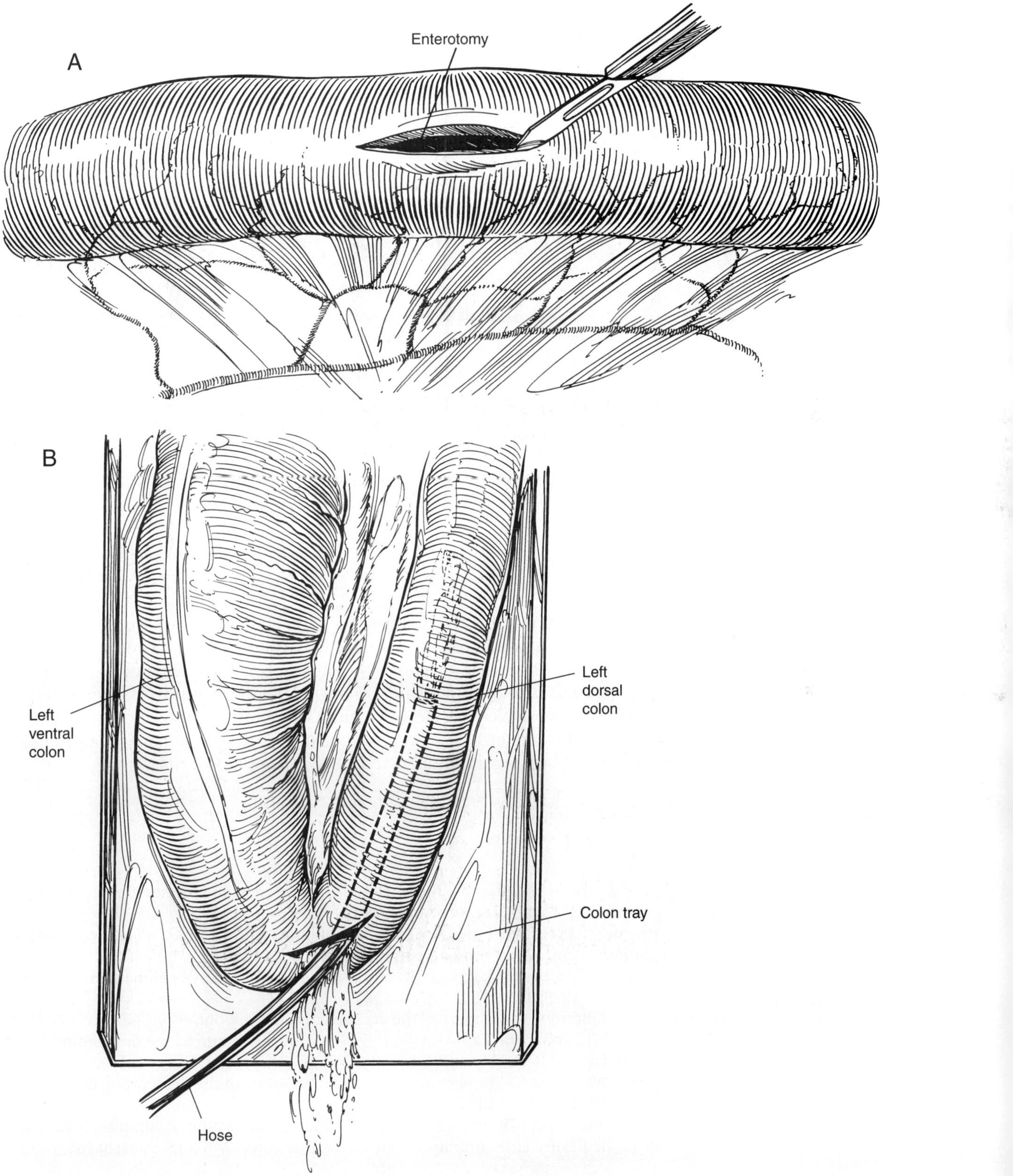

FIGURE 7.5. Enterotomies. **A.** In antimesenteric border of small intestine. **B.** In area of pelvic flexure with irrigation hose in left dorsal colon.

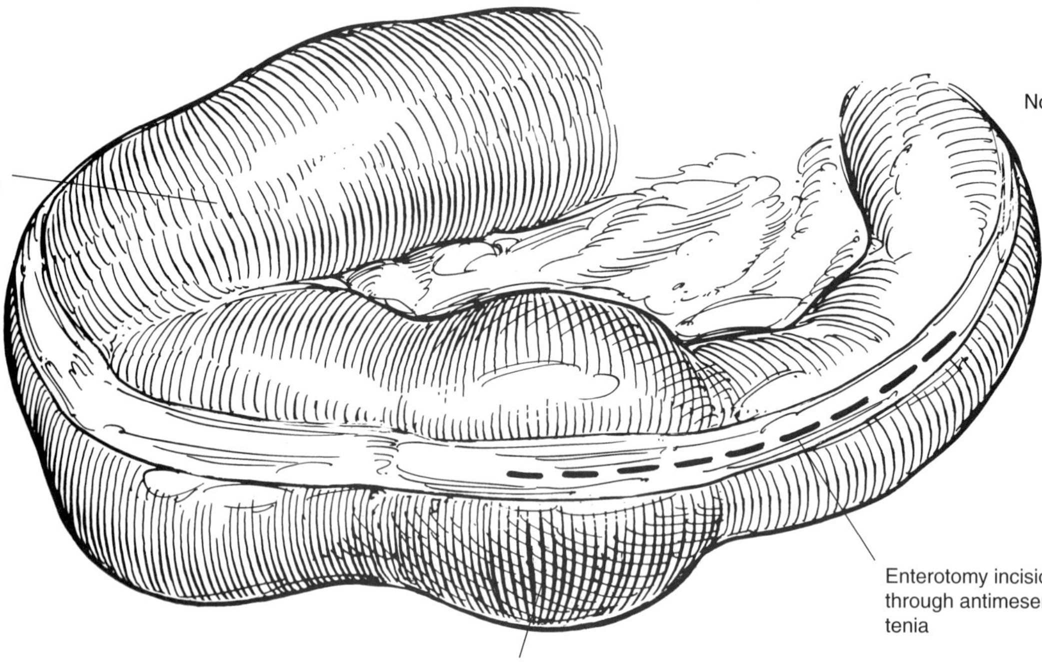

Figure 7.5. *(continued)* C. In small colon through the antimesenteric tenia.

Stomach enterotomy (gastrotomy) is rare but may be performed midway between the greater and lesser curvature with the incision placed parallel to the segmental gastric vessels. Because the stomach is relatively inaccessible and cannot be exteriorized, contamination is a problem. Decompression with a tube is preferred, if possible. The stomach has a rich blood supply and heals rapidly, but because it secretes pepsin, a synthetic absorbable or nonabsorbable suture material has been recommended with a two-layer closure (1).

REFERENCES

1. Stashak TS. Techniques for enterotomy, decompression and intestinal resection-anastomosis. Vet Clin North Am Large Animal Pract 1982;4:147.
2. Foerner JJ. Diseases of the large intestine: differential diagnosis and surgical management. Vet Clin North Am Large Animal Pract 1982;4:129.
3. Markel MD, Stover SM, Pascoe JR, et al. Evacuation of the large colon in horses. Comp Cont Edu 1988;10:96.
4. Hardy J, Bertone AL. Surgery of the equine large colon. Comp Cont Edu 1992;14:1501.
5. Beard WL, Robertson JT, Getzy DM. Enterotomy technique in the descending colon of the horse. Effect of location and suture pattern. Vet Surg 1989;18:135.
6. Beard WL, Lohse CL, Robertson JT. Vascular anatomy of the descending colon of the horse. Vet Surg 1989;18:130.
7. Young RL, Snyder JR, Pascoe JR, et al. A comparison of three techniques for closure of pelvic flexure enterotomies in normal equine colon. Vet Surg 1991;20:185.

Intestinal Resection, Anastomosis, and Stapling: General Considerations

The initial problems with any intestinal resection are in evaluating intestinal integrity or viability and in defining the margins of viability. Evaluation of the color of the intestines and mesentery, peristalsis, pulsation of the mesenteric vessels, and enterotomy to visualize mucosal color is still the most frequently used means to assess intestinal viability.

Newer, sophisticated means of quantitative assessment of both small and large bowel viability have been reported experimentally and clinically. These include fluorescein dye injection with examination of fluorescence, surface oximetry for estimation of tissue oxygenation, and Doppler ultrasound to detect arterial flow (1–3). The use of intravenous infusion of fluorescein dye did not prove to be equal to its anticipated value in the horse (4). Studies have shown bowel segments remaining viable after fluorescent patterns indicated a nonviable state. The situation is further complicated by the fact that, in the horse, unacceptable adhesion formation occurs after temporary ischemia despite the bowel remaining viable (4). A general principle is that if the viability of a segment, particularly the ileum, is questionable, resection is indicated. The principles of resection technique will be illustrated when discussing resection of the small intestine and end-to-end anastomosis.

Intestinal healing can be divided into three phases. Phase 1, the lag phase, lasts from 0 to 4 days and is characterized by inflammatory edema. There is some tissue strength on day 1 and 2 because of the formation of fibrin clots, but by the third postoperative day the sutured intestine is functionally weakest because of the transition of fibrin breakdown (fibrinolysis) to the deposition of immature collagen (5). Phase 2, the proliferative phase, lasts from 3 to 14 days and is characterized by formation of fibrous tissue and mucosal union. A rapid gain in tissue strength is associated with this phase. Phase 3, the remodeling phase, begins approximately day 10 and lasts until day 180. This period is characterized by a gradual increase in tissue strength as a result of collagen remodeling. It takes approximately 17 to 21 days for the anastomotic site to reach the tensile strength of normal adjacent bowel.

Rates and strengths of healing vary somewhat, depending on the location of the intestinal anastomosis and the suture material selected. The small intestine provides the ideal set of circumstances because it has an abundant blood supply, a strong mucosal layer, minimal intraluminal bacterial counts (compared with the large bowel), semiliquid feces, and a mucosal layer capable of rapid regeneration (5). In comparison, the colon has a relatively poor blood supply, high intraluminal bacterial counts, an increased level of collagenase, and more solid fecal material.

When considering anastomosis of the equine small intestine as a typical example, postoperative complications can result from anastomotic leakage, stenosis, or adhesions. Formation of an impervious seal, first-intention healing with minimal fibrosis and good alignment of tissue layers, and maintenance of an adequate luminal diameter are among the goals when trying to minimize the potential for such complications (6).

Three general techniques of intestinal anastomosis are available: end-to-end, end-to-side, and side-to-side. End-to-end anastomosis is performed when sections of intestine of similar diameter are to be anastomosed. The technique is used for anastomosis of the small intestine and small colon and will be detailed here, using small intestine as an example. End-to-side anastomosis has been frequently used for ileocecal or jejunocecal anastomosis. Side-to-side anastomosis is used in anastomosing the large colon and is an alternative technique for jejunocecal anastomosis. It is also used in gastro-jejunostomy.

Suture Techniques

Various suture patterns can be used with these different anastomotic techniques. Suture placement is important with regard to the strength and healing of an intestinal anastomosis in that suture placement should not compromise the vascular supply, and the submucosa must be engaged by each suture (7). To minimize any vascular compromise, it has been proposed that sutures placed in an interrupted fashion perpendicular to the cut surface and parallel to the bowel's long axis are preferable (5). Sutures placed in a continuous pattern with the bites parallel to the cut surface of the bowel and perpendicular to the long axis of the intestines (such as Cushing or Connell sutures) have a tendency to reduce the blood supply to the healing edge (5). However, experimental work has shown that although such interrupted suture patterns result in good histologic healing, adhesions develop in 50% of cases, whereas adhesions were not found in association with continuous inverting suture patterns (6).

Intestinal anastomotic techniques can be classified according to whether they oppose, invert, or evert the incised edge of the bowel and whether they are performed in single or double rows.

Opposing Sutures

End-to-end opposing sutures include the simple interrupted approximating suture that approximates all layers of the intestine (Fig. 7.6*A*); a crushing suture that is placed in the same fashion as above but tied tightly enough to cut through the serosa, muscularis, and mucosa and snugly hold the submucosal tunics (8); and the Gambee suture pattern placed so that the suture selectively picks up the mucosa and prevents its eversion (Fig. 7.6*B*). These sutures all provide good anatomic alignment of all intestinal layers, the lumen of the bowel is not compromised, minimal vascular compromise is noted, and the surgeon can be sure that the submucosa is engaged by the sutures. Also, rapid healing with mucosal union is noted, the techniques are simple to perform, distensibility is superior to other patterns, and there is early return to intestinal mobility (5, 9). The only detracting feature of such suture patterns is the potential for adhesion formation. Although one report found adhesions not to be a problem with the Gambee pattern (9), another study demonstrated adhesions associated with 50% of the Gambee and crushing anastomoses (6).

Inverting Suture Patterns

A double-layer inverting suture pattern still used by many surgeons includes the use of interrupted or continuous Cushing, Connell, Lembert, or Halsted techniques. Single-layer inverting suture patterns can also be done in interrupted or continuous fashion, but the continuous is the most common (Fig. 7.6*C*). Two-layer inverting patterns have a high initial tensile and bursting strength. There are fewer adhesions and, because two layers are formed, the bowel can be adequately sealed and cleaned before placement of the second layer. However, internal cuff formation (from inverted tissues) may cause intraluminal obstruction. In addition, there is poor apposition of layers and kinking of the blood vessels, which will decrease blood flow, causing retarded intestinal healing, delayed return to normal motility, and increased incidence of anastomotic failure. The ability of the intestine to distend is also reduced. The one-layer inverting closure has similar problems but can be more rapidly applied and has less tissue reaction, earlier revascularization, and more rapid healing compared with the two-layer pattern (5).

A two-layer inverting anastomosis composed of a simple continuous mucosal layer and a continuous Lembert seromuscular layer has been described for end-to-side jejunocecal anastomosis in the horse (10) and has been studied with

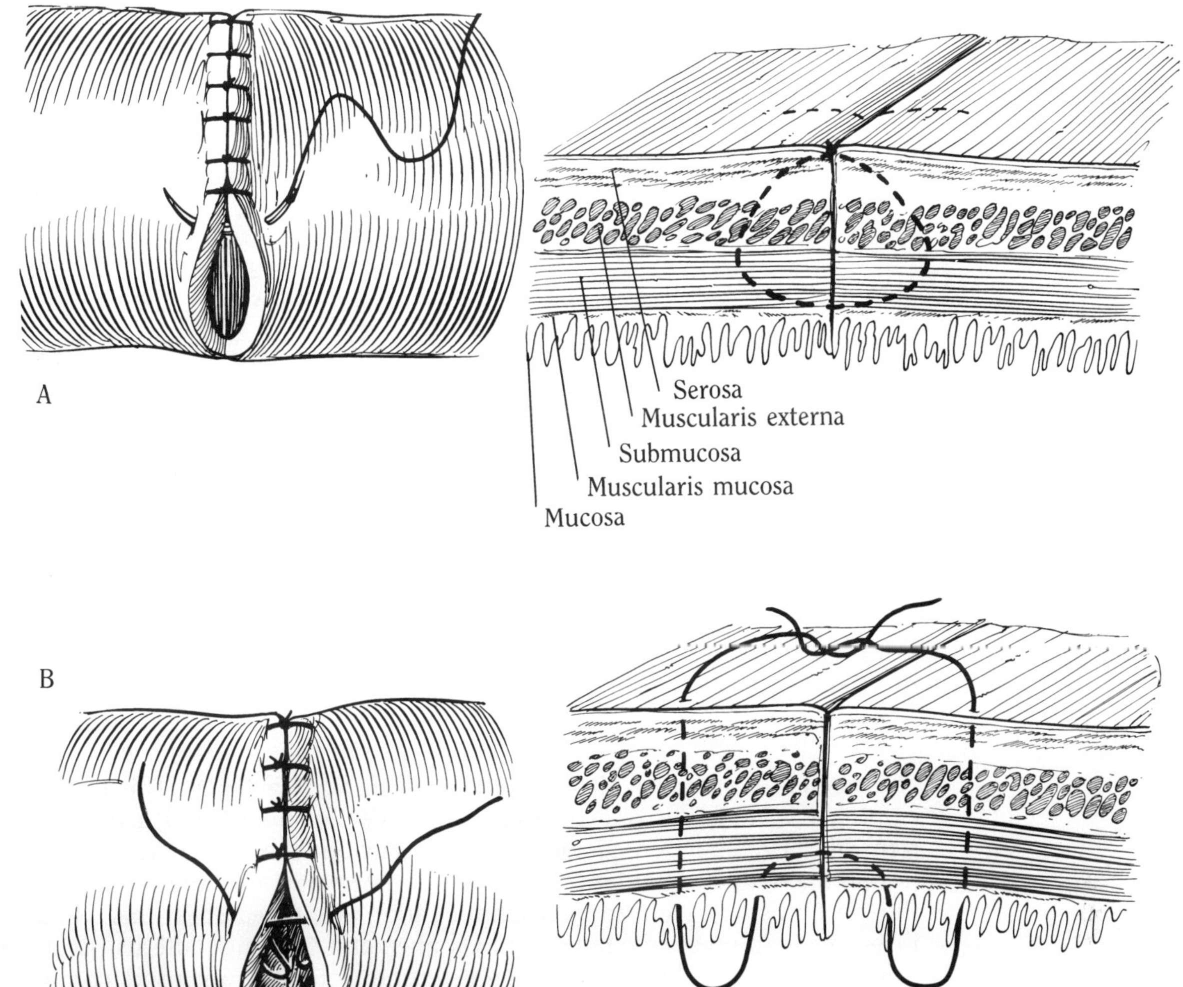

FIGURE 7.6. Intestinal anastomosis. A. Simple interrupted approximating suture. B. Gambee suture (interrupted). C. Continuous inverting (Cushing) suture pattern.

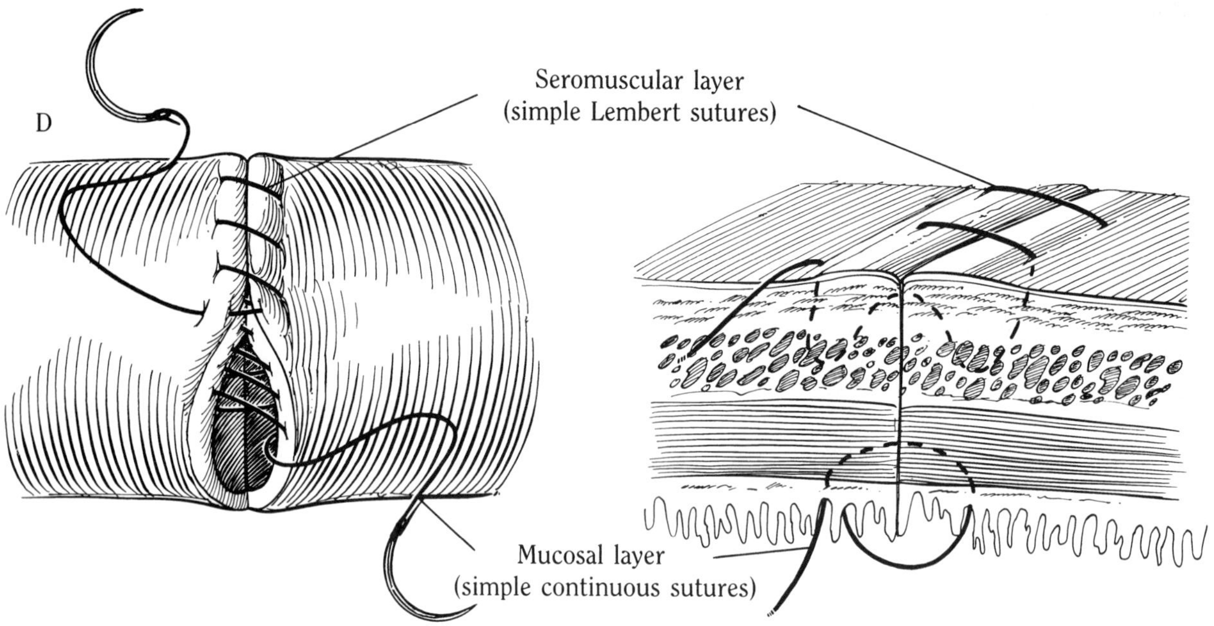

Figure 7.6. *(continued)* D. Two-layer inverting suture with simple continuous mucosal layer and continuous Lembert seromuscular layer.

end-to-end anastomosis of the small intestine (6) (Fig. 7.6*D*). This technique eliminates some of the drawbacks of the conventional two-layer inverting patterns because the mucosa is opposed and only one layer is inverted, resulting in minimal reduction of luminal diameter. Comparative studies show that although fibrosis and suture tract inflammation are increased in this two-layer inverting technique, compared with Gambee and Cushing patterns, no adhesions formed in six horses when the inverting technique was used, compared with 50% adhesion incidence with the other two techniques (6).

In the same controlled study, the crushing anastomoses had the largest percentage of normal diameter (72 ± 15%), followed by the Gambee anastomoses (69 ± 19%). The two-layer inverting anastomoses had the smallest percentage of normal diameter (66 ± 16%); however, there was no significant difference in the mean percentage of normal diameter among the three techniques. These authors concluded that the two-layer inverting technique of closure of the small intestine was superior to the single-layer techniques in that experiment because of its reduced incidence of adhesions and maintenance of adequate lumen diameter (6).

Inverting patterns are still used with side-to-side anastomotic techniques using suture material.

Everting Patterns

The authors do not recommend everting patterns for intestinal anastomosis. The incidence of inflammation, adhesions, strictures, and peritonitis is higher than with the opposing and inverting techniques (5, 9). The everted bacteria-laden mucosa forms a nidus for infection and microabscesses (9).

Obviously, the ideal suture pattern does not exist, but either the opposing or the modified inverting types, which are illustrated in Figure 7.6, are considered satisfactory. Although it is acknowledged that, with tissue remodeling, the long-term result is probably the same, any interim problems such as stenosis or adhesion formation can be significant morbidity factors postoperatively because temporary bowel dysfunction can have marked clinical effects. The selection of suture material also merits consideration and is discussed below. With regard to suture patterns, recognize that suture material acts as a foreign body in the abdominal cavity and that more suture material is exposed to the peritoneum in single-layer interrupted patterns than in continuous patterns. In dogs, it has also been shown that the Cushing technique demonstrated greater avascular widths of tissue adjacent to the anastomosis than did a continuous approximating pattern (11). This study also showed less mucosal eversion and adhesion formation than with either crushing or approximating interrupted patterns. While it would seem that the opposing interrupted techniques offer the best apposition and healing, adhesion formation is of concern. A continuous approximating pattern may be an excellent compromise. Presently, the two-layer inverting technique with a continuous outer layer has the best results in terms of minimal adhesion formation (6).

Suture material used for gastrointestinal anastomosis should have the qualities of easy handling with minimal tissue friction, reactivity, and capillarity. It is difficult to find one that fulfills all these criteria. Chromic catgut was once the standard suture for gastrointestinal surgery, but the cellular inflammatory response and edema are undesirable, especially for circular closure of the intestine. Polyglactin 910 (Vicryl), a synthetic multifilament absorbable suture, is now commonly used in the horse (5). Polydioxanone (PDS) offers the advantages of a monofilament suture with less inflammatory response, and it retains strength longer and has a slower rate of absorption than do the synthetic multifilament materials (12). It is, however, somewhat more difficult to handle because it kinks.

A controlled study with the modified two-layer anastomotic technique demonstrates that suture pattern is a more critical factor than are differences between monofilament and multifilament material (12). Four different anastomoses were compared using combinations of polyglactin 910 and polydioxanone, with continuous and interrupted suture patterns in the seromuscular layer of a two-layer inverting technique. The mean diameter percentages following anastomoses were not significantly different between techniques. However, the pyogranulomatous suture tract inflammation previously reported with polyglactin 910 was reduced with polydioxanone. The major finding of significance was that the use of an interrupted suture pattern in the seromuscular layer resulted in a greater than 50% incidence of anastomotic adhesions, regardless the suture material used, which is unacceptable for anastomosis of the small intestine in the horse (12).

When anastomosis of the large colon is considered, the use of a synthetic absorbable material is critical because of the slower healing rate of this section of the alimentary tract.

Intestinal Stapling Devices

The intestinal stapling instruments were originally developed in Russia and are now readily available in the United States. The staples are stainless steel and are nonreactive in the intestine. When inserted, the staple is shaped into the form of a "B" configuration, allowing capillary flow through the tissue clasped within the staple. The staple units also have a double row of staples, which alternates the staple placement. The intestinal staplers have the advantages of speeding the resection of intestine and can be used for rapid execution of an anastomosis (saving valuable surgical time); a nonreactive suture with less inflammation; and rapid healing of the incision. The units also can be used to reach relatively inaccessible regions with less chance of contamination, compared with suturing. Disadvantages of the intestinal staplers are eversion of the tissue with the TA-55 and TA-90 (Auto Suture, U.S. Surgical Corp., Norwalk, CT) units and other units like them, which tend to promote adhesion formation;

tearing or pulling of staples because of tension on the anastomotic site; and inadequate closure if the tissue is too thick. The expense of the staples also requires consideration.

There are several types of stapling devices. The devices may be completely disposable, or nondisposable with disposable loading units. Two types used for intestinal anastomosis are illustrated in the description of jejunocecal anastomosis. An example of the first type goes under the designation of thoracoabdominal (TA-90 or TA-55, the number representing the length of the staple row). They are used to make a blind stump of intestine and also to close an enterotomy, but produce an everted tissue apposition. The other instrument is called a gastrointestinal anastomosis instrument, or a GIA (Auto Suture, U.S. Surgical Corp., Norwalk, CT), which produces two rows of double staples with a cutting blade between the rows. The two parts of the stapling apparatus are inserted into adjacent segments of bowel to produce a closure of the two bowel segments with a stoma within the closure. This results in inversion of the tissue edges. A similar instrument, the ILA-100 (Auto Suture, U.S. Surgical Corp., Norwalk, CT), is used in the same fashion. There are GIA instruments available that create stomas of 48 mm (GIA-50 and GIA-50 Premium), 75 mm (Multifire GIA-80), and 85 mm (GIA-90 Premium). Only the Multifire GIA-80 offers a disposable loading unit with staples that are 4.85 mm in length. The staple leg length with the other models is 3.85 mm. When closed, the 4.85-mm staple is approximately 2.0 mm, as compared with 1.5 mm with the 3.85 staple. Obviously, this is advantageous when the stapler is applied to equine gut. The ILA-100 creates a stoma of 96 mm and also has cartridges with staples that have a 4.8-mm leg length and close to 2.0 mm. The authors currently use the ILA-100 because of the advantages of the long stoma length and staple size. The GIA or ILA are routinely used for performing jejunocecal, ileocecal, or colic-colic anastomoses. The TA-90 is also used for creating a blind stump in the ileum with a jejunocecal anastomosis. These techniques are specifically demonstrated in the sections on jejunocecal anastomosis and large colon resection and anastomosis.

A third instrument called a ligator stapling device (LDS) (Auto Suture, U.S. Surgical Corp, Norwalk, CT) is used to ligate mesenteric vessels with two staples and cut between them to complete the removal. This device uses a crescent-shaped staple to close the vessel. It also can greatly decrease surgical time for bowel resections. When the mesentery is devitalized or there is excessive mesenteric fat, double ligation is recommended (13). A fourth instrument, the EEA stapling device, is not currently used in the horse.

Some other rules that must be followed when using the stapling equipment include use of tension-relieving sutures at each end of the suture line to prevent tension on the staples to avoid failure of the anastomoses and making certain the tissues are not too thick to allow for proper staple penetration and staple closure in the completed "B" form (14).

The authors' experiences in the horse would generally agree with human studies reporting that if the technical details of surgical stapling are mastered, the stapling technique appears to be as safe as suturing in the performance of anastomoses in the GI tract. However, the authors also believe that the indications are *more limited* in the horse than in man, such as in the small intestine, where we consider the use of presently available stapling devices inappropriate for end-to-end anastomosis (the reasons are given in the next section). Conversely, the stapling devices have increased our capabilities in colonic anastomoses and our speed in closing jejunocecal anastomoses.

REFERENCES

1. Freeman DE, Gentile DG, Richardson DW, et al. Comparison of clinical judgment, Doppler ultrasound, and fluorescein fluorescence as methods for predicting intestinal viability in the pony. Am J Vet Res 1988;49:895–900.

2. Snyder JR, Pascoe JR, Meagher DM, et al. Surface oximetry for intraoperative assessment of colonic viability in horses. JAVMA 1994;204:1786–1789.
3. Brusic RW, Sullins KE, Silverman DG, et al. Fluorometric evaluation of large and small intestinal ischemia in the horse. Equine Vet J 1989;21:358–363.
4. Sullins KE, Stashak TS, Mero KN. Evaluation of fluorescein as an indicator of small intestinal viability in the horse. JAVMA 1985;186:257.
5. Stashak TS. Enterotomy, decompression, and intestinal anastomosis. Vet Clin North Am Large Animal Pract 1982;4:147.
6. Dean PW, Robertson JT. Comparison of three suture techniques for anastomosis of the small intestine in the horse. Am J Vet Res 1985;46:1282.
7. Jansen A, Becker AE, Brummelkamp WH, et al. The importance of the apposition of the submucosal intestinal layers for primary wound healing of intestinal anastomosis. Surg Gynecol Obstet 1981;152:51.
8. Herthel DJ. Technique of intestinal anastomosis utilizing the crushing type suture. Proceedings of the Annual Convention of the American Association of Equine Practitioners 1972, San Francisco, CA, 1983:303–306.
9. Reinertson EL. Comparison of three techniques for intestinal anastomosis in Equidae. JAVMA 1976;169:208.
10. Donawick WJ, Christie BA, Stewart JV. Resection of diseased ileum in the horse. JAVMA 1971;159:1146.
11. Ellison GW, Jokinen MP, Park RD. End-to-end approximating intestinal anastomosis in the dog: a comparative fluorescein dye angiographic and histopathologic evaluation. J Am Animal Hosp Assoc 1982;18:729.
12. Dean PW, Robertson JT, Jacobs RM. A comparison of suture materials and suture patterns for inverting intestinal anastomosis in the horse. Am J Vet Res 1985;46:2072.
13. White NA. Intestinal stapling in the horse. ACVS Forum, 1984.
14. Chassin JL, Rifkind KM, Sussman B, et al. The stapled gastrointestinal tract anastomosis: incidence of postoperative complications compared with the sutured anastomosis. Ann Surg 1978;188:689.

Resection and End-to-End Anastomosis of Small Intestine

Surgical Technique

The segment of intestine to be resected is exteriorized and isolated from the abdominal cavity and other normal viscera. The entire segment to be resected should include at least 10 to 20 cm of normal bowel at each end of the lesion to ensure normal vascularity at the anastomotic site. Impervious draping is used. Any exposed normal viscera are kept moist with saline or balanced electrolyte solution during this procedure. If possible, intestinal occlusion clamps should be placed across the borders of the fluid-filled ischemic bowel to prevent reflux of toxic fluids into normal adjacent intestines (Fig. 7.7*A*). The rationale for this is that toxic fluids can otherwise be absorbed through normal intestine and contribute to endotoxemia. Following this, the contents in the normal bowel are hand-stripped away from the occlusion clamps to a position approximately 20 cm beyond the proposed site of resection. A Penrose drain is placed through a small hole in the mesentery between segmental vessels to encircle the intestine and is pulled up snug and fixed with forceps to occlude the lumen (Fig. 7.7*A*). This procedure is repeated at the other resection location. Penrose drains and not intestinal clamps are used because (*a*) they do not slip, (*b*) they do not interfere with bowel manipulations at the anastomotic site, (*c*) they effectively occlude the intestine, and (*d*) they do not cause the vascular compromise potentially possible with intestinal clamps. Having an assistant occlude the bowel lumen manually with a gauze sponge is an alternative, but is not recommended.

Following placement of the Penrose drains, the resection site in the decompressed normal segment is selected based on its having a good segmental arterial supply to the antimesenteric surface. If possible, this site will be selected close to a major mesenteric artery that remains uninterrupted. Intestinal clamps may then be placed across the bowel at the proposed line of resection (but on the discarded side of resection). These clamps are placed at an oblique angle of 60° to the mesenteric surface. Such angulation of the line of resection ensures an adequate antimesenteric blood supply and a slightly increased luminal diameter at the anastomosis (Fig. 7.7*A*). Mesenteric vessels to the portion to be resected are bluntly dissected free of the mesentery with a hemostat, doubly ligated or stapled, and cut. The bowel is then resected immediately adjacent to the forceps and on the side that is being retained. No clamps are placed on the bowel that is to be retained and anastomosed. After transection of the bowel, the mesentery is incised, and the resected intestine is discarded.

Stay sutures are placed at the mesenteric and antimesenteric borders, and an assistant holds them under slight tension to keep the ends of the intestine somewhat stretched and in apposition while the anastomosis is performed (Fig. 7.7, *B* and *C*). The technique for the anastomosis will be based on personal preference. The choices of suture pattern and material have been discussed in the previous section. On the basis of current knowledge, an apposing anastomosis or a double-layered technique with *minimal inversion* should be used with synthetic absorbable suture material (1, 2). If the double-layered technique is used, the single continuous layer in the mucosa should be interrupted and tied at 180°. Make sure that normal alignment of the ends of the intestine is maintained so that there is no rotation of segments. Following completion of the intestinal anastomosis, the mesenteric defect is sutured in a simple continuous pattern. Care must be taken not to penetrate or occlude vital mesenteric vessels (Fig. 7.7*D*).

Comments

The use of staples is not considered appropriate for end-to-end anastomosis of the small intestine in the horse. Although a triangulating technique using a TA-

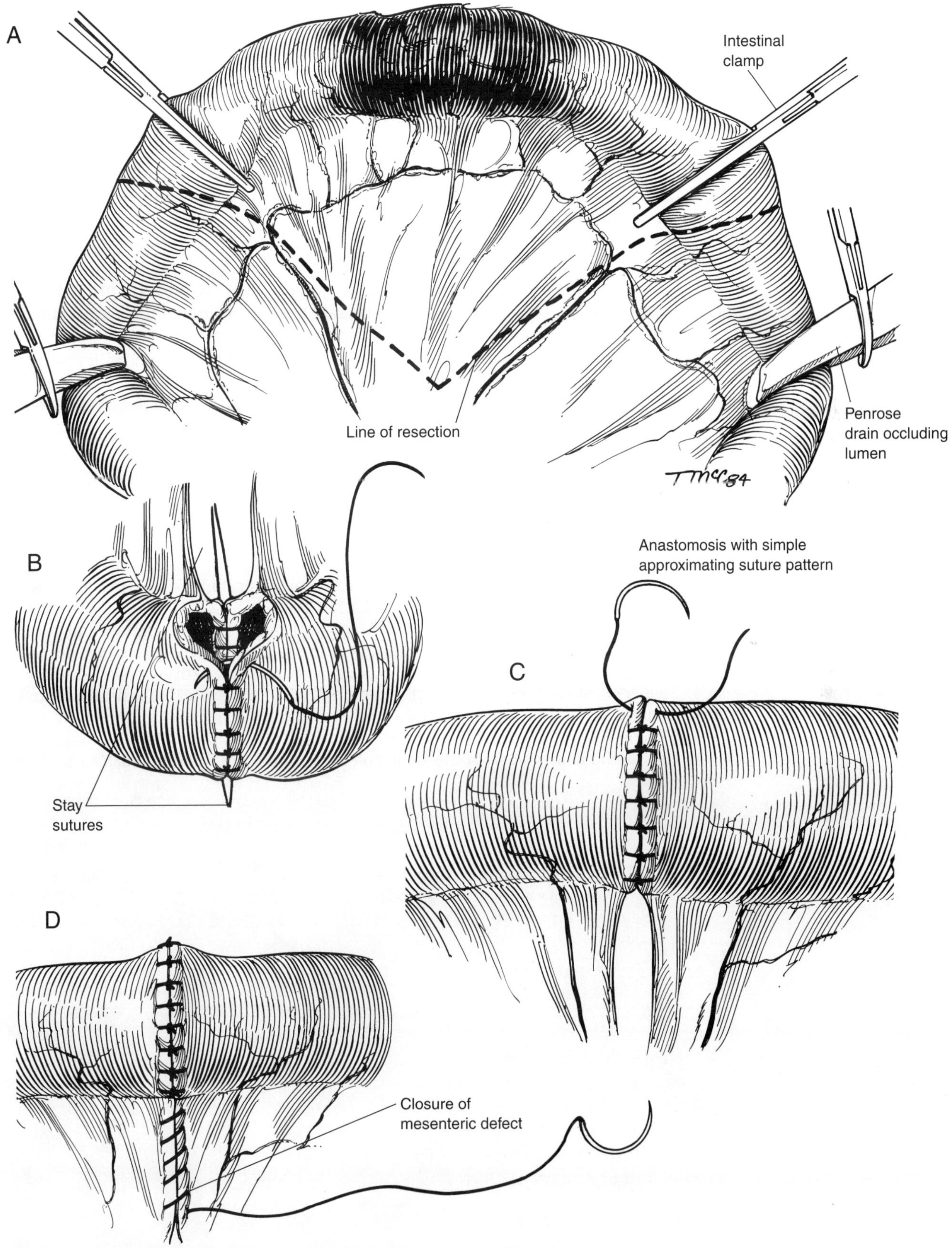

FIGURE 7.7, A–D. Resection and end-to-end anastomosis of small intestine.

55 or TA-90 stapling device can be performed (3), it results in undesirable mucosal eversion. Studies in the horse have confirmed that such a technique will result in extensive adhesion and stricture formation associated with the anastomosis and problems with colic postoperatively (4). Another alternative would be to perform a side-to-side anastomosis of the small intestine with the two ends of the bowel stumped off. Such a technique could be performed with the GIA, ILA, or TA staplers. However, in the authors' experience, the use of such a side-to-side anastomosis can result in pocketing of intestinal contents and is not recommended. Also, if the ends or "stumps" are sutured closed by hand, no appreciable time is saved.

Anastomosis of the small colon can be made using the same principles as described above for the small intestine. However, the mesocolon contains considerable fat, making identification of the vessels difficult, and the procedure is consequently harder. Care also must be taken not to damage the blood supply to normal small colon, particularly if the margin for resection is adjacent to a segment that cannot be exteriorized and excessive tension could inflict permanent vascular damage.

Different techniques for end-to-end anastomosis of the small colon have been evaluated experimentally. A two-layer closure is recommended, and excessive inversion of tissue at the anastomotic site should be avoided (5).

REFERENCES

1. Dean PW, Robertson JT. Comparison of three suture techniques for anastomosis of the small intestine in the horse. Am J Vet Res 1985;46:1282.
2. Dean PW, Robertson JT, Jacobs RM. A comparison of suture materials and suture patterns for inverting intestinal anastomosis in the horse. Am J Vet Res 1985;46:2072.
3. Reiling RB. Staplers in gastrointestinal surgery. Surg Clin North Am 1981;60:381.
4. Sullins KE, Stashak TS, Mero KM. Evaluation of intestinal staples for end-to-end anastomosis of the small intestine in the horse. Vet Surg 1985;14:87.
5. Hanson RR, Nixon AJ, Calderwood-Mays M, et al. Evaluation of three techniques for end-to-end anastomosis of the small colon in horses. Am J Vet Res 1988;49:1613.

Jejunocecal Anastomosis

When any part of the ileum is to be resected, a jejunocecal anastomosis is recommended because the ileum has a single blood supply that would make any form of end-to-end anastomosis a risk; in addition, the ileocecal valve is inaccessible to surgery (the only possible exception to this statement is if the TA-90 is used in a blind fashion to resect ileum at the level of the ileocecal valve). Jejunocecal anastomosis was initially described in the English literature as an end-to-side anastomosis using suture material (1). Its successful use has been subsequently documented by other authors (2–4). The time-honored end-to-side technique using sutures as initially described by Donawick and his co-workers will be described and illustrated here (1). Alternatives and the use of stapling equipment will also be addressed.

Surgical Technique

The technique is illustrated in Figure 7.8. The basic principle is that a blind stump is made of the ileum, and viable small intestine (the site will vary depending on the amount of ileum and jejunum resected) is anastomosed into the cecum between its medial and dorsal bands in an end-to-side fashion. One author has reported better results with a side-to-side anastomosis (5), and this technique also will be illustrated. A perceived advantage of a side-to-side anastomosis is that the size of the stoma can be selected.

The cecum is brought out of the ventral midline incision, and the apex is pulled caudad to expose the dorsal band of the cecum. The dorsal band of the cecum is followed to the ileocecal fold and the ileum (Fig. 7.8*A*). Two intestinal clamps are then placed across the ileum close to the ileocecal junction but in an appropriately accessible place, and a scalpel is used to divide between them. The ileal stump is then closed with a continuous or interrupted Lembert oversew using 0 synthetic absorbable suture (Fig. 7.8, *B* and *C*). Suturing can be extremely difficult if the ileum is edematous or swollen, and in this situation a two-layer inverting pattern is recommended. It is important to obtain as much inversion as possible with compromised ileum.

An alternative means of blind-stumping the ileum is provided by using the TA-90 as illustrated in Figure 7.8, *D* and *E*. The TA-90 is positioned and clamped shut. A bowel clamp is placed to prevent loss of bowel contents at the time of transection (Fig. 7.8*D*). The TA-90 is then fired, a scalpel is used to transect the bowel immediately proximal to the TA-90, and the TA-90 is then removed (Fig. 7.8*E*). The stapling device also provides a means of resecting ileum closer to the ileocecal junction, a definite advantage when the terminal ileum is considered nonviable. The staple line can be oversewn with a continuous suture for additional security. Once closure of the ileal stump has been completed, it is released back into the abdominal cavity.

The portion of bowel to be resected is then attended to. Before resection, this portion of terminal small intestine can be used as a conduit to evacuate proximal bowel contents into a container after ligation of mesenteric vessels and division of the mesentery. Resection of the compromised piece of bowel is then completed in the same fashion as described in the previous section for end-to-end anastomosis of small intestine.

The portion of jejunum to be anastomosed to the cecum is occluded by Penrose drains and/or fingers, rather than clamps, and is placed in an accessible position distal (approximately 20 cm) to the ileocecal junction and between the medial and dorsal bands of the cecum. The long axis of the jejunum is perpendicular to the long axis of the cecum. Care is taken that the jejunum is not rotated 180° because this can occlude the jejunal lumen or compromise the mesentery. Interrupted stay sutures are then placed at the mesenteric and

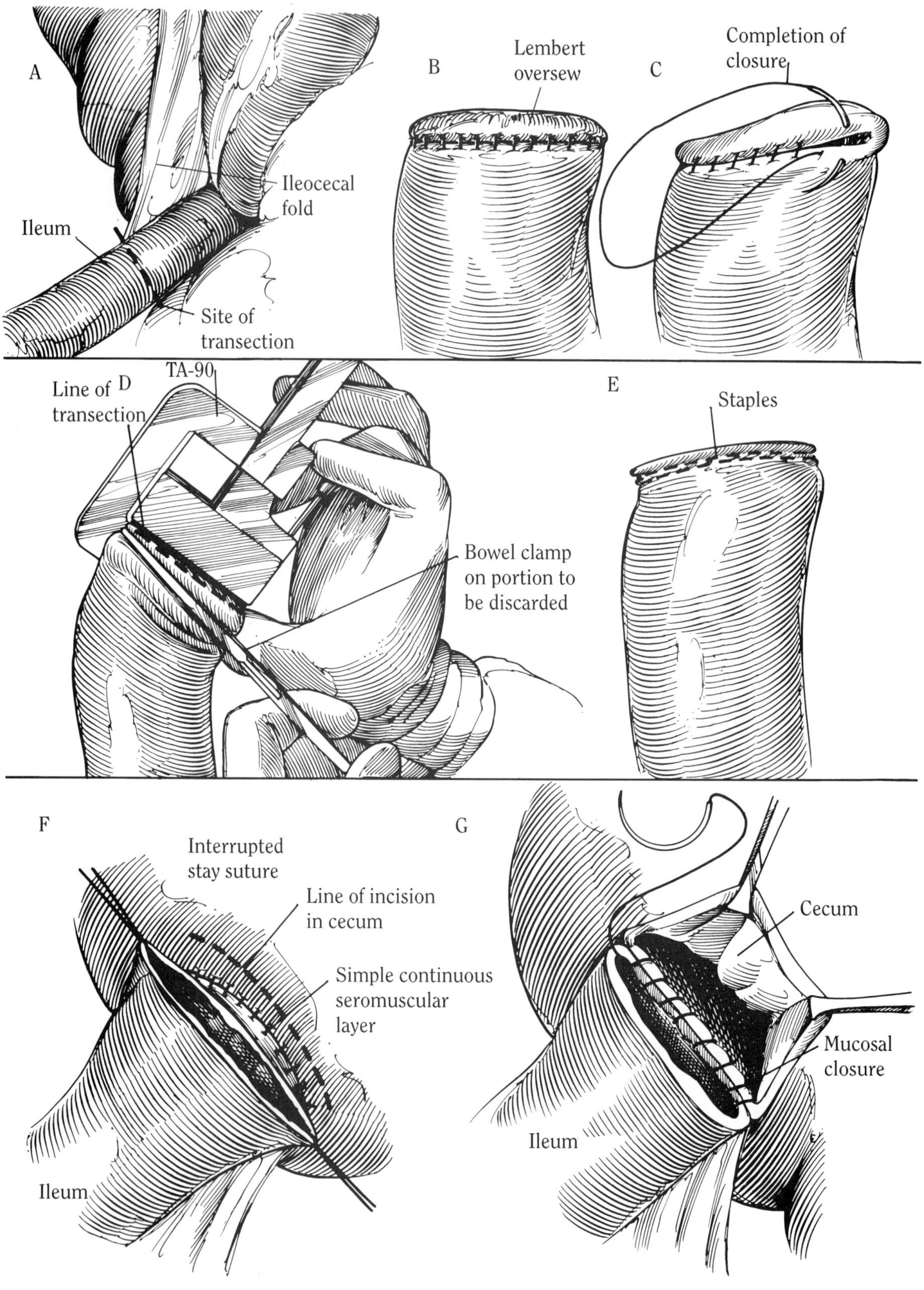

Figure 7.8, A–G. Jejunocecal anastomosis.

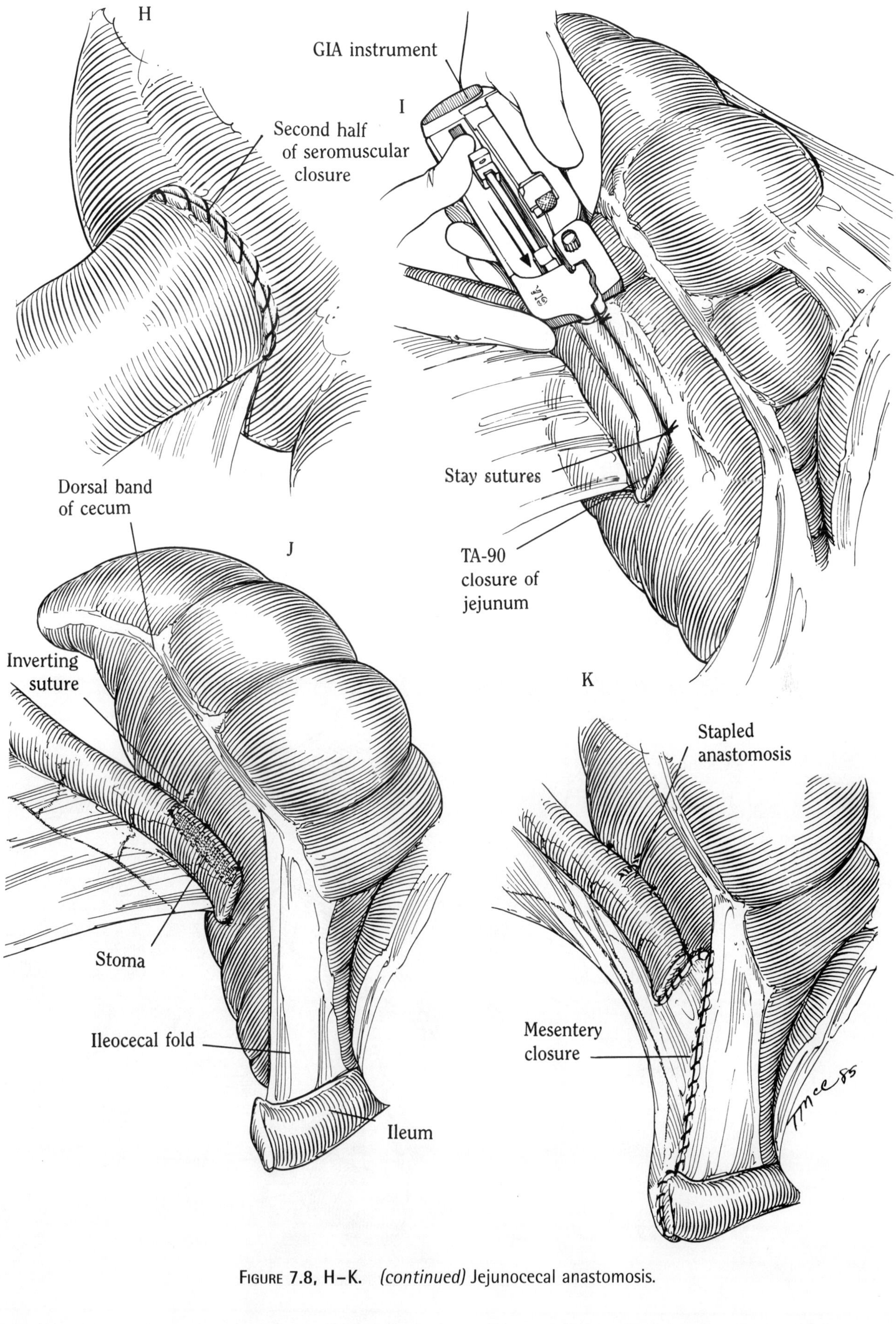

Figure 7.8, H–K. *(continued)* Jejunocecal anastomosis.

antimesenteric borders of the jejunum to fix the open end of the jejunum to the cecum in a stretched-out position with as wide a diameter as possible (Fig. 7.8*F*). The seromuscular layer of jejunum on the side adjacent to the cecum is then attached to the cecum in a simple continuous pattern using 2/0 synthetic absorbable suture material on a taper needle (Fig. 7.8*F*). An incision is then made in the cecum alongside the previous aligned suture line (Fig. 7.8*F*). The mucosa of the jejunum and cecum are then apposed in a simple continuous pattern around the entire circumference, interrupted with a knot at 180° (Fig. 7.8*G*). The remaining sides of the seromuscular incisions in the cecum and jejunum are then closed in a continuous Lembert pattern (Fig. 7.8*H*).

It has been reported that better results might be obtained using a side-to-side anastomosis (5). The advantage of a side-to-side anastomosis is that the size of the jejunocecal stoma can be selected and any risk of stomal edema and occlusion obviated. However, with careful attention to stretching of the jejunal end and not inverting mucosa, stomal occlusion does not seem to be a problem with the end-to-side technique.

The jejunocecal anastomosis can also be performed using stapling equipment in a side-to-side technique. The end of the jejunum to be anastomosed to the cecum is closed using the TA-90. The end of the jejunum is then placed on the cecum and tacked to the cecum using two stay sutures. Holes are then made in the jejunum and cecum, and the arm of the GIA or ILA instrument is inserted into one lumen and the anvil into the other (Fig. 7.8*I*). The instrument is then clamped together, the cartridge is fired, and the blade is pushed into position

L

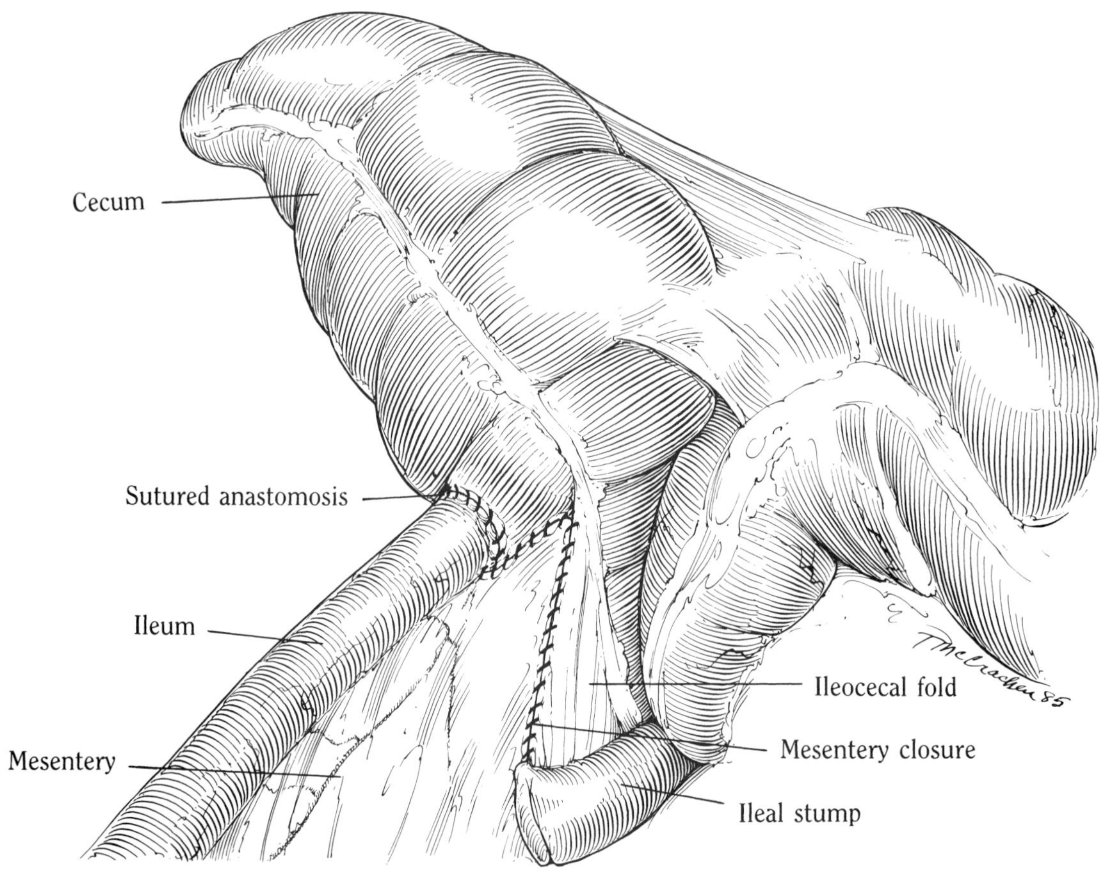

Figure 7.8, L. *(continued)* Jejunocecal anastomosis.

to create the stoma (Fig. 7.8*I*). The GIA is then unlocked and removed, and the holes are closed with an inverting suture (Fig. 7.8*J*). If a larger stoma is desired, the GIA can be applied twice. In a controlled study comparing the stapled side-to-side technique with the conventional sutured end-to-side anastomosis, the former was considered superior, based on both the postoperative course of the experimental animals and the necropsy findings (6).

The jejunal mesentery must be apposed to the cecum to prevent postoperative internal herniation. The jejunal mesentery is sutured to the ileal stump, ileocecal fold, and dorsal band of the cecum. This closure is illustrated for a staple and a suture anastomosis in Fig. 7.8, *K* and *L*, respectively.

Comments

There is a critical amount of small intestine that can be resected beyond which the patient can suffer permanent gastrointestinal compromise. These limits have been somewhat defined by the experimental work of Tate et al., which showed that at a point between resection of 40 and 60% of the small intestine, malabsorption, weight loss, and liver damage will develop (7). An unexpected finding of this work was an altered D-xylose absorption curve when ileocecal bypass (without resection) was performed.

An alternative technique, jejunocecal bypass, can be performed when there is obstruction but viable bowel, such as in ileum impaction (obstipation), ileal muscular hypertrophy (8), or chronic ileal intussusception (9). The bypass is created as a side-to-side anastomosis and leaves the normal ileal pathway open (8).

REFERENCES

1. Donawick WJ, Christie BA, Stewart JV. Resection of diseased ileum in the horse. JAVMA 1971;159:1145.
2. Owen R ap R, Physick-Sheard PW, Hilbert BJ, et al. Jejuno- or ileocecal anastomosis performed in seven horses exhibiting colic. Can Vet J 1975;165:1645.
3. Robertson JT. Conditions of the stomach and small intestine. Vet Clin North Am Large Animal Pract 1982;4:105.
4. Stashak TS. Techniques for enterotomy, decompression and intestinal resection-anastomosis. Vet Clin North Am Large Animal Pract 1982;4:147.
5. Huskamp B. The various types and frequency as seen in the Animal Hospital in Hochmoor. In: Proceedings of the Equine Colic Research Symposium. Georgia: University of Georgia, 1982:261–272.
6. Blackwell RB. Jejunocecostomy in the horse: a comparison of two techniques. In: Proceedings of the Equine Colic Research Symposium. Georgia: University of Georgia, 1982:288–289.
7. Tate LP, Ralston SL, Koch CM, et al. Effects of extensive resection of the small intestine in the pony. Am J Vet Res 1983;44:1187.
8. Kersjes AW, Nemeth F, Rutgers LJE. Atlas of Large Animal Surgery. Baltimore: Williams & Wilkins, 1985.
9. Scott EA, Todhunter R. Chronic intestinal intussusception in two horses. JAVMA 1985; 186:383.

Large Colon Resection and Anastomosis

Resection and anastomosis of the large colon is now a commonly performed procedure (1–5). The indications for colon resection are significant in number, including strangulation obstruction of the mobile portions of the large colon, large intramural lesions, focal stricture, intussusception, and mural devitalization caused by long-standing obstructions (1, 2, 5, 6).

Resection of the dorsal and ventral large colon at the sternal and diaphragmatic flexures can be performed successfully in clinical cases without long-term nutritional compromise (1, 7, 8). More extensive resections can also be accomplished (2–4). Resection of the entire large colon is not practical because of the inability to surgically expose it. Localized lesions such as a focal stricture or an infarcted area may be amenable to selective resection and end-to-end anastomosis with sutures (2, 9, 10). When greater amounts of bowel (left dorsal and ventral colon, or parts of the right dorsal and ventral colon) require resection, a side-to-side anastomosis with closure of the ends of each colon is performed.

Closure and transection of adjacent colons followed by a side-to-side colocolostomy can be performed with suturing or stapling equipment. Both techniques are described.

Additional Instrumentation

If stapling techniques are used, both the TA-90 and GIA or ILA instruments are necessary. In a typical case of 60% colon resection with closure and resection of the adjacent colons and their side-to-side anastomosis, four to six cartridges of 4.8-mm staples for the TA-90, four cartridges for the GIA, and two cartridges for the ILA will be used.

Surgical Technique

Focal Resection with End-to-End Anastomosis

This technique is only used for focal lesions as illustrated in Figure 7.9*A* (11). Contents are milked out of the region of bowel to be resected. The artery and vein at either end of the segment to be removed are doubly ligated and transected. The mesocolon adjacent to the segment of colon to be removed is separated from the colon. Intestinal clamps are placed on the colon to be removed as illustrated in simple end-to-end anastomosis of the small intestine. The colon is transected with a scalpel at either end of the lesion and removed. An end-to-end anastomosis is then performed using a suture pattern of the surgeon's preference. A double-layer (simple continuous oversewn with a continuous Lembert) pattern is illustrated in Figure 7.9*B*. The anastomotic site is rinsed off thoroughly, and the colon is returned to the abdomen.

Resection of Adjacent Arms of Colon and Side-to-Side Anastomosis Using Sutures

If a significant amount of colon is to be resected and stapling equipment is unavailable, the following technique can be used. Resection of the left dorsal and left ventral colon at the level of the sternal and diaphragmatic flexure is used as an example. Both the left ventral and dorsal colons are sectioned transversely with a scalpel and sutured closed with a double-inverting suture pattern (Fig. 7.9*C*). Occlusion of the left ventral colon and the right ventral colon is important during this procedure. A 15- to 20-cm length of adjacent left ventral and left dorsal colon is apposed using a simple continuous seromuscular suture,

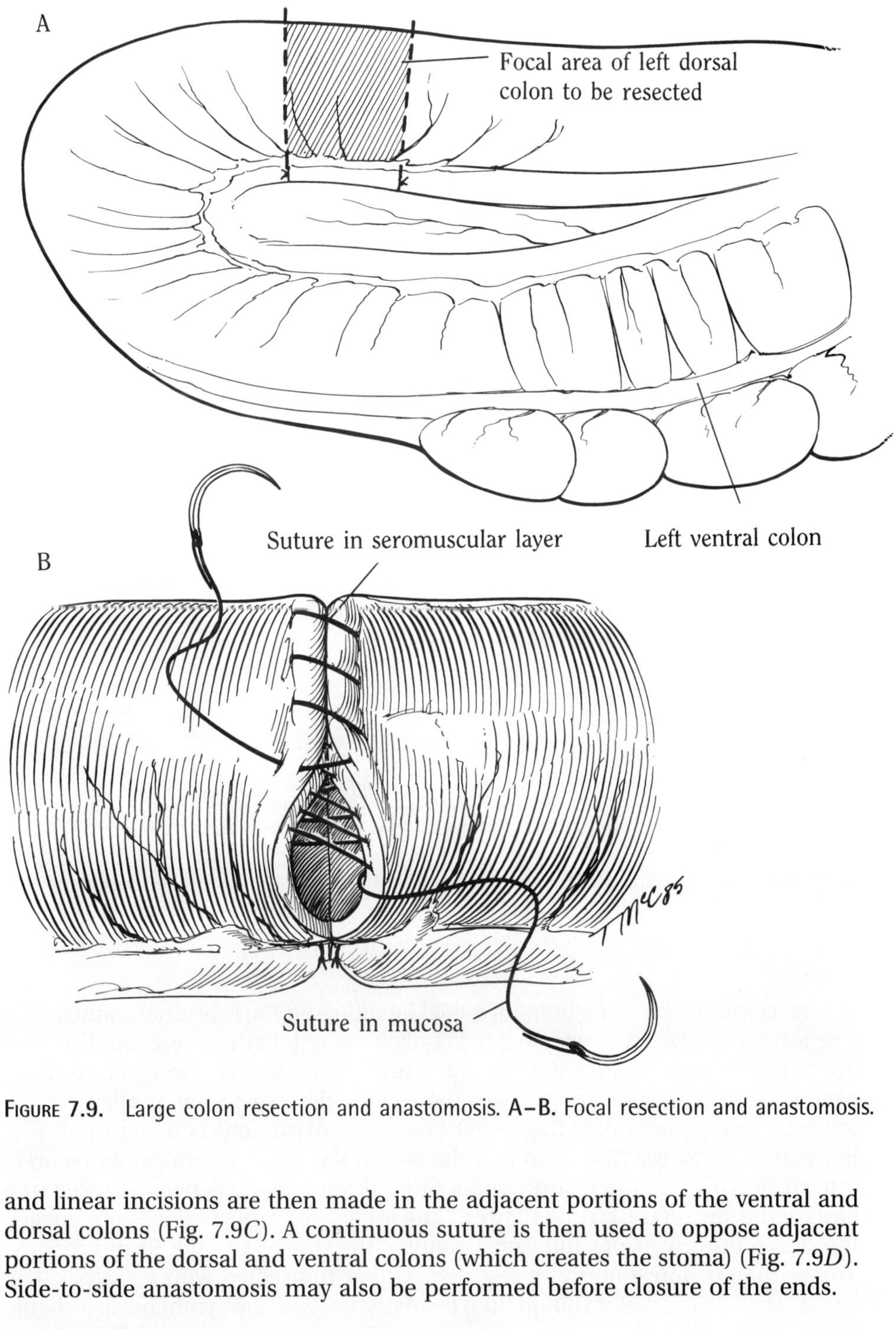

FIGURE 7.9. Large colon resection and anastomosis. A–B. Focal resection and anastomosis.

and linear incisions are then made in the adjacent portions of the ventral and dorsal colons (Fig. 7.9*C*). A continuous suture is then used to oppose adjacent portions of the dorsal and ventral colons (which creates the stoma) (Fig. 7.9*D*). Side-to-side anastomosis may also be performed before closure of the ends.

Resection and Side-to-Side Anastomosis with Stapling Equipment

Transection at the level of the sternal and diaphragmatic flexure (approximately 60% resection) is illustrated in Figure 7.9*E* (1). The dorsal and ventral colons are occluded with bowel clamps to prevent ingesta from reaching the anastomotic sites. These clamps are placed directly opposite each other and distal to a prominent intramural vessel (Fig. 7.9*F*). The dorsal and ventral colic vessels (right colic vessel and colic branches of the ileocolic vessels, respectively) are dissected from the mesentery and doubly ligated. The TA-90 stapler is then used to place a double-staggered row of stainless steel staples across the dorsal and

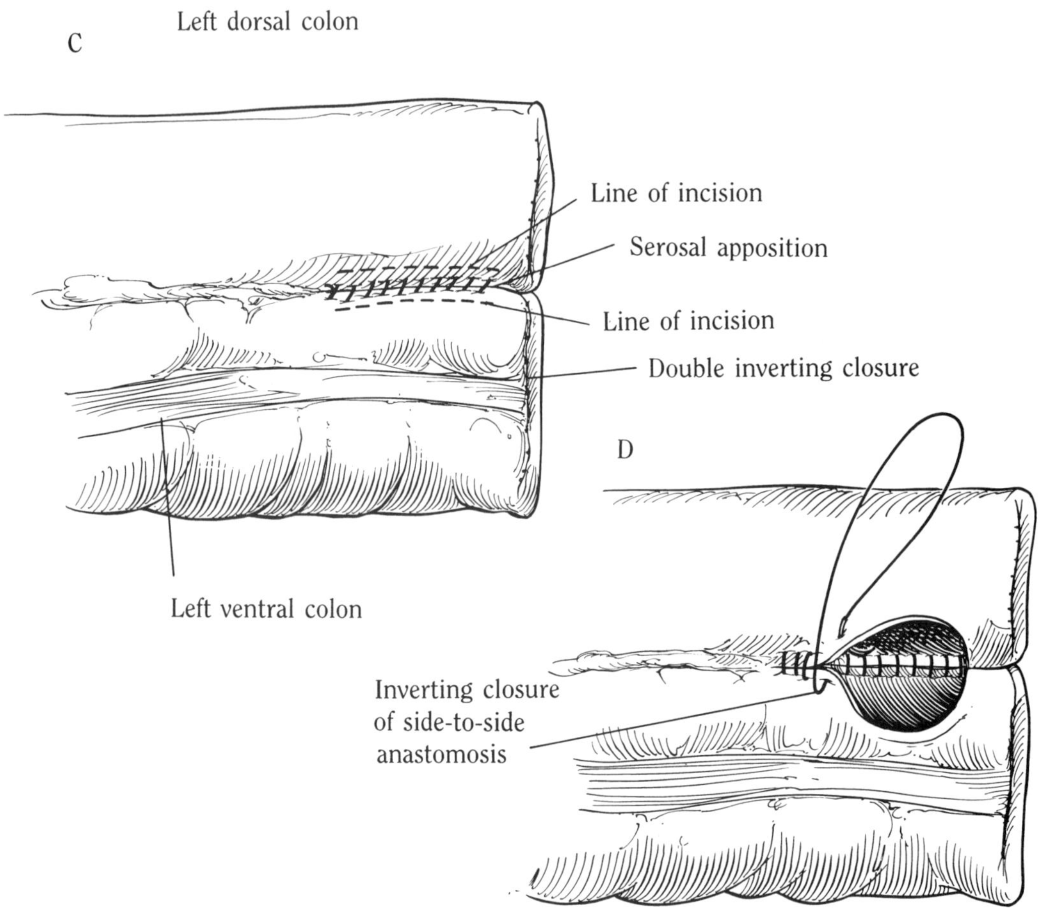

Figure 7.9, C–D. *(continued)* Resection of adjacent arms of colon and side-to-side anastomosis.

ventral colon between the point of vessel ligation and the intestinal clamps (Fig. 7.9*F*). Because the TA-90 staple line is only 9 cm in length, several applications are required to close the colons in the adult horse. Care is also taken to make each sequential staple row overlap the end of the previously applied row to ensure a complete seal. If the TA-90 Premium instrument is being used, it is imperative to ensure that the pin at the end of the staple cartridge fits securely into the anvil when the instrument is fired. If thick tissue is being stapled, the ends of the jaws of the stapler may not line up properly, the pin does not engage the slot in the anvil side, and, subsequently, the staples will not form properly. The portion of intestine to be resected is then transected with a scalpel (Fig. 7.9*G*). The line of staples should then be oversewn with 2/0 synthetic absorbable suture material in a continuous Lembert pattern (5).

A side-to-side anastomosis between the right dorsal and right ventral colons is then performed commencing 1.5 cm from the distal extremity of the stapled intestinal stumps. The stoma is placed on the juxtaparietal side of the colons and parallel to their longitudinal axes. Five simple interrupted sutures of no. 2/0 polyglactin 910 are placed 5 cm apart to appose the dorsal and ventral colons so that the distal and proximal sutures are 20 cm apart (Fig. 7.9*H*). A 1-cm stab incision is then made into the lumina of both colons 5 cm from the distal stay suture. The GIA or GIA-50 Premium stapler is then inserted along this line between the two stay sutures and closed, and the staples are applied (Fig. 7.9*H*). This procedure is performed both cranial and caudal to the stab incision and

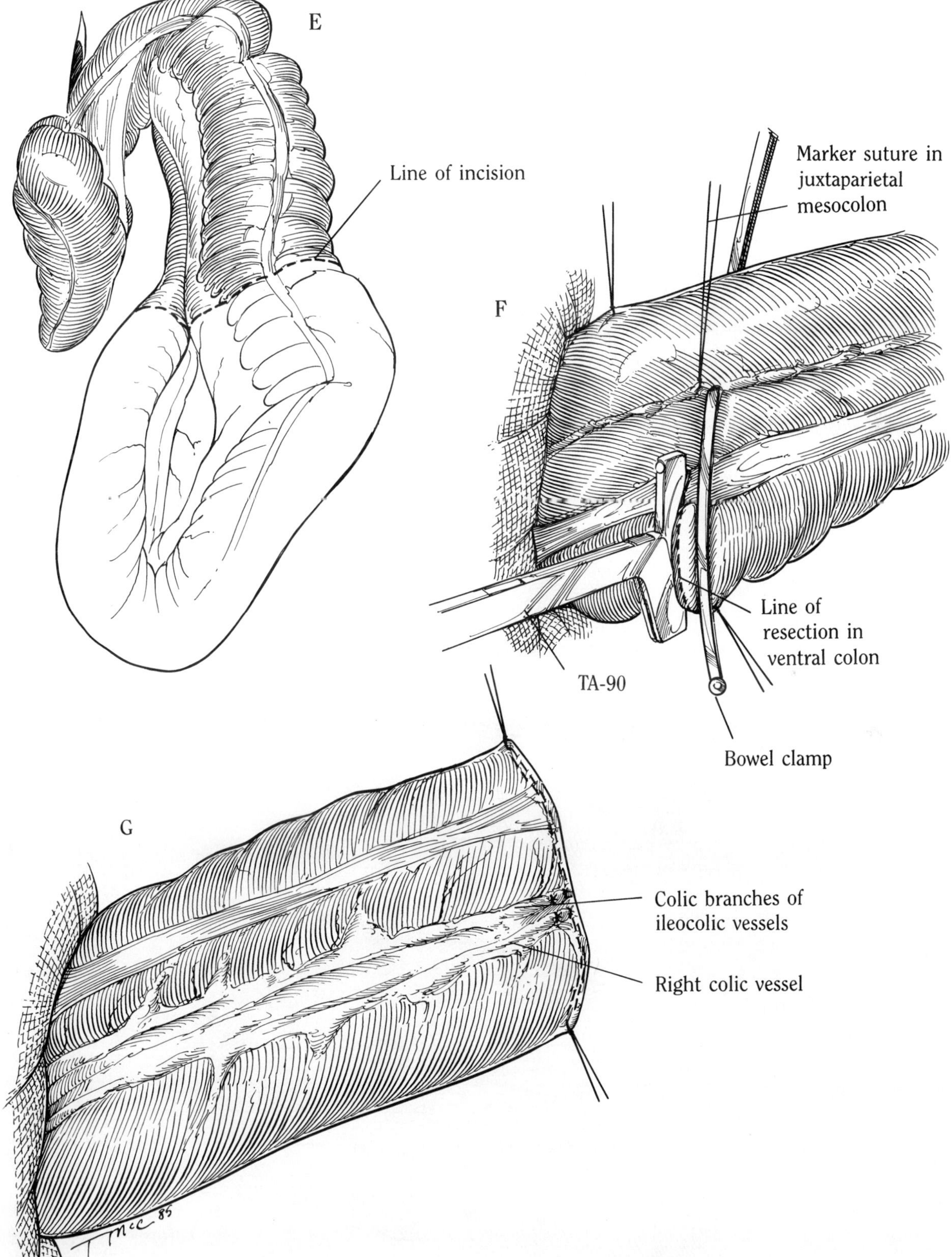

FIGURE 7.9, E–G. *(continued)* Resection and side-to-side anastomosis with stapling equipment.

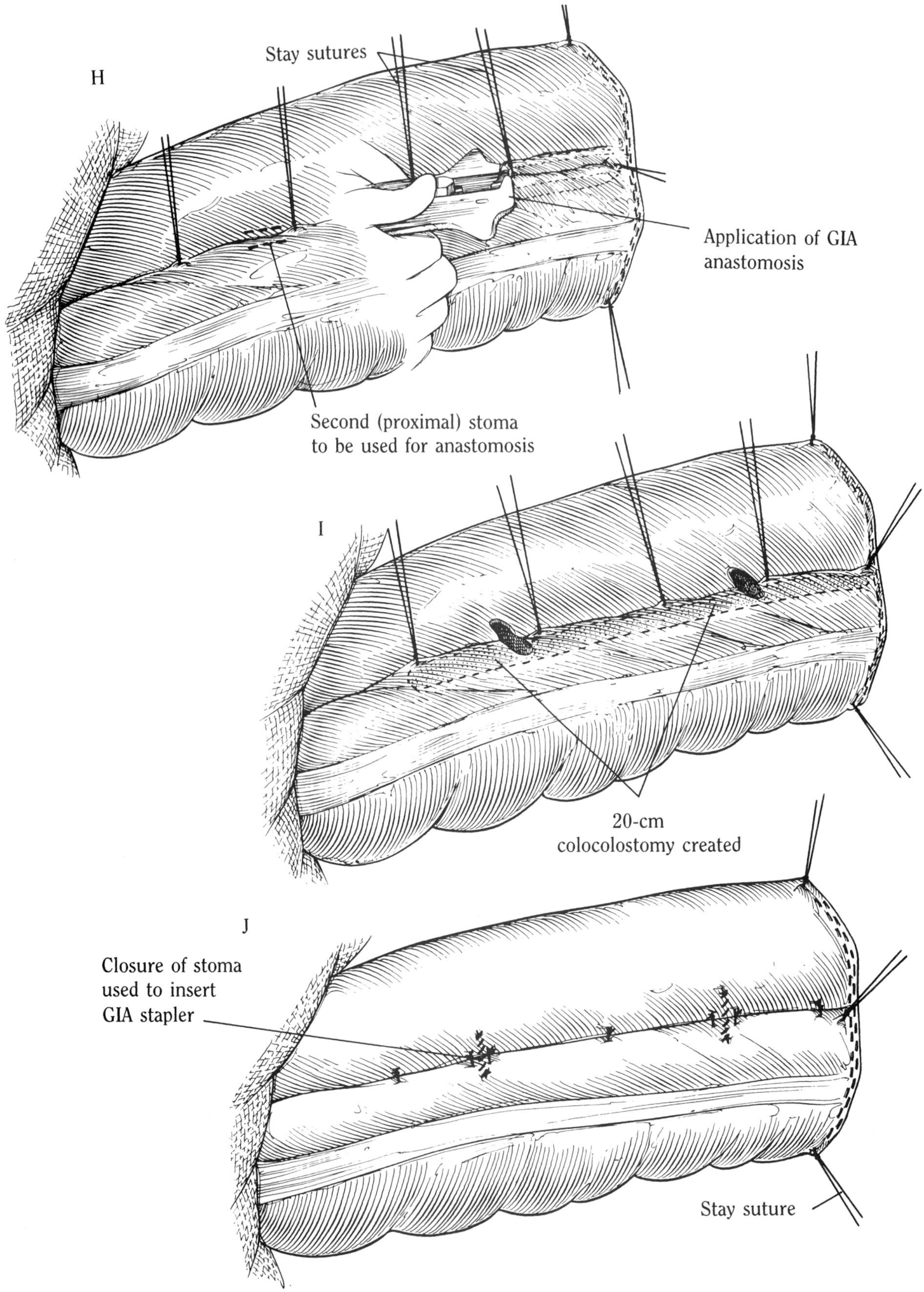

Figure 7.9, H–J. *(continued)* Resection and side-to-side anastomosis with stapling equipment.

is repeated through a second stab incision 5 cm from the cranial stay suture. In this way, the instrument applications effect a continuous 20-cm side-to-side anastomosis (Fig. 7.9*I*). Alternatively, two applications of the ILA-100 stapler or the GIA-90 Premium or the Multifire GIA-80, cranial and caudal through a single stab incision, create an appropriately sized stoma. As mentioned previously, both of these instruments have the advantage of creating a longer stoma than the GIA-50 and have cartridges with staples that have a leg length of 4.8 mm. Also, with only two applications required, there is less likelihood of technical error. The incisions used for entry of the GIA or ILA instrument are closed with a double-inverting layer of continuous sutures in a Lembert pattern using no. 2/0 polyglactin 910 (Fig. 7.9*J*). Defects at the junction of the double rows of staples must be closed carefully (12). Reinforcing sutures of the same material are placed at the cranial and caudal limits of the stapled anastomosis. The resection-anastomosis site is then cleansed by rinsing and returned to the abdomen.

If cost is a concern, the side-to-side anastomosis can be performed with sutures after the transection with the TA-90 stapler (10). A 20-cm continuous Lembert pattern using no. 2/0 polyglactin 910 is placed in the seromuscular layers to appose the dorsal and ventral colons approximately 1 cm from their attachments to the mesocolon and starting 1.5 cm from the distal extremity of the stapled intestinal stumps. The lumens of the colon are opened adjacent to the suture line, and a simple continuous suture pattern, interrupted at 180°, is used to appose the mucosa in a stoma. The original Lembert pattern is then continued to complete a second anastomotic layer.

EXTENSIVE RESECTION WITH END-TO-END ANASTOMOSIS

An alternative method for extensive large colon resection and anastomosis was recently described (13). Rather than a side-to-side anastomosis following resection, an end-to-end anastomosis of the dorsal and ventral colon is performed. The purported advantage of this anastomosis is an improved stoma size (12–14 cm).

In preparation for resection, the large colon is exteriorized and the mesocolon is bluntly separated from the right dorsal and ventral colon. The line of resection is approximately 10–12 cm distal to the cecocolic fold. Using the TA-90 Premium stapling device, the mesocolon is ligated and transected. The right ventral colon is sharply transected perpendicular to its long axis, while the right dorsal colon is transected at an oblique angle, 30° from perpendicular, leaving the antimesenteric border shorter and increasing the circumference of the right dorsal colon so it approximates that of the right ventral colon. The GIA Premium 55 is then applied along the adjacent mesenteric borders of the right dorsal and ventral colon to create a V-shaped stoma that increases the stomal size of the completed anastomosis. The staple lines are reinforced with sutures. An end-to-end anastomosis of the dorsal and ventral colon is performed in two layers, using size 0-polydioxanone. The initial layer, a continuous Connell pattern, is oversewn with a continuous Lembert. Wider bites are taken in the ventral colon to assure proper alignment.

Postoperative Management

Feed is withheld overnight and one gallon of mineral oil is administered by nasogastric tube before access to feed is allowed. Broad-spectrum antibiotic administration is continued for 3 to 5 days following surgery.

Comments

Extensive large colon resection can be performed in the horse at the cecocolic junction. The use of this technique, removing approximately 95% of the length of the large colon as measured from the cecocolic orifice and transverse colon to the pelvic flexure, has been described in 10 normal horses (3). Four horses died, and three of these had failure or contamination of the transection staple line. Clinically, it is questionable whether such a resection can be successful in a horse with a volvulus of the large colon that involves the cecocolic ligament and the base of the cecum (14).

Resection of a segment of the right dorsal colon may be indicated for treatment of horses with right dorsal ulcerative colitis if the ulceration is found to be severe and is associated with ongoing protein loss (15). It can be determined at the time of a ventral midline exploratory laparotomy whether the involved segment is amenable to resection and anastomosis and a second surgery can be performed.

The junction of the right dorsal colon and transverse colon is approached with the horse in left lateral recumbency using 16th rib resection technique (15). It is the authors' experience that the costal attachment of the diaphragm can vary between horses, and with an incision at the level of the 16th rib, the diaphragm may be incised. If this occurs, pneumothorax will develop and positive-pressure ventilation will be required. The large colon is exteriorized and placed in a colon tray and the affected right dorsal colon is resected. The remaining right dorsal colon is anastomosed to the proximal transverse colon in an end-to-end fashion (15).

REFERENCES

1. Sullins KE, Stashak TS, Ralston SL. Evaluation of 60% resection of the large colon in the horse and comparison of stapled vs. sutured techniques. Vet Surg 1985;14:67.
2. Bertone AL, Stashak TS, Sullins KE. Large colon resection and anastomosis in horses. JAVMA 1986;188:612–617.
3. Bertone AL, Stashak TS, Sullins KE, et al. Experimental large colon resection at the cecocolic ligament in the horse. Vet Surg 1987;16:5–12.
4. Ducharme NG, Horney FD, Baird JD, et al. Extensive large colon resection in the pony. I. Surgical procedures and clinical results. Can J Vet Res 1987;51:66–75.
5. Rose PL, Bradley WM. Resection and anastomosis for treatment of strangulating volvulus of the large colon of horses. JAVMA 1992;201:454–456.
6. Robertson JT, Tate LP Jr. Resection of intussuscepted large colon in a horse. JAVMA 1982;181:927.
7. Bertone AL, Cockerell GL, Lee RE, et al. Alteration in intestinal morphologic features associated with extensive large colon resection in horses. Am J Vet Res 1990;51:1471–1475.
8. Bertone AL. Large colon resection. In: Snyder JR, Markel MD, eds. Advances in Equine Abdominal Surgery. Philadelphia: WB Saunders, 1989;5:377.
9. Embertson RM, Schneider RK, Granstedt M. Partial resection and anastomosis of the large colon in a horse. JAVMA 1982;180:1230.
10. Stashak TS. Techniques for enterotomy, decompression and intestinal resection/anastomosis. Vet Clin North Am Large Animal Pract 1982;4:147.
11. Wilson DG, Wilson WD. Intussusception of the left dorsal colon in a horse. JAVMA 1983;183:464.
12. Mackey VS, Pascoe JR, Peterson PR. A potential technique error in stapled side-to-side anastomosis of the small intestine of the horse. Vet Surg 1987;16:189–192.
13. Hughes FE, Slone DE. A modified technique for extensive large colon resection and anastomosis in horses. Vet Surg 1998;27:127–131.
14. Ross MW, Hanson RR Jr. Large intestine. In: Auer JA, ed. Equine Surgery. Philadelphia: WB Saunders, 1992:400.
15. Simmons TR, Gaughan EM, Ducharme NG, et al. Treatment of right dorsal ulcerative colitis in a horse. JAVMA 1990;196:455–458.

Jejunocolic Anastomosis

Complete cecal bypass (ileocolostomy or jejunocolostomy) is now generally considered to be the most effective procedure for treatment of horses with cecal impaction (1, 2). Although many cecal impactions will resolve with medical treatment, surgery is frequently required in more severe, prolonged, or recurrent cases to prevent cecal rupture (3, 4). Previously reported techniques have included infusion and manual massage to soften cecal contents, typhlotomy and evacuation of cecal contents, cecocolic anastomosis, and incomplete cecal bypass with an ileocolostomy (1, 5, 6). Most of these techniques have been found to be less successful than complete bypass for achieving a permanent cure.

Anesthesia and Surgical Preparation

The surgery is done under general anesthesia using a conventional ventral midline laparotomy. As in most cases of intestinal anastomosis, the decision to perform this surgical technique is an intraoperative one. Perioperative, broad-spectrum antibiotics are administered, as well as tetanus toxoid.

Additional Instrumentation

Surgical stapling instruments such as the TA-90 and the GIA may be used during the resection and anastomosis. The appropriate number of staple cartridges must be available.

Surgical Technique

The impacted cecum is exteriorized and packed off. An enterotomy incision is made in the cecal apex between the lateral and ventral cecal taenia, and the cecal contents are manually evacuated. Following a thorough lavage, the enterotomy incision is closed with two continuous inverting layers using 2/0 absorbable synthetic suture material. Alternatively, if there is a great deal of serosal contamination, the cecal apex can be amputated quickly using the TA-90 staple instrument. The staple line should then be oversewn with a continuous layer of 2/0 synthetic suture material and inverted with a second continuous suture line.

In the initial report of ileocolostomy as a technique for management of cecal impaction, the ileum was transected using a stapling instrument, but none of the ileum was resected (1). In a more recent report of nine cases of ileo- or jejunocolostomy, all horses had either a 15- to 30-cm segment of ileum or the entire ileum and a portion of distal jejunum resected (2). It would appear that the need to resect is based on surgeon choice. Some surgeons prefer to resect back to a point where the distal jejunum is supplied by a complete vascular arcade, ensuring adequate blood supply at the anastomosis. The free end of the ileum or distal jejunum can be stapled and oversewn in a fashion similar to the ileal stump (see "Jejunocecostomy"). The side-to-side anastomosis will be performed in the most proximal, exteriorized portion of right ventral colon between the medial and lateral free taeniae. The blind end of the small intestine must be directed orally (1, 2). Two stay sutures are used to attach the distal 15 cm of small intestine to the right ventral colon and a 10-cm long, hand-sutured or stapled anastomotic stoma is created (see "Jejunocecal Technique"). The

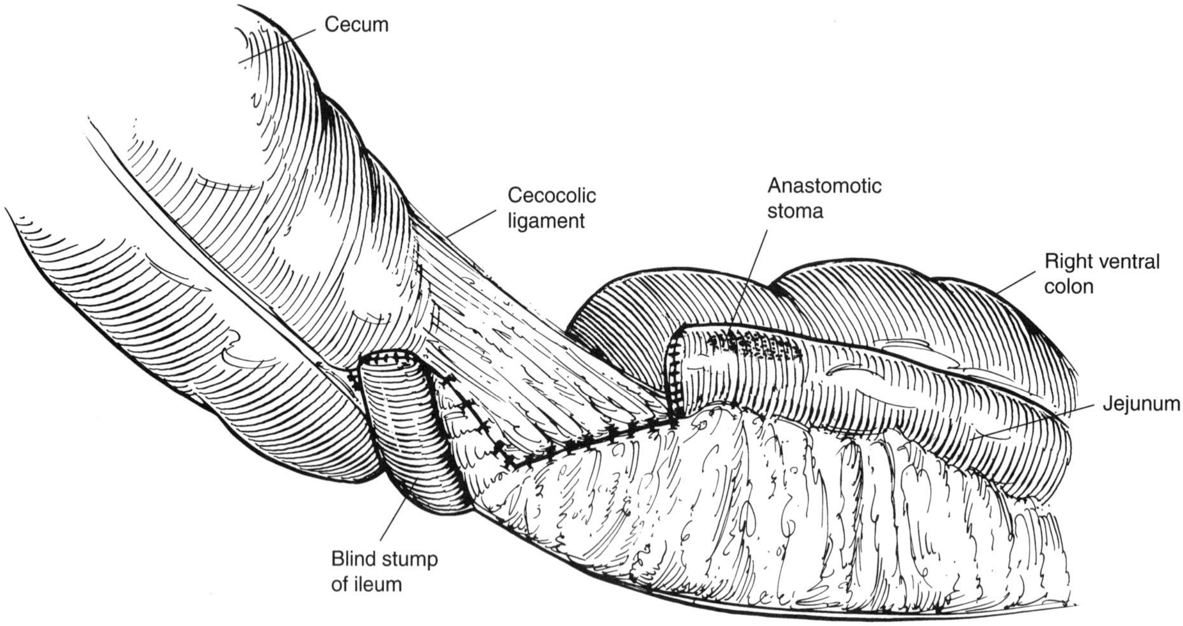

Figure 7.10. Jejunocolic anastomosis.

mesenteric defect created after ileal transection and resection must be closed to prevent internal herniation (Fig. 7.10).

Comments

The blind end of the small intestine at the anastomotic site must be directed orally (1, 2). Placing it in an aboral direction may predispose to postoperative ileus and may also result in a failure to close the mesenteric defect (2).

Ileocolostomy in conjunction with partial typhlectomy has been used successfully for treatment of a nonreducible cecocolic intussusception in a horse (7). Total typhlectomy and ileocolostomy have been described, but a right flank approach with a rib resection is required. Because of the rare demand for this technique, it is not described or illustrated in this text, and interested readers should consult the original reference (8).

REFERENCES

1. Craig DR, Pankowski RL, Car BD, et al. Ileocolostomy: a technique for surgical management of equine cecal impaction. Vet Surg 1987;16:451.
2. Gerard MP, Bowman KF, Blikslager AT, et al. Jejunocolostomy or ileocolostomy for treatment of cecal impaction in horses: nine cases (1985–1995). JAVMA 1996;209:1287.
3. Campbell ML, Colahan PC, Brown MP, et al. Cecal impaction in the horse. JAVMA 1984;184:95.
4. Ross MW, Martin BB, Donawick WJ. Cecal perforation in the horse. JAVMA 1985;187:249.
5. Ross MW, Tate LP, Donawick WJ. Cecocolic anastomosis for the surgical management of cecal impaction in horses. Vet Surg 1986;15:85.
6. Ross MW, Orsini JA, Ehnen S. Jejunocolic anastomosis for surgical management of recurrent cecal impaction in a horse. Vet Surg 1987;16:265.
7. Ward JL, Fubini SL. Partial typhlectomy and ileocolostomy for treatment of nonreducible cecocolic intussusception in a horse. JAVMA 1994;205:325.
8. Huskamp B. Some problems associated with intestinal surgery in the horse. Equine Vet J 1977;9:111.

Temporary Diverting Colostomy for the Management of Rectal Tears

Rectal tears are a relatively common accident and are typically iatrogenic in association with rectal examination (1). There are reports of noniatrogenic causes of rectal perforation, including thrombosis or ischemic vascular disease (2). The consequences of a rectal tear depend on its size and position, the tissue layers penetrated, the time between injury and initiation of treatment, and the effectiveness of treatment. Rectal tears have been classified according to the tissue layers penetrated at the time of injury (3).

An attempt is made to manage most mucosal tears by medical means. More significant tears that have penetrated the mucosal, submucosal, and muscularis layers are not usually amenable to such conservative treatment. There is a great risk of development of a complete tear and fatal peritonitis if some form of surgical treatment is not initiated. Suture repair of a tear can be attempted per rectum in either the standing or recumbent animal (1, 4–6). This can be extremely difficult because of the relative inaccessibility of the tear. Special long instruments and an expandable rectal speculum have been developed to facilitate direct surgical repair of rectal tears (5). Surgical stapling for repair of a rectal tear has also been reported (6). Suturing of the rectal tear may also be attempted through a ventral midline laparotomy incision. Dorsal tears are relatively inaccessible but may be accessed by creating a enterotomy in the ventral aspect of the small colon or proximal rectum (1). In addition to direct suturing, or if direct suturing is not attempted, some form of fecal diversion must be accomplished.

A temporary indwelling rectal liner (TIRL) can be placed within the involved rectum with an anchoring attachment cranial to the tear, thereby preventing direct fecal contact with the tear (1, 7, 8). This can be performed via a ventral midline celiotomy. Suture closure of the rectal tear is advocated in conjunction with placement of a TIRL to prevent peritoneal contamination with fecal material should an incomplete tear progress to a complete tear. This combination of suture closure of the tear and implantation of a TIRL resulted in a 60 to 70% success rate for rectal tears that involved laceration of all layers of the rectum except the serosa or mesorectum (7). A distinct advantage of the use of a TIRL is that the surgery is a one-stage procedure compared with a two-stage colostomy. Colostomy is advised, however, if the rectal tear involves greater than 25% of the circumference of the rectum; if the rectum is too small to accommodate the TIRL device; and if the tear is more than 50 cm cranial to the anus (7). A detailed description of how to construct and place a TIRL can be found in the literature (8).

Both end colostomies (transection of the small colon with closure of the distal segment) (9–12) and loop colostomies (continuity of colon maintained with diversion through a stoma on the antimesenteric aspect of the small colon) (11, 13–16) have been used. End colostomy ensures *complete* diversion of feces from the caudal colon (3). A major drawback of this technique is the difficulty encountered during reanastomosis as a result of marked atrophy of the distal segment of colon. The loop colostomy is quicker and easier to construct and revise later. Both techniques will be illustrated. A "low flank" approach is used for the colostomy. This approach is preferable to a ventral abdominal approach in the prevention of herniation of the small colon out through the colostomy site and also stricturing of the lumen by tight fascial bands ventrally.

If management of the tear is medically attempted, feed is withheld and a laxative agent is given until the feces are soft. Enemas in the initial period are indicated. Tears are often compounded by the animal straining to defecate, and there is a tendency for fecal material to lodge in the tissue defect. Periodic cleaning of the area of the rectal defect can be indicated, and this offers an opportunity to assess additional tearing or separation. The tear can be viewed directly with an endoscope. If in 3 to 4 days the wound margins are thickened and granulating without progression of the tear, medical management will probably be adequate. When there is any tendency for walling off of an abscess, the region must be kept open to drain. Periodic evaluation of peritoneal fluid samples is also helpful in monitoring the condition. If a partial tear is approaching complete penetration, a diverting colostomy should be performed. If a complete tear is present, the tear must first be sutured directly before the colostomy is done.

Anesthesia and Surgical Preparation

Palpation of the rectal tear itself should be done only after the animal is sedated and restrained to minimize any additional damage. A lidocaine enema may be beneficial, and rectal passage of an endoscope will sometimes allow direct viewing of the tear. Both end and loop colostomies can be created under local analgesia with the sedated animal standing. If the patient is not suited for standing surgery, an exploratory laparotomy is necessary, or if contamination of the peritoneal cavity is considered to be a problem and the peritoneum is going to be irrigated, then general anesthesia is required. The patient should be placed on broad-spectrum antibiotics as soon as the problem is ascertained. The colostomy is performed with the anesthetized patient in right lateral recumbency.

The colostomy is performed low in the left flank cranial to and at the level of the fold of the flank. If the technique will be done under general anesthesia, the proposed site should be marked with a suture before anesthesia because the anatomy of the region can become distorted when the horse is stretched out in lateral recumbency. If the horse was being examined for colic when the tear occurred, a ventral midline exploratory celiotomy should be performed before doing a colostomy.

Surgical Technique

End Colostomy

A low paralumbar flank incision is made through the skin, incising the external abdominal oblique fascia in the same direction (Fig. 7.11*A*). The internal abdominal oblique muscle, transversus abdominis aponeurosis, and peritoneum are bluntly perforated. The small colon is exteriorized, and the area of rectal damage may be evaluated more directly at this stage with palpation. The small colon should be transected at least 1 meter cranial to the area of the tear to allow adequate manipulation of the small colon at the time of repair (Fig. 7.11*B*). The mesentery of the small colon is divided for half its distance to allow mobility of the two ends. The transected portion of the caudal segment of small colon is evacuated, and the end is oversewn with a double-inverting layer of suture material using no. 2/0 polyglactin 910 (Fig. 7.11*C*). At this stage, the surgeon has the choice of placing the transected end of the cranial segment in the ventral portion of the flank incision or positioning it through a *separate* stoma located ventrally to the laparotomy incision. If a separate stoma is made, the transected end of the cranial segment of small colon is oversewn prior to its being pulled through the stoma. The stoma is created by making a circular incision of slightly smaller diameter than that of the small colon through skin and fascia of the external abdominal oblique muscle. The muscle layers of the internal abdominal oblique and transversus abdominis are separated along the fiber planes, but short perpendicular incisions are made in these two layers to reduce the constricting effect of the muscles (12).

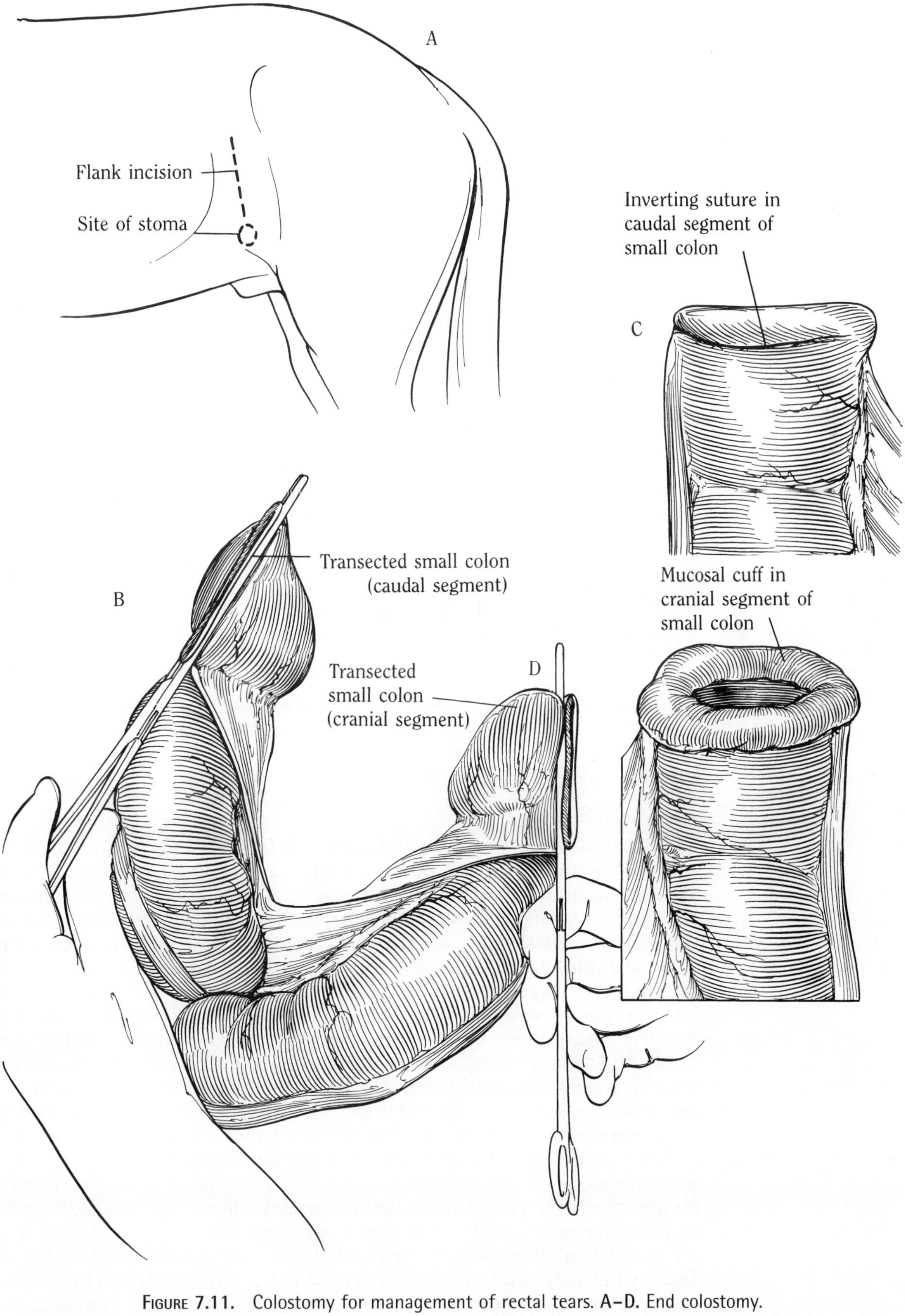

Figure 7.11. Colostomy for management of rectal tears. A–D. End colostomy.

Reanastomosis of the Colon

Before final positioning of the transected end of the cranial portion of the small colon, the transected end is prepared into a cuff. The mucosa of the transected end (stoma) is folded back and sutured to the serosa in a simple continuous pattern with two to three ties (Fig. 7.11*D*). The cut stoma is placed in position so the cuff is outside of the skin (Fig. 7.11*E*), and four to five simple interrupted sutures are placed between the transversus abdominis muscle and the serosa of the small colon to tack it in place. Similarly, other simple interrupted sutures are placed between the internal abdominal oblique muscle and the small colon, and these layers are closed dorsally to the colostomy stoma if the colostomy is being placed within the initial laparotomy incision (Fig. 7.11*E*) (9). If sutures are at 1 and 3 o'clock in one layer, they are placed at 2 and 4 o'clock in the next layer. Simple interrupted sutures are then placed between the external abdominal oblique fascia and the small colon (this is the principal stabilizing layer), and the dorsal aspects of the laparotomy incision are closed. Subcutaneous tissue is then pulled in immediately behind and adjacent to the margins of the reflected mucosal cuff and sutured to the small colon. The skin is not sutured to the small colon at the stoma but is closed dorsally to the stoma.

If the cranial small colon is placed through a separate stoma, it is tacked in place in the deeper layers and positioned in the same fashion relative to the skin as previously described (Fig. 7.11*F*). The flank laparotomy incision is closed routinely. One surgeon has also performed a colostomy by creating a circular stoma alone of sufficient size to place a hand through and grasp the small colon. This technique is appropriate only when there is no contamination of the peritoneal cavity to deal with and therefore limited surgical exposure is required (Boles CL, Herthel DJ, personal communication, 1975).

If a ventral midline exploratory laparotomy is done under general anesthesia before performing the colostomy, it is beneficial to evacuate the contents of the large colon through a pelvic enterotomy. Obviously, this greatly reduces the fecal material presented to the colostomy site in the immediate postoperative period. This can be done before construction of either an end or a loop colostomy. If necessary, the abdomen can be lavaged and ventral abdominal drains placed for the postoperative period.

Loop Colostomy

The principle behind the loop colostomy is to retain the caudal segment of small colon at the surgical site and through regular gentle retroflushing of the caudal segment retain its size and partial function. At the same time, the fecal material is diverted. The loop colostomy can be created using either a single or a double incision approach (15) (Fig. 7.11*G*). If the procedure is attempted in the standing position, the double incision approach is necessary. A loop of small colon, situated at least 1 meter cranial to the peritoneal reflection, is selected and an attempt is made to manually strip fecal material proximal to this site so that the loop is free of feces. One group of surgeons has recommended that both arms of the loop of small colon be joined using absorbable suture material for a distance of approximately 8 cm (15). As the suture line approaches the folded end of the small colon, it should be brought closer to the mesentery to allow the antimesenteric tenia to be exposed through the abdominal incision.

The positioning of the loop in the incision does not appear to be a critical factor for success. Some surgeons recommend that the cranial end of the colonic loop be situated ventral to the caudal loop; others orient the cranial end dorsally as well as ventrally (15, 16). The loop of small colon is tacked to the edges of the peritoneum, internal abdominal oblique, and external abdominal oblique fascia with no. 0 polyglactin 910 in a simple interrupted pattern with the sutures not penetrating the lumen of the colon (Fig. 7.11*H*). Care should be taken not to incorporate the mesentery. The laparotomy incision dorsal to the colostomy

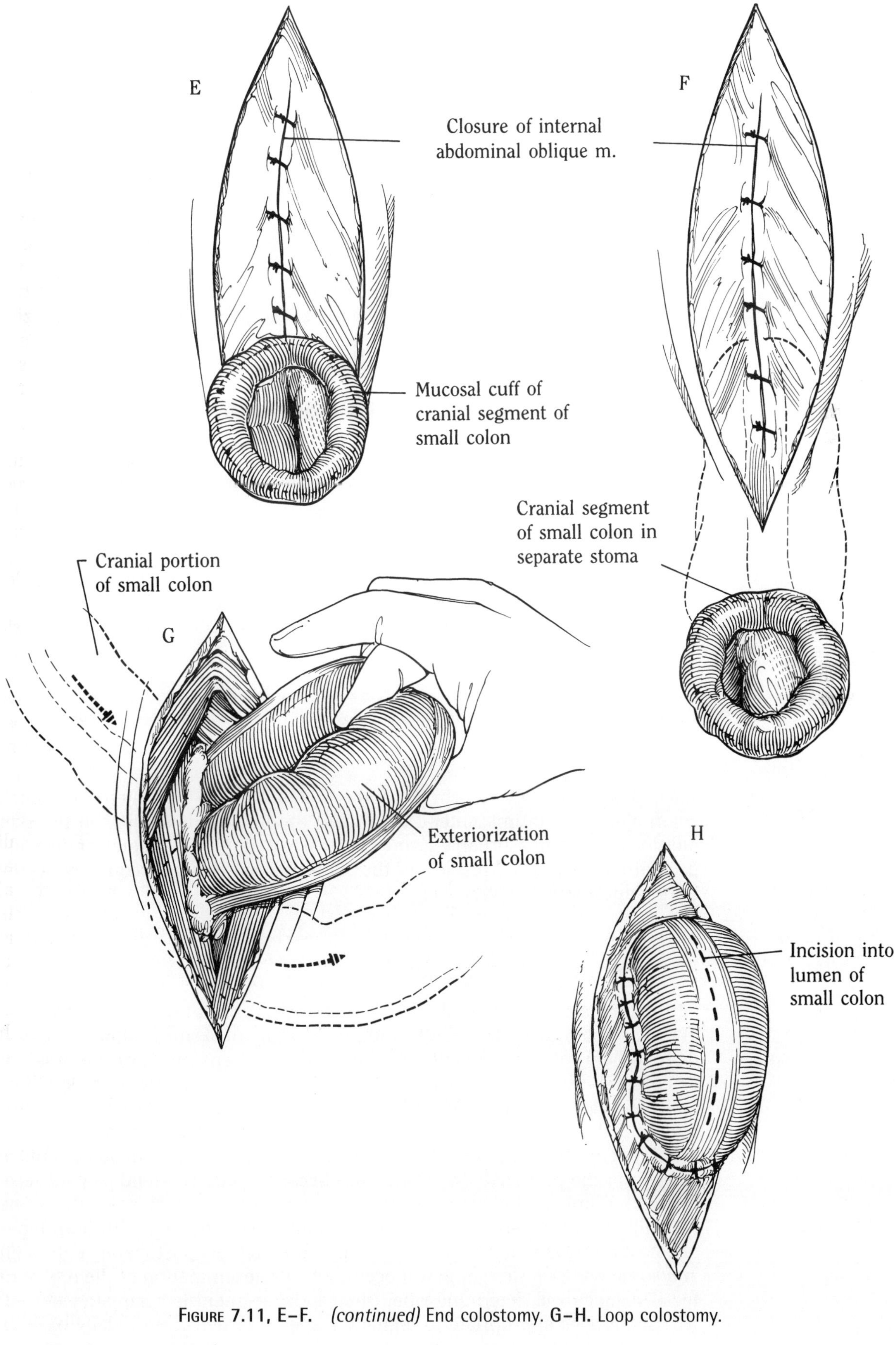

Figure 7.11, E–F. *(continued)* End colostomy. **G–H.** Loop colostomy.

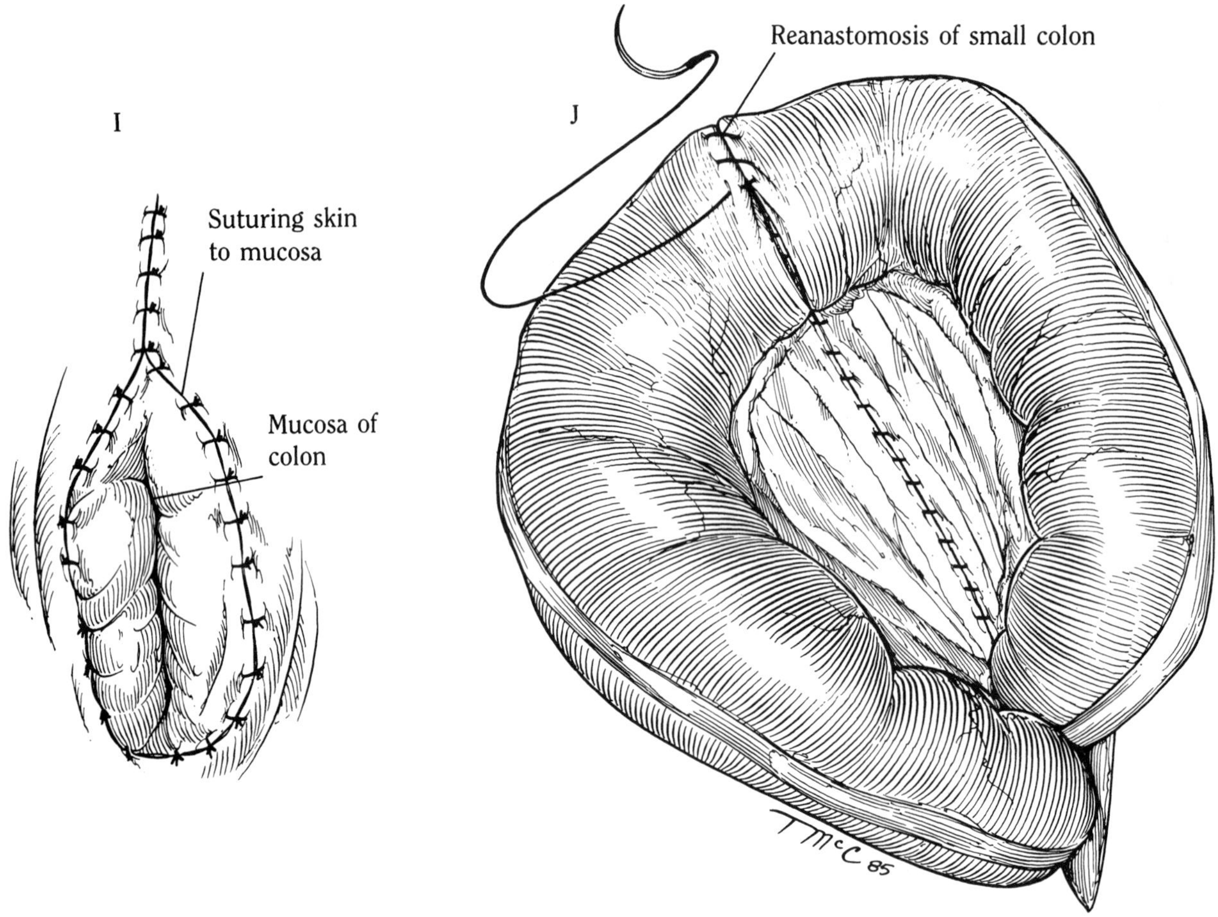

Figure 7.11, *(continued)* **I.** Loop colostomy. **J.** Reanastomosis of colon.

site is closed routinely. A 6-cm incision is then made into the lumen of the small colon along the antimesenteric band, and the mucosa is sutured to the skin incision using nonabsorbable suture material in a simple interrupted or mattress pattern (Fig. 7.11*I*). Disruption of the skin-mucosal closure frequently occurs during anesthetic recovery (16).

Postoperative Management

Petrolatum is applied ventral to the colostomy to prevent scalding. In the case of the loop colostomy, the rectum and caudal segment of small colon are flushed daily to help maintain function of the caudal segment (this procedure is not essential). With the end colostomy this is not done. Broad-spectrum systemic antibiotics are continued for at least 5 postoperative days. The horse is also maintained on a laxative diet (fresh green grass is ideal), and the colostomy site is kept clean. With a loop colostomy it may be necessary to digitally remove feces from the proximal arm of the loop because there is a tendency for fecal material to impact during the first few postoperative days. This must be done carefully to avoid disrupting the mucocutaneous suture line. With both types of colostomy, the mucosal cuff will swell in the first few postoperative days (9) and some mucosal sloughing will occur. Periodic examination of the region of rectal damage will determine when the caudal segment is adequately healed. It is sometimes appropriate to digitally inspect the defect on a daily basis to prevent an abscess or to keep an abscess open. Generally in clinical cases, reanastomosis should be performed, if possible, by 14 days following the initial surgery. If the surgeon waits 30 days, problems with atrophy of the caudal segment of small colon will be experienced, particularly with an end colostomy. Abdominal wall infection or cellulitis around the colostomy stoma may necessitate a delay in performing the reanastomosis.

Reanastomosis of Small Colon

In the case of the end colostomy, if reanastomosis is performed 12 to 14 days after the colostomy, end-to-end anastomosis is feasible. The left flank laparotomy is repeated and the cranial portion of small colon is removed from the incision and the end transected. The oversewn stump of the caudal end is similarly transected, and an end-to-end anastomosis is performed using a simple continuous pattern in the mucosa followed by a continuous inverting Lembert pattern in the seromuscular layers (Fig. 7.11*J*). If reanastomosis is performed at a later time and atrophy of the caudal segment is significant, an end-to-side anastomosis is necessary.

If a loop colostomy has been performed, the temporary colostomy is separated from its attachment to the skin incision and body wall, a portion of the colon is resected, if necessary, and an end-to-end anastomosis is performed. The small colon is replaced in the abdomen and the laparotomy incision is then closed routinely in the appropriate layers.

In either case, the animal is maintained on a laxative diet after reanastomosis. Normal diet can be resumed gradually over the following 2 weeks.

Comments

Possible complications of colostomy include detachment of the small colon, prolapse, herniation, retraction, and stenosis (10, 16, 17). These can be obviated by good technique and positioning of the colostomy site in the ventral part of the flank. If reanastomosis can be accomplished within 2 weeks, some of the complications can be avoided. Unfortunately, most rectal tears require more than 14 days to heal.

REFERENCES

1. Sayegh AI, Adams SB, Peter AT, et al. Equine rectal tears: causes and management. Compend Con Edu October 1996:1131.
2. Guglick MA, MacAllister G, Ewing PJ, et al. Thrombosis resulting in rectal perforation in a horse. JAVMA 1996;209:1125–1127.
3. Arnold JS, Meagher DM. Management of rectal tears in the horse. J Equine Med Surg 1978;2:64.
4. Rick MC. Management of rectal tears. Vet Clin North Am Equine Pract 1989;5:415.
5. Spensley MS, Meagher DM, Hughes JP. Instrumentation to facilitate surgical repair of rectal tears in the horse: a preliminary report. Proceedings of the 31st Annual Convention of the AAEP, Toronto, Ontario, Canada, 1985:553–562.
6. Stewart RH, Robertson JT. Surgical stapling for repair of a rectal tear in a horse. JAVMA 1990;197:746.
7. Watkins JP, Taylor TS, Schumaker J, et al. Rectal tears in the horse: an analysis of 35 cases. Equine Vet J 1989;21:186.
8. Taylor TS, Watkins JP, Schumaker J. Temporary indwelling rectal liner for use in horses with rectal tears. JAVMA 1987;191:677.
9. Boles CL. Rectal tears and colostomies. American College of Veterinary Surgeons Annual Forum, 1984.

10. Herthel DJ. Colostomy in the mare. Proceedings of the 20th Annual Convention of the AAEP, 1974, Las Vegas, NV, 1975:187.
11. Spiers VC, Christie BA, Van Veenendaal JC. The management of rectal tears in horses. Aust Vet J 1980;56:313.
12. Stashak TS, Knight AP. Temporary diverting colostomy of the management of small colon tears in the horse: a case report. J Equine Med Surg 1978;2:196.
13. Azzie MAJ. Temporary colostomy in the management of rectal tumors in the horse. J Afr Vet Assoc 1975;46:121.
14. Shires M. The temporary loop colostomy—another choice. Proceedings of the Equine Colic Research Symposium. Georgia: University of Georgia, 1982:293.
15. Freeman DE, Richardson DW, Tulleners EP, et al. Loop colostomy for management of rectal tears and small-colon injuries in horses: 10 cases (1976–1989). JAVMA 1992; 200:1365–1371.
16. Blikslager AT, Bristol DG, Bowman KF, et al. Loop colostomy for treatment of grade-3 rectal tears in horses: seven cases (1983–1994). JAVMA 1995;207:1201–1205.
17. Brown M. Rectal tears. LA Pract 1982;4:185.

Inguinal Herniorrhaphy

Inguinal and scrotal hernias usually occur in two situations in the horse: in the adult stallion and in the young foal. As in most domestic animals, inguinal hernias in the horse are usually *indirect*, whereby viscera (usually jejunum or ileum) pass through the vaginal ring into the vaginal process or tunica vaginalis, which forms the hernial sac (1, 2). The adult stallion usually shows signs of colic as a result of the hernia shortly after breeding a mare or some other strenuous activity such as racing or jumping a fence (1–4). Such activities presumably result in stretching of the inguinal rings, as well as an increase in intra-abdominal pressure and the occurrence of the hernia (2, 3). Rectal examination of such a patient will reveal intestine descending into the ring, confirming the diagnosis. The testicle and scrotum on that side may feel enlarged and tense, although in the initial stages there may be no obvious scrotal swelling. This is why it is so important to perform a rectal examination on an intact male horse showing signs of colic (1). The hernia must be differentiated from torsion of the testicle and thrombosis of the testicular artery, which are rare (1). Occasionally, adult males will develop a reducible scrotal hernia that does not produce signs of colic.

Shortly after its occurrence, an inguinal hernia in a stallion sometimes can be manually reduced per rectum. This technique of reduction should be discouraged because of the risk of tearing the intestine or rectum and the chance of recurrence of the hernia. In addition, the entrapped bowel may have undergone irreversible morphologic changes requiring resection that will not be evident, clinically, for several days. Inguinal or scrotal hernia in the mature horse is therefore best thought of as a surgical emergency. The key to successful treatment is an early diagnosis (1, 5).

In the young colt, inguinal and scrotal hernias occur at birth or shortly thereafter. Descent of the testicle occurs at or near birth; thereafter, the relatively large ring begins to close and becomes relatively smaller. Many of these hernias in foals can be treated conservatively by manually reducing the hernia ("buying time" for the ring to become smaller). Many spontaneously reduce by 3 to 6 months of age (1). Conversely, surgery is indicated if the swelling suddenly enlarges, the skin of the inguinal area becomes edematous, manual reduction becomes impossible, or the foal begins to show signs of colic—an indication of incarceration of bowel and likely rupture of the parietal tunic (6, 7). In very large hernias in which the external inguinal ring is greater than 10 to 12 cm, spontaneous closure is unlikely and immediate elective surgery is indicated.

Anesthesia and Surgical Preparation

Attention must be given to the overall hydration and acid-base status of the stallion or colt before surgery. Broad-spectrum perioperative antibiotics are administered, as well as tetanus toxoid. If the animal has an acute intestinal obstruction, appropriate supportive treatment must be administered, including placement of a nasogastric tube to drain the stomach. Protracted cases of inguinal hernia will require intense monitoring and management while under general anesthesia.

The herniorrhaphy is done under general anesthesia with the patient in dorsal recumbency. The scrotal and inguinal areas usually require some clipping, although hair in this region is usually scant. The surgeon should always be prepared for a *supplementary midline or paramedian laparotomy incision.* The authors prefer the ventral midline approach, cranial to the prepuce and directed through the linea alba. Therefore, *both* the scrotal region and the ventral midline region should always be simultaneously prepared for sterile surgery in a routine manner. These regions are draped in anticipation of using both procedures so that the surgeon can use them without risking a break in aseptic technique.

Additional Instrumentation

Malleable or Balfour retractors may be used.

Surgical Technique

A straight incision (approximately 10 cm long in foals and 15 cm long in adults) is made directly over the external inguinal ring, in a location similar to what would be made with an inguinal approach to cryptorchidism (Fig. 7.12*A*). Larger hernias may require even longer incisions. In foals with a ruptured tunic, loops of intestine may be located quite superficially. The incision is made only through the skin, subcutaneous tissues, and fascia over the inguinal ring. A number of methods can be used for management of the hernia from this point. In the first method (only applicable for a nonincarcerated hernia in a foal), the common vaginal tunic is freed from surrounding tissues by blunt dissection (Fig. 7.12*B*). The contents of the hernia are then milked into the abdominal cavity while steady traction is exerted on the testis, tunics, and spermatic cord. The freed vaginal hernia is not incised. The entire structure is then twisted several times on its long axis, aiding in the passage of the herniated intestine into the peritoneal cavity. The spermatic cord is transfixed with a ligature just distal to the inguinal ring, using no. 1 or no. 2 synthetic absorbable suture material of the surgeon's choice, and then emasculated distal to the ligature. This technique resembles the method used to correct an inguinal hernia in a piglet (8). The superficial inguinal ring is then sutured with three or four preplaced simple interrupted sutures by the method outlined below. It is obviously important to see that all the intestine has been replaced into the abdominal cavity when using this method.

A variation of this technique is preferred by the authors for handling a reducible inguinal hernia in a horse of any age. The common vaginal tunic is bluntly separated from its surrounding fascial attachments down to the level of the external inguinal ring. Care must be taken not to tear the common vaginal tunic during this dissection, particularly in young foals. The cremaster muscle is bluntly separated from the common tunic at a level close to the external inguinal ring. The cremaster is then emasculated. After ensuring the hernia is reduced by stripping any contents back into the abdominal cavity, a transfixation ligature is placed across the spermatic cord as close to the inguinal ring as possible, and the cord is emasculated a safe distance below the ligature. The external inguinal ring can be closed or the inguinal canal can be packed with gauze to help prevent against the possibility of evisceration. This is practically impossible if the cord has been transfixed and emasculated properly.

In foals wherein the common vaginal tunic has ruptured allowing intestine to become localized subcutaneously, one must be extremely careful when incising the skin and bluntly separating the underlying fascia to avoid damage to the bowel or its mesentery. If the condition is treated soon after the tunic ruptures, the intestine is in good condition and a simple reduction is all that is required. Reducing a large herniation of small intestine can be difficult but requires patience because the young foal's bowel is easily traumatized and friable. If the condition has existed for a prolonged period of time, the serosa of the bowel may be inflamed and invested in a layer of fibrin. A resection and anastomosis should be considered because of the high susceptibility of such bowel to adhesions. Following reduction of the hernia, the external inguinal ring can be sutured closed with simple interrupted sutures of no. 1 synthetic

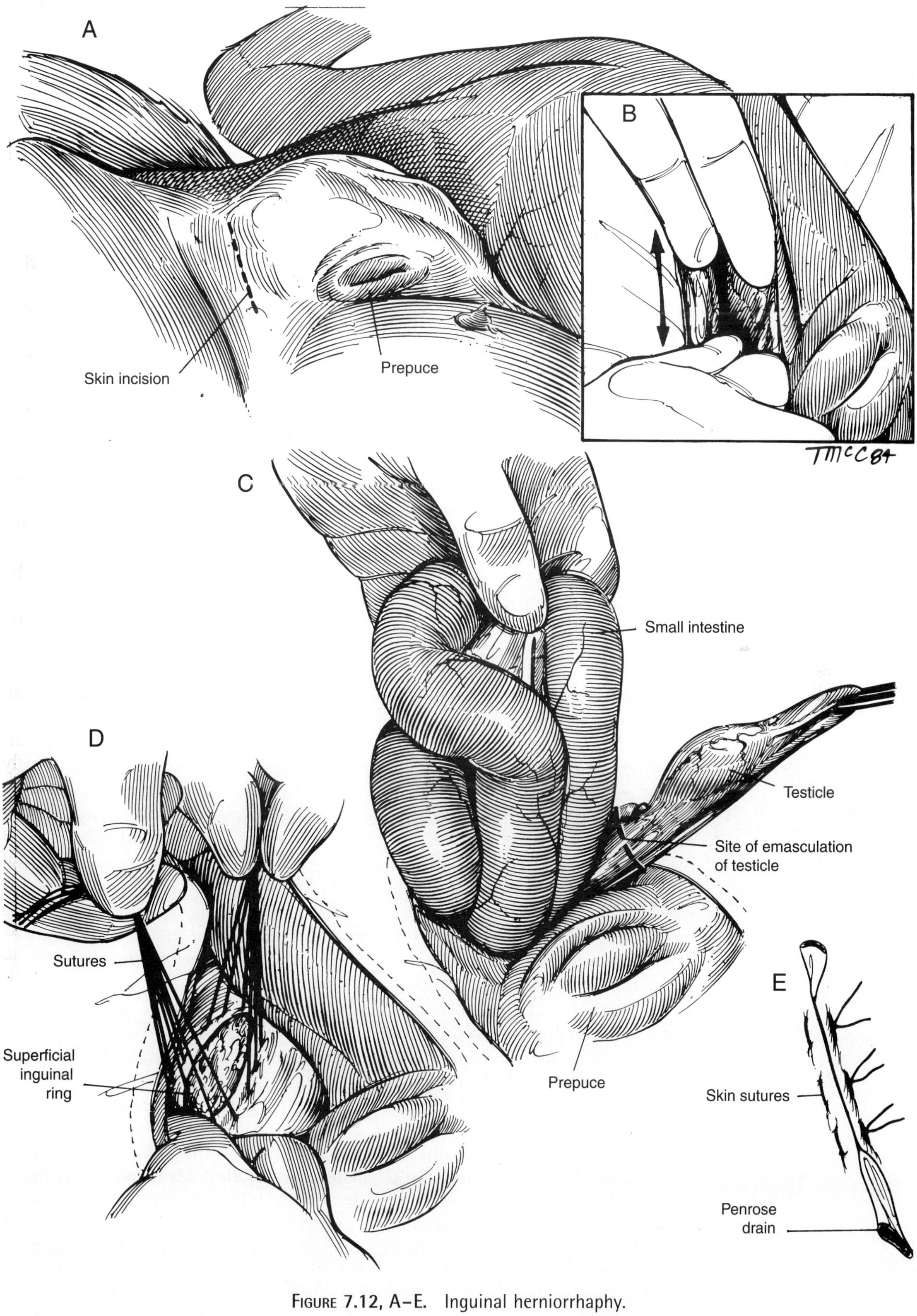

FIGURE 7.12, A–E. Inguinal herniorrhaphy.

absorbable suture material. The remaining inguinal dead space can then be packed with gauze to support the external inguinal ring closure, closed primarily with sutures, including the skin, or closed leaving a Penrose drain that exits through a small incision adjacent to the median raphe to provide ventral drainage. The anesthetic recovery should be assisted to prevent the foal from doing the splits and tearing the sutures in the ring.

An incarcerated and possibly strangulated inguinal hernia is approached with a 15-cm skin incision made through the skin and subcutaneous tissues directly over the external inguinal ring and extending over the neck of the scrotum. The common tunic is exposed by blunt dissection and carefully incised along its longitudinal axis to expose the underlying intestine (Fig. 7.12*C*). A small initial incision can be made with a scalpel, being careful not to incise the underlying intestine, and then extended using scissors. The bowel is exteriorized and inspected. If the surgeon is convinced that the bowel is viable (a difficult decision in some horses!), the bowel can be returned to the abdomen through the inguinal ring. If intestinal resection and anastomosis is necessary, it can be accomplished via the inguinal approach provided only the jejunum is involved. It is much easier, however, to reduce the hernia and exteriorize the affected bowel through a ventral midline incision. If the distal jejunum and ileum are involved and resection is required, it must be done through a ventral midline approach to accomplish a jejunocecostomy. Additional benefits of performing a ventral midline laparotomy in conjunction with the inguinal approach are that hernia reduction is facilitated by manual traction on the intestine from within the abdomen, and distended small intestine proximal to the obstruction can be decompressed. In one report of 24 operations, 14 patients required a ventral midline laparotomy in addition to the inguinal approach (1).

It may be impossible to mobilize the incarcerated bowel unless the common tunic is opened almost up to the level of the vaginal ring. This can be accomplished with scissors and with a finger inside the vaginal cavity to guide the ends of the scissors as the incision is extended into the inguinal ring on the cranial aspect of the tunic. It is usually not necessary to incise the vaginal ring per se, although many authors describe incision of the vaginal ring (5; Huskamp B, personal communication, 1996). When the constricting tissue within the inguinal canal is incised, it will become apparent because the surgeon's finger(s) will slip freely into the abdominal cavity. The hernia can then be reduced or the bowel exteriorized at this point. If a ventral midline incision has been made, the surgeon can pass an arm into the abdominal cavity and reduce the hernia by pulling from within and pushing the bowel into the abdomen from the inguinal side. Decompression at several sites with the aid of suction and an 18-gauge needle may be necessary. Once the hernia is reduced, the affected intestine can then be exteriorized through the ventral midline incision for further assessment or for resection and anastomosis.

The testicle and common vaginal tunic are dissected free, and the cord is transfixed and emasculated distal to the ligature and removed.

Following reduction of the hernia, the superficial (external) inguinal ring is closed. The superficial inguinal ring is a slit in the aponeurosis of the external abdominal oblique muscle. Its medial border is usually well-defined and easily identified. Its lateral border is made up of dense fascia on the medial side of the thigh. Anywhere from three to seven preplaced simple interrupted sutures are used to close the ring (Fig. 7.12*D*). The suture material is usually a synthetic absorbable material of the surgeon's choice and USP no. 2 (metric no. 5) in size. Care is taken to avoid the external pudendal artery and vein. Slight adduction of the limb as the sutures are tied reduces the distances between the edges of the ring and facilitates closure.

In the foal, a layer of inguinal fascia is usually available and should be sutured over the external inguinal ring to provide further strength to the closure. A Penrose drain can be placed in the wound but must exit through a small incision made in the scrotum, adjacent to the median raphe (Fig. 7.12*E*). This ensures ventral drainage. The skin can be partially closed to facilitate rapid healing. The sutures in the skin should not be tied too tightly because swelling rapidly ensues, making removal difficult. The ends of the skin sutures should be long to facilitate their retrieval at the time of removal.

In the mature stallion, the authors prefer to pack the subcutaneous area with a length of sterile cotton gauze. This is used in lieu of a Penrose drain. The gauze should not be forced down the inguinal canal but merely placed in the subcutaneous space in an accordion-like fashion, and brought out through an incision made in the scrotum, adjacent and parallel to the medial raphe. The subcutaneous tissue of the inguinal incision is closed with a simple continuous layer of size 0 synthetic absorbable suture material. Using no. 0 polypropylene, three or four large mattress sutures are used to close the skin of the scrotum. A small length of gauze is left to protrude from the scrotal incision and is incorporated in one of the skin sutures. The ends of the skin sutures are left long to facilitate removal.

The inguinal canal on the opposite side should always be checked for size, and the cord should be transfixed above the level of emasculation if bilateral castration is requested. The inguinal canal can then be packed to help prevent evisceration. The inguinal packing is removed in 48 hours through the scrotal incisions.

Most stallions will continue to breed satisfactorily following removal of one testicle, provided the remaining testicle is normal. Occasionally, the surgeon will be faced with a request to preserve the testicle on the herniated side. Any owner making such a request must be informed of the risks of such a decision, which include reherniation, strangulation of bowel, avascular necrosis of the testicle, infection at the surgical site, chronic orchitis, etc. If the testicle is considered viable, albeit edematous, and salvage is desired, the surgeon should make every effort to preserve the integrity of the common vaginal tunic. Once the hernia is reduced, a purse string, imbricating type of suture can be carefully placed circumferentially around the tunic as close to the vaginal ring as possible. The surgeon places an index finger into the lumen of the tunic through the incision. With this finger in place, the surgeon can place the purse string suture taking 3 to 4 small bites through the tunic, avoiding the structures of the spermatic cord within the tunic. A size 1 absorbable synthetic suture material on a taper needle is used and, once the suture is placed, the first throw is made and tightened. It must be tightened enough to prevent reherniation but not so tight that the blood supply to the testicle is compromised. The tightness can be digitally assessed from within the tunic. The suture is then tied. The common vaginal tunic is closed with a simple continuous layer of 2/0 synthetic absorbable suture material. The external inguinal ring is then closed around the cord and the subcutaneous tissues and skin are closed.

If a ventral midline incision has been used, it should be closed using a synthetic absorbable suture material of the surgeon's choice and of the appropriate size. The subcutaneous fascia and skin of this wound should also be closed.

Postoperative Management

Immediately following surgery, while the horse is under anesthesia, horses that are large enough to permit rectal examination can be examined to assure that there has been complete reduction of the hernia. This examination can be repeated after recovery, if the surgeon is concerned. A violent recovery from anesthesia can potentially disrupt the sutures in the external inguinal ring.

Attention must be paid to the fluid, electrolyte, and acid-base balance of the horse. Careful postoperative monitoring in those critical cases is essential for a successful outcome. Postoperative broad-spectrum antibiotics are recommended, especially if there was a break in aseptic technique or there was an intestinal anastomosis. The horse (or foal) should be confined for 3 to 4 weeks following surgery.

If a Penrose drain has been placed, it should be gently manipulated to encourage drainage. It should be removed 3 to 4 days after surgery. If gauze packing has been used, it is removed in 48 to 72 hours, depending on surgeon preference. It should not be removed unless a rectal examination reveals that the inguinal rings are free of bowel.

Following removal of the gauze or Penrose drain, the horse should be hand-walked to help minimize postoperative swelling. Hand-walking should be done twice daily and gradually increased as the animal becomes more comfortable. The normal playful physical activities of foals themselves will provide sufficient exercise to minimize swelling.

At no stage during the first 3 to 4 weeks after surgery should the animal be turned out with other horses. Excessive activity is likely to disrupt the suture line and lead to recurrence of the hernia.

REFERENCES

1. Schneider RK, Milne DW, Kohn CW. Acquired inguinal hernia in the horse: a review of 27 cases. JAVMA 1982;180:317.
2. Vasey JR. Simultaneous presence of a direct and indirect inguinal hernia in a stallion. Aust Vet J 1981;57:481.
3. Goetz TE, Boulton CH, Coffman JR. Inguinal and scrotal hernias in colts and stallions. Compend Con Edu Pract Vet 1981;3:272.
4. Vaughan JT. Surgery of the male equine reproductive system. In: Jennings P, ed. Textbook of Large Animal Surgery. Philadelphia: WB Saunders, 1984.
5. Van der Velden MA. Surgical treatment of acquired inguinal hernia in the horse: a review of 51 cases. Equine Vet J 1988;20:173–177.
6. Spurlock GH, Robertson JT. Congenital inguinal hernias associated with a rent in the common vaginal tunic in five foals. JAVMA 1988;193:1087–1088.
7. Van der Velden MA. Ruptured inguinal hernia in new-born foals: a review of 14 cases. Equine Vet J 1988;20:178–181.
8. Turner AS, McIlwraith CW. Inguinal herniorrhaphy in the piglet. In: Techniques in Large Animal Surgery. Philadelphia: Lea & Febiger, 1982:312.

Herniorrhaphy Using Synthetic Mesh and a Fascial Overlay

An abdominal hernia requiring a synthetic mesh is usually acquired and may be the result of previous abdominal surgery, an unusual case of a failed umbilical herniorrhaphy, or trauma to the lower flank area. In the authors' experience, incisional hernias are most likely to occur if a postoperative colic patient has abdominal distension and abdominal pain, if the laparotomy incision becomes infected, or if the horse is afflicted with a concurrent infection in another organ system (1, 2). A concurrent peritonitis resulting in a hypoproteinemia frequently produces "delayed" wound healing. Complications such as postoperative diarrhea (e.g, salmonellosis) or pneumonia may exacerbate weight loss and what is termed a "catabolic state" (3).

Because herniorrhaphy with mesh implantation can usually be done on an elective basis, the horse should be in the best physical condition possible, that is, an anabolic state before commencement of surgery. Horses that are thin and recovering from a protracted postoperative convalescence following intestinal surgery should receive the appropriate nutritional therapy before attempting surgery of this magnitude. Certainly, a horse that is coughing because of pneumonia would be a poor risk for mesh implantation because of the tension placed on the suture line during coughing episodes.

Candidates for herniorrhaphy with mesh implantation may have suture abscesses and fistulae as a result of previous surgery. Sepsis and edema at the surgical site *must* be attended to before mesh implantation. The surgeon should be prepared to remove offending suture material to resolve this condition in a separate operation. Ideally, a well-defined fibrous ring should be palpable. Frequently, the edges of the hernia are indistinct, and rather than being one continuous defect, there exists a series of smaller holes in the linea alba. An ultrasound examination of the region may give more information about tissue thickness.

Whether to repair the hernia routinely with a suture closure or to use a synthetic mesh is clearly a matter of surgical judgment. Incisional hernias may be referred for mesh implantation when it is feasible to close the defect with standard techniques. Sometimes in these situations, the authors advise that the abdominal wall be closed using a meticulously applied Mayo overlap (vest-over-pants) or a near-far–far-near suture pattern with heavy (e.g, no. 2) synthetic absorbable suture material. If the surgeon is absolutely confident that sepsis has been eliminated from the surgical site, then one of the braided synthetics may be used.

Anesthesia and Surgical Preparation

The herniorrhaphy must be done under as ideal facilities as available and under strict aseptic techniques. Because the procedure is time-consuming and tedious, general anesthesia using inhalation agents such as halothane is mandatory. Because of the long surgery time and the fact that the surgery involves implantation of a large foreign body that may potentiate infection, perioperative antibiotics are indicated. Even though the surgery is performed under aseptic conditions, tissue handling and its subsequent devitalization, as well as hemorrhage, are more than for most operations. This, combined with the prospect of having undetectable sepsis at the surgical site from previous surgery, indicates mandatory broad-spectrum antibiotic coverage.

Before induction of anesthesia, the ventral midline and hernial sac are clipped. Following anesthetic induction, the horse is placed in dorsal recumbency and any areas that were not clipped while the horse was standing are now attended to. The area is shaved and prepared for surgery in a routine manner. The method described was first applied to the horse by Scott and termed a "fascial overlay" technique (4).

Additional Instrumentation

Several synthetic meshes are available for herniorrhaphy in both people and domestic animals. Metallic meshes (e.g, tantalum and stainless steel) were used initially, but these tended to fragment and better alternatives now exist (3, 4). A frequently used material is knitted polypropylene mesh (Marlex Mesh #1266, Dowd Inc, Providence, RI). This mesh is easily handled, does not fragment with time, has low reactivity (inertness), and has a high tensile strength (3–5). It is also tolerated well in the face of infection (6). The cut edges resist fraying, and capillaries can grow through the mesh (3). Woven plastic (nylon) (Proxplast, Goshen Laboratory, Goshen, NY) mesh (used by the author) has the same desirable characteristics as polypropylene. Because it is woven and not knitted, there is less sagging, but it does fray when cut (3). Its main advantage is its cost relative to polypropylene, and for this reason it has become the implant of choice for some surgeons, especially in food animals where cost is a factor (3).

Also available to the surgeon should be an unlimited supply of a compatible suture material with an atraumatic noncutting needle (so as not to lacerate the mesh) to anchor the mesh to the body wall. The author prefers using a no. 5 braided synthetic material such as Ethibond (Ethicon, Somerville NJ) to anchor the mesh. A monofilament such as nylon or polypropylene can also be used.

Surgical Technique

Following draping, the extent of the hernia (including any smaller holes in the linea alba) is palpated. A semi-elliptical incision extending beyond the cranial and caudal margins of the hernia is made (Fig. 7.13*A*). The skin border is grasped with Allis tissue forceps or Backhaus towel clamps, and the skin flap and subcutaneous tissue are reflected to one side (Fig. 7.13*B*). Hemostasis should be attended to at this point. The hernial sac is incised carefully along the fascial margins of the hernia, except at the base, which is left attached (Fig. 7.13*B*). The hernial sac (fibrous sac and peritoneum) is then reflected toward its opposite attached base (Fig. 7.13*C*). It is essential that a peritoneal closure be accomplished before mesh placement; otherwise, intestinal adhesions to the mesh are likely to ensue. Even with very large ventral hernias, the peritoneum adhered to the hernial sac can be dissected free, undermined to relieve tension, and closed with a simple continuous line of 2/0 synthetic absorbable suture. The peritoneum is undermined around the margins of the hernial ring to expose approximately 4 to 5 cm of fascia, which allows for suture placement through the mesh and hernial ring.

A double layer of the synthetic mesh, trimmed to shape, is placed deep to the exposed fascial margin of the hernia but superficial to the retroperitoneal fat and closed peritoneum. The mesh is initially anchored on the side of the hernia that corresponds to the attached edge of the fascial flap. The mesh is anchored to this fascial border by simple interrupted mattress sutures. The sutures should be preplaced (using hemostats to secure the free ends) around half of the fascial border using nonabsorbable synthetic suture material. Each suture passes from exterior to interior, is looped longitudinally through the mesh, then exits from interior to exterior. The bites through the fascial ring should be placed at right angles to the edge of the hernia, and each suture should be 1 to 2 cm apart. The suture should enter the fascial ring approximately 3 to 4 cm from

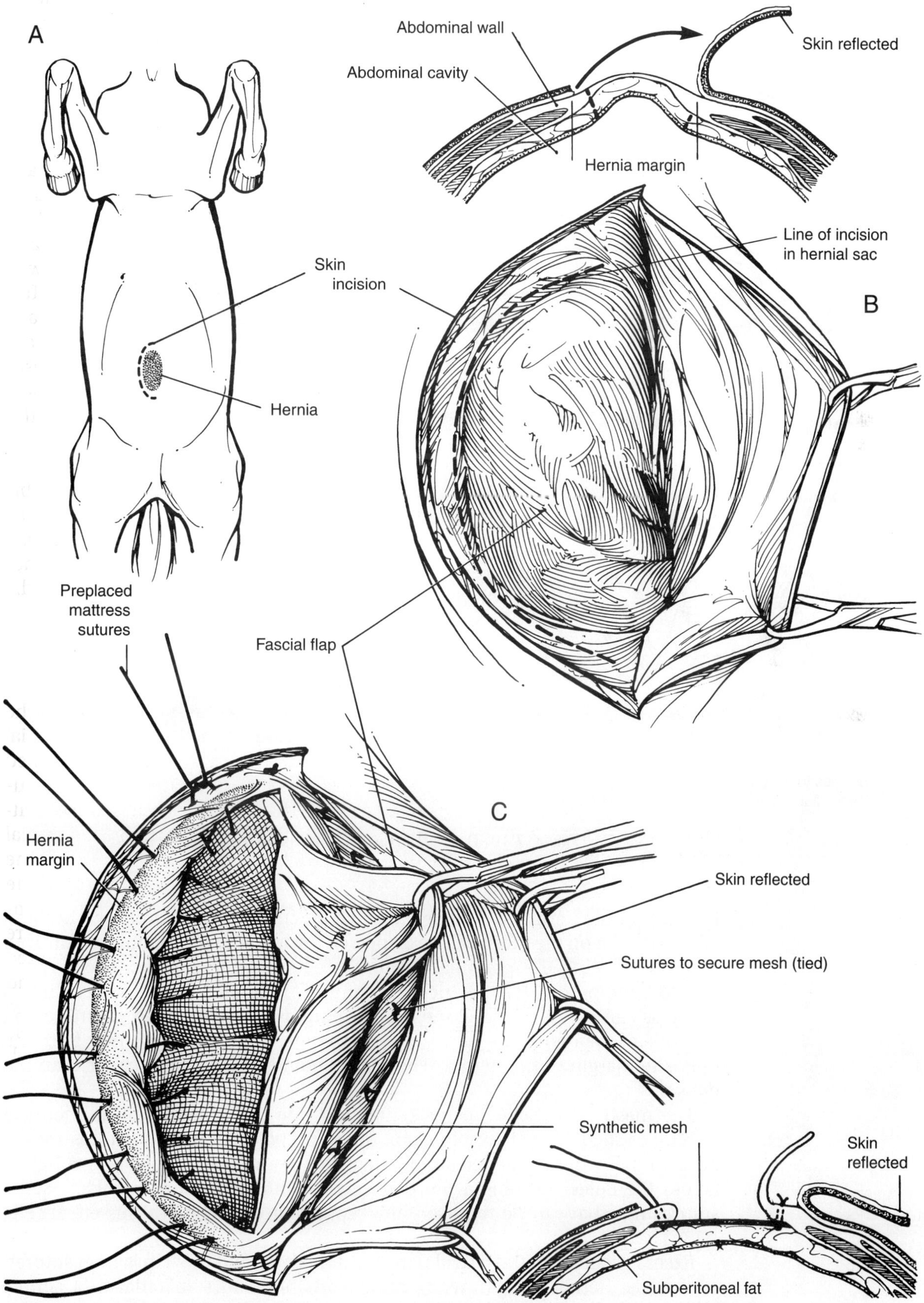

Figure 7.13, A–C. Herniorrhaphy using synthetic mesh.

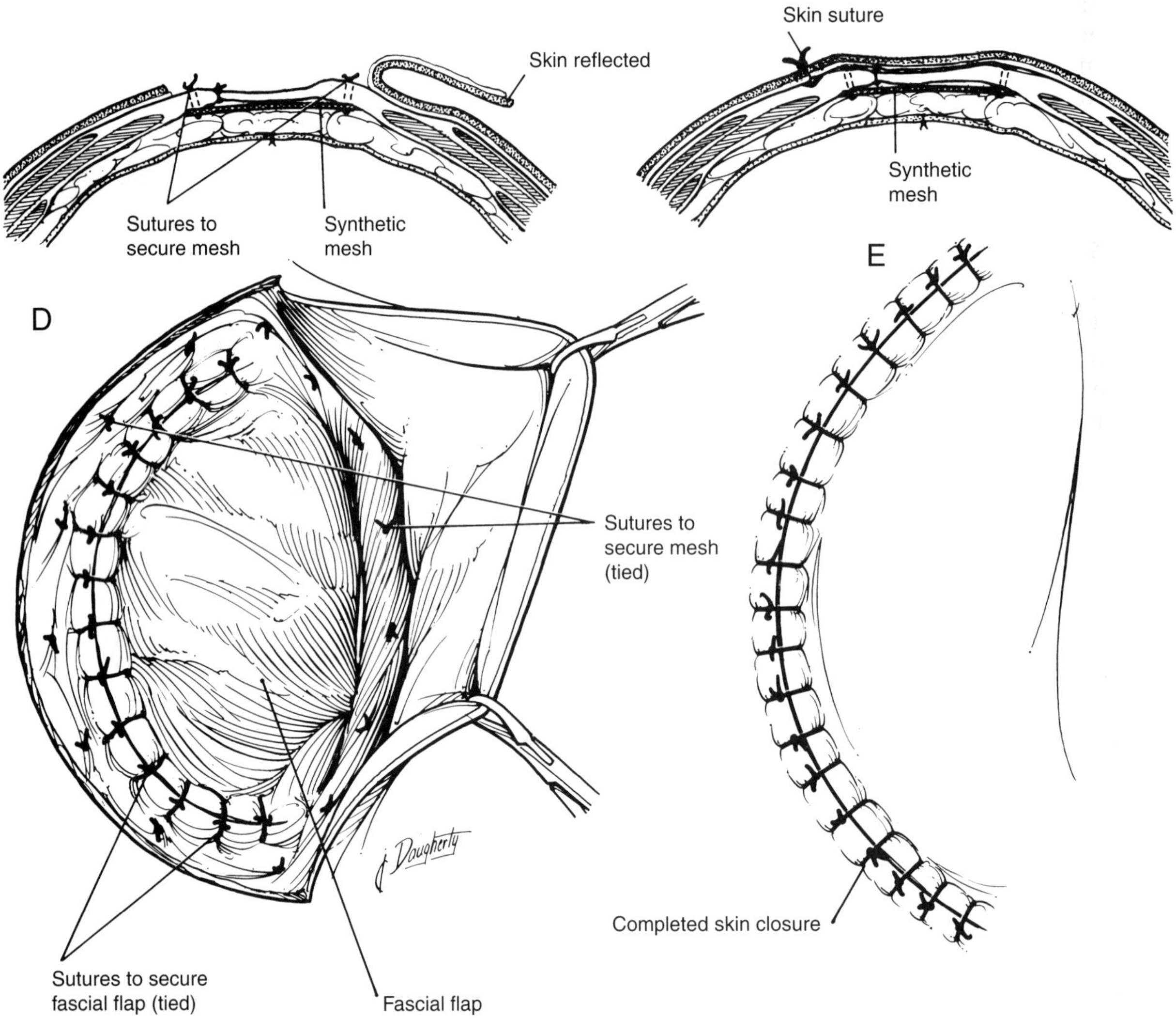

Figure 7.13, D–E. Herniorrhaphy using synthetic mesh.

the edge of the hernia and enter the mesh an equal distance from the hernia's edge. Tension on the mesh will be dispersed through the use of multiple sutures, thereby reducing the potential necrosing effect of the sutures. The surgeon should attempt to place the anchoring sutures in as dense and mature fibrous tissue as can be found along the hernia margins. The preplaced sutures along this side of the hernia are now tied, and the mesh is trimmed further to fit the opposite margin of the hernia. The mesh should be 2 to 3 cm larger than the defect.

The mesh is anchored in the remaining side of the hernia in an identical fashion as the first side. The location of the preplaced mattress sutures should be such that when tightened simultaneously the mesh should be drawn tightly across the defect forming a *flat* diaphragm, without folds or wrinkles. Some sutures may have to be removed and repositioned to achieve this effect (Fig. 7.13*C*).

Excess tissue from the fascial flap is trimmed off, and the flap is then sutured to the free hernia margin, using nonabsorbable suture material in a simple interrupted pattern (Fig. 7.13*D*). The mesh now lies deep to the fascial margins and is covered by the fascial tissues that once comprised the hernial sac. By keeping the hernial sac attached at one edge and suturing it over the implant, tension on the mesh is reduced and drainage of abdominal fluid and subsequent seroma formation are virtually eliminated.

Subcutaneous tissues are approximated with absorbable sutures in a simple continuous pattern. Any excess skin (found in the more pendulous hernias) is resected. The skin is either sutured with nonabsorbable monofilament suture in a simple interrupted pattern or apposed with stainless steel staples (Fig. 7.13*E*).

Postoperative Management

Antibiotics are continued for 3 to 5 days. Nonsteroidal anti-inflammatory drugs such as phenylbutazone can be administered for the first 2 days to reduce incisional pain and minimize swelling. We recommend a "belly bandage" or corset arrangement to help support the surgical repair. Another benefit of these devices is their ability to keep the surgical site free of dirt, straw, urine, and feces if the horse lies down. Another method of protection is to secure a stent bandage such as a folded hand towel over the incision.

Comments

The fascial overlay method has been previously described for use in the horse (4). It offers some obvious advantages to earlier methods that involved removal of the hernial sac. By preserving the flap and suturing it over the mesh, tension, drainage, and seroma formation are reduced (4). Equally as important, the technique provides a substantial additional layer of tissue between the implant and the external environment. This decreases the chances of infection gaining access to the mesh by way of the skin incision and establishing infection. Nevertheless, attention must still be paid to asepsis, gentle tissue handling, and hemostasis. We strongly advocate that all evidence of sepsis be controlled before mesh implantation. If monofilament suture materials are used, attention must be given to proper knotting techniques.

When the abdomen is entered, care must be taken to avoid incising bowel that may be adhered to the abdominal wall. This would result in inadvertent spillage of bowel contents, with a risk of fatal peritonitis. If this were to happen, the offending bowel should be repaired and extensive lavage of the abdomen performed. The mesh implantation would have to be abandoned until the horse has made a complete recovery.

After the horse is anesthetized and placed in dorsal recumbency, it may become evident that the hernia can be closed directly without having to use a fascial graft overlay. Mesh can still be used, however, to provide reinforcement for this closure (7). The mesh is used as a means to coapt the hernial margins and to absorb some of the tension across the suture line when the hernial edges are apposed. With this method, the entire hernial sac is resected. The peritoneum is closed and the mesh is placed in the retroperitoneal, subfascial space. The mesh is secured to the hernial ring on the near side with mattress sutures as previously described for the fascial graft overlay technique. Sutures are then preplaced along the far side in such a fashion that when these sutures are gathered together and simultaneously retracted toward the near side, the hernial margins are drawn into apposition. Each of these preplaced sutures are tied while tension is maintained on the untied sutures. The edges of the hernia ring are then sutured with no. 2 absorbable synthetic suture material in a vertical mattress or a near-far-far-near suture pattern. This technique of a reinforced direct repair should only be used in patients with a hernial ring that is less than 10 cm in width and where there is a thick fibrous hernial ring (7).

Other authors have reported using a double application of a mesh for herniorrhaphy (5). One layer is placed deep to the hernia ring, and the other is placed superficial to it. With this method it is technically more difficult to suture the meshes to the hernia margins, either independently or together. Also with this method, one of the mesh layers is much closer to the external environment, making infection a greater risk. In addition, it has been observed that adhesions of bowel to the mesh are more likely to form with the mesh placed intraperitoneally. Adhesions seem to occur more frequently when the mesh is placed on the abdominal floor in contrast to the use of the mesh for flank herniorrhaphy.

The use of synthetic meshes for hernias in other locations in horses is well established (3). Hernias of the flank of the horse are usually large, and primary apposition of the edges of the hernia is usually accompanied by excessive tension. With flank hernias in horses, the use of a neatly constructed fascial flap as described previously is impossible, as is reconstruction of the peritoneum. However, the principles of mesh implantation are the same. As much soft tissue as possible should be placed between the mesh and subcutaneous and skin layers to minimize the possibility of infection becoming established around the mesh. In many of these repairs in the flank or the caudal abdominal wall region, the mesh is exposed to the abdominal cavity because it is impossible to close the peritoneum. Subsequently, there is a greater likelihood of adhesions forming to the mesh.

It has been demonstrated in human surgery that synthetic meshes such as polypropylene tolerate infection well. They are sometimes used to provide a scaffolding for granulation tissue ingrowth in patients with massive abdominal wall defects (eg., extensive trauma with tissue loss or resection of malignant tumors). As the granulation tissue grows into the mesh, it cleans the mesh of bacteria even when there is gross purulence and allows the mesh to remain intact, instead of requiring removal (8). However, managing such a case of open granulation over mesh is much more difficult in the equine patient than in humans. The authors cannot overemphasize the need to avoid infection around the implant. If drainage and fistulation begin, several options are available. In some cases, drainage can be traced to one or two offending anchoring sutures that can be manually removed without necessitating removal of the entire implant. If the entire implant requires removal, the surgeon has no choice but to remove it and wait until the infection has resolved before implanting another mesh. All signs of drainage must be eliminated before a second surgical procedure is considered.

Adhesions and subsequent intestinal obstruction have been observed with mesh implantation in horses (3), although polypropylene mesh is as well-tolerated intraperitoneally as any material currently available. Adhesions are treated by laparotomy and intestinal resection as appropriate.

REFERENCES

1. Ingle-Feher JE, Baxter GM, Howard RD, et al. Bacterial culturing of ventral median celiotomies for prediction of postoperative incisional complications in horses. Vet Surg 1997;26:7–13.
2. Honnas CM, Cohen ND. Risk factors for wound infection following celiotomy in horses. JAVMA 1997;210:78–81.
3. Tulleners EP, Fretz PB. Prosthetic repair of large abdominal wall defects in horses and food animals. JAVMA 1983;182:258.
4. Scott EA. Repair of incisional hernias on the horse. JAVMA 1979;175:1203.
5. Hilbert BJ, Slatter DH, McDermott JD. Repair of a massive abdominal hernia in a horse using polypropylene mesh. Aust Vet J 1978;54:588.
6. McCarthy JD, Twiest MW. Intraperitoneal polypropylene mesh support of incisional herniorrhaphy. Am J Surg 1981;142:707.
7. Robertson JT. Abdominal closure in the equine acute abdomen. In: White NA, ed. The Equine Acute Abdomen. Philadelphia: Lea & Febiger, 1990:293–307.
8. Voyles CR, Richardson JD, Bland KI, et al. Emergency abdominal wall reconstruction with polypropylene mesh. Ann Surg 1981;194:219.

8

SURGERY OF THE UROGENITAL SYSTEM

Ovariectomy (Tumor Removal)

One or both ovaries have been removed in the mare for surgical correction of various ovarian conditions (1–4). The most frequent indication for removal of a pathologic ovary is a granulosa cell tumor. Other ovarian tumors (teratoma, cystadenoma, adenocarcinoma, dysgerminoma, arrhenoblastoma, and ovarian lymphosarcoma) occur in mares but are much less common (5). The surgical removal would be handled in the same fashion as discussed here for an ovary with a granulosa cell tumor. Less common indications for ovariectomy include ovarian abscess and hematoma, ovarian cysts, nymphomania, and prevention of estrus (4, 6). Bilateral ovariectomy is more commonly done to alter the mare physiologically than to remove a pathologic ovary. The prognosis following ovariectomy in cases of severe nymphomania is unpredictable because the problem may not be attributable to ovarian dysfunction (4). Despite bilateral ovariectomy, some mares will still continue to show behavioral estrus (7).

For the removal of normal-sized ovaries, many surgical approaches are available, including colpotomy (removal *per vaginam*); flank with the mare standing; or flank, ventral midline, paramedian, or diagonal paramedian with the animal under general anesthesia (6–9). The surgical situation of greatest clinical importance and the one that presents special problems and potential complications is removal of an enlarged tumorous ovary (granulosa cell tumor is usually the problem). This is the surgical technique that will be described.

The midline or paramedian approaches are the most versatile, not only for removal of a tumorous ovary but also for a bilateral ovariectomy. Although a tumorous ovary can be removed and transfixion ligation performed through a flank approach, exposure can be difficult with a severely enlarged ovary because of the limitations in size of the paralumbar fossa. In these situations, the ventral midline and the diagonal paramedian approaches provide improved access, and the size of the incision is flexible. They are also logical approaches when the ovarian size cannot be completely determined on rectal palpation (10). The technique using a ventral midline incision located just cranial to the mammary gland and the diagonal paramedian approach will be described.

Mares afflicted with a granulosa cell tumor of the ovary can have different clinical signs varying from anestrus, masculine or stallion-like behavior and continuous estrus, to asymptomatic, with the tumor being found on a routine rectal examination. The diagnosis of granulosa cell tumor is based on clinical signs, presence of an enlarged ovary that has no distinct ovulation fossa, and an ultrasonographic examination of the enlarged ovary per rectum. Usually the uninvolved ovary is suppressed in its activity and palpates as small and firm (2,

11). It is believed that the clinical signs can be related to abnormal hormone production within the ovary. The tumor fluid generally contains higher levels of progesterone and testosterone than of estrogen (11). However, there is no apparent correlation between the hormone levels and the mares' behavioral patterns. Concentrations of inhibin, a hormone produced in granulosa cells, are usually elevated and are an accurate indicator of the presence of a granulosa cell tumor (12).

Although removal of a granulosa cell tumor may be considered as an elective procedure, it is one that carries a number of potential complications that have been experienced by the authors and recognized by other surgeons (1, 2, 13). These complications are discussed later; the technique presented here is intended to minimize these potential complications as much as possible.

Anesthesia and Surgical Preparation

An ovariectomy is best done under inhalation anesthesia. Flunixin meglumine and broad-spectrum antibiotics are administered preoperatively. Hypotensive premedicants should be avoided with this operation because of concerns with low blood pressure and postoperative rhabdomyolysis and nerve paresis (2). During the surgical procedure, careful attention should be paid to direct arterial blood pressure monitoring, as well as other routine monitoring devices. The surgical site is prepared for aseptic surgery.

Surgical Technique

With a ventral midline approach, the skin and subcutaneous tissues are incised on the ventral midline, beginning immediately cranial to the mammary gland and extending a variable distance beyond the umbilicus depending on the size of the ovary (Fig 8.1*A*). The incision is continued through the linea alba and peritoneum in a routine fashion. Some mares have considerable subcutaneous

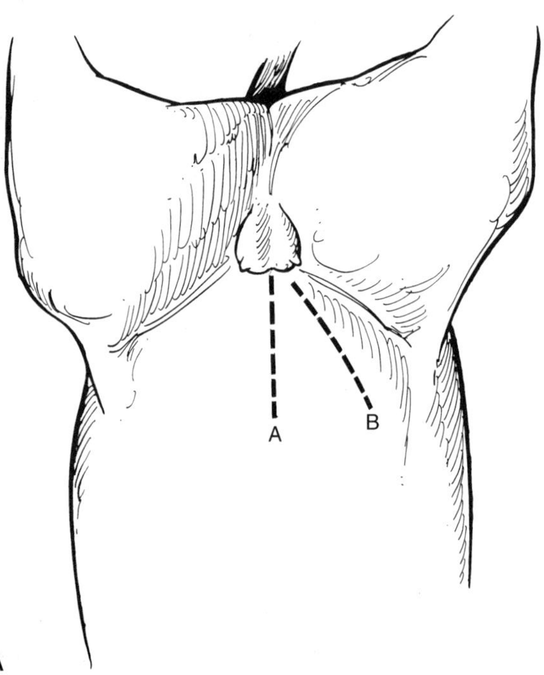

A

Figure 8.1, A. Ventral view of a mare with the ventral midline (*A*) and diagonal paramedian (*B*) incisions indicated by dotted lines.

fat immediately cranial to the mammary gland. The affected ovary is located and exteriorized as much as possible (Fig. 8.1*B*). Exteriorization can be difficult with a large ovary because of the short nature of the pedicle and the breadth of the attachments. If the ovary contains a large volume of fluid, the fluid can be removed by needle aspiration and suction to reduce its size. The fluid content of the ovary can usually be estimated during the preoperative ultrasound examination. Balfour or Finochietto retractors may be helpful with small ovaries but not with large ovaries whereby manual retraction and pressure on the body wall adjacent to the incision are necessary.

Before ligation of the ovary, 8 mL of 2% lidocaine is injected into the pedicle using a 20-gauge needle attached to an intravenous set. The pedicle is then relaxed for a few minutes before commencing ligation. This procedure is done in an attempt to minimize intraoperative as well as postoperative complications. Performing this technique in clinical cases may prevent the marked drop in blood pressure that can be associated with traction or ligation.

Transfixion ligation of segments of the pedicle is performed in the fashion illustrated in Figure 8.1*C*, using no. 1 or 2 synthetic absorbable suture material. These sutures are also overlapped so that no vessels escape ligation. All portions of the pedicle are ligated, and following ligation of a portion, the ovary can be severed from that portion of the pedicle. This maneuver can help provide increased exposure to the remaining pedicle, although once the ovary is removed there is a tendency for the pedicle to retract back into the abdomen. The extensive blood supply associated with pathologic ovaries provides the greatest surgical challenge with this technique. It is important to remember the effect of tension and relaxation when placing ligatures. A ligature that may seem to be secure and tight on a stretched pedicle may loosen and slip after release. Although tension is usually necessary for placement of the individual sutures, it is important to relax this tension on the pedicle when the knot is actually tied. Failure to do so probably accounts for the considerable postoperative hemorrhage experienced in some cases. The authors' experience with removal of a teratomatous ovary has been that fibrosis around the vessels can make effective ligation particularly difficult. When ligation is completed, the ovary is severed (Fig. 8.1*D*) and the stump is carefully evaluated for hemorrhage. Some authors consider that the cut edge should be oversewn at this stage to prevent adhesion formation (1, 5). The oversew can be done with an inverting suture pattern using no. 00 suture material.

An alternative technique for large tumors difficult to exteriorize is to use the TA-90 surgical stapling equipment with the largest available staples for ligation across the pedicle (14). Some surgeons routinely use stapling equipment for pedicle ligation. The use of this instrument is described in the section on gastrointestinal surgery.

After the ovary has been removed and carefully checked to ensure that no hemorrhage is occurring, the ventral midline incision is closed with interrupted or far-near, near-far sutures of no. 2 synthetic absorbable material in the linea alba or a simple continuous suture using no. 2 polyglycolic acid suture. A simple continuous suture of no. 0 synthetic absorbable material is used in the subcutaneous tissue, and the skin is closed with simple interrupted sutures or a continuous lock stitch. If surgical staples are used in the skin, they can be difficult to remove postoperatively.

The diagonal paramedian approach for ovarian tumor removal allows for good exteriorization of most granulosa cell tumors (8) (Fig. 8.1*A*). The advantages of this approach are that the incision is closer to the ovary than a ventral midline incision; there is minimal hemorrhage because the rectus abdominis muscle is separated longitudinally and not transected; and the body wall in this area is thin and flexible. The closure is secure and, although there can be considerable postoperative swelling, there is a relatively low rate of incisional complications.

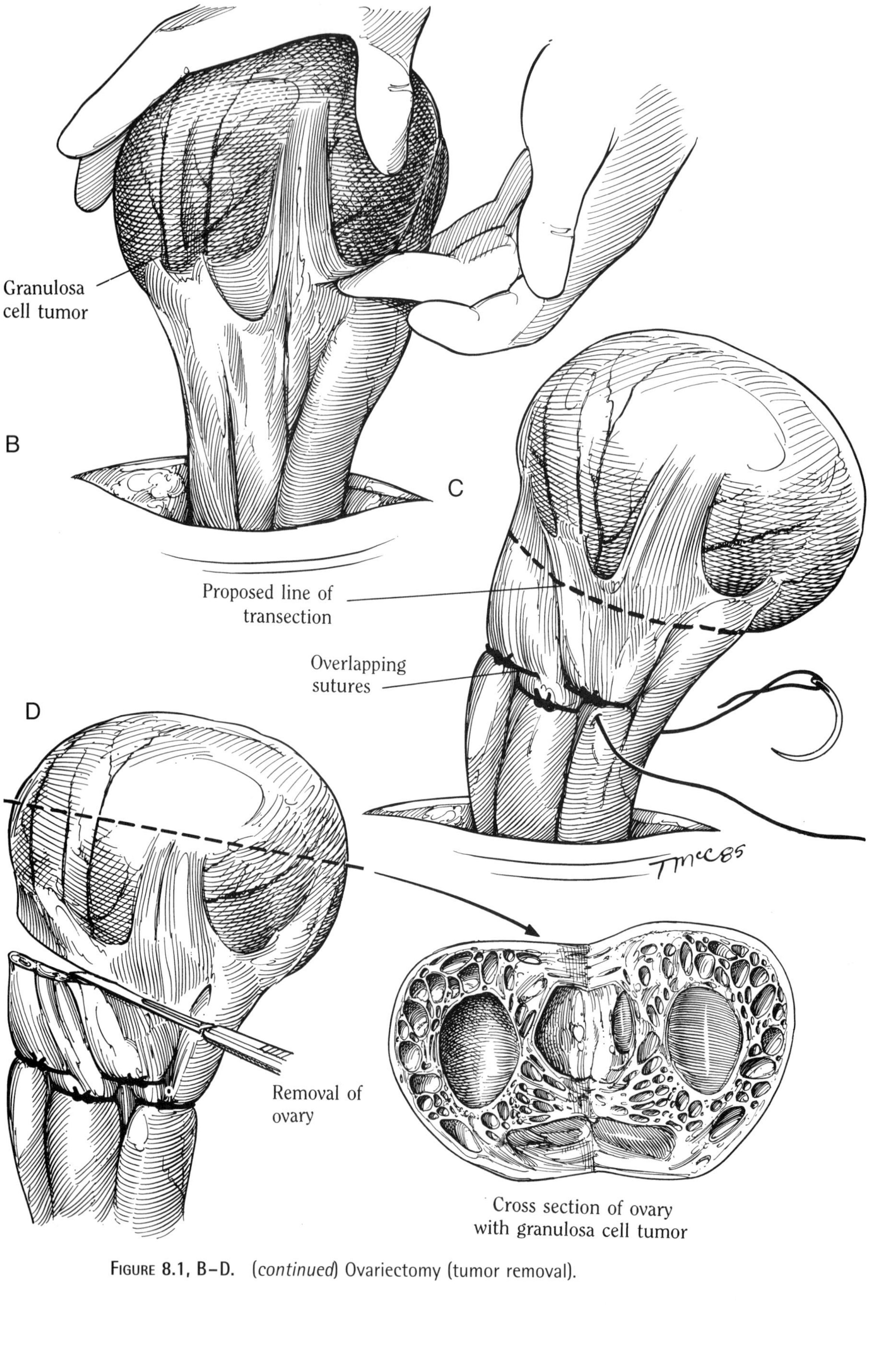

FIGURE 8.1, B–D. (*continued*) Ovariectomy (tumor removal).

The mare is placed in dorsal recumbency and a skin incision is made on a line between the cranial border of the ipsilateral mammary gland and the cranial end of the fold of the flank (8). The incision is started approximately 5 cm cranial to the mammary gland and extended for 20 cm or more toward the flank, depending on the anticipated needs for exposure. The cutaneous trunci muscle may be encountered as the incision approaches the flank. The incision is continued through the subcutaneous tissues and the cutaneous trunci muscle to the level of the external sheath of the rectus abdominis. The external sheath is incised sharply along the length of the incision, exposing the muscle fibers of the rectus abdominis. These fibers run nearly parallel to the line of the incision and can be bluntly separated. The internal sheath is incised as is the peritoneum. The ovary is then exteriorized and removed as previously described.

Closure of the diagonal paramedian incision following ovariectomy can be accomplished by apposing the peritoneum and internal rectus sheath with interrupted sutures of no. 0 synthetic absorbable suture material. The rectus muscle is apposed with no. 1 synthetic suture material in an interrupted pattern, and the external rectus sheath is closed with a simple interrupted or a simple continuous pattern using no. 2 synthetic absorbable suture material. The subcutaneous tissue is closed with a simple continuous layer of 2/0 synthetic absorbable suture, and the skin can be closed with a nonabsorbable suture material or closed with staples.

Postoperative Management and Complications

Postoperative antibiotics are administered by some surgeons. Intensive care, including fluid therapy and close monitoring, may be important depending on the status of the animal postoperatively. Ovariectomy is attended by various degrees of pain, and the routine use of an analgesic such as flunixin meglumine during the first 24 to 48 hours after surgery will enhance postsurgical recovery. Severe intractable abdominal pain is suggestive of a more serious problem. Ileus can develop in some of these patients and will require appropriate management. It has been suggested that very large hematomas of the right ovary or ovarian pedicle may place extramural pressure on the terminal ileum or proximal jejunum, interrupt the flow of ingesta, and produce signs of colic (13). The pain often seen in these cases may be associated with some degree of postoperative hemorrhage. Major hemorrhage requiring surgical reintervention should not occur. Formation of adhesions and hematoma around the pedicle are all potential developments that should be minimized by good technique. Manual massage per rectum to break down adhesions has been described (13) but is not usually necessary.

In one report of 78 cases, 19 mares experienced complications (2). These included formation of a seroma or hematoma at the incision site, superficial infection at the incision site, nerve paresis following recovery from anesthesia (including femoral, peroneal, or radial nerves), generalized rhabdomyolysis following recovery from anesthesia, postoperative shock, wound dehiscence, herniation, peritonitis, and postsurgical diarrhea. Six mares died in this study (2). It has been suggested that this high incidence of postanesthetic complications is related to a decrease in arterial pressure when tension is placed on the ovarian pedicle, but this has not been proven (1, 2). Any degree of peritonitis is generally localized to adhesions around the pedicle site.

Comments

Given that no immediate complications develop, ovariectomy is associated with a reasonably high percentage of mares resuming normal reproductive activity

(2, 10). In one report, regular estrus returned in 42 of 57 mares that were followed up, and the time from surgery to the return of the regular estrus cycle ranged from 2 to 16 months (2). In another report there was a 64% resumption of normal reproductive activity (10).

Laparoscopic ovariectomy has been described in both the standing and anesthetized mare. In one study of five mares, standing laparoscopic laser ovariectomy of normal ovaries resulted in good hemostasis, minimal postoperative pain, and rapid recovery (15). In another clinical report, two mares with granulosa cell tumors were anesthetized, placed in dorsal recumbency, and successfully ovariectomized using laparoscopic equipment. Those authors stated that granulosa cell tumors as large as 20 cm in diameter can be removed by laparoscopic ovariectomy (16).

REFERENCES

1. Colahan PT. Female urogenital surgery. In: Mansmann RA, McAllister ES, Pratt PW, eds. Equine Medicine and Surgery. 3rd ed. Santa Barbara, CA: American Veterinary Publications, 1982:1367.
2. Meagher DM, Wheat JD, Hughes JP, et al. Granulosa cell tumors of mares—a review of 78 cases. In: Proceedings of the 1977 Meeting of the American Association of Equine Practitioners, Vancouver, British Columbia, Canada, 1977:133.
3. Pearson H, Pinsent PJN, Denny HR, et al. The indications for equine laparotomy—analysis of 140 cases. Equine Vet J 1975;7:131.
4. Walker DF, Vaughan JT. Bovine and Equine Urogenital Surgery. Philadelphia: Lea & Febiger, 1980.
5. Pugh DG, Bowen JM. Equine ovarian tumors. Compend Cont Edu 1985;12:5710.
6. Trotter GW, Embertson RM. Surgical diseases of the cranial reproductive tract. In: Auer JA, ed. Equine Surgery. Philadelphia: WB Saunders, 1992:750.
7. Hooper RN, Taylor TS, Varner DD, et al. Effects of bilateral ovariectomy via colpotomy in mares: 23 cases (1984–1990). JAVMA 1993;203:1043–1046.
8. Moll HD, Slone DE, Juzwiak JS, et al. Diagonal-paramedian approach for removal of ovarian tumors in the mare. Vet Surg 1987;16:451–458.
9. Colbern GT, Reagan WJ. Ovariectomy by colpotomy in mares. Compend Cont Edu 1987;9:1035–1039.
10. Bosu WTK, Van Camp SC, Miller RB, et al. Ovarian disorders: clinical and morphological observations in 30 mares. Can Vet J 1982;23:6.
11. Stickle RL, Erb RE, Fessler JF, et al. Equine granulosa cell tumors. JAVMA 1975;167:148.
12. McCue PM. Equine granulosa cell tumor. In: Proceedings of the 38th Annual Convention of the AAEP, Orlando, FL, 1992:587–593.
13. Scott EA, Kunze DJ. Ovariectomy in the mare: presurgical, surgical and postsurgical considerations. Equine Med Surg 1977;1:5.
14. Doran R, Allen D, Gordon B. Use of stapling instruments to aid in the removal of ovarian tumors in mares. Equine Vet J 1988;20:37–40.
15. Palmer SE. Standing laparoscopic laser techniques for ovariectomy in five mares. JAVMA 1993;203:279–293.
16. Ragle CA, Southwood IL, Hopper SA, et al. Laparoscopic ovariectomy in two horses with granulosa cell tumors. JAVMA 1996;209:1121–1124.

Urethroplasty (Urethral Extension)

Urethroplasty is a surgical technique that provides caudal extension of the urethra. It is performed in mares that have retention of voided urine in the vaginal fornix (and consequent cervicitis and endometritis). These mares are generally barren multiparous mares, and the condition results from poor vaginal muscle tone and elongated ligamentous support, allowing the vagina to fall below the level of the pelvic floor (1–3). Sloping of the cranial pelvis ventrad, prominent ischiatic tuberosities, poor physical condition, a sunken perineum, and pneumovagina may be associated with the syndrome (1, 4).

Urethroplasty is designed to surgically create a mucosal shelf from the urethra to the mucocutaneous junction so that urine is voided to the exterior and not into the vestibule. It is an alternative technique to that previously developed by Monin (4), whereby the transverse fold over the external urethral orifice is used to provide a caudal extension. Monin's technique has been described in a previous textbook (5). The urethral extension techniques described here are considered to be preferred for urine pooling in the vagina. In one study, an extension technique was successful in 16 of 18 mares (1); in another study, 32 of 34 mares were successfully corrected with a modified urethral extension technique (1, 6). The correction of the problem should be attempted early, not late, since in prolonged cases permanent endometrial degeneration with persistent infertility can occur.

Anesthesia and Surgical Preparation

Before surgery, the mare's reproductive capability should be thoroughly evaluated by rectal and ultrasonographic examinations and by taking a uterine biopsy to help determine the extent of degenerative uterine changes that may have occurred (1, 6). A tranquilizer should be administered preoperatively. Tetanus toxoid should be given, as are perioperative broad-spectrum antibiotics.

Surgery is done with the mare standing and restrained in the stocks. Epidural anesthesia using 2% lidocaine hydrochloride, alone or in combination with xylazine, usually provides adequate anesthesia for the procedure (7). However, when previous epidural anesthesia has been given, supplemental local analgesia may be necessary. Fecal material in the rectum is manually evacuated, and the tail is wrapped and tied out of the way. The perineal area is prepared surgically and a no. 30 French Foley catheter (Rusch, Duluth, GA) is placed in the bladder to prevent urine contamination of the surgical field during the procedure (Fig. 8.2*A*). Retraction of the vulvar lips is provided by Balfour retractors or stay sutures in the vulva.

Surgical Technique

Urethral Extension as Reported by Brown, et al. (1)

The transverse fold overlying the external urethral orifice is grasped with thumb forceps, and the thin caudal edge of the fold is split into dorsal and ventral layers with a scalpel (Fig. 8.2*B*). This incision is continued caudad along the left and right ventrolateral walls of the vestibule to approximately 2 cm from the mucocutaneous junction of the vulvar labia. The mucosa along the incision is then undermined dorsad and ventrad to create two mucosal layers. This submucosal dissection is continued until the edges of the mucosal shelves can be readily apposed in the midline. The mucosal layers are then apposed right side to left side with three layers of suture.

The right ventral mucosal layer is apposed to the left ventral mucosal layer by a continuous horizontal mattress pattern of no. 2/0 nylon or polypropylene

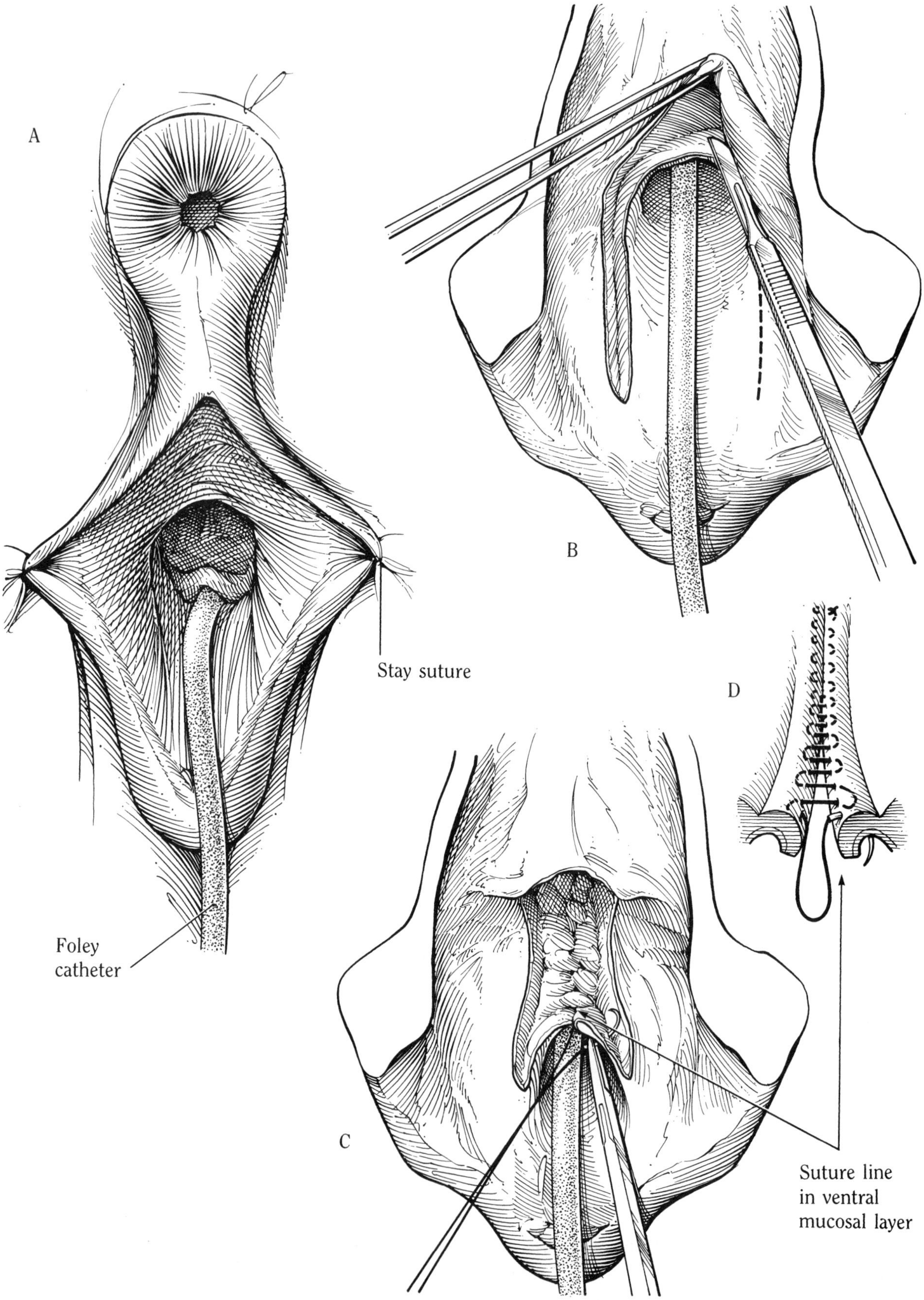

Figure 8.2, A–D. Urethroplasty.

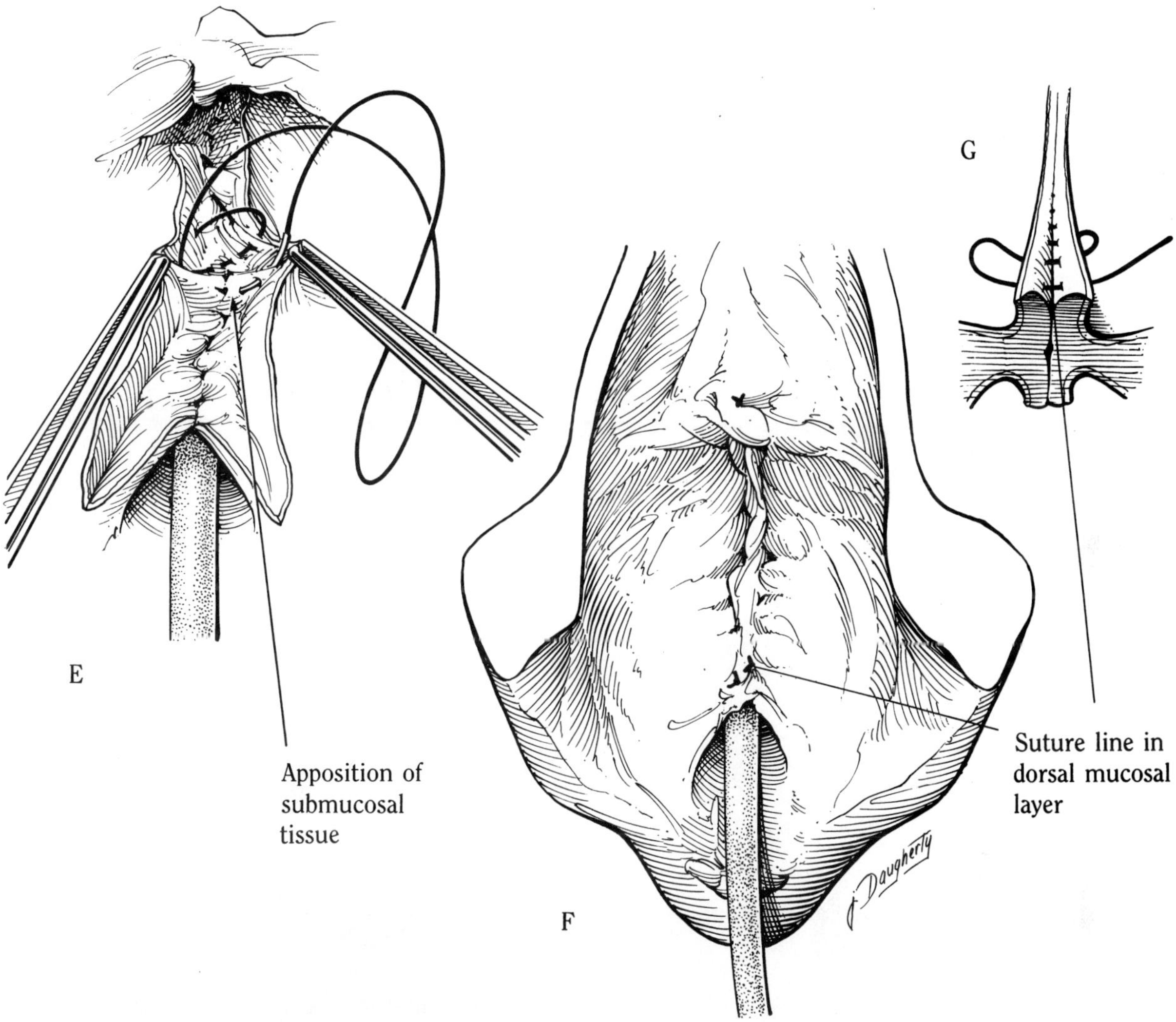

Figure 8.2, E–G. (*continued*) Urethroplasty.

(Prolene Ethicon, Somerville, NJ). The suture line is kept tight to ensure apposition throughout its entire length, and the mucosal surface is thus everted ventrad (Fig. 8.2, *C* and *D*). The submucosal tissue between the two mucosal shelves is then apposed, using a simple continuous suture pattern of no. 2/0 nylon polypropylene (Fig. 8.2*E*). (This suture line is optional and can be omitted.) The right dorsal mucosal shelf is then apposed to the left dorsal mucosal shelf with no. 2/0 nylon or polypropylene sutures in a continuous horizontal mattress pattern such that the mucosal surface is everted dorsad (Fig. 8.2, *F* and *G*). Synthetic absorbable monofilament suture material may be substituted in all layers.

The Foley catheter is removed after completion of the procedure.

Urethral Extension as Reported by McKinnon, et al. (6)

The caudal border of the transverse fold is grasped on midline with Allis tissue forceps and is retracted caudally. Using a no. 12 blade, the mucosa is incised transversely approximately 2 to 4 cm cranial from the caudal border of the transverse fold. This mucosal incision is extended laterally and slightly dorsally to the lateral border of the transverse fold. The incision is then continued caudally along the wall of the vagina with a no. 10 blade. This incision is made

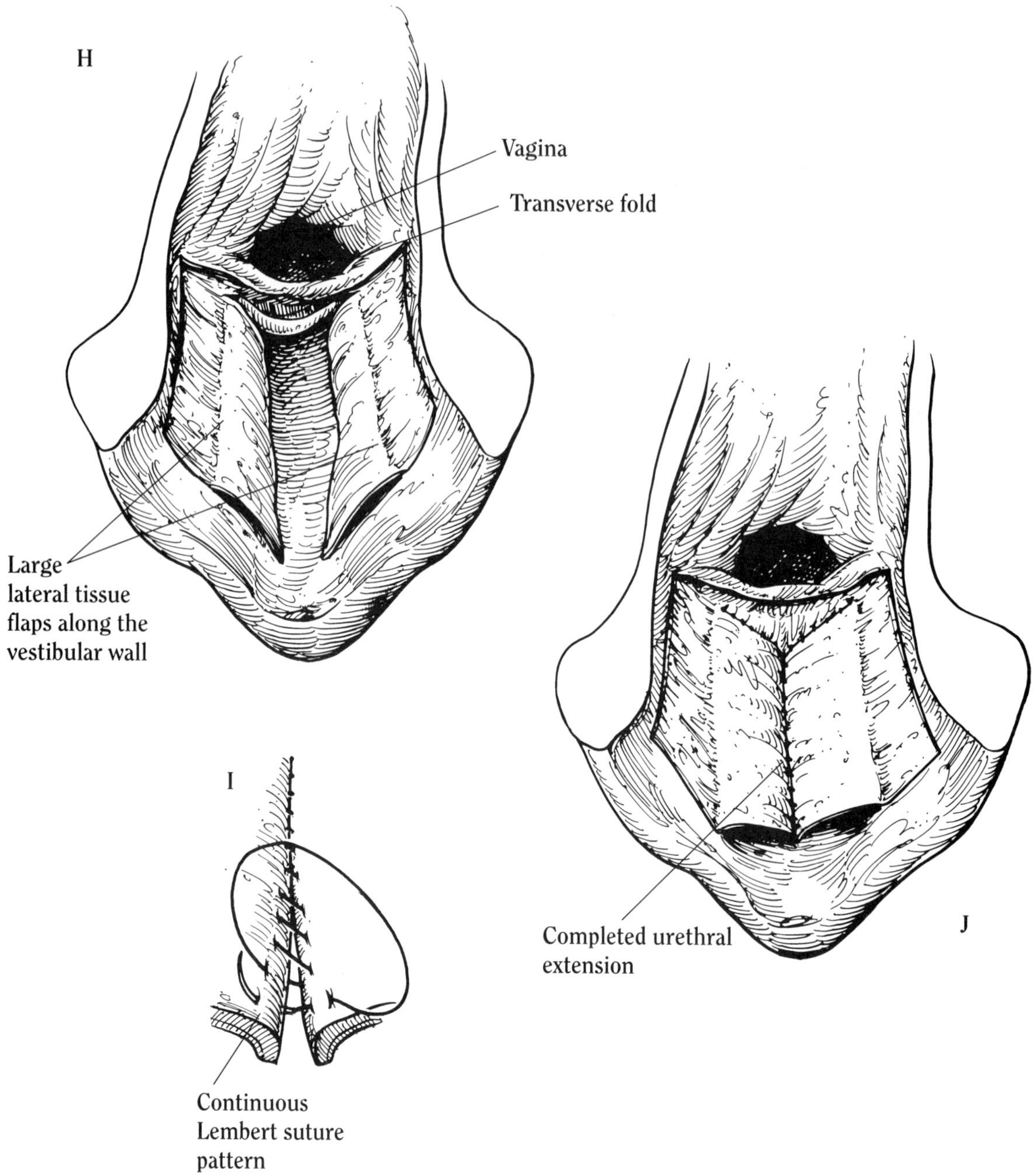

Figure 8.2, H–J. (*continued*) Modified urethroplasty. (Adapted from Trotter GW. Female reproductive system. In: Auer JA, ed. Equine Surgery. Philadelphia: WB Saunders, 1992.)

approximately one-half the distance between the vaginal floor and roof and is extended caudally to the vulvar labia. A similar incision is created on the opposite side. The mucosa over the transverse fold is freed enough to allow caudal retraction of that flap approximately 3 to 6 cm, and vaginal flaps are created that allow the cut edges to be reflected past midline without tension (Fig. 8.2*H*).

Using 2/0 synthetic absorbable suture, the submucosa at the lateral border of the transverse fold is apposed to submucosa of the rostral vaginal mucosa using a continuous, inverting (modified Connell or Lembert) suture line. The suture line starts laterally and ends at the middle of the transverse fold. The other side is sutured in a similar fashion producing a mucosal closure in a Y configuration. The vaginal flaps are then apposed with a similar suture pattern starting cranially at the juncture of the transverse fold and the vaginal mucosa and extending to the caudal end of the vaginal flaps (Fig. 8.2, *I* and *J*).

Postoperative Management

Anti-inflammatory medication may help minimize local irritation. Nonabsorbable sutures are not removed, but their retention has not been associated with adverse consequences.

Comments

In the initial report of the urethral extension technique, urine pooling was no longer observed in 16 (89%) of the 18 mares in which urethroplasty was performed. Failure in the remaining two cases was caused by formation of a fistula in the cranial extremity of the suture line. Of the 16 successful cases, 11 mares were known to have been rebred and 7 (64%) conceived (determined by rectal palpation or delivery of a live foal). In most mares, the mucosa and submucosa of the vaginal walls have sufficient elasticity and lend themselves well to surgical manipulation and satisfactory postoperative healing. When vaginal atrophy or scarring of the vaginal wall (because of advanced age, dystocia, or previously unsuccessful attempts at urethral extension) are present, these patients are poor candidates for the procedure. This was the situation in the two cases reported by Brown et al., in which fistulae had formed (both mares had had unsuccessful urethral extensions previously) (1).

The second submucosal suture line can be omitted (1). It has been suggested that it may be used when there is excessive tension on the suture line in an attempt to decrease the likelihood of fistula formation. Local anesthesia should be infiltrated into the vaginal wall only if absolutely necessary, as it can potentially delay healing. The polypropylene sutures were not removed in any of the mares reported by Brown et al., and no complications have been seen as a result (1). It is recommended that mares be bred by artificial insemination to prevent trauma to the urethral extension on insertion of the penis (1). However, mares have been bred naturally with no reported problems.

The modified urethral extension technique was used to correct urine pooling in 32 of 34 mares. This technique is easier to perform and requires less surgical time than the original technique. A more spacious urethral tunnel can be created, therefore the suture lines are under less stress. However, as with the original procedure, fistulae can still form, particularly at the Y juncture of the transverse fold and the reflections of the vaginal wall mucosa (6).

REFERENCES

1. Brown MP, Colahan PT, Hawkins DL. Urethral extension for treatment of urine pooling in mares. JAVMA 1978;173:1005.
2. Colahan PT. Female urogenital surgery. In: Mansmann RA, McAllister ES, Pratt PW, eds. Equine Medicine and Surgery. 3rd ed. Santa Barbara, CA: American Veterinary Publications, 1982:1367.
3. Vaughan JT. Equine urogenital system. In: Jennings PB, ed. The Practice of Large Animal Surgery. Philadelphia: WB Saunders, 1984:1122.
4. Monin T. Vaginoplasty: a surgical treatment for urine pooling in the mare. In: Proceedings of the 19th Meeting of the AAEP, San Francisco, CA, 1972:99–102.

5. Turner AS, McIlwraith CW. Techniques in Large Animal Surgery. Philadelphia: Lea & Febiger, 1989.
6. McKinnon AO, Belden JO. A urethral extension technique to correct urine pooling (vesiculovaginal reflux) in mares. JAVMA 1988;192:647–650.
7. Grubb TL, Riebold TW, Huber MJ. Comparison of lidocaine, xylazine, and xylazine/lidocaine for caudal epidural analgesia in horses. JAVMA 1992;201:1187–1190.

Episioplasty (Perineal Body Reconstruction)

Episioplasty is an extension of the concept of Caslick's operation and was initially introduced as a means of reducing the size of the vulva to prevent aspiration of air associated with ascending reproductive tract infections. The Caslick's technique has been described in a previous textbook (1).

Episioplasty provides a method of repairing compromised function of the constrictor muscles of the vulva and vestibule, which serve—together with the labia—as a defense against environmental contamination of the reproductive tract. The general situation is represented by a case of chronic pneumovagina in which no effective valvular action remains in the vestibule. This situation is in contrast to that in the normal mare, in which, after parting the labia (overriding the constrictor vulvae muscle), the constrictor vestibule muscle still provides closure of the vestibule. The vulvar and vestibular sphincters can become incompetent as a result of repeated stretching during foalings or second-degree lacerations (2, 3). The circular muscles that form the sphincters of the anus, vulva, and vestibule intersect in the perineal body, and any disruption in this region will cause loss of function.

Such advanced cases of pneumovagina are more of a problem of the aged than of the young animal. In some situations, sagging viscera (splanchnoptosis) associated with gradual stretching of the mesometrium and enlargement of the abdominal cavity also can be present. It may be necessary to perform urethroplasty (separately described) for vesicovaginal reflux of urine, along with the episioplasty (3). The technique described requires special dissection and reconstruction of the perineal body and ceiling of the vestibule as well as the dorsal commissure of the vulva.

Anesthesia and Surgical Preparation

The episioplasty is done on the standing animal restrained in stocks. Some degree of sedation is usually necessary (the combined use of xylazine and butorphanol has been useful). Tetanus toxoid and broad-spectrum antibiotics are administered before surgery. Epidural anesthesia using 2% lidocaine or a combination of 2% lidocaine and xylazine will provide analgesia to the level of the transverse fold over the external urethral orifice. If any additional anesthesia in the deeper tissues is required, local infiltration of the ischiorectal region can be performed. The tail is bandaged and tied out of the way, and the rectum is manually evacuated before surgery. The perineum and vulva are surgically prepared.

Surgical Technique

The labia are retracted using stay sutures in the vulva or long-jawed Balfour retractors. An incision is made along the mucocutaneous junction of the labia in a dorsoventral direction and extended craniad along the dorsal commissure of the vestibule to the vicinity of the vaginovestibular junction (approximately 15 cm craniad from the edge of the labium) (Fig. 8.3*A*). The lines of incision are best demonstrated on the sagittal view represented diagrammatically in Figure 8.3*B* and are in the shape of a triangle. This triangular section of mucosa is then dissected submucosally from the dorsum and dorsolateral aspect of the vestibule, and removed (Fig. 8.3*C*). Care is used in the submucosal dissection to ensure that the rectum is not penetrated. The incised edge of the mucosa of the right side of the vestibule is then sutured to the incised edge of the left side of the vestibule using a simple continuous pattern of no. 0 polydioxanone (PDS) (Fig. 8.3*D*). The raw triangular surface dorsal to this suture line is apposed with

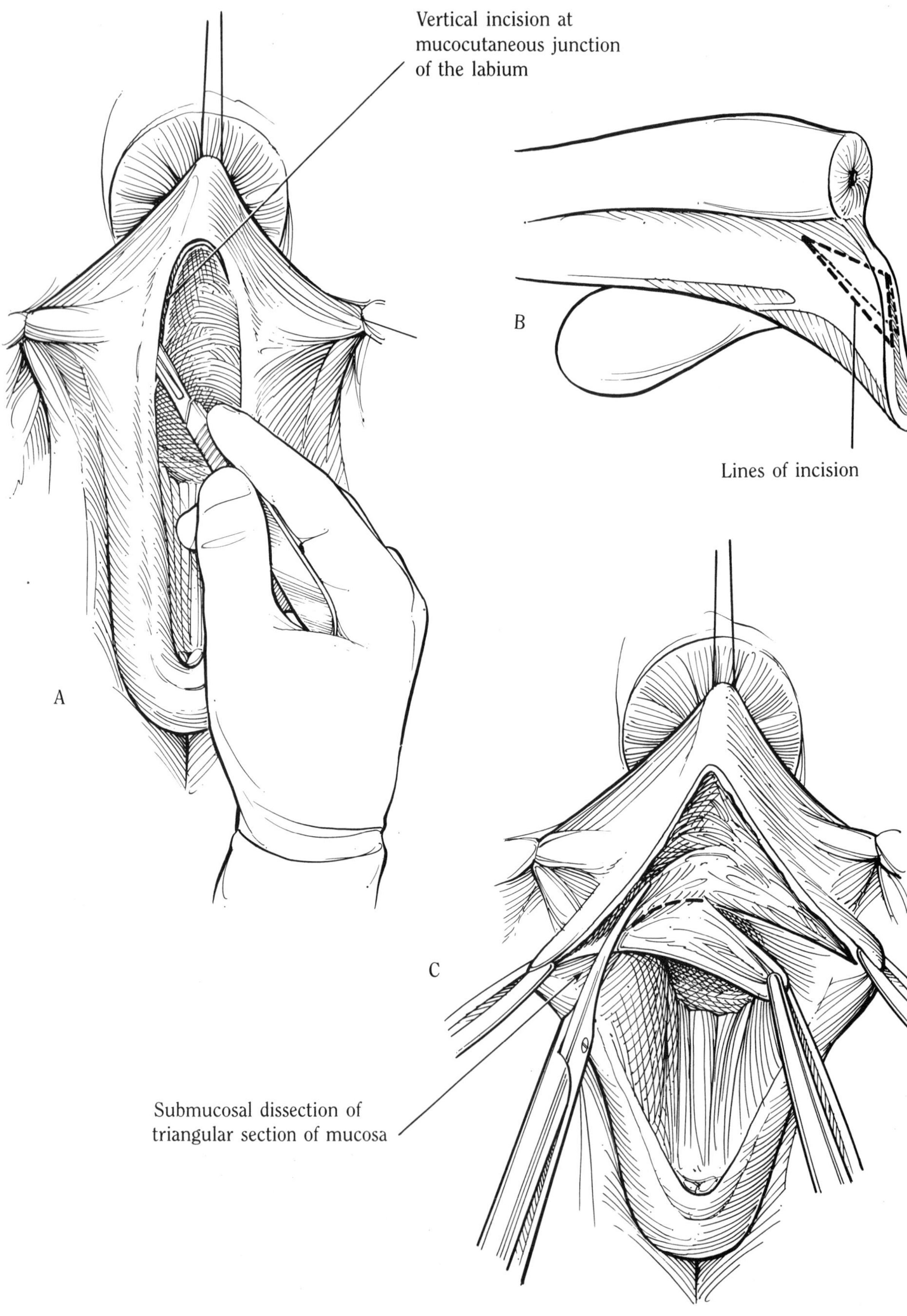

Figure 8.3, A–C. Episioplasty.

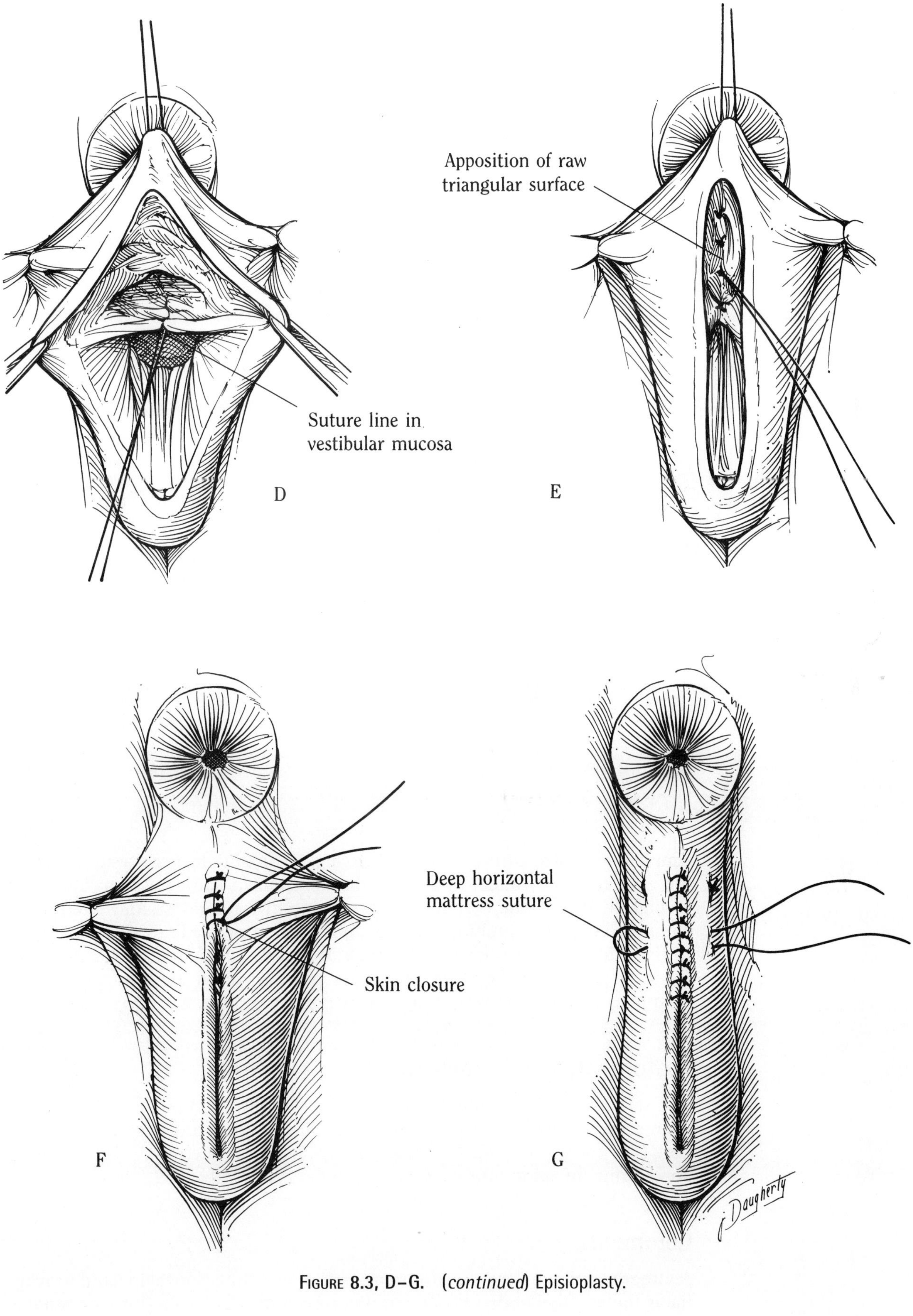

FIGURE 8.3, D–G. (*continued*) Episioplasty.

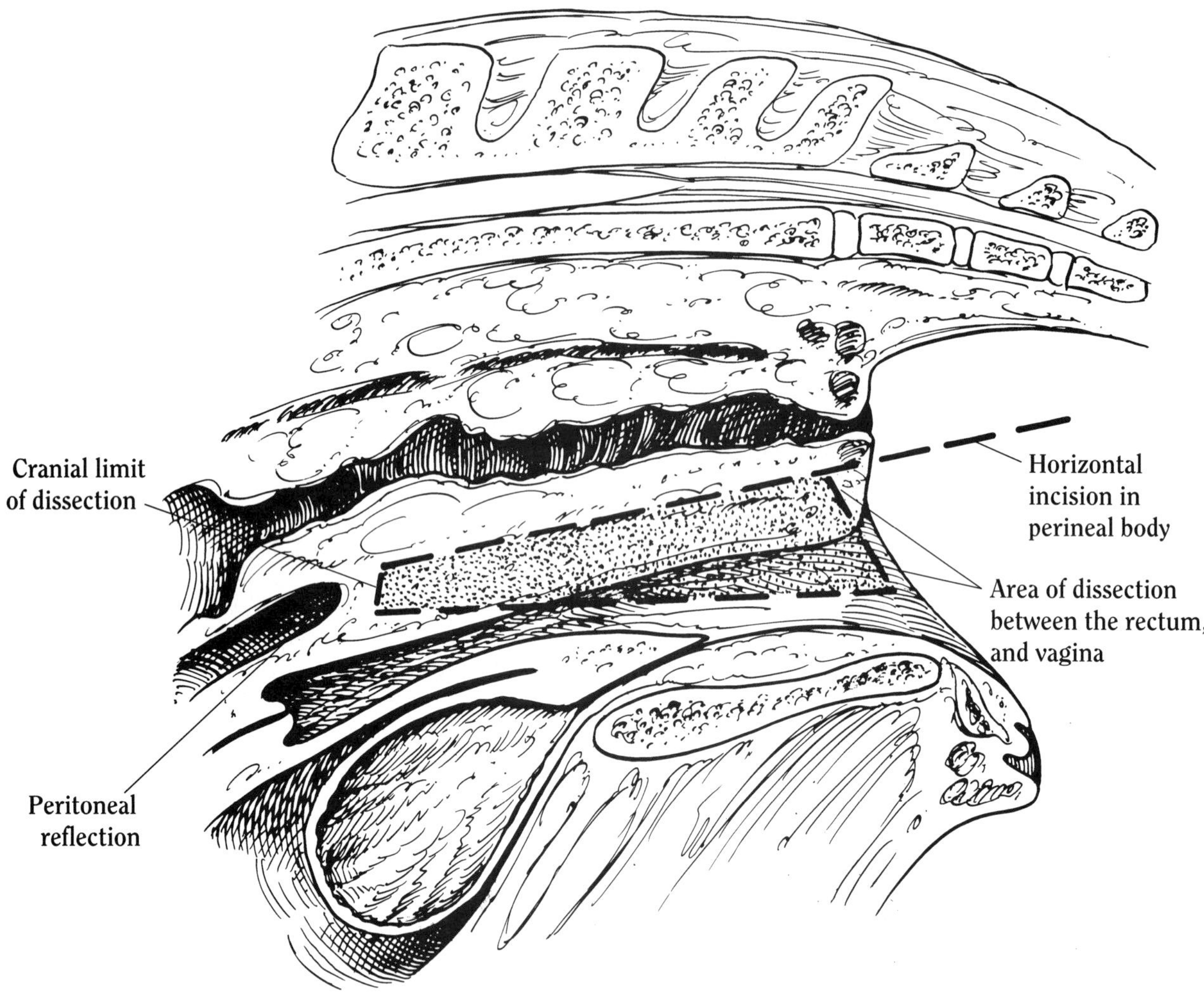

Figure 8.4. Pouret's procedure. (Adapted from Trotter GW. Female reproductive system. In: Auer JA, ed. Equine Surgery. Philadelphia: WB Saunders, 1992.)

simple interrupted sutures of no. 0 PDS (Fig. 8.3*E*). Both layers are sutured from the cranial to the caudal aspects of the incision. In some cases having deep cranial dissection, the continuous suture line in the mucosa may need to be alternated with the "quilting" sutures above. These suture lines are brought out to the skin, and the skin of the perineum and vulva is then closed as in the Caslick's procedure (Fig. 8.3*F*). Some deeper horizontal mattress sutures are then placed across the reconstructed perineal body (Fig. 8.3*G*).

Postoperative Management

The skin sutures are removed at 10 to 12 days, but complete healing of the deeper tissues will take 4 to 8 weeks. Complete sexual rest is essential at this time (1). Any return to natural breeding will also be related to the resolution of any uterine infection (4).

Comments

Another technique described for treatment of both pneumovagina and urovagina is the perineal body transection (Pouret's procedure) (5). This technique is recommended for mares with poor perineal conformation in which the anus is sunken and the vulva is sloped forward (5, 6). This procedure may be more beneficial for correcting pneumovagina than urovagina (6). An advantage of this technique is that the vulvular and vestibular openings are not constricted as a result of surgery.

The principle of the surgery is to separate the muscular and ligamentous attachments between the rectum and the caudal vagina, thereby allowing the vulva to assume a more vertical position (6). The surgical approach is similar to that described for the dissection required for repair of a rectovaginal fistula (7). The surgery is done with the mare standing in stocks and with epidural anesthesia. The skin and perineal body are incised horizontally midway between the anus and dorsal commissure of the vulva. Laterally, the incision is continued ventrally 3 to 4 cm on each side of the lips of the vulva. The horizontal component of the dissection is extended up to 14 cm cranially or as far as is necessary to free the caudal vagina (6). It is necessary to use a scalpel to incise through the perineal body, but, cranial to the perineal body, long-handled Metzenbaum scissors are used to separate between the rectum and vagina. A hand can be placed in the vagina to ensure that the horizontal plane of dissection is maintained and neither the rectum nor the vagina are perforated. The dissection should not extend so far forward that it perforates the peritoneal reflection (Fig. 8.41).

It has been recommended that no skin closure be performed and that the entire wound be allowed to heal by second intention. It is also recommended that the feces be soft following surgery because some of these mares find it painful to defecate and may become constipated.

REFERENCES

1. Turner AS, McIlwraith CW. Techniques in Large Animal Surgery. Philadelphia: Lea & Febiger, 1989.
2. Colahan PT. Female urogenital surgery. In: Mansmann RA, McAllister ES, Pratt PW, eds. Equine Medicine and Surgery. Santa Barbara, CA: American Veterinary Publications, 1982:1367–1384.
3. Vaughan JT. Equine urogenital system. In: Jennings PB, ed. The Practice of Large Animal Surgery. Philadelphia: WB Saunders, 1984:1122–1150.
4. Gadd JD. The relationship of bacterial cultures, microscopic smear examination and medical treatment to surgical correction of barren mares. In: Proceedings of the 21st Meeting of the AAEP, Boston, MA, 1975:362–368.
5. Pouret EJM. Surgical technique for the correction of pneumo- and urovagina. Equine Vet J 1982;14:249.
6. Trotter GW, McKinnon AO. Surgery for abnormal vulvar and perineal conformation in the mare. Vet Clin North Am Equine Pract 1988;4:389.
7. Embertson RM, Robertson JT. Parturient perineal and rectovestibular injuries. In: Robinson NE, ed. Current Therapy in Equine Medicine. 2nd ed. Philadelphia: WB Saunders, 1987:550–555.

Repair of Third-Degree Perineal Laceration

Perineal lacerations in the mare occur during parturition, when the foal's limb(s) or head is forced caudad and dorsad. The injury is seen predominantly in primiparous mares and is usually caused by violent expulsive efforts by the mare in combination with some degree of malposition of the fetus. The injury is also seen following forced extraction of a large fetus or extraction before full dilatation of the birth canal (1). First-degree lacerations occur when only the mucosa of the vestibule and vulva is involved. Second-degree lacerations occur when the submucosa and the muscularis of the vulva, anal sphincter, and perineal body are involved, but there is no damage to the rectal mucosa. Third-degree perineal lacerations occur when there is tearing through the rectovestibular septum, musculature of the rectum and vestibule, and the perineal body (Fig. 8.5*A*) (2). Most tears are situated caudal to the vestibular sphincter (level of the transverse fold) and therefore should be classified as rectovestibular tears and not as rectovaginal tears. Occasionally, severe tears will involve the caudal vagina as well as the vestibule. Because the vestibular sphincter is usually intact, most mares have little fecal contamination of the cranial vagina. However, reconstruction of third-degree perineal lacerations is necessary to return the mare to breeding soundness. The communication between the rectum and vestibule results in the constant presence of fecal material in the vestibule. Reconstruction is done occasionally in riding horses to eliminate the unpleasant sound made by air aspirated into the vestibule.

Generally, surgery is not done on an emergency basis. On discovery of the injury, tetanus immunization should be administered. Some cases may require a course of antibiotics. The torn tissues are edematous, necrotic, and grossly contaminated, and it is advisable to wait a minimum of 8 weeks before attempting repair. Repairs attempted earlier than this are unsuccessful. While waiting for repair, the mare should remain under close observation. The excessive straining caused by the injury can lead to prolapse of the viscera, including eversion of the urinary bladder (3).

The cervix should also be examined for lacerations before repair because lacerations of the cervix result in a poor prognosis for return to breeding soundness. Mares with lacerations of the cervix are more susceptible to endometritis and early abortion (2).

The Aanes' technique, as described in a previous text, was performed in two stages. In the first operation, a rectovestibular shelf is constructed; the second operation involves reconstruction of the perineal body (1, 2, 4). The aim of two-stage repair is reduction of the incidence of straining and subsequent tearing of sutures. Delaying reconstruction of the perineal body avoids reduction in the size of the rectal lumen, minimizes the accumulation of feces, and reduces the number of muscular contractions necessary to void feces. The author, however, prefers a one-stage repair in which reconstruction of the rectovestibular shelf and the perineal body are completed in one operation (5, 6). The author's technique differs from the Aanes' technique and will be described in this text.

The success of the surgery is dependent on proper preoperative preparation of the mare. The feces must be soft and must remain soft for at least 2 weeks following the repair. If the mare starts to strain following surgery and repeated manual evacuation of feces is required, the surgery will fail. The best way to prepare these mares is to put them in a pasture with lush grass, and feed them nothing else. In a few days, the feces are generally soft. Immediately following surgery they are returned to the pasture for at least 2 weeks. There may be some weight loss during this time, particularly if a foal is at the mare's side. Clients should be encouraged to wean the foal early, before surgery.

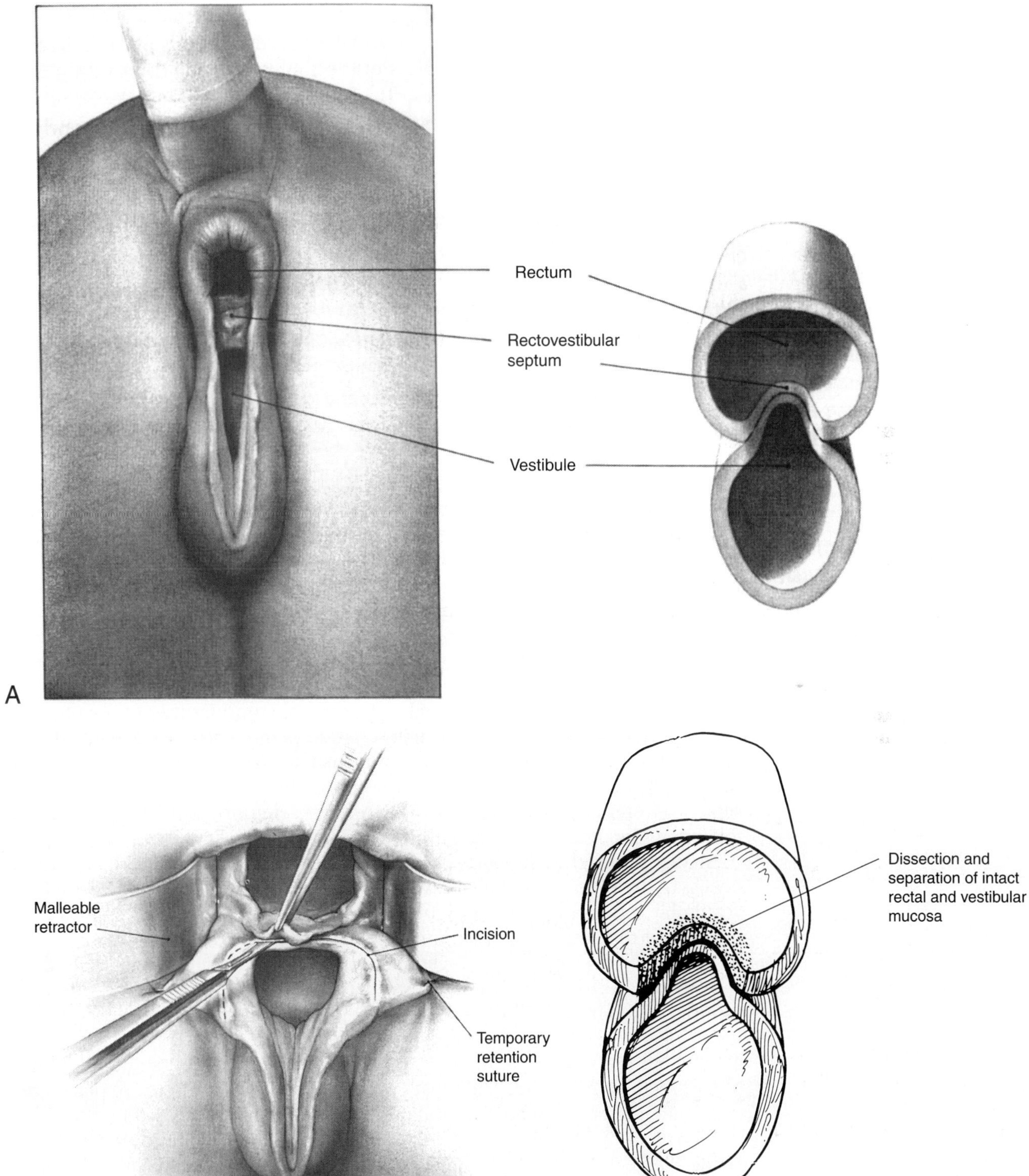

FIGURE 8.5, A–B. Repair of third-degree perineal laceration. (Adapted from Turner AS, McIlwraith CW. Techniques in Large Animal Surgery. 2nd ed. Philadelphia: Lea & Febiger, 1989.)

Anesthesia and Surgical Preparation

An intravenous catheter is placed, the mare is sedated and placed in stocks, and an epidural anesthetic is administered (7). A combination of lidocaine and xylazine is preferred by the author. The tail is wrapped and tied (with a quick-release knot) over the top of the stocks. Feces in the rectum, vagina, and vestibule are removed manually and the perineal region scrubbed with mild soap and water. The rectum and vestibular region are then cleansed with a very dilute povidone-iodine solution (Betadine), and excess fluids are absorbed with moistened cotton. Tetanus toxoid and perioperative, broad-spectrum antibiotics are administered prior to surgery.

Additional Instrumentation

The surgery is greatly facilitated by using long-handled Metzenbaum scissors, needle holders, thumb forceps, and scalpel handles. An assistant can hold a portable light behind the surgeon, or the surgeon can wear a head lamp to illuminate the surgical site.

Surgical Technique

Two temporary retaining sutures are placed on each side of the laceration—one at the level of the anal sphincter and one near the dorsal commissure of the vulva. These sutures are tied to the skin 8 to 10 cm lateral to the normal position of the anus and vulva.

An incision is made along the scar tissue at the junction of the rectal and vestibular mucosa, commencing at the cranial end of the shelf and moving caudad toward the operator (Fig. 8.5*B*). The completed incision should extend from the shelf formed by the intact rectum and vestibule, along the scar tissue margin in the vestibule, to the level of the dorsal commissure of the vulva.

The rectal and vestibular layers will separate as the incision is deepened. The vestibular mucous membrane and submucosa will reflect ventrad from the line of the incision. At the shelf, the rectum and vestibular (or vaginal) mucosa are separated cranial for a distance of 2 to 3 cm. Hemorrhage from the tissues following this incision is usually minimal.

At this point, the surgeon should determine whether further dissection is necessary by estimating the ease with which the rectovestibular tissue and the vestibular mucosa can be brought into apposition. The mucosa should form the roof of the vestibule with minimal tension on the suture material.

The repair consists of two layers of sutures. The crucial layer is that which sutures the perivestibular tissue from each side into apposition. There are a number of different techniques for suture placement that have been described featuring 4-or 6-bite, purse string-type sutures (1, 2, 4–6). This author prefers a 4-bite suture technique incorporating the perivestibular tissue and a small bite of rectal submucosa. The most cranial two or three sutures are placed between the intact rectal and vestibular layers in the space created by the initial incision and dissection between these layers at the cranial end of the defect. Using a large taper-point needle, sweged on to no. 2 synthetic absorbable suture material, a substantial bite is taken in the left perivestibular tissue (Fig. 8.5*C*). A second bite is taken through the rectal mucosa at the edge of the defect, a third bite through the opposite rectal submucosa, and the fourth and final bite through the right perivestibular tissue. A surgeon's throw is placed on the suture and the suture is pulled tightly by hand and tied. The knot is therefore situated ventrally, not beneath the rectal mucosa, so there is less suture material exposed to potential contamination. This pattern tightly apposes and slightly inverts the rectal mucosa into the rectal lumen. These sutures are placed approximately 1 cm apart. After a number of these sutures are placed, a second layer in the

Order of purse string type suture placement

1) Left side perivestibular tissue, large bite
2) Left rectal submucosa, small bite
3) Right rectal submucosa, small bite
4) right perivestibular tissue, large bite

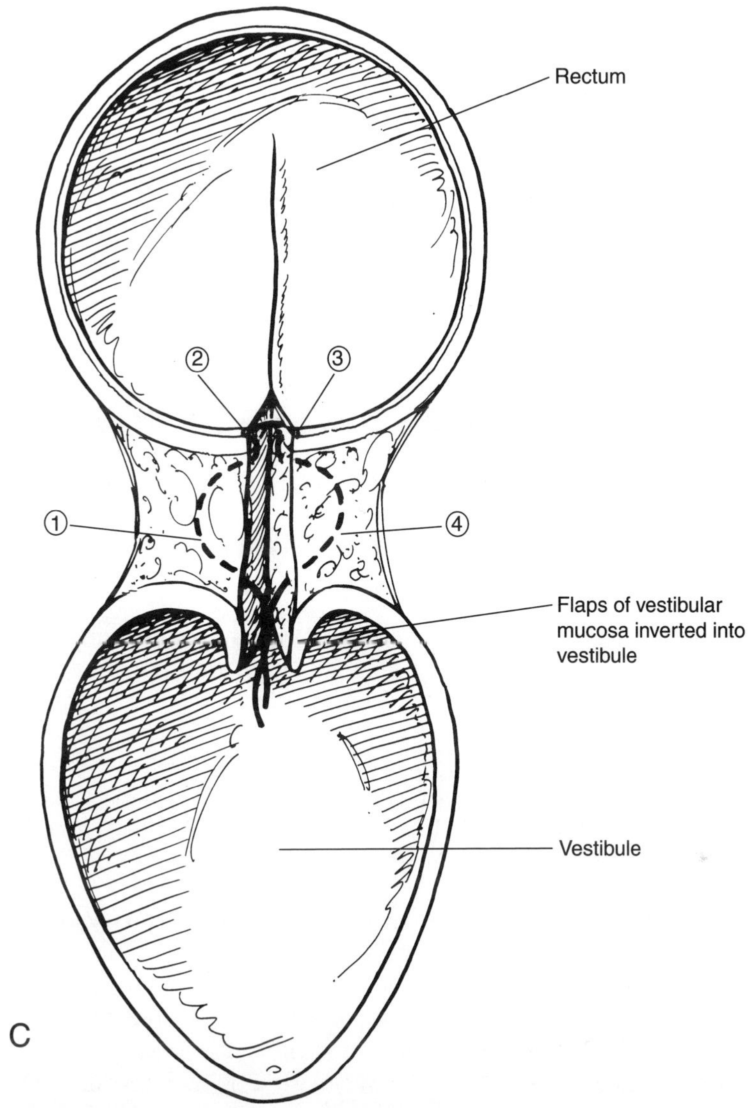

FIGURE 8.5, C. (*continued*) Reconstruction of the rectovestibular shelf.

vestibule is started. Horizontal mattress sutures of no. 1 synthetic absorbable material are placed across the vestibular mucosa to invert that mucosa into the lumen of the vestibule (Fig. 8.5*D*). Fairly large bites can be taken to eliminate dead space between the first layer of closure and the vestibular layer. A taper needle is used so as not to inadvertently cut the sutures in the first layer. The repair of the rectovestibular shelf then continues, pausing to place sutures in the vestibular layer. Once reconstruction of the shelf is completed, perineal body repair is initiated.

To obtain fresh surfaces for reconstruction and healing of the perineal body, epithelialized tissue must be removed. An incision that commences at the cranial margin of the perineal body is made; it extends peripherally along the scar tissue margin and ends at the dorsal commissure of the vulva, forming two sides of a triangle. An incision is made on the opposite side and a superficial layer of epithelium is removed, creating two raw, triangular surfaces that will be sutured together (Fig. 8.5*E*).

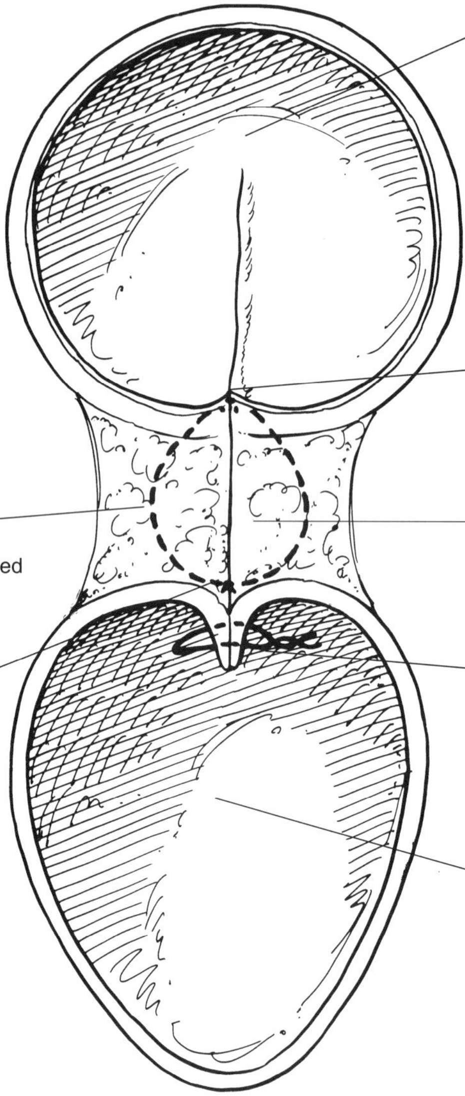

Figure 8.5, D. (*continued*) Reconstruction of the rectovestibular shelf.

Closure of the deep layers of the perineal body should commence cranially with simple interrupted sutures of no. 1 polyglactin 910 (Vicryl). This closure is completed with simple interrupted sutures of 2/0 nylon placed within the epithelial edges of the anus (Fig. 8.5*F*). The nylon and Vicryl sutures are placed alternately until reconstruction of the perineal body is completed. No attempt is made to locate and suture the ends of the anal sphincter muscle because they are usually surrounded by scar tissue. The dorsal portion of the vulvar lips is removed just as in Caslick's operation for pneumovagina. The skin of the perineum and lips of the vulva are closed with interrupted sutures of 2/0 nylon.

Postoperative Management

The mare is put back to pasture immediately after the operation. The nylon sutures in the epithelium of the anus, skin of the perineum, and lips of the vulva are removed 14 days after surgery.

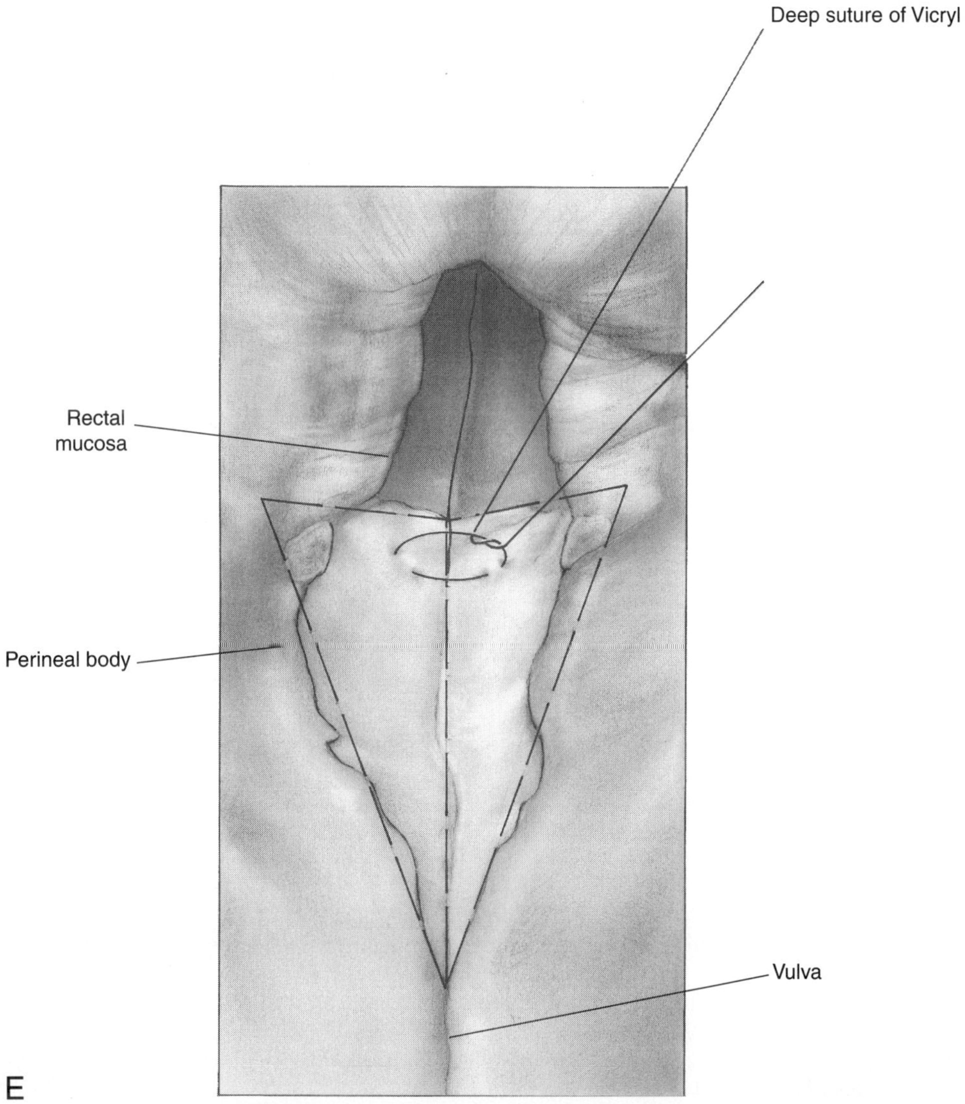

FIGURE 8.5, E. (*continued*) Perineal body reconstruction. (Reprinted with permission from Turner AS, McIlwraith CW. Techniques in Large Animal Surgery. 2nd ed. Philadelphia: Lea & Febiger, 1989.)

Following healing, the mare should be examined for endometritis and treated accordingly. Natural service should be postponed for at least 60 days to allow the region to attain some strength. The author has had some mares that conceived when bred by artificial insemination within 30 days of repair. Some mares require artificial insemination because of a marked reduction in the size of the vulvar opening.

In most cases, the prognosis for future pregnancies following successful repair of a third-degree perineal laceration is excellent. Endometrial inflammation has been shown to subside within 2 weeks of repair (8). At subsequent parturitions, the amount of trauma and subsequent injury is variable, ranging from no injury to another third-degree perineal laceration. It is advisable to have an attendant present during future foalings to minimize the severity of damage if a dystocia should occur.

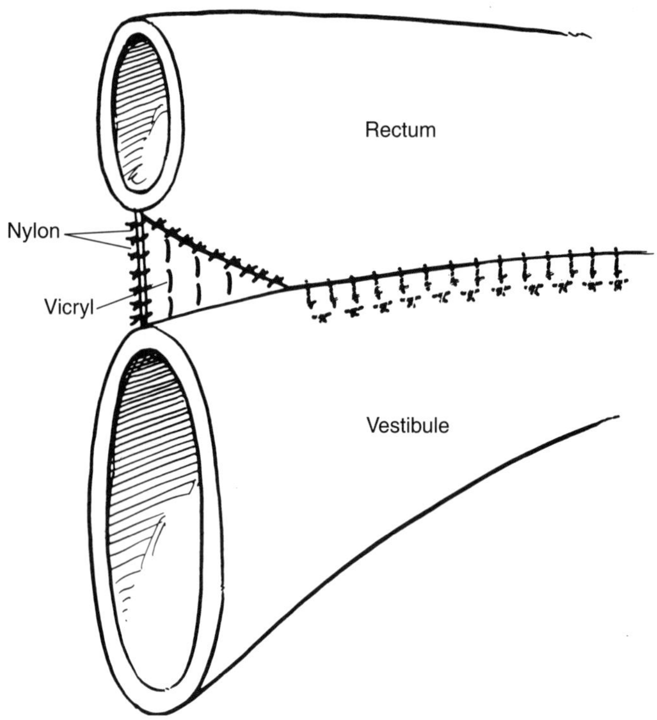

F

Figure 8.5, F. (*continued*) Sutures in perineal body reconstruction.

REFERENCES

1. Colbern GT, Aanes WA, Stashak TS. Surgical management of perineal lacerations and rectovestibular fistulae in the mare: a retrospective of 47 cases. JAVMA 1985;186: 265–269.
2. Aanes WA. Surgical repair of third-degree perineal laceration and rectovestibular fistula in the mare. JAVMA 1964;144:485–491.
3. Haynes PF, McClure JR. Eversion of the urinary bladder: a sequel to third-degree perineal laceration in the mare. Vet Surg 1980;9:66.
4. Turner AS, McIlwraith CW, eds. Techniques in Large Animal Surgery. 2nd ed. Philadelphia: Lea & Febiger, 1989:211–217.
5. Belknap JK, Nickels FA. A one-stage repair of third-degree perineal lacerations and rectovestibular fistulae in 17 mares. Vet Surg 1992;21:378–381.
6. Embertson RM, Robertson JT. Parturient perineal and rectovestibular injuries. In: Robinson NE, ed. Current Therapy in Equine Medicine. 2nd ed. Philadelphia: WB Saunders, 1987:550–555.
7. Grubb TL, Riebold TW, Huber MJ. Comparison of lidocaine, xylazine, and xylazine/lidocaine for caudal epidural analgesia in horses. JAVMA 1992;201:1187–1190.
8. Schumaker J, Schumaker J, Blanchard T. Comparison of endometrium before and after repair of third-degree rectovestibular lacerations in mares. JAVMA 1992;200: 1336–1338.

Repair of a Rectovestibular Fistula

During parturition, the same circumstances that contribute to a third-degree perineal laceration also are factors in producing a rectovestibular fistula. The difference, however, is that once the foal's foot perforates through the vestibule and into the rectum, it is then withdrawn by the foal or pushed back into the vestibule by an attendant. This leaves a communication or fistula between the vestibule and the rectum, but the perineal body remains intact. Some rectovestibular fistulae will heal spontaneously but most require surgical repair. The immediate management of this injury is similar to that described for third-degree perineal lacerations, and the fistula is allowed to heal by second intention before attempting a repair.

The anesthesia, surgical preparation, and additional instrumentation are the same as for repair of a third-degree perineal laceration.

Surgical Technique

Some surgeons advocate converting a rectovestibular fistula to a third-degree perineal laceration and repairing it as has been previously described. The author prefers to preserve the integrity of the tissues caudal to the fistula and repair the fistula through a perineal body transection approach (1). A 4 to 5 cm horizontal incision is made through the skin just below the anal sphincter and above the dorsal commissure of the vulva. Using sharp dissection, this horizontal incision is continued through the muscular perineal body and into the rectovestibular septum. The rectum and the vestibular mucosa are then bluntly separated with long scissors up to the level of the fistula. The operator can place a hand into the vestibule or rectum to help guide the points of scissors so that the mucosa of the vestibule or rectum is not perforated. The scar along the caudal margin of the fistula can then be perforated sharply with a long-handled scalpel, thereby separating the rectal and vestibular mucosa. This sharp incision is carried around the full circumference of the fistula, along the scar line between the rectum and the vestibule. Then, using the long-handled Metzenbaum scissors for blunt dissection, the horizontal incision is extended cranial to the fistula into the intact rectovestibular shelf for a distance of 3 to 4 cm (Fig. 8.6*A*).

The rectum is closed transversely (front to back) while the vestibular mucosa is closed longitudinally (side to side). Both the rectum and vestibule are closed with interrupted Lembert sutures using size 1 synthetic suture material (Fig. 8.6, *B* and *C*). The rectal closure is the most critical of the two layers of closure of the fistula, and rectal sutures are placed in the submucosa with care taken not to penetrate the rectal mucosa. The Lembert sutures are placed in such a fashion that there is minimal inversion of the rectal mucosa into the lumen of the rectum. The dead space between the rectum and the vestibule is then packed with nitrofurazone-soaked gauze. The lateral margins of the horizontal skin incision are closed with interrupted sutures of 2/0 polypropylene. The central portion of the skin incision is left open for gauze removal and subsequent drainage. Alternatively, the dead space can be closed with simple interrupted sutures of 0-Vicryl apposing the rectal and vestibular submucosal tissue. The horizontal skin incision is sutured, leaving a central opening to allow for drainage.

Postoperative Management

The mare is observed for straining and signs of constipation in the immediate postoperative period. The laxative diet is maintained for 2 weeks following surgery. The gauze packing is removed 3 to 4 days after surgery, and the incisional area can be cleaned daily until drainage ceases. Some mares resent any manipu-

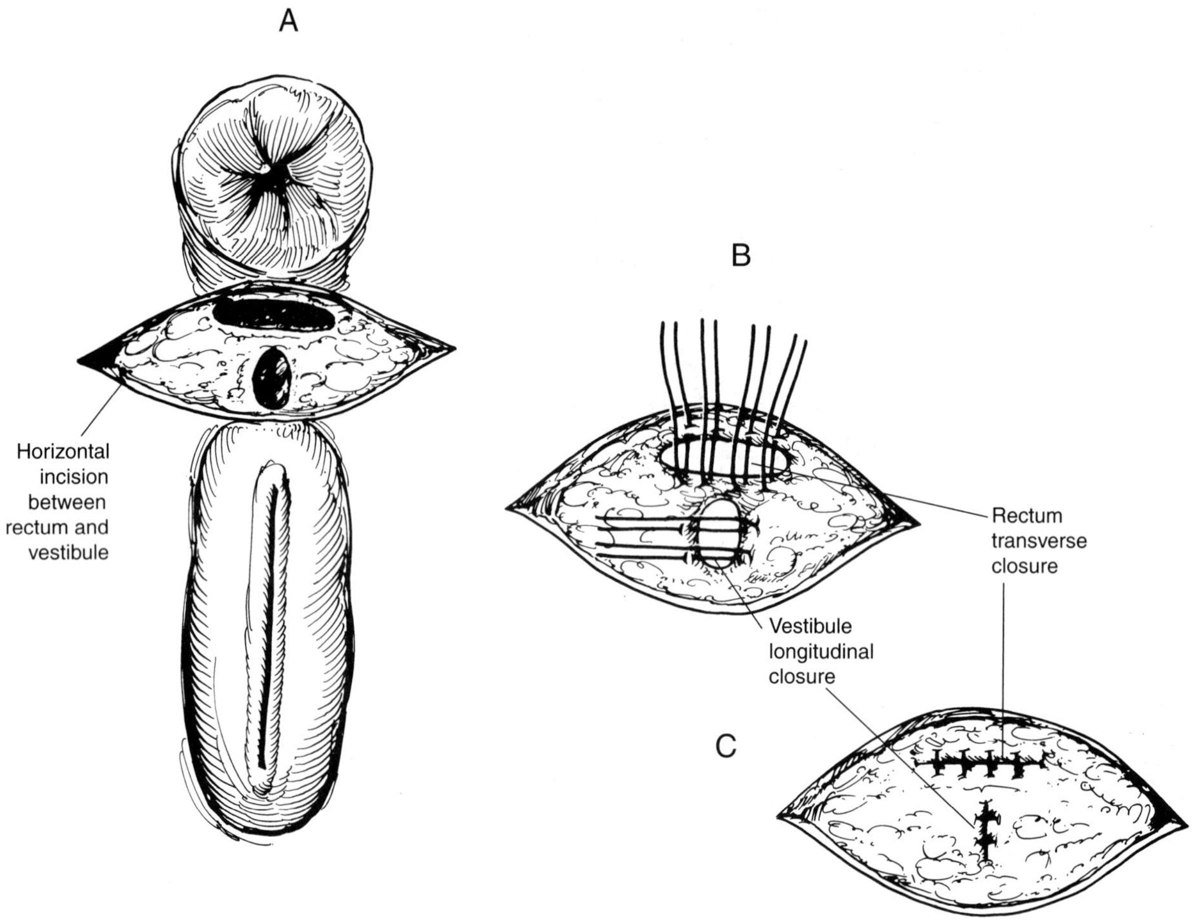

FIGURE 8.6, A–C. Rectovestibular fistula repair. (Adapted from Embertson RM, Robertson JT. Parturient perineal and rectovestibular injuries. In: Robinson NE, ed. Current Therapy in Equine Medicine. 2nd ed. Philadelphia: WB Saunders, 1987.)

lation of the area and are best left alone. The skin sutures are removed 2 weeks after surgery.

The prognosis for reproductive soundness following successful repair of a rectovestibular fistula is excellent, and there is little chance of reinjury at subsequent parturitions.

REFERENCES

1. Embertson RH, Robertson JT. Parturient perineal and rectovestibular injuries. In: Robinson NE, ed. Current Therapy in Equine Medicine. 2nd ed. Philadelphia: WB Saunders, 1987:550.

Repair of a Cervical Laceration

Cervical tears usually occur as a result of excessive stretching of the cervix during delivery of a foal and are frequently associated with dystocias that require a great deal of obstetric manipulation or a fetotomy. Cervical tears can, however, occur during an uneventful delivery or during an abortion of a relatively small fetus (1–4). Most lacerations involve only that portion of the cervix that projects into the vagina, although severe lacerations can involve the entire length of the cervix. The tear can involve just the mucosa of the cervix or can involve the mucosal and muscular layers, producing a wedgelike defect with its base at the cervical os and the apex at the reflection of the vestibular mucosa (1). A complete tear through the mucosal and muscular layers that involves greater than 50% of the vestibular portion of the cervix usually produces cervical incompetence (2, 4). Occasionally, the cervical musculature will be torn without disrupting the mucosa, producing a cervical incompetence. There may be more than one tear around the circumference of the cervical os, although additional tears tend to be less severe.

Some cervical tears heal spontaneously and require no repair. When a cervical tear is found on a postpartum examination, it should be allowed to heal by second intention. A reevaluation at 30 to 60 days following parturition will determine whether surgical repair is necessary. At that time, in addition to performing a routine speculum examination, a digital examination of the cervix should be performed to fully evaluate the cervix for any defects, weaknesses, or adhesions of the cervical and vestibular mucosa. This examination is best done when the cervix is under the influence of progesterone and the cervical muscle tone is at its greatest. If it is apparent on digital examination that the cervix is not closed tightly, and the cervix muscle tone does not provide resistance when an index finger is introduced into the lumen of the cervix, cervical incompetence should be suspected. If the cervix is not able to close tightly under the influence of progesterone, the resultant chronic uterine contamination and endometritis will lead to a failure to conceive or maintain pregnancy. Before doing a surgical repair of the cervix, a complete reproductive assessment of the reproductive tract, including a uterine culture and biopsy, should be carried out to establish a prognosis for future fertility (5). The surgical repair can be done any time during the estrus cycle.

Anesthesia and Surgical Preparation

An intravenous catheter is placed and the mare is put in stocks. Perioperative antibiotics are administered, as well as tetanus toxoid. A small amount of a sedative (such as a xylazine and butorphanol combination) is given intravenously. An epidural anesthetic is administered, with the author preferring to use a combination of xylazine and 2% lidocaine in saline (6). The rectum is evacuated of feces and the perineal region and vulvar area are cleaned with mild soap and water. When the epidural has taken effect, the vestibule and vagina can be cleansed as well.

Additional Instrumentation

Long-handled (12-inch) Metzenbaum scissors, thumb forceps, Allis tissue forceps, and needle holders are required. Large, broad-bladed retractors or a vaginal speculum are also needed for retraction of the walls of the vestibule. A head lamp can be used for illumination.

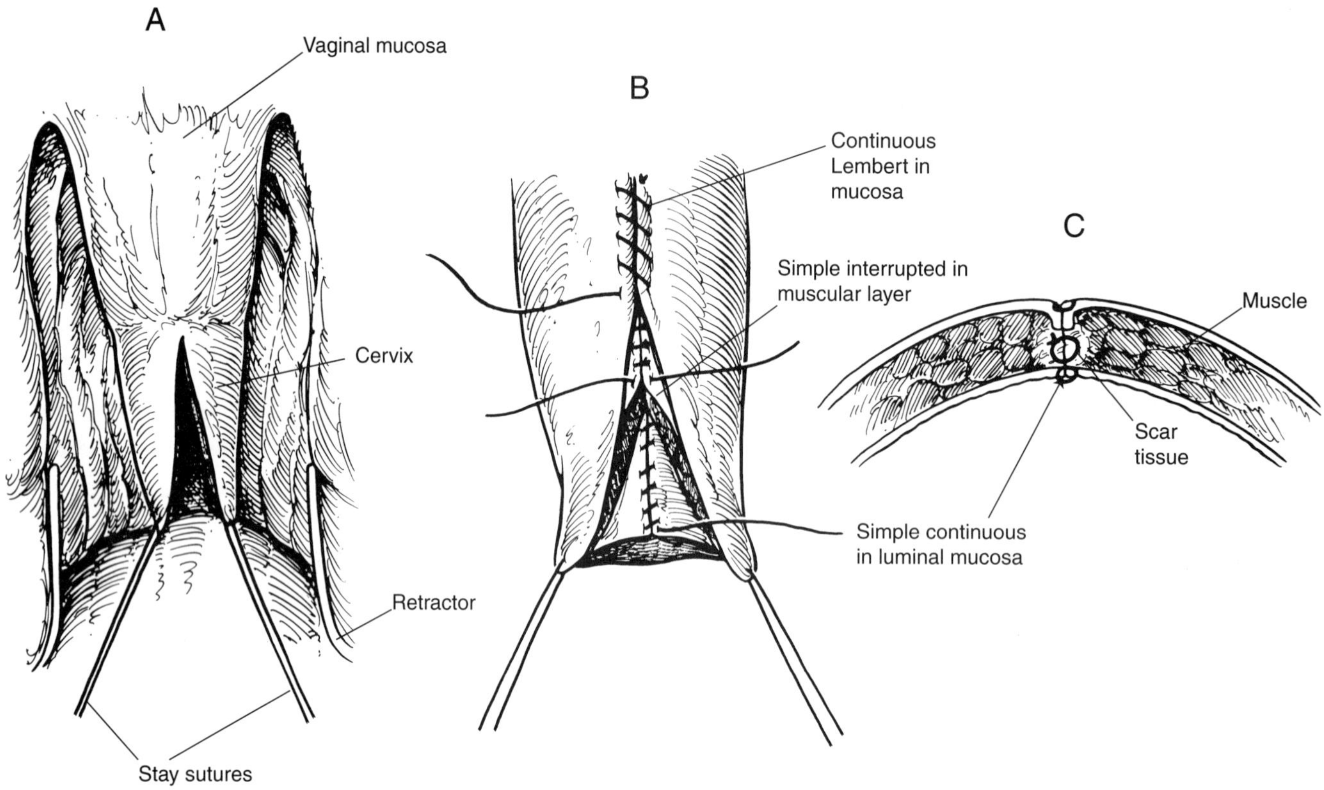

Figure 8.7, A–C. Repair of cervix laceration. (Adapted from Robertson JT. Cervical lacerations. In: White NA, Moore JN, eds. Current Practice of Equine Surgery. Philadelphia: JB Lippincott, 1990.)

Surgical Technique

Two long stay sutures of no. 2 Braunamid, (Jorgenson Laboratories, Loveland, CO) are placed through the most caudal part of the cervix on each side of, and immediately adjacent to, the edges of the tear. This requires that the surgeon pass both lubricated arms into the vagina and, palpating the defect with one hand, pass each suture through the cervix using a large cutting needle. The ends of these stay sutures are tied and tagged with a hemostat. Retractors are placed or held in the vestibule by assistants, and the cervix is retracted caudally to the level of the vestibule with strong traction on the stay sutures (Fig. 8.7*A*). Most mares will tolerate this only if the epidural anesthesia is completely effective.

Using the long-handled scissors, the scar tissue and redundant mucosa along both sides of the defect are resected, leaving a wedge-shaped defect for closure. Most of the palpable scar tissue is resected, although it is difficult to differentiate the muscular tissue from scar tissue. If a muscular defect exists but there is a mucosa bridging the defect, a wedge-shaped piece of mucosa is removed, exposing the edges of the muscular layers.

A three-layer closure is optimal (Fig. 8.7, *B* and *C*). Each layer of closure starts at the cranial end of the defect (apex of the wedge) and ends at the most caudal aspect, immediately adjacent to the stay sutures. The luminal mucosa is simply apposed with a continuous layer of 2/0 Vicryl. The muscular layer is the most important layer of closure. Because there is still some residual scar tissue along the freshened edges, it may be necessary to use a cutting needle for suturing this layer. Simple interrupted sutures of 0-Vicryl are used to close this layer. If a cutting needle is used, care must be taken not to cut other previously placed sutures. The mucosa on the vaginal side is closed with a continuous Lembert suture pattern using 2/0 Vicryl. Inverting this mucosa covers the knots of the sutures in the muscular layer and reduces the likelihood of formation of cervical adhesions. Any additional tears are repaired in a similar fashion.

Severe lacerations involving the entire length of the cervix may be impossible to repair successfully. The author has attempted repair of these types of tears under general anesthesia, with the mare positioned in sternal recumbency and her rear quarters off the surgery table (1). General anesthesia is necessary to retract the cervix far enough into the vestibule to allow intraluminal dissection and suturing and to maintain it in that position for the entire duration of the surgery.

Postoperative Management

A nonsteroidal, anti-inflammatory agent can be administered for 3 to 4 days following surgery. On speculum examination, the cervix will appear edematous and hyperemic for at least 2 weeks after surgery. Manual examination of the cervix is not recommended during this time, except in those rare cases in which the surgeon might wish to inspect for adhesions and break them down. At least 30 days of sexual rest are recommended following surgery.

Comments

The prognosis given for reproductive soundness following surgery is based on the surgeon's assessment of the quality of the repair and on the results of the preoperative reproductive examination, which includes an endometrial biopsy. In a mare with a grade I-II endometrium and a single cervical defect that has been successfully reconstructed, a 50 to 60% chance of delivering a live foal can be given (1–5). It may take two breeding seasons to get these mares in foal. Owners should be warned of the possibility of reinjury to the cervix at the time of foaling and the need for further reconstruction.

Postbreeding repair of cervical lacerations has been reported in five mares (7). These mares were bred with artificial insemination and were repaired 2 to 3 days after ovulation. The margins of the laceration were trimmed and the defect was closed with size 0 PDS in a simple continuous pattern. The sutures penetrated the external mucous membrane and the fibromuscular layer but did not incorporate the internal mucosal layer. All mares received perisurgical anti-inflammatory therapy. There were two failures out of these five mares; however, performing the repair shortly after breeding allowed for a more timely return to production.

For mares with a severely damaged cervix in which it is apparent that surgical reconstruction will not successfully restore cervical function, a nonabsorbable purse string retention suture can be placed submucosally around the circumference of the vaginal portion of the cervix to close it (1, 3, 4). The author recommends using size 2 polypropylene suture. The suture can be placed in the standing mare either before or after breeding. If the suture is placed before breeding, a small luminal opening must be left to allow for passage of an insemination pipette. Pyometra may develop if the uterus becomes infected. Also, if the mare successfully carries a foal to term, the purse string suture must be removed before foaling.

REFERENCES

1. Robertson JT. Cervical Laceration. In: White NA, Moore JM, eds. Current Practice of Equine Surgery. Philadelphia: JB Lippincott, 1990:696–699.

2. Brown JS, Varner DD, Hinrichs K, et al. Surgical repair of the lacerated cervix in the mare. Theriogenology 1984;22:351–359.
3. Evans LJ, Tate LP, Cooper WL, et al. Surgical repair of cervical lacerations and the incompetent cervix. In: Proceedings of the AAEP Annual Convention, Miami Beach, FL, 1979:483–486.
4. Fraunfelder HC. Cervical abnormalities. In: Robinson NE, ed. Current Therapy in Equine Medicine. 2nd ed. Philadelphia: WB Saunders, 1987:516–518.
5. Kenney RM. Cyclic and pathologic changes of the mare endometrium as detected by biopsy, with a note on early embryonic death. JAVMA 1978;172:241–262.
6. Grubb TL, Riebold TW, Huber MJ. Comparison of lidocaine, xylazine, and xylazine/lidocaine for caudal epidural analgesia in horses. JAVMA 1992;201:1187–1190.
7. Foss RR, Wirth NR, Kutz RR. Post-breeding repair of cervical lacerations. In: Proceedings of the 4th Annual Conference of the AAEP. 1994:11–12.

Removal of Cystic Calculi (Laparocystotomy)

Cystic calculi in the horse are caused by precipitation of urine salts on a nidus. Such calculi are usually solitary although calculi can occur at several sites. The nidi for calculi formation include exposed suture material, fibrin, leukocytes, whole blood, albumin, or urinary mucoproteins. Two types of calculi are seen in horses. One type is rough and spiculated, relatively soft (they can be fragmented), and abrasive to the wall of the bladder—often producing traumatic cystitis. The other type is a smooth, hard, whitish-appearing calculus. Both types are similar chemically, consisting of calcium carbonate with magnesium, ammonium, and phosphate making up other constituents (1).

A horse with a cystic calculus will exhibit dysuria, stranguria, pollakiuria, and hematuria. Less common signs include mild colic, loss of condition, and a stilted gait. The horse will adopt the urinating stance for some time before and after micturition. Soiling and scalding of the perineum and between the legs may also be seen.

The condition is suspected on the basis of clinical signs; a more definitive diagnosis is based on rectal examination. Since cystic calculi usually do not produce clinical signs until they have reached a certain size, they are fairly obvious on rectal palpation. Their presence can be confirmed by cystoscopy using a flexible endoscope, as well as with an ultrasound examination done per rectum (1). Urinalysis will show a concurrent cystitis with crystalluria, red blood cells, white blood cells, and bacteria.

Various surgical approaches are available for removal of cystic calculi. Other than laparocystotomy described here, urethrostomy, pararectal cystotomy (Goekel's operation) in males (2), and urethral sphincterotomy in mares have all been described (1). Laparocystotomy is the approach that is most widely applicable, is less traumatic, and is the most commonly used for larger calculi. Recurrence of urolithiasis is lower following laparocystotomy than following perineal urethrostomy (3).

Anesthesia and Surgical Preparation

The horse should be off feed for at least 24 hours before surgery to allow as much emptying of the intestinal tract (particularly the cecum and colon) as possible. This will reduce interference by the bowel during exteriorization of the bladder. Before surgery, the horse should be started on broad-spectrum intravenous antibiotics. This will minimize the risk of postoperative peritonitis because spillage of some urine into the abdominal cavity is frequently unavoidable as the stone is being manipulated out of the bladder.

The operation is done under general anesthesia with the horse in dorsal recumbency. After the horse is positioned for surgery (with slight elevation of the hindquarters), a urinary catheter is passed into the bladder to provide urine drainage. The prepuce should be packed with dry cotton gauzes and held closed with two or three Backhaus towel clamps and the catheter directed to the side of the abdomen opposite the incision. The caudal ventral abdomen and prepuce in males are prepared for aseptic surgery.

Additional Instrumentation

Laparocystotomy requires a suitable suction apparatus to remove urine, an abdominal surgery suction tip (e.g., Yankauer), narrow umbilical tape (e.g., ⅛-inch), Babcock forceps, and Balfour retractors.

Surgical Technique

A ventral paramedian incision is used in the male and a ventral midline incision in the female. For the paramedian approach, a 20-cm incision is made between the midline (prepuce) and the inguinal ring. The incision is carried through the superficial and deep abdominal fascia, rectus abdominis muscle, and peritoneum. The large pudendal and superficial abdominal vessels are ligated. In the mare, the midline incision should extend from the umbilicus, caudal to the prepubic tendon. Considerable fat and areolar tissue will be encountered as the incision is extended between the mammary glands. When the abdomen is entered, a large Balfour retractor is inserted to help keep the incision apart and facilitate exteriorization of the bladder.

When performing this operation, even the experienced surgeon is always impressed at just how far caudally in the pelvic cavity the bladder is located. It will feel small and contracted. The bladder is located by inserting a hand into the abdomen caudad and dorsad into the pelvic canal. The contracted bladder and calculus are grasped behind the calculus, as with a clenched fist (4). Steady traction is begun in an attempt to fatigue the musculature of the bladder. Eventually, relaxation will occur, but it may take several minutes. When the bladder and stone are exteriorized as much as possible, the bladder will occupy a good proportion of the incision, and this will help prevent exposure of the bowel (Fig. 8.8*A*) (5). The bladder is then isolated with moist towels. Two stay sutures of narrow cotton umbilical tape or heavy suture material are placed through the bladder wall at each end of the proposed incision (Fig. 8.8*A*). The length of the incision will be somewhat variable, depending on the size of the calculus. The incision is made directly onto the stone. The edges of the incision are then grasped with Babcock forceps at its midpoint. Additional points of fixation such as this will help manipulate the wound edges and prevent spillage of any residual

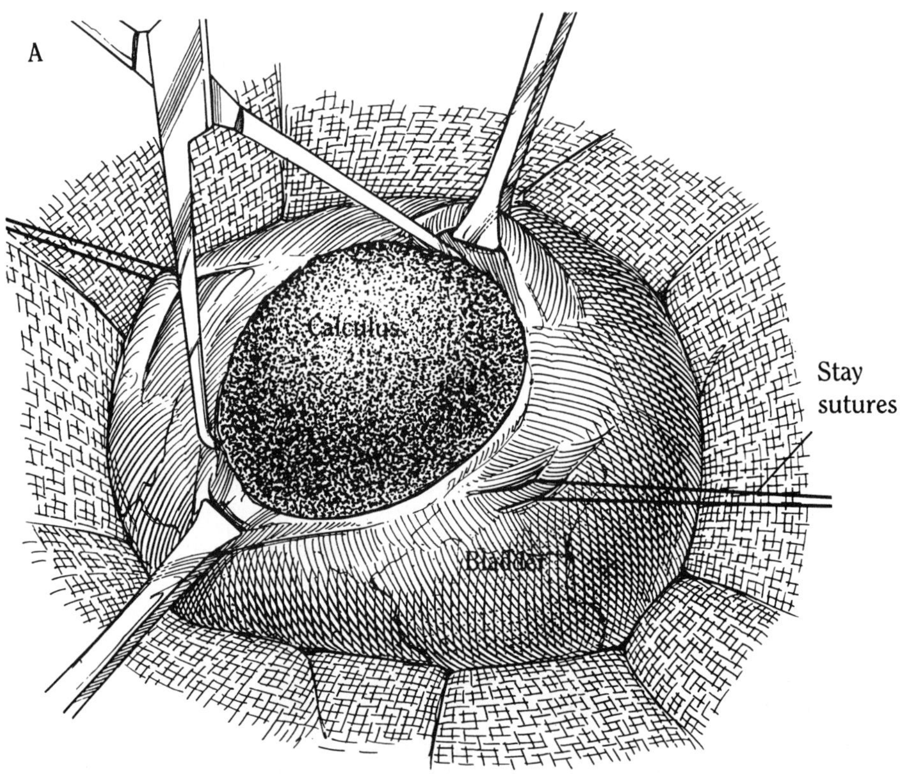

Figure 8.8, A. Laparocystotomy for removal of cystic calculus.

B

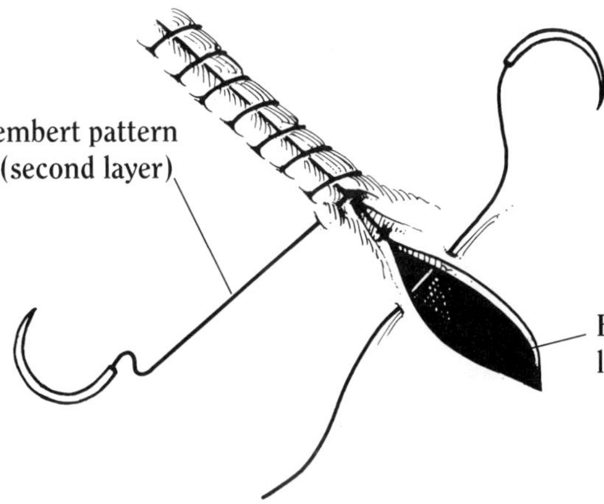

Figure 8.8, B. (*continued*) Laparocystotomy for removal of cystic calculus.

urine into the abdominal cavity. It is frequently difficult to extract the stone (especially the rough-surfaced type) because the bladder mucosa is firmly adhered and interdigitates with the rough surface of the stone. To remove the stone, the bladder mucosa must be peeled slowly away from the mucosa much as the bovine placental caruncle and uterine cotyledon are separated (4). When the stone has been removed, any debris (sand) that remains in the bladder must be removed. Dry gauzes are useful for manual removal of the larger fragments, and saline lavage and suction can be used to get smaller fragments and any blood clots.

The closure of the bladder should be in two layers, using a synthetic absorbable suture material (2/0 or 0 gauge) such as polyglycolic acid (Dexon), Vicryl, or PDS. The first layer of sutures can be a simple interrupted or simple continuous pattern that closes the mucosa, but the second layer should be one of the inverting patterns (such as a continuous Lembert pattern) that is placed in the seromuscular layer (Fig. 8.8*B*). The isolated field of the surgery should be lavaged with warm, balanced electrolyte solution and as much retrieved by suction as possible. Any towels used to pack off the bladder are now removed, and a new pair of outer gloves are donned by the surgeon.

Closure of the midline incision on the mare is routinely done in three or four layers, depending on the surgeon's choice. Closure of the paramedian incision is usually a little more tedious. Here the superficial and deep rectus sheaths of the rectus abdominis muscle are closed separately (the superficial rectus sheath is the critical layer).

Postoperative Management

Postoperative antibiotics are continued for several days following surgery. Penicillin is a good choice because it is excreted in the urine in an active form. The duration of postoperative antibiotic administration is dependent on many variables. These include the degree of cystitis present and the amount of spillage of urine into the abdominal cavity during surgery. A rectal examination can be performed during the first 36 hours to "brush off" any bowel that may be beginning to adhere to the incision in the bladder. Obviously this should be done with some caution, but it can prevent adhesions of bowel to the bladder from forming postoperatively if done several times during the first 36 hours postoperatively. The authors do not maintain a urinary catheter following surgery. Urinary acidification and reduction of dietary calcium intake after surgery may reduce the likelihood of recurrence of a cystic calculus (6).

Comments

The main advantage of laparocystotomy over other approaches for stone removal is that it is possible to ensure that all fragments of calculus have been removed (7, 8). Any fragments remaining can act as a potential nidus for future stone formation or potentially move down the urinary tract and cause urethral obstruction. Subischial urethrostomy and crushing the stone with a lithotrite can be done with the horse standing with little risk of peritonitis and because the incision heals rapidly, the horse can return to work quickly. Disadvantages of the technique, however, are the trauma sustained by the urethra and bladder during stone crushing and removal, and the high rate of calculus recurrence (3, 8). The surgery can be protracted and frustrating if it is necessary to use a lithotrite to crush the stone, and urethral stricture or persistent fistula formation can occur at the urethrostomy site if there has been a great deal of trauma. The long-range prognosis following removal of cystic calculi should always be guarded because these horses are probably predisposed to recurrence of stone formation.

REFERENCES

1. DeBowes RM, Nyrop KA, Boulton CH. Cystic calculi in the horse. Symposium Cont Edu 1984;6:5268.
2. Kersjes AW, Nemeth F, Rutgers LJE. Pararectal cystotomy and urethrotomy. In: Atlas of Large Animal Surgery. Bunge, Utrecht: 1985:68–69.
3. Laverty S, Pascoe JR, Ling GU, et al. Urolithiasis in 68 horses. Vet Surg 1992;21:56–62.
4. Hackett RP, Vaughan JT, Tennant BC. Diseases of the urinary bladder. In: Mansmann RA, McAllister ES, Pratt PW, eds. Equine Medicine and Surgery. 3rd ed. Santa Barbara, CA: American Veterinary Publications, 1983:912.
5. Reed DG. Suprapubic cystotomy in a stallion. Can J Comp Med Vet Sci 1964;28:95.
6. Remillard RL, Modransky PD, Welker FH, et al. Dietary management of cystic calculi in a horse. J Equine Vet Sci 1992;12:359–363.
7. Lowe JE. Suprapubic cystotomy in a gelding. Cornell Vet 1960;50:510.
8. Robertson JT, Buffington CA. Surgical removal of uroliths. In: White NA, Moore JN, eds. Current Practice of Equine Surgery. Philadelphia: JB Lippincott, 1990:734–739.

Resection of the Diseased Urachus in Foals

In utero, the urachus is a connection between the urinary bladder and the allantoic cavity (1). Normally the urachus closes at or soon after birth and is eventually reduced to a scar at the apex of the bladder. The urachus may persist as a fistula between the umbilicus and the urinary bladder, allowing urine to escape. More importantly, it can act as an avenue for bacterial infection and lead to infections elsewhere in the foal's body (1–6). It has been suggested also that infection of the umbilicus can lead to a reopening of the urachus, instead of infection being the result of a patent urachus (1). Infection and abscessation of the umbilical vein or umbilical arteries can occur, and this can also act as a nidus of infection.

The sequelae to an unattended infection in this area are well documented and can be devastating to the animal. These sequelae include retrograde cystitis, osteomyelitis, infectious arthritis, meningitis, and hypopyon (2, 5, 6). Neonatal foals that are hospitalized for neonatal maladjustment syndrome, septicemia, or weakness often develop a patent urachus and occasionally, tears in the urachus that cause accumulation of urine in the abdomen or into the subcutaneous tissues (7). For these reasons, early resection of the infected urachus, a portion of the bladder, and the associated umbilical vessel remnants is indicated. Resection is indicated in cases of patent urachus that do not respond to the more conservative methods of treatment, which usually include cauterization with silver nitrate or strong iodine solutions. Ultrasound examination of the umbilical area is useful for evaluating whether the umbilical remnants are enlarged or abscessed (6). Surgical exploration and removal of infected remnants is indicated if abscesses are present or if the remnants are enlarged and the foal is septicemic or develops arthritis. Occasionally, foals with enlarged umbilical structures will respond well to antibiotic therapy and surgical intervention is not necessary. An ultrasonographic examination should be performed daily to monitor the effectiveness of medical treatment.

Anesthesia and Surgical Preparation

Perioperative treatment of the foal with intravenous broad-spectrum antibiotics is always indicated to minimize the chances of bacteremia at the time of surgical manipulation. They are also indicated if the area is abscessed because there is a risk of spilling septic contents into the abdomen during surgery. Gram-negative and Gram-positive aerobic bacteria, as well as anaerobic bacteria, may be cultured from infected umbilical cord remnants. The most frequently cultured group of organisms are Gram-negative enterics and B-hemolytic streptococcal species. These same organisms are commonly associated with septicemia in neonates (6). Foals that are bacteremic/septicemic may require more aggressive medical therapy before risking general anesthesia.

Inhalation anesthesia such as halothane induced by mask, followed by endotracheal intubation, is the preferred technique. The foal is positioned in dorsal recumbency, and a soft rubber urinary catheter is inserted into the bladder to evacuate its contents. In male foals, the penis should be catheterized to prevent urine spilling into the surgical site. The penis is then sutured into the prepuce with a 2/0 polypropylene purse string suture and the catheter is taken off to one side. The urachal area is frequently moist and should be cleaned when the hair in this area has been clipped. Before the surgical scrub is initiated, the opening in the urachal stump is closed with interrupted Lembert sutures placed in the skin (1). The entire ventral abdomen is then clipped and prepared for aseptic surgery in a routine manner. It is important to prepare the foal for the possibility of extending the ventral midline incision as far cranial as the xiphoid cartilage if an umbilical vein resection is required.

Surgical Technique

The skin incision on the ventral midline is started approximately 4 to 5 cm cranial to the umbilicus and extends caudally around each side of the umbilicus in an elliptical fashion, connecting caudal to the umbilicus and continuing approximately another 2 cm to the cranial margin of the prepuce (Fig. 8.9*A*). The skin and the subcutaneous tissue are then dissected free of the body wall, leaving the umbilicus still attached (Fig. 8.9*B*). The linea alba is incised cranial to the umbilicus, and the surgeon is able to insert an index finger to feel the dimensions of the urachus, umbilical vessels, and assess for the presence of an abscess or adhesions to other viscera. Using Metzenbaum scissors, with digital guidance, the abdominal wall incision is continued around either side of the umbilicus to allow for a complete en bloc resection (Fig. 8.9*B*). The ventral midline body wall incision is then continued caudal to the umbilicus for approximately 2 cm using a scalpel.

The excised portion of skin attached to the umbilicus, the urachus, the apex of the bladder, and the umbilical vessels is carefully dissected free of the body wall in preparation for amputation. If the urachus is not abscessed and the junction of the urachus with the bladder is obvious and palpable, the urachus can be simply double-ligated and transected. Frequently it is difficult to distinguish the bladder from the urachus. The urachus will be enlarged and inflamed because of fibrosis, and amputation must be made further caudad, along with a portion of the apex of the bladder (3).

In preparation for resection of a portion of the apex of the bladder, stay sutures are placed around the umbilical arteries immediately adjacent to the bladder at the proposed site of amputation. These sutures are used to maintain traction on the bladder during resection and bladder closure. The umbilical arteries distal to the level of the stay sutures, as well as the umbilical vein, are double-ligated and transected. Doyen intestinal clamps are placed across the apex of the bladder at the proposed site of amputation. The bladder should be transected through healthy-appearing wall. The Doyen clamps prevent spillage of septic contents from an infected urachus or a urachal abscess. The area is packed off with moist towels and, using a scalpel, the bladder is incised using the caudal edge of the Doyen forceps as a cutting guide. The amputated umbilical structures, apex of the bladder, and Doyen clamps are then removed from the surgical field. It is not necessary to place an additional clamp across the bladder to prevent urine spillage from the bladder because the urinary catheter placed before surgery will ensure that the bladder is empty (Fig. 8.9*C*).

The bladder is closed in two layers. The authors prefer an initial simple interrupted layer of sutures (Fig. 8.9*D*) followed by an inverting layer, such as a continuous Lembert pattern, that ensures a watertight seal. Synthetic absorbable suture material such as 2/0 polyglycolic acid (Dexon) or polyglactin 910 (Vicryl) is recommended. Nonabsorbable suture material or stainless steel surgical staples are contraindicated because of their predisposition to calculus formation when exposed to urine.

Abscessation or extensive infection of the umbilical arteries or umbilical vein necessitates a more aggressive resection of the affected vessel(s) than that just described. The condition of these vessels should be assessed at the time of surgery by visual inspection and digital palpation. The umbilical arteries extend caudally to the iliac arteries, while the umbilical vein extends cranially to the liver (1, 2, 5). Attempts should be made to resect the entire abscessed portion of the vessel. The umbilical vein should be double-ligated; otherwise, there is a possibility of bleeding back from the liver because there are no valves in the

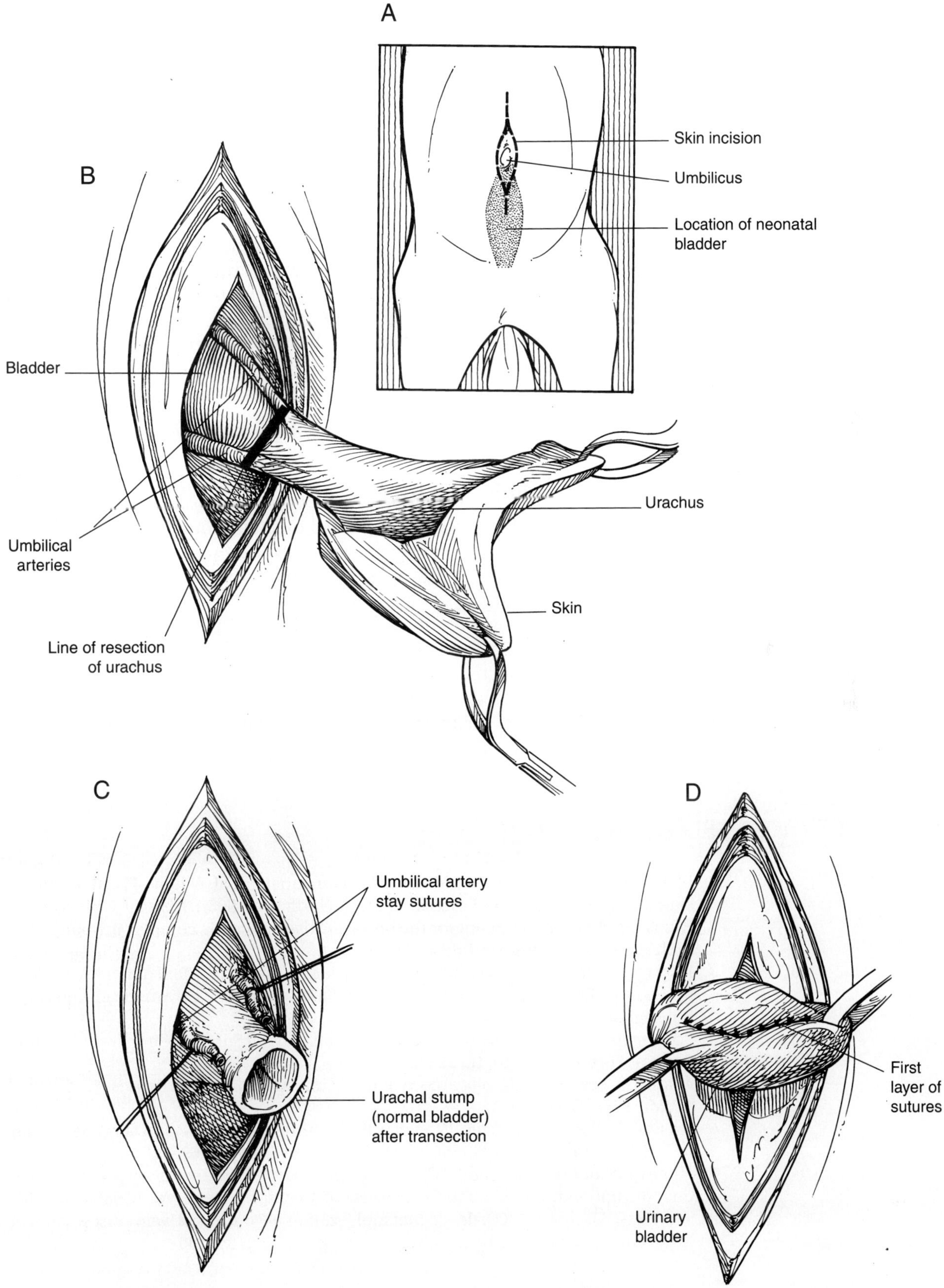

FIGURE 8.9, A–D. Resection of a diseased urachus in the foal.

vessel. The authors have encountered foals where this vein was thickened to 2 cm in diameter and filled with exudate extending craniad to the liver. In such cases there are two surgical options. Resection of the umbilical vein as close to the liver as possible can be attempted, but the risk of spillage of exudate or uncontrollable hemorrhage is high. An alternative is to remove the caudal portion of the umbilical vein and marsupialize the remaining portion through a small ventral abdominal incision adjacent to the ventral midline incision. This allows for chronic drainage of the infected umbilical vein tissues (8). If the umbilical vein is marsupialized through the ventral midline incision, a postoperative incisional hernia may develop.

Following the resection of these diseased tissues, the surgical area should be rinsed with warm, balanced polyionic solution. This procedure should be done several times if purulent material spilled during dissection. The abdominal wall should be closed in three layers. A simple continuous or simple interrupted layer of one of the synthetic absorbable suture materials (no. 1 or no. 2) is used to close the linea alba. A simple continuous layer of a similar suture material (no. 2/0) is used in the subcutaneous tissues. The skin can be closed with skin staples or nonabsorbable suture material of the surgeon's choice.

Postoperative Management

Intensive medical support including intravenous antibiotics and fluids is indicated in foals that are compromised, particularly foals that are febrile or toxemic before surgery. Postoperative intravenous antibiotics should be maintained for 5 to 7 days following surgery.

The clinician must pay attention to signs of incisional infection or metastatic bacterial localization. This means aggressive ancillary treatment for foals that develop infections, arthritis, and meningitis. Any acute joint swelling or lameness should be investigated immediately and treated as an emergency situation, if necessary. The surgical treatment for infectious arthritis is discussed elsewhere in this book.

REFERENCES

1. Richardson DW. Urogenital problems in the neonatal foal. Equine Practice Symposium on Neonatal Equine Disease. Vet Clin North Am 1985;1:179.
2. Evans LH. Surgical treatment for the polyarthritis-septicemia complex in young foals. Arch Am Coll Vet Surg 1977;6:44.
3. Hackett RP, Vaughan JT, Tennant BC. The urinary system. In: Mansmann RA, McAllister ES, eds. Equine Medicine and Surgery. Santa Barbara, CA: American Veterinary Publications, 1982.
4. Robertson JT. In: The Proceedings of the Equine General Surgery Seminar. 12th Annual Surgical Forum, Chicago, IL, 1984:93.
5. Adams SB, Fessler JF. Umbilical cord remnant infections in foals: 16 cases (1975–1985). JAVMA 1987;190:316–321.
6. Reef VB, Collatos C, Spencer PA, et al. Clinical ultrasonographic and surgical findings in foals with umbilical remnant infections. JAVMA 1989;195:69–72.
7. Adams R, Koterba AM, Cudd TC, et al. Exploratory celiotomy for suspected urinary tract disruption in neonatal foals: a review of 18 cases. Equine Vet J 1988;20:13–17.
8. Steiner A, Lischer CJ, Oertle C. Marsupialization of umbilical vein abscesses with involvement of the liver in 13 calves. Vet Surg 1993;22:184–189.

Cystorrhaphy For Ruptured Bladder in Foals

Rupture of the urinary bladder occurs most frequently in newborn male foals. It is rarely seen in adults (1–7). The cause of the condition is unknown, although it is believed that strong forceful abdominal contractions at the time of parturition are the major contributing factor (5). Occasionally, defects of the bladder wall, and not traumatic ruptures, are seen (6).

The clinical signs of ruptured bladder in a foal may be subtle in the initial stages. This leads to a delay in diagnosis that can be life-threatening because of the associated electrolyte abnormalities that ensue. For this reason, most of these foals are referred for surgery at 3 to 7 days of age. The foals will be depressed and anorexic and have an increased heart rate and respiratory rate. They will strain intermittently and attempt unsuccessfully to urinate. The abdomen will be distended, and ballottement produces a fluid wave. Abdominal paracentesis will reveal a clear odorless fluid (usually voluminous) that froths when shaken and emits an ammonia odor when heated (5). The concentration of creatinine in the abdominal fluid is at least twice that of the serum concentration in foals with uroperitoneum (8). To obtain additional confirmation of the diagnosis, a suitable dye such as methylene blue can be injected through a urinary catheter and then checked to see if it readily flows out an indwelling abdominocentesis catheter. Positive-contrast cystography as an aid to diagnosis is popular with other species such as the dog but is not used routinely. It can be useful for helping to localize the defect (i.e., bladder vs. urachus). Tears in the urachus can cause uroperitoneum or an accumulation of urine into the subcutaneous tissues around the umbilicus, depending on the extent of the tear. Also, if there is a uroperitoneum, and there is no evidence of a bladder or urachal defect, a ruptured ureter should be suspected (9). The differential diagnosis for uroperitoneum in a foal also includes retained meconium, colic resulting from impending enteritis, and the rare case of atresia of portions of the intestinal tract.

Anesthesia and Surgical Preparation

Anesthesia should not be induced until the severe electrolyte abnormalities that occur with this condition have been corrected. Typically these foals are hyponatremic and perhaps hypochloremic, resulting from an inability to excrete urine. More significantly, they are hyperkalemic because of failure to effectively excrete potassium (1–4). There may also be a slight to moderate metabolic acidosis. This array of metabolic derangements can lead to life-threatening cardiac arrhythmias, including premature ventricular contractions, ventricular fibrillation, third-degree A-V block, and cardiac arrest, because of potentiation of the cardiotoxicity of the general anesthesia (3, 4).

Some foals with marked abdominal distension as a result of uroperitoneum will have free fluid in the thoracic cavity (6). A preoperative radiograph or ultrasonographic examination of the chest can be performed to identify these foals. If a significant volume of pleural effusion persists despite preoperative abdominal drainage, thoracocentesis may be necessary before anesthesia.

Although surgery should be scheduled as soon as possible, it is highly recommended that some degree of preoperative stabilization be achieved. Intravenous catheterization and administration of 0.9% saline solution should be performed. Bicarbonate should be administered in 5% dextrose if metabolic acidosis exists. It has also been suggested that dextrose and insulin be given because of their hypokalemic effect (3, 4). The dose is 0.5 g of dextrose/kg/per body weight and 0.1 unit of crystalline insulin/kg per body weight intravenously (3, 4). This can also be administered during anesthesia if arrhythmias occur. Care should be taken to see that the foal does not become hypothermic. Body heat can be lost by using cold saline solutions to flush the abdomen. Tilting the animal toward the hindquarters will minimize the pressure on the diaphragm from the fluid in the abdomen.

Decompression of the abdomen before inducing anesthesia is also beneficial. As well as removing toxic metabolites, it will minimize the respiratory embarrassment caused by the distension. The midline should be clipped and scrubbed. A suitable catheter of the surgeon's choice should be inserted after the appropriate local skin analgesic has been applied. Suitable catheters include Foley, sump, or de Pezzer types, although a blunt teat cannula can be used for short-term drainage.

Foals with severe metabolic changes can be peritoneally dialyzed for as long as 12 hours preoperatively to make them a safer anesthetic risk (2). Once the diagnosis of uroperitoneum is made, the foal should be started on intravenous broad-spectrum antibiotics. The foal should also be checked for failure of passive transfer and given a plasma transfusion if necessary. Anesthesia is induced by mask, using halothane or isoflurane (6). A soft rubber catheter is inserted aseptically through the penis into the bladder and directed to one side. The preputial area should be sealed with towel clamps or sutured closed with a purse string suture to exclude this potentially contaminated area from the surgical site. The foal is placed in dorsal recumbency, and the ventral midline is prepared for aseptic surgery in a routine manner.

Additional Instrumentation

Balfour retractors, soft rubber urinary catheters, and warmed normal (0.9%) saline solution are needed.

Surgical Technique

A narrow elliptical skin incision that is pointed at both ends is made around the urachus. The incision is extended back to the anterior margin of the prepuce as illustrated in the approach for the diseased urachus (Fig. 8.9*A*). This approach will allow adequate access to the bladder and allows the urachus itself to be freed and attended to, if necessary. When the incision is made through the linea alba, urine will flow from the abdominal cavity. Much of the urine can be removed from the abdominal cavity at this time with a suction apparatus.

The urachal stump is then dissected free by continuing the elliptical incision through the abdominal wall at its midline. The incision in the linea alba should be extended caudad several centimeters in the direction of the prepuce as necessary. The urachus should be freed from the ventral body wall (where it is still attached at this age) using sharp dissection as illustrated previously (Fig. 8.9*B*). Providing the tissue is healthy, it can be used to maintain traction on the bladder as it is repaired. Later the urachus will be removed completely from the bladder and either ligated or transected and oversewn because this area may be a potential source of leakage during the postoperative period.

If it is necessary to get access to the more caudal portion of the bladder, the skin incision can be extended caudally and laterally around the prepuce. The prepuce can be mobilized with subcutaneous dissection and retracted to expose the ventral midline. The abdominal wall incision can then be extended caudally to the level of the pubis. Alternatively, the entire approach can be made through a paramedian incision. Hemorrhage is more likely to be a problem with a paramedian approach than with a ventral midline incision approach.

The craniodorsal wall of the bladder should be inspected first because this is where smaller traumatic tears are most often found (4). The ventral aspect

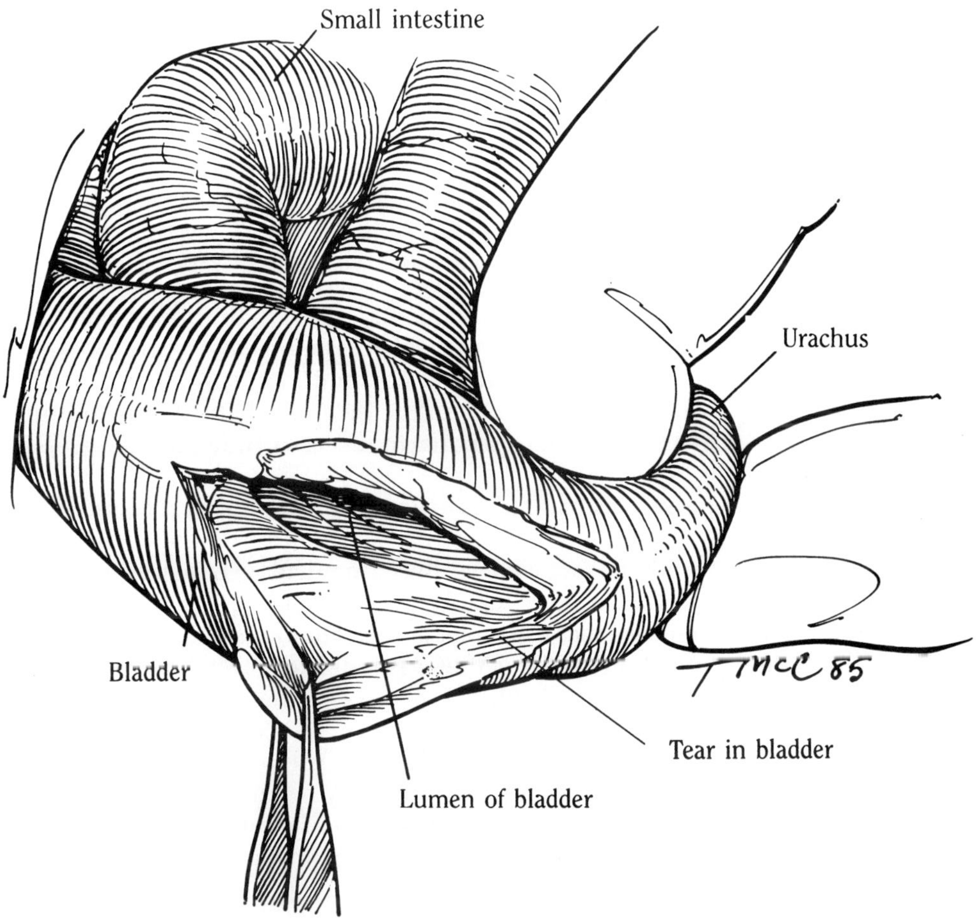

Figure 8.10. Cystorrhaphy for ruptured bladder.

of the bladder should be examined also because larger defects have been reported in this region (Fig. 8.10). These more ventral tears frequently extend far into the pelvic canal, making it extremely difficult to locate and securely suture the caudal end of the defect. To assist exploration, a Balfour retractor can be inserted and the intestines packed off with moist towels.

When the tear has been found, the edges should be examined. If the tissues appear devitalized, debridement with a good sharp pair of Metzenbaum scissors is recommended. A variety of suture patterns can be used for closure. The first layer consists of a simple interrupted pattern followed by an inverting layer, such as a continuous Lembert as illustrated previously (Fig. 8.9*D*). Some surgeons prefer two layers of inverting patterns. The suture material must be absorbable material such as Dexon, Vicryl, or PDS. No. 2/0 or 3/0 suture material is generally satisfactory for most foals. Tapered (not cutting-edged) needles are recommended. Regardless the pattern or material used for the closure, the important points are to invert the final layer and ensure a watertight closure. The bladder should be checked for leaks by distending it with saline solution. Any partial tears should be attended to immediately (by inverting suture lines) because they are potential sources of leakage during the postoperative period. The urachus and umbilical vessel remnants are then resected as described in "Resection of the Diseased Urachus in Foals."

Following repair of the bladder, the abdominal cavity can be lavaged with warm isotonic saline solution. This dialysis will aid in removing toxic urinary products remaining in the abdominal cavity.

The ventral midline closure is routine. The authors use no. 1 or no. 2 synthetic absorbable sutures in a simple interrupted pattern or a simple continuous pattern to close the linear alba. In the subcutaneous layer, 2/0 or 3/0 simple continuous sutures of a synthetic absorbable material are recommended. The skin is closed with a nonabsorbable material of the surgeon's choice or with stainless steel skin staples.

Postoperative Management

Despite large volumes of urine being frequently found in the abdominal cavity, peritonitis is unusual. If concurrent urachal abscessation has occurred, however, septic peritonitis may pose a threat. The authors routinely continue intravenous antibiotics for 3 to 4 days after the operation; however there are no controlled studies to show that antibiotics are essential to successful outcome of uncomplicated bladder rupture in foals.

Insertion of an indwelling catheter to keep the bladder decompressed following the repair has been recommended (2–5). The authors do not advocate routine use of such a catheter; we believe that a meticulously placed watertight closure of the bladder wall is more important. There may be situations, however, when the surgeon believes that the repair appears tenuous because the bladder tissue is friable, and an indwelling catheter is indicated. This type of bladder is usually found in septicemic foals (6).

Intravenous fluids of normal saline solution should continue until urination is noticed. If the foal has been adequately hydrated before and throughout surgery, then a strong forceful urination will usually occur shortly after the foal recovers from the anesthesia and stands. Failure to do so may mean recurrence of the uroperitoneum (i.e., further unseen leaks in the bladder). Electrolyte balance should be monitored, and any corrections in therapy are made as necessary.

Comments

The prognosis for uncomplicated rupture of the urinary bladder is generally good if repair is attempted early and severe electrolyte abnormalities have not developed. Cases that have progressed for several days frequently experience complications related to anesthetic management, such as third-degree A-V block that is relatively resistant to atropine (4). Surgical complications are usually the result of inadequate repair or failure to recognize additional leaks in the bladder or to attend to the urachus. Postoperative adhesions of bowel to the bladder have been observed. Leaks can also occur if the sutures in the bladder have been placed in unhealthy tissues, resulting in shredding of the tissue and separation of the suture line.

REFERENCES

1. Behr MJ, Hackett RP, Bentinck-Smith J, et al. Metabolic abnormalities associated with rupture of the urinary bladder in neonatal foals. JAVMA 1981;178:263.
2. Kritchevsky JE, Stevens DL, Christopher J, et al. Peritoneal dialysis for presurgical management of a ruptured bladder in a foal. JAVMA 1984;185:81.
3. Richardson DW, Kohn CW. Uroperitoneum in the foal. JAVMA 1983;182:267.
4. Richardson DW. Urogenital problems in the neonatal foal. Vet Clin North Am 1985; 1:179.
5. Walker DF, Vaughan JT. Bovine and Equine Urogenital Surgery. Philadelphia: Lea & Febiger, 1980.

6. Adams R, Koterba AM, Cudd TC, et al. Exploratory celiotomy for suspected urinary tract disruption in neonatal foals: a review of 18 cases. Equine Vet J 1988;20:13–17.
7. Gibson KT, Trotter GW, Gustafson SB. Conservative management of uroperitoneum in a gelding. JAVMA 1992;200:1692–1694.
8. Hackett RP. Rupture of the urinary bladder in neonatal foals. Compend Cont Edu 1984;6:S491–494.
9. Robertson JT, Spurlock GH, Bramlage LL, et al. Repair of ureteral defect in a foal. JAVMA 1983;183:799–800.

9

REMOVAL OF A DENTIGEROUS CYST (AURAL FISTULA)

A dentigerous cyst represents a special form of dental teratoma characterized by the presence of dental tissue at the base of a draining tract. The lesion appears as a fluctuant swelling at the base of the ear in a young horse, often accompanied by a discharging fistula that may open some distance up the margin of the pinna (1). The tooth is usually associated with the temporal bone. The condition is also known as heterotopic polyodontia (2). This condition is treated by complete removal of the tract and the cyst.

ANESTHESIA AND SURGICAL PREPARATION

The operation is done under general anesthesia with the horse in lateral recumbency and the affected side up. Before induction of anesthesia, perioperative antibiotics are administered and the temporal area is clipped. Shaving and routine surgical preparation are performed after induction of anesthesia.

SURGICAL TECHNIQUE

The skin incision is made over the central part of the lesion from the fistula craniad (Fig. 9.1*A*). The direction of the tract may be better defined if a probe can be placed through the fistula. Radiographs can also be used to ascertain the presence of a dental tissue and its position. The tract and the cyst are separated by blunt dissection at the base (Fig. 9.1*B*). The tooth is usually attached to the temporal bone, and the attachments need to be cut or broken down using an osteotome if necessary (Fig. 9.1*C*). This should be done carefully because the attachment may be firm, and fracture in the temporal bone must be avoided. If possible, the cyst and its associated tract are removed unopened (Fig. 9.1*C*). Following removal, the cyst can be opened to confirm the presence of dental tissue.

The dead space left by removal of the cyst is closed as well as possible using subcutaneous sutures of absorbable material, and a Penrose drain may be placed (Fig. 9.1*D*). The skin is closed with simple interrupted sutures of nonabsorbable material or skin staples. A stent bandage using a 4-inch roll of gauze (Kling) may also be sutured over the incision to help prevent formation of a postoperative seroma.

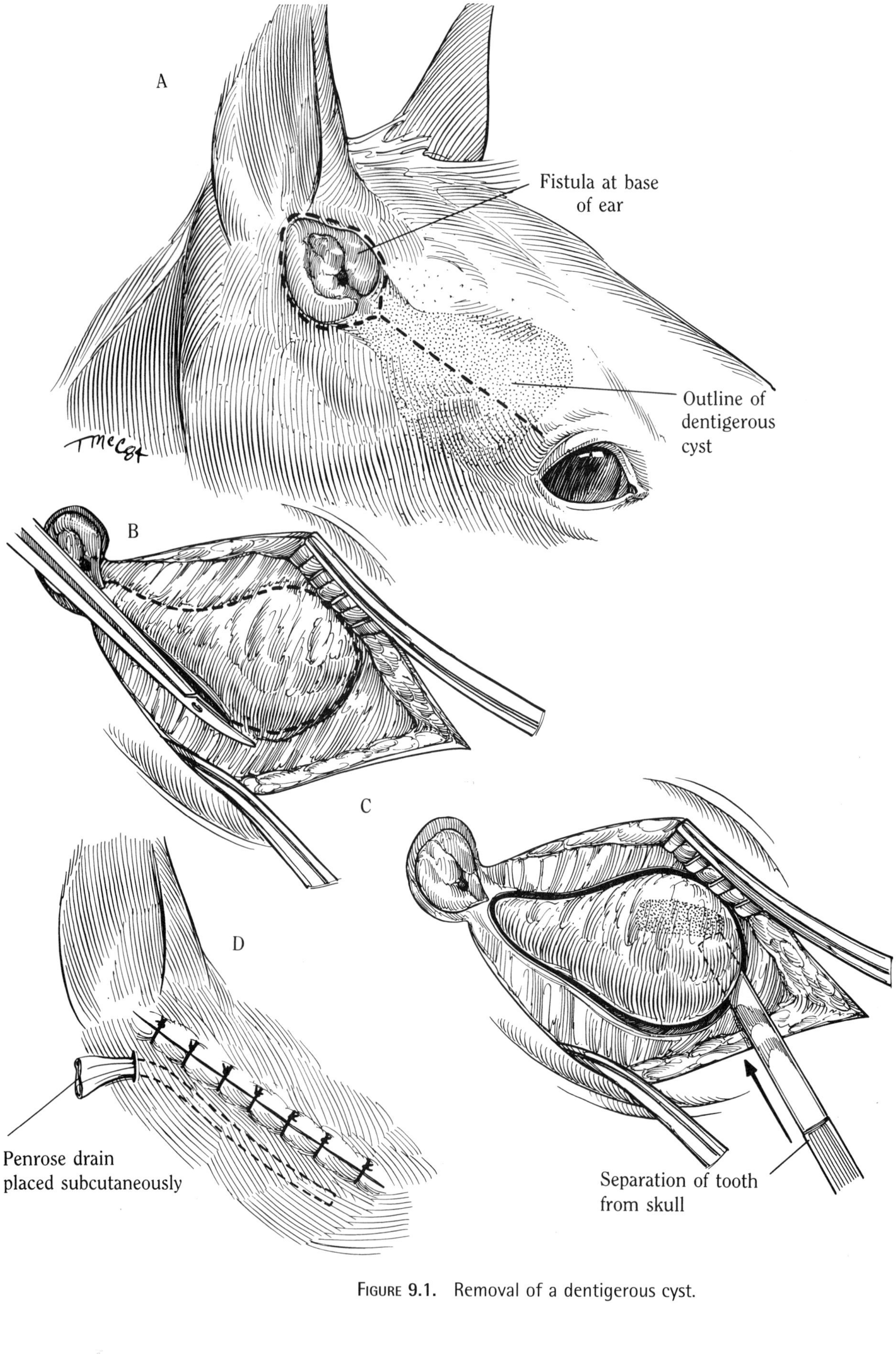

Figure 9.1. Removal of a dentigerous cyst.

POSTOPERATIVE MANAGEMENT

The drain is removed at 4 to 5 days, and the skin sutures or staples are removed at approximately 12 days. No other special care is necessary.

COMMENTS

It is necessary to resect the entire secreting membrane and enamel components to prevent against recurrence of the fistula. Surgeons should be cautioned against overzealous chiseling to remove the enamel, which could cause temporal bone trauma and fracture of the cranium. Additional structures at risk of trauma include the rostral auricular artery, the auriculopalpebral nerve, and the auricular muscles (2).

REFERENCES

1. McIlwraith CW. Equine digestive system. In: Jennings PB, ed. The Practice of Large Animal Surgery. Philadelphia: WB Saunders, 1984.
2. Fessler JF. Heterotopic polyodontia in horses: nine cases (1969–1986). JAVMA 1988; 192:535.

APPENDIX I

Equipment Required for Lag Screw Fixation with 4.5-mm Cortical Bone Screws

1. ASIF screwdriver
2. 4.5-mm drill bit
3. 3.2-mm drill bit
4. 4.5-mm cortical bone tap
5. 4.5-mm tap sleeve
6. 3.2-mm drill guide
7. ASIF compressed nitrogen or similar drill
8. ASIF cortical bone screws (4.5-mm outside diameter)
9. Countersink
10. Depth gauge

APPENDIX II[a]

Equipment Appropriate for Bone Plate Application

1. Countersink
2. Depth gauge
3. Tap handle and 4.5-mm taps (regular and extra long)
4. 6.5-mm cancellous tap
5. Standard screwdriver and screwdriver for quick coupling
6. Ruler
7. 8-mm hexagonal open-end wrench (for nuts)
8. Small air drill
9. Cortical and cancellous bone screw supplies
10. 4.5-mm drill bit—extra long (170 mm)
11. 4.5-mm drill bit (120 mm)
12. 3.2-mm drill bit—extra long (170 mm)
13. 3.2-mm drill bit (120 mm)
14. 2-mm drill bit
15. 6.5-mm cancellous tap sleeve
16. 3.5-mm tap sleeve
17. 4.5-mm tap sleeve and plate protector
18. 3.2-mm drill sleeve
19. 22-mm wide-tipped Hohmann retractor
20. 18-mm narrow-tipped Hohmann retractor
21. Sharp hook
22. 35-mm wide-tipped Hohmann retractor
23. 43-mm narrow-tipped Hohmann retractor
24. Drill sleeve for tension device
25. Tension device—span 16 mm
26. Pin wrench
27. Socket wrench
28. Open-end and box wrench—11 mm
29. DCP neutral drill guide, green
30. DCP load drill guide, yellow
31. Bending irons (2)
32. Bending press
33. Bending pliers for plates
34. Bending templates
35. 1.2-mm cerclage wire
36. Wire passer
37. Wire tightener with handle
38. Wire cutters
39. ASIF bone reduction forceps (large)
40. Verbrugge bone-holding forceps

---

[a] Adapted from Fackelman GE, Nunamaker DM. Manual of Internal Fixation in the Horse. Berlin: Springer-Verlag, 1982.

Inventory of ASIF Dynamic Compression Plates

(Plate supply that would allow repair of most equine long bone fractures)

	Narrow	*Broad*
8 hole	–	2
9 hole	2	2
10 hole	2	2
11 hole	2	2
12 hole	2	2
13 hole	–	2
14 hole	–	2
16 hole	–	2
18 hole	–	2

APPENDIX III

Equipment Required for Fiberglass Cast Application

Casting tape (4′, 5′, and 6′ widths)
Stockinette
Orthopaedic felt
1 towel clamp
Acrylic for the cap (e.g., Technovit)
Bailing wire
Hand drill and drill bit
Water at room temp. (70–75°F)
3-M casting tape (optional)

APPENDIX IV

Equipment Required for Arthroscopic Surgery

25 and 30° 4-mm arthroscope
5-mm arthroscopic sleeve
Sharp trocar and blunt obturator for insertion of sleeve
Fiberoptic cable
Fiberoptic light source
Video camera (optional)
Probe
Egress cannula (2.3-mm and 4.5-mm)
McIlwraith arthroscopy rongeur (Sontec)
Ferris-Smith intervertebral disc rongeurs, 4 × 10-mm cup (Sontec)
5-mm ethmoid forceps (Sontec)
Malleable fragment forceps (Sontec)
Periosteal elevator
4-mm osteotome
Curettes (2/0 and 1)
Curved curette (Sontec)
Motorized burr (Dyonics or Wolf)
Sesamoid knife (Sontec)
Curved Foerner elevator (Sontec)

INDEX

Note: Page numbers in *italics* denote figures; those followed by a "t" denote tables.